Grant's ATLAS OF ANATOMY

NINTH EDITION

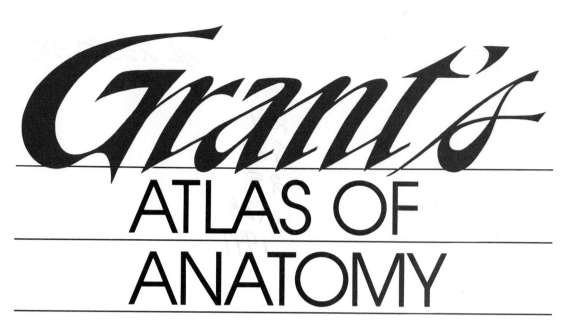

Grant's
ATLAS OF
ANATOMY

NINTH EDITION

Anne M. R. Agur, B.Sc. (OT), M.Sc.

Associate Professor of Anatomy and Cell Biology
Rehabilitation Medicine
Biomedical Communications
Faculty of Medicine
University of Toronto
Toronto, Ontario
Canada

with the assistance of

Ming J. Lee, M.D.

Senior Tutor in Anatomy and Cell Biology
Faculty of Medicine
University of Toronto
Toronto, Ontario
Canada

Williams & Wilkins

BALTIMORE • PHILADELPHIA • HONG KONG
LONDON • MUNICH • SYDNEY • TOKYO

A WAVERLY COMPANY

Editor: John N. Gardner
Managing Editor: Victoria M. Vaughn
Copy Editor: Shelley Potler
Production Coordinator: Barbara J. Felton
Cover Design: Amy Sweet

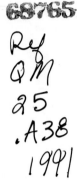

68765

Ref
QM
25
.A38
1991

#23081983

$6.54

Copyright © 1991
Williams & Wilkins
428 East Preston Street
Baltimore, Maryland 21202, USA

Printed in the United States of America

First Edition 1943

Library of Congress Cataloging-in-Publication Data

Agur, A. M. R.
    Grant's atlas of anatomy. — 9th ed. / Anne M.R. Agur; with the
assistance of Ming J. Lee.
        p.   cm.
    Rev. ed. of: Grant's atlas of anatomy. 8th ed. / James E.
Anderson. c1983.
    Includes index.
    ISBN 0-683-03701-3
    1. Human anatomy—Atlases.   I. Lee, Ming J.   II. Anderson, James
E. (James Edward), 1926-   Grant's atlas of anatomy.   III. Title.
IV. Title: Atlas of anatomy.
    [DNLM: 1. Anatomy, Regional—atlases.   QS 17 A284g]
    QM25.A38   1991
    611'.0022'2—dc20
    DNLM/DLC
    for Library of Congress   91-7251
                                                              CIP

97 98 99
11 12 13 14 15

To my husband, Enno,
And for my children, Erik and Kristina

Preface

Grant's Atlas of Anatomy is:

1. A companion in the dissecting room, guiding the dissector through each step of exploring and exposing structures; rather than providing an idealized view of human anatomy, it represents real dissections that are readily related to the actual specimen being studied;

2. A portable "anatomical museum" useful in determining relationships when deep dissection has destroyed superficial structures; review regions (at home) by studying the illustrations guided by the brief text; and prepare for practical examination (cover the reader labels and practice identifying structures);

3. One of the trio of books designed by Dr. Grant particularly for beginning students; the other two are *Grant's Method of Anatomy: A Clinical Problem-Solving Approach* by John V. Basmajian and Charles E. Slonecker, and *Grant's Dissector* by Eberhardt K. Sauerland.

4. A lifetime companion as a reference book in all fields of medicine; the first edition of *Grant's Atlas of Anatomy* appeared in two volumes in 1943 and met with immediate success; the second edition appeared in 1947 with 200 new illustrations, the addition of color, and the useful schemes of distribution of cranial nerves; the third edition followed in 1951, and the fourth in 1956; the fifth edition appeared in 1962 at which time the plates were re-engraved and the small diagrams from *Grant's Method* were added as secondary or supporting figures; the sixth edition followed in 1972.

Following Dr. Grant's death in 1973, Dr. J.E. Anderson became the editor of *Grant's Atlas of Anatomy*. Under Dr. Anderson's capable direction, the seventh and eighth editions were published in 1978 and 1983, respectively. The *Atlas* was resequenced to conform with *Grant's Dissector* and divided into ten color-coded sections for easier reference. Also, the text was rewritten with emphasis on clinical applications and 91 new figures were added. For the first time, radiographs and photographs of living anatomy were included.

The accuracy and simplicity of the halftone illustrations prepared by Dr. Grant and his assistants has always been one of the acclaimed features of the *Atlas*.

The challenge in planning this revision was to safeguard the historical strengths of the *Atlas* while, at the same time, to bring the work up to date and in line with changes in anatomical education in the medical, dental, physical and occupational therapy and other programs where this book has been used and respected over its long history. This, the ninth edition of *Grant's Atlas of Anatomy*, is a major revision. At first glance, the most noticeable change is the coloring of the artwork. This improvement was instituted in order to enhance further the usefulness and clarity of the classic illustrations. Photoretouch dyes were used on photographic prints of all the halftone illustrations, making it possible to add colors without modifying the original drawings. Numerous new halftone drawings have been added to make some of the dissection sequences more complete and easier to follow sequentially from superficial to deep. Some of the new halftone drawings were prepared from dissected specimens and continue in the original spirit of unmodified exactitude. Other new drawings temper this approach by providing an *overview* showing the relationship of more superficially and deeply located structures. The intent of these drawings is to supplement the illustrations of the specific dissections by providing an understanding of the region as a whole.

Most of the original line illustrations have been redrawn; new ones have been added where needed for orientation and/or clarification of basic anatomical concepts. The overall consistency of style, color, and simplicity of the new line figures has been maintained throughout the *Atlas*.

The line drawings, radiographic images, and surface anatomy photographs have been placed, whenever possible, alongside the appropriate halftone illustrations. Also, more emphasis has been placed on sectional anatomy with the inclusion of magnetic resonance images (MRIs) and corresponding illustrations of the body sectioned in various planes.

Finally, the terminology throughout the present edition has been modified to conform with the sixth edition of the *Nomina Anatomica* (1989).

Anne M.R. Agur
Toronto

Acknowledgments

The ninth edition of *Grant's Atlas of Anatomy* has been built upon the strengths of its preceding editions. Over the nearly 50-year history of this work, many people have given generously of their talents and expertise and I acknowledge their participation with heartfelt gratitude. Most of the original carbon dust halftones on which this book is based were created by Dorothy Foster Chubb, a pupil of Max Brodel, and one of Canada's first professionally trained medical artists. She was later joined by Nancy Joy, who is presently Professor Emeritus in the Department of Art as Applied to Medicine, University of Toronto. Mrs. Chubb was mainly responsible for the artwork of the first two editions and the sixth edition; Miss Joy for those in between. In subsequent editions, additional line and halftone illustrations by Elizabeth Blackstock, Elia Hopper Ross, Marguerite Drummond, and Joseph Bottos were added. Much credit is also due to Charles E. Storton for his role in the preparation of the majority of the original dissections and preliminary photographic work. I also wish to acknowledge the work of Dr. James Anderson, a pupil of Dr. Grant, under whose stewardship the seventh and eighth editions were published. The individuals listed below also provided invaluable contributions to the previous editions of the *Atlas*, and are gratefully acknowledged:

C.A. Armstrong	B.S. Jaden
P.G. Ashmore	G.F. Lewis
D. Baker	I.B. MacDonald
D.A. Barr	D.L. MacIntosh
J.V. Basmajian	R.G. MacKenzie
S. Bensley	K.O. McCuaig
D. Bilbey	W.R. Mitchell
W. Boyd	K. Nancekivell
J. Callagan	A.J.A. Noronha
H.A. Cates	W. Pallie
S.A. Crooks	W.M. Paul
M. Dickie	C.H. Sawyer
J.W.A. Duckworth	A.I. Scott
F.B. Fallis	J.S. Simpkins
J.B. Francis	J.S. Simpson
J.S. Fraser	C.G. Smith
R.K. George	I.M. Thompson
M.G. Gray	J.S. Thompson
B.L. Guyatt	N.A. Watters
C.W. Hill	R.W. Wilson
W.J. Horsey	

This ninth edition of *Grant's Atlas of Anatomy* would not have been possible without the dedication and commitment of the medical artists: David Mazierski, Stephen Mader, Bart Vallecoccia, Sari O'Sullivan, and Kam Yu of IMS Creative Communications, University of Toronto. David Mazierski coordinated the production and the coloring of the artwork, and also created most of the new halftone illustrations. A large number of the existing line illustrations have been redrawn and many new line drawings have been created. Much of this work was coordinated and expertly performed by Stephen Mader. The coloring of the halftones was skillfully carried out by Peter George. Many thanks to Bart Vallecoccia for his patience in the coloring of the line drawings.

I offer my sincerest gratitude to Tiiu Kask and Ann Eastwood, project coordinators; Paul Schwartz, medical photographer; Lesia Olexandra and Linda van der Beek, electronic page assembly; and the rest of the IMS Creative Communications team for their role in the production of this *Atlas*. Many thanks to Richard Minns and Osmo Monomen for the page layout design, and to Angela Cluer for her help in the initial phases of the project.

I am indebted to my former professors and to my colleagues in the Department of Anatomy at the University of Toronto for their encouragement. A very special thank you to Dr. Keith L. Moore for his expert advice and assistance in reading the manuscript. Also, my appreciation to Dr. M. Lee for his daily support, advice, and assistance in all aspects of the project. I extend my gratitude to Drs. M.J. Wiley, E. Sauerland, K.O. McCuaig, B. Liebgott, and Mr. S. Toussaint for their invaluable input; to Drs. E.L. Lansdown, J. Heslin, W. Kucharczyk, E. Becker, and D. Armstrong for their enthusiastic support in providing most of the radiological material; and to Sylvia Davidson and Danny Uy for their dissections of the back and upper and lower limbs.

As an undergraduate student in 1972 taking my first course in Anatomy, I remember using *Grant's Atlas* as an integral part of my studies. Also, I recall several of my professors, who had worked with Dr. Grant, relating many of his anecdotes and providing the students with study hints that Dr. Grant had used in his lectures. The Anatomy Museum at the University of Toronto was instituted by Dr. Grant. For several years now, it has been called the J.C.B. Grant Museum, and it is still used extensively by the students. It is a tribute to Dr. Grant that his name lives on with the museum and this *Atlas*.

I would like to express my gratitude to Williams & Wilkins for asking me to edit this ninth edition of *Grant's Atlas of Anatomy*. It has been an honor and enjoyable experience carrying out this work. I am especially thankful to John N. Gardner, Editor-in-Chief; Timothy Satterfield, Senior Editor; Laurel Craven, Editor; Victoria M. Vaughn, Managing Editor; Barbara J. Felton, Production Coordinator; Shelley Potler, Copy Editor; and Wayne Hubbel, Illustration Planner, all of Williams & Wilkins. I would also like to thank the reviewers who provided expert advice on the development of this edition, especially Margaret Hines, B. Peter Austin, Leonard L. Seelig, Brian L. O'Connor, Michael Wiley, Charles P. Barrett, and Ron Philo. Finally, I would like to thank the hundreds of instructors and students who have, over the years, communicated via the publisher their suggestions and advice as to how this *Atlas* might be improved. These suggestions have been passed on to me and I have tried to consider all of them. I hope readers will find many of these suggestions incorporated and will continue to provide their input.

Anne M.R. Agur
Toronto

Contents

1 The Thorax

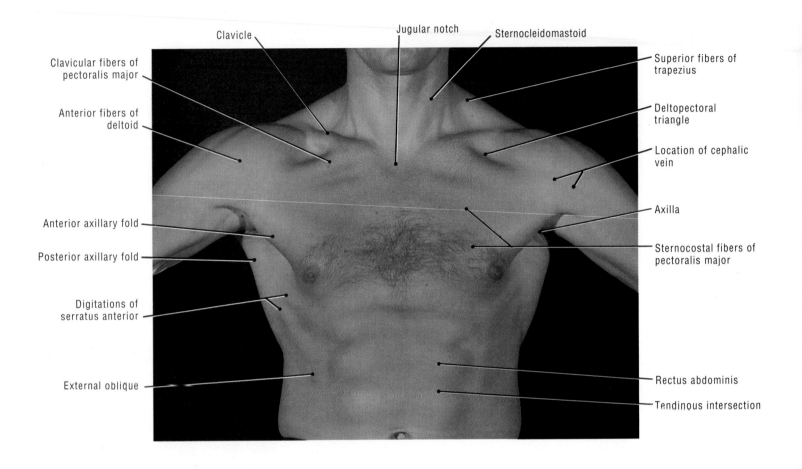

Clavicle

Jugular notch

Sternocleidomastoid

Clavicular fibers of
pectoralis major

Anterior fibers of
deltoid

Anterior axillary fold

Posterior axillary fold

Digitations of
serratus anterior

External oblique

Superior fibers of
trapezius

Deltopectoral
triangle

Location of cephalic
vein

Axilla

Sternocostal fibers of
pectoralis major

Rectus abdominis

Tendinous intersection

1.1
Surface anatomy of the pectoral region of the male

The photograph was taken with the subject adducting the shoulders against resistance to demonstrate the pectoralis major muscle and the anterior fibers of the deltoid muscle.

Observe:
1. The sternal part of the sternocostal head of the pectoralis major muscle originating from the manubrium and body of the sternum;

2. The clavicular fibers of the pectoralis major muscle originating from the medial half of the anterior surface of the clavicle;

3. The anterior axillary fold formed by the inferior border of the pectoralis major muscle;

4. The deltopectoral triangle (infraclavicular fossa) bounded by the clavicle superiorly, the deltoid muscle laterally, and the pectoralis major muscle medially;

5. The subcutaneous cephalic vein that drains into the deep venous system at the deltopectoral triangle.

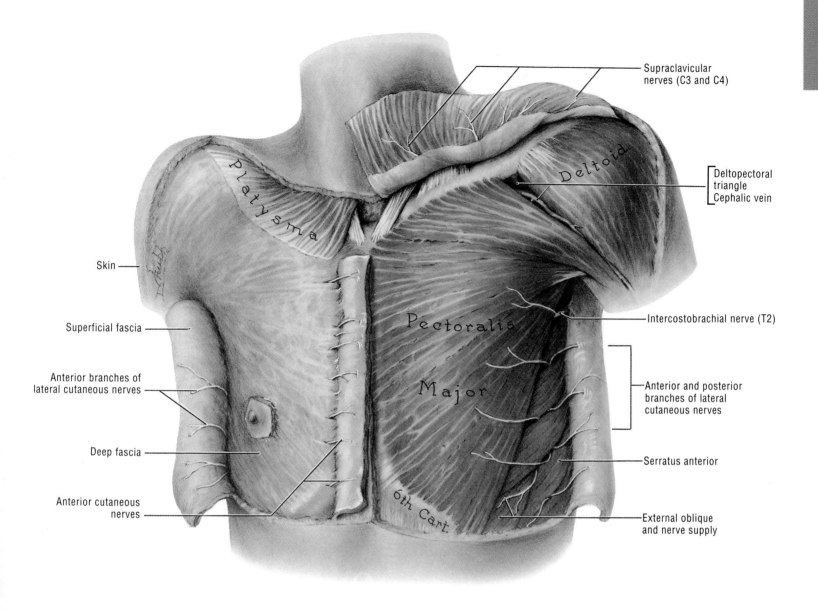

Supraclavicular nerves (C3 and C4)

Deltoid

Deltopectoral triangle
Cephalic vein

Skin

Platysma

Superficial fascia

Pectoralis

Intercostobrachial nerve (T2)

Anterior branches of lateral cutaneous nerves

Major

Anterior and posterior branches of lateral cutaneous nerves

Deep fascia

Serratus anterior

Anterior cutaneous nerves

6th Cart.

External oblique and nerve supply

1.2
Superficial dissection of the pectoral region of the male

The platysma muscle, which descends to the 2nd or 3rd rib, is cut short on the right side; it, together with the supraclavicular nerves, is reflected on the left side.

Observe:

1. The deep fascia covering the pectoralis major muscle is filmy;

2. The intermuscular bony strip running along the clavicle is both subcutaneous and subplatysmal;

3. The two heads of pectoralis major muscle meet at the sternoclavicular joint;

4. The cephalic vein passing deeply, to join the axillary vein, in the deltopectoral triangle;

5. The cutaneous innervation of the pectoral region by the supraclavicular nerves (C3 and C4) and upper thoracic nerves (T2 to T6); the brachial plexus (C5, C6, C7, C8, and T1) does not supply cutaneous branches to the pectoral region.

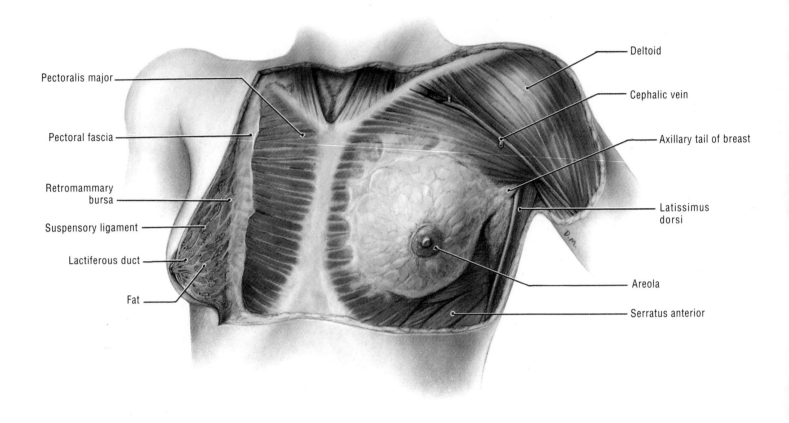

Pectoralis major

Pectoral fascia

Retromammary bursa

Suspensory ligament

Lactiferous duct

Fat

Deltoid

Cephalic vein

Axillary tail of breast

Latissimus dorsi

Areola

Serratus anterior

1.3
Superficial dissection of the pectoral region of the female

Observe on the left side:
1. The breast extending from the 2nd to the 6th rib and the axillary tail projecting into the axilla;

2. The pectoralis major muscle forming the anterior axillary fold and the latissimus dorsi muscle and the teres major muscle (not visible) forming the posterior axillary fold;

3. The cephalic vein draining deeply into the axillary vein at the deltopectoral triangle;

Observe on the right side:
1. The deep pectoral fascia covering the pectoralis major muscle;

2. The suspensory ligaments, in the sagittally sectioned breast, extending from the deep fascia to the skin;

3. The region of loose connective tissue between the deep fascia and the deep surface of the breast (the retromammary bursa) permitting the breast to move on the deep fascia;

4. The lactiferous ducts (usually 15 to 20 in number) running at first dorsally in the long axis of the nipple, enveloped in an areolar cuff, and then spreading radially and draining the glandular tissue.

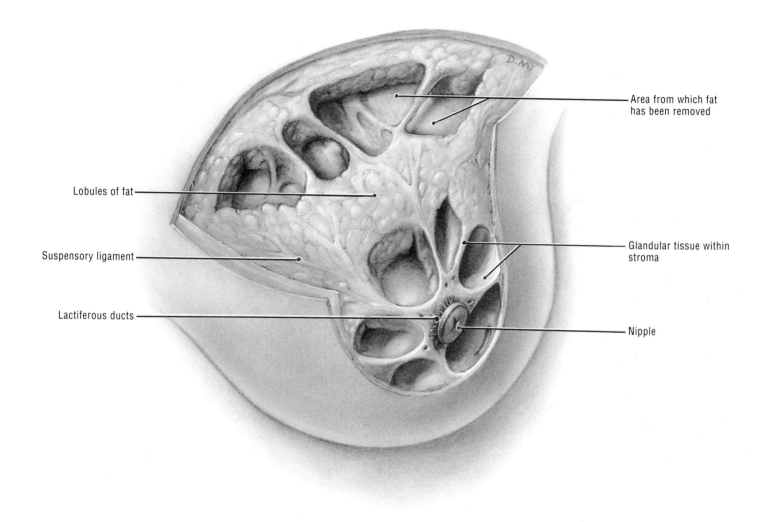

Lobules of fat

Suspensory ligament

Lactiferous ducts

Area from which fat has been removed

Glandular tissue within stroma

Nipple

1.4
Mammary gland of the female

The breast or mammary gland lies in the superficial fascia and varies considerably in size and shape. The nonlactating breast consists primarily of fat compartmentalized in connective and glandular tissue septa.

With the rounded handle of the scalpel, collections of superficial fat were scooped out of their compartments between septa.

Observe:
1. The lactiferous ducts opening on the nipple;

2. The glandular tissue within a dense (fibro-) areolar stroma from which septa (suspensory ligaments) extend to the deeper layers of the skin; cancer of the breast may result in fibrosis of the suspensory ligaments and subsequent retraction and pitting of the skin of the breast; the cancerous breast may lose its mobility and adhere to the underlying pectoralis major muscle if the tumor invades the deep fascia.

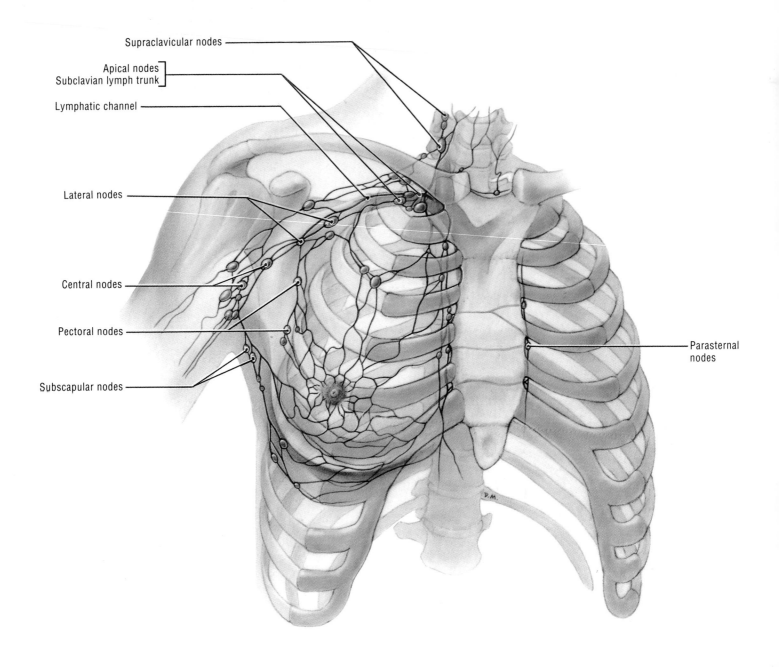

Supraclavicular nodes

Apical nodes
Subclavian lymph trunk

Lymphatic channel

Lateral nodes

Central nodes

Pectoral nodes

Subscapular nodes

Parasternal nodes

1.5
Lymphatic drainage of the breast

Drainage of lymph from the upper limb and breast passes through nodes arranged irregularly in groups: *pectoral*, along the inferior border of the pectoralis minor muscle; *subscapular*, along the subscapular artery and veins; *lateral*, along the distal part of the axillary vein; *central*, at the base of the axilla embedded in axillary fat; *apical*, along the axillary vein between the clavicle and the pectoralis minor muscle. Most of the breast is drained through this system to the *subclavian lymph trunk* that joins the venous system at the junction of the subclavian and internal jugular veins. The medial part of the breast drains to the *parasternal nodes* that follow the internal thoracic vessels and are much less accessible surgically. When blockage of the lymphatic system occurs, as in cancer, drainage may go to the opposite breast and its nodes or inferiorly along the anterior abdominal wall to the inguinal nodes.

1.6
Lymphogram of the nodes involved in the lymphatic drainage of the breast

On this anteroposterior postmastectomy lymphogram, observe the supraclavicular, parasternal, and axillary lymph nodes. (From Clouse ME, Wallace S. *Lymphatic imaging.* Baltimore: Williams & Wilkins, 1985.)

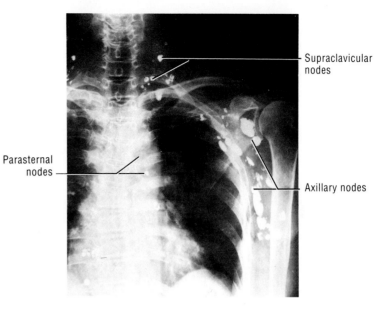

Supraclavicular nodes

Parasternal nodes

Axillary nodes

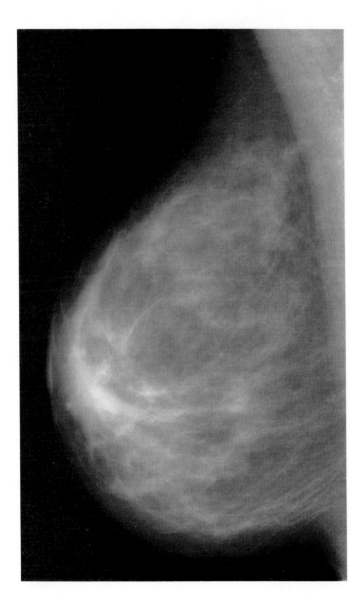

1.7
Normal lateral mammogram

Observe the connective tissue network of the breast. The fatty tissue of the breast provides a natural contrast medium for the connective tissue and glandular stroma. The stroma of the breast is radiopaque and changes with age and during lactation. (Courtesy of Dr. E.L. Lansdown, Professor of Radiology, University of Toronto, Toronto, Ontario, Canada.)

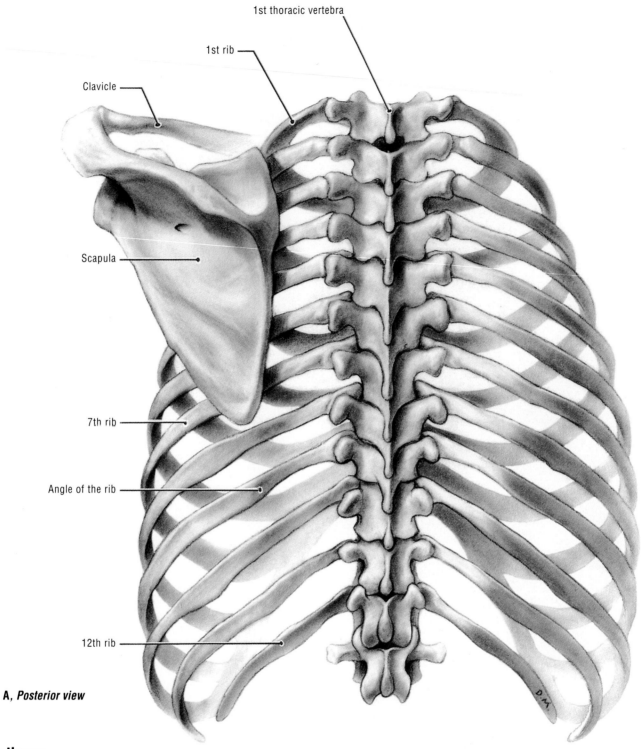

1st thoracic vertebra

1st rib

Clavicle

Scapula

7th rib

Angle of the rib

12th rib

A, *Posterior view*

1.8
Bony thorax

Study both views of the bony thorax (**A** and **B**) and observe that:
1. The skeleton of the thorax consists of 12 thoracic vertebrae, 12 pairs of ribs and costal cartilages, and the sternum;

2. Each rib articulates posteriorly with the vertebral column;

3. Anteriorly, the superior seven costal cartilages articulate with the sternum; the 8th, 9th, and 10th cartilages articulate with the cartilages next above; the 11th and 12th are "floating" ribs; their cartilages do not articulate anteriorly;

4. Posteriorly, all ribs incline inferiorly; anteriorly, the 3rd to 10th costal cartilages incline superiorly;

5. The superior thoracic aperture (thoracic inlet) is the doorway between the thoracic cavity and the neck region; it is bounded by the 1st thoracic vertebra, the 1st ribs and their cartilages, and the manubrium of the sternum.

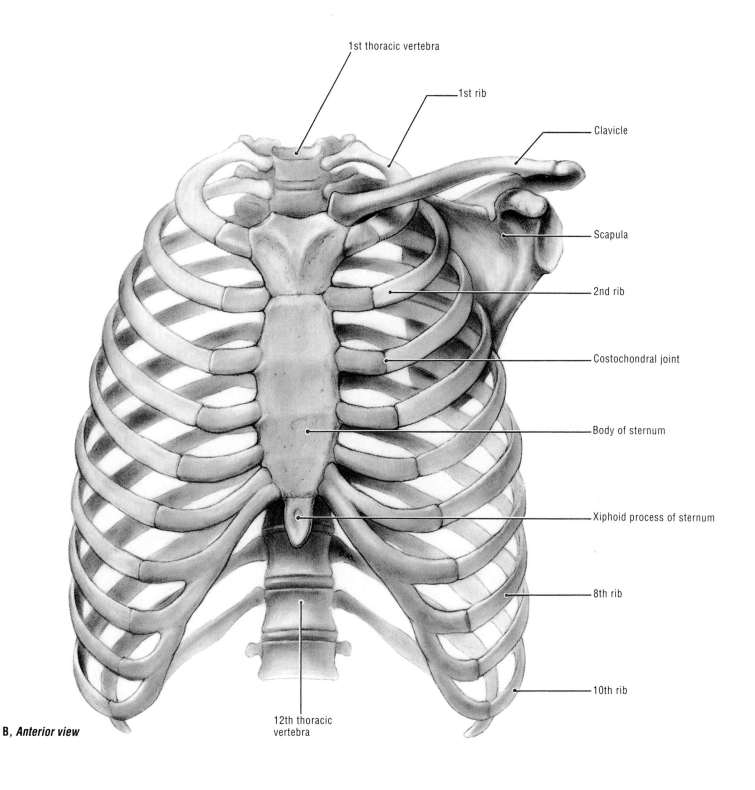

1st thoracic vertebra

1st rib

Clavicle

Scapula

2nd rib

Costochondral joint

Body of sternum

Xiphoid process of sternum

8th rib

10th rib

12th thoracic vertebra

B, *Anterior view*

1.8
Bony thorax *(continued)*

6. The clavicle lies over the anterosuperior aspect of the 1st rib, making it difficult to palpate;

7. The 2nd rib is easy to locate because its costal cartilage articulates with the sternum at the *sternal angle;* find this important bony elevation at the junction of manubrium and body of the sternum (Fig. 1.11**B**);

8. The 3rd to 10th ribs can be palpated in sequence inferolaterally from the 2nd rib; the fused costal cartilages of the 7th to the 10th ribs form the costal arch (margin) and the tips of the 11th and 12th can be palpated posterolaterally;

9. The scapula is suspended from the clavicle and crosses the 2nd to the 7th ribs.

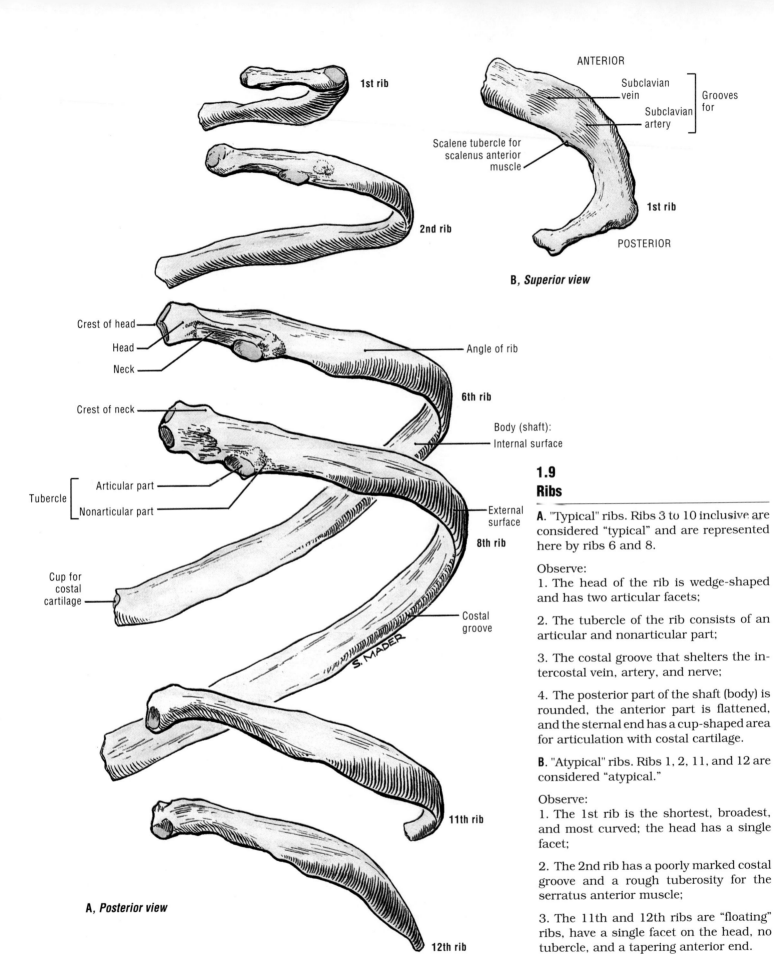

1st rib

2nd rib

B, _Superior view_

ANTERIOR

Subclavian
vein
} Grooves
for
Subclavian
artery

Scalene tubercle for
scalenus anterior
muscle

1st rib

POSTERIOR

Crest of head

Head

Neck

Angle of rib

6th rib

Crest of neck

Body (shaft):
Internal surface

Tubercle {
Articular part

Nonarticular part

External
surface

8th rib

Cup for
costal
cartilage

Costal
groove

S. MADER

11th rib

A, _Posterior view_

12th rib

1.9
Ribs

A. "Typical" ribs. Ribs 3 to 10 inclusive are considered "typical" and are represented here by ribs 6 and 8.

Observe:

1. The head of the rib is wedge-shaped and has two articular facets;

2. The tubercle of the rib consists of an articular and nonarticular part;

3. The costal groove that shelters the intercostal vein, artery, and nerve;

4. The posterior part of the shaft (body) is rounded, the anterior part is flattened, and the sternal end has a cup-shaped area for articulation with costal cartilage.

B. "Atypical" ribs. Ribs 1, 2, 11, and 12 are considered "atypical."

Observe:

1. The 1st rib is the shortest, broadest, and most curved; the head has a single facet;

2. The 2nd rib has a poorly marked costal groove and a rough tuberosity for the serratus anterior muscle;

3. The 11th and 12th ribs are "floating" ribs, have a single facet on the head, no tubercle, and a tapering anterior end.

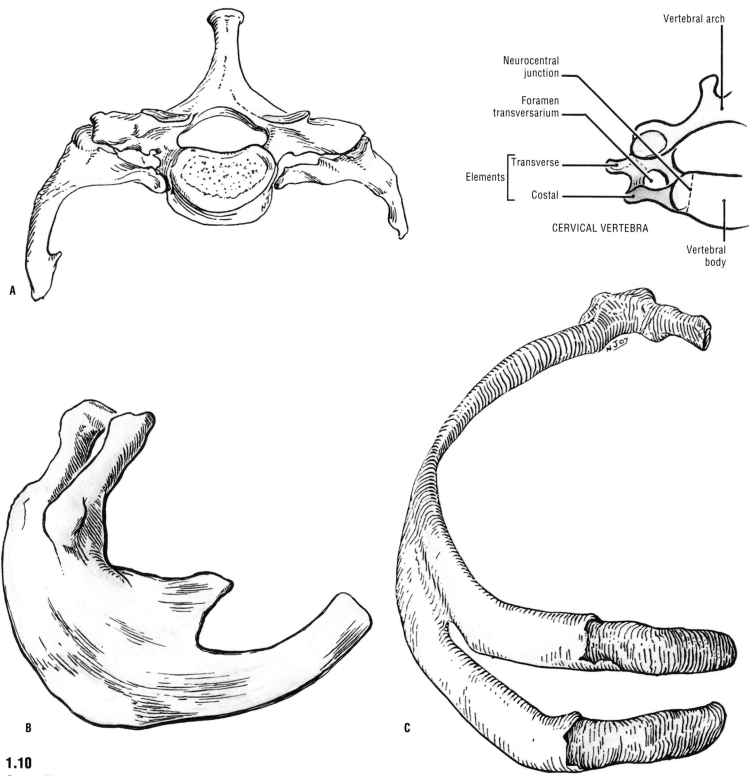

Vertebral arch

Neurocentral
junction

Foramen
transversarium

Elements { Transverse

Costal

CERVICAL VERTEBRA

Vertebral
body

A

B

C

1.10
Anomalies of the ribs

A. Cervical ribs. A cervical rib is an enlarged costal element of the 7th cervical vertebra. It may be large and palpable or detectable only radiologically; unilateral or bilateral; asymptomatic or through pressure on the most inferior root of the brachial plexus may produce sensory and motor changes over the distribution of the ulnar nerve.

B. Bicipital rib. In this specimen, there has been partial fusion of the first two thoracic ribs. A similar condition results from the partial fusion of a cervical rib with the 1st thoracic rib.

C. Bifid rib. The superior component of this 3rd rib is supernumerary and articulated with the lateral aspect of the 1st sternebra of the body of the sternum. The inferior component articulated at the junction of the 1st and 2nd sternebrae.

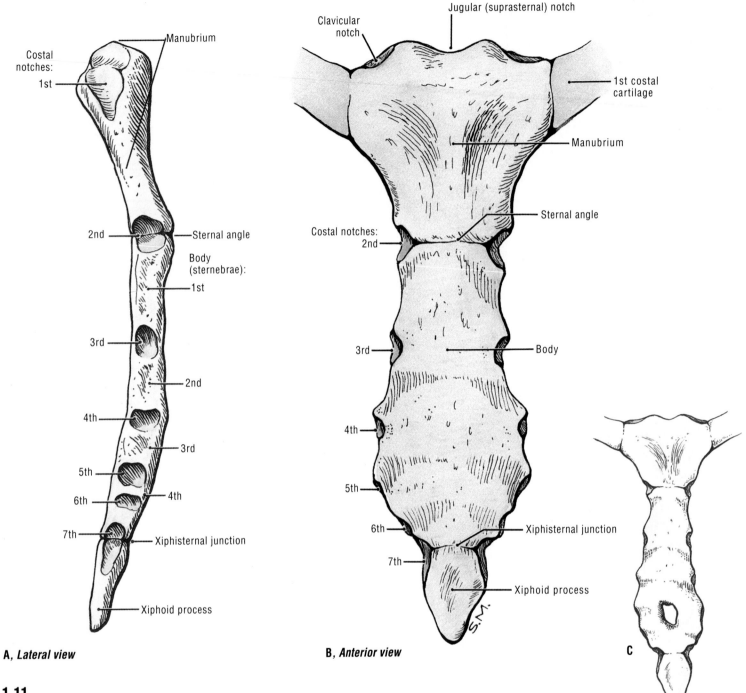

A, *Lateral view*

B, *Anterior view*

C

1.11
Sternum

Observe in **A** and **B**:

1. The great thickness of the superior third of the manubrium, between the clavicular notches;

2. The medial ends of the clavicles deepen the jugular (suprasternal) notch; a finger placed in this notch palpates the trachea;

3. The sternal angle, at the junction of the manubrium and body, is a palpable landmark guiding your fingers to the 2nd costal cartilage;

4. The sharp inferior edge of the body at the xiphisternal junction is palpable; forceful displacement of the xiphoid endangers the underlying liver;

5. Seven costal cartilages articulate with the sternum: the 1st with the manubrium and the 6th with the lateral aspect of the 4th sternebra; all others articulate at junctions of the six elements of the sternum: the manubrium, the four sternebrae, and the xiphoid process.

C. Sternal foramen. This relatively common malformation results from a defect of ossification and is diagnosed as a bullet wound by the unwary. This specimen also shows synostosis of the xiphisternal joint.

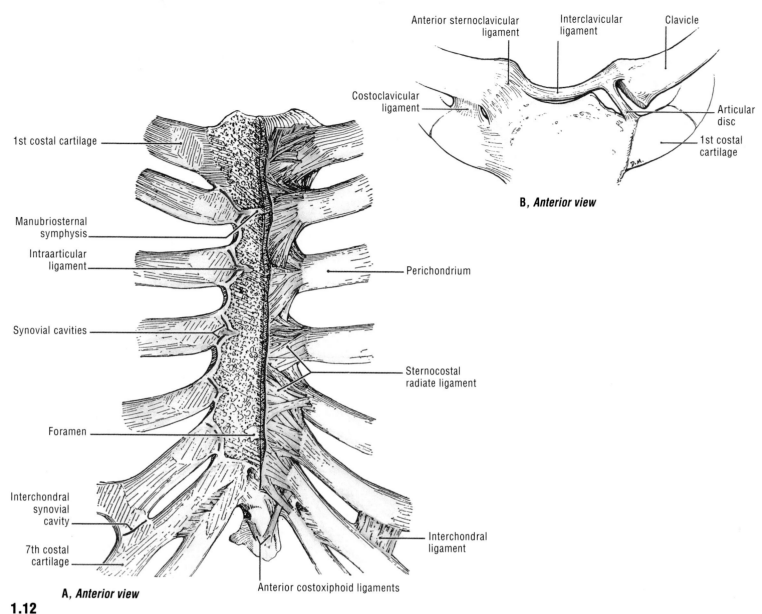

1st costal cartilage

Manubriosternal symphysis

Intraarticular ligament

Synovial cavities

Foramen

Interchondral synovial cavity

7th costal cartilage

Perichondrium

Sternocostal radiate ligament

Interchondral ligament

Anterior costoxiphoid ligaments

A, *Anterior view*

Anterior sternoclavicular ligament

Interclavicular ligament

Clavicle

Costoclavicular ligament

Articular disc

1st costal cartilage

B, *Anterior view*

1.12

Sternocostal, interchondral, and sternoclavicular joints

A. Sternocostal and interchondral joints.
Observe:

1. On the right side, the cortex of the sternum and costal cartilages has been shaved away; to obtain a specimen of bone marrow, a sternal puncture is done through the thin cortical bone into the area of spongy bone;

2. On the left side, dissection shows that the fibers of the perichondrium terminate as sternocostal radiate ligaments;

3. Three types of joints are demonstrated: *synchondroses* between the 1st costal cartilage and manubrium, and between the 7th costal cartilage and the sternum (in this case); *symphysis* at the manubriosternal joint; *synovial joints* at the other sternocostal joints and the interchondral joints.

B. Sternoclavicular joint. The sternoclavicular joint is the only articulation between the appendicular skeleton of the upper limb and the axial skeleton of the trunk. Fractures of the clavicle are more common than dislocation of the medial end of the clavicle,

due to the strength of the articular disc within the joint and the surrounding ligaments.

Observe on the right side:
1. The anterior sternoclavicular ligament reinforces the joint capsule anteriorly;

2. The interclavicular ligament connects the medial ends of the clavicles and reinforces the superior aspect of the joint;

3. The short, fibrous costoclavicular ligament joins the 1st rib and costal cartilage to the inferior surface of the clavicle.

Observe on the left side:
1. The joint capsule is removed revealing the articular disc, which attaches superiorly to the clavicle and inferiorly to the 1st costal cartilage;

2. The articular surface of the clavicle is larger than that of the manubrium.

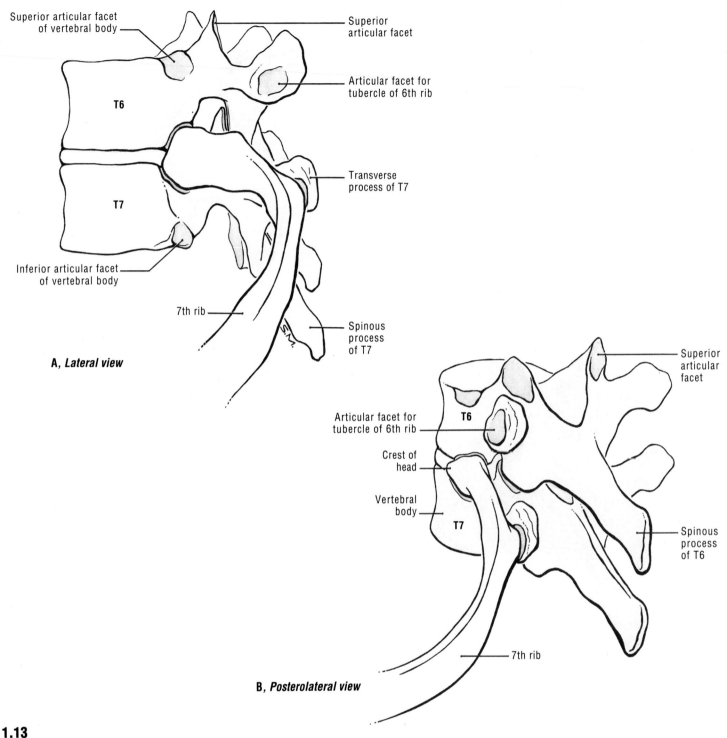

Superior articular facet of vertebral body

Superior articular facet

Articular facet for tubercle of 6th rib

T6

Transverse process of T7

T7

Inferior articular facet of vertebral body

7th rib

Spinous process of T7

A, *Lateral view*

Superior articular facet

Articular facet for tubercle of 6th rib

T6

Crest of head

Vertebral body

T7

Spinous process of T6

7th rib

B, *Posterolateral view*

1.13
Costovertebral articulations of a typical rib

Study both views (**A** and **B**) of the costovertebral articulations and observe that:

1. The costovertebral articulations (joints) include the articulation of the head of the rib with two adjacent vertebral bodies, and the articulation of the tubercle of the rib with the transverse process of a vertebra;

2. There are two articular facets on the head of the rib: a larger, inferior one for articulation with the vertebral body of its own number, and a smaller superior facet for the vertebral body above;

3. The crest of the head of the rib separates the two articular facets;

4. The smooth articular part of the tubercle of the rib articulates with the transverse process of its own numbered vertebra at the costotransverse joint.

1.14
Costovertebral joints

A and **B**. Ligaments of the costovertebral articulations.

Observe in **A**:

1. The radiate ligament joining the head of the rib to two vertebral bodies and the interposed intervertebral disc;

2. The superior costotransverse ligament joining the crest of the neck of the rib to the transverse process above;

3. The crest of the head of the rib is joined to the intervertebral disc by the intraarticular ligament.

Observe **B**:

1. The vertebral body, transverse processes, superior articulating processes, and the posterior elements of the articulating ribs have been transversely sectioned to enhance visualization of the joint surfaces and ligaments;

2. The costotransverse ligament joining the posterior aspect of the neck of the rib to the adjacent transverse process;

3. The lateral costotransverse ligament joining the nonarticulating part of the tubercle of the rib to the tip (apex) of the transverse process;

4. The articular surfaces (blue) of the synovial plane costovertebral joints.

C. Costotransverse joints. This diagram shows that at the 1st to the 7th costotransverse joints the ribs rotate; at the 8th, 9th, and 10th they glide, increasing the transverse diameter of the upper abdomen.

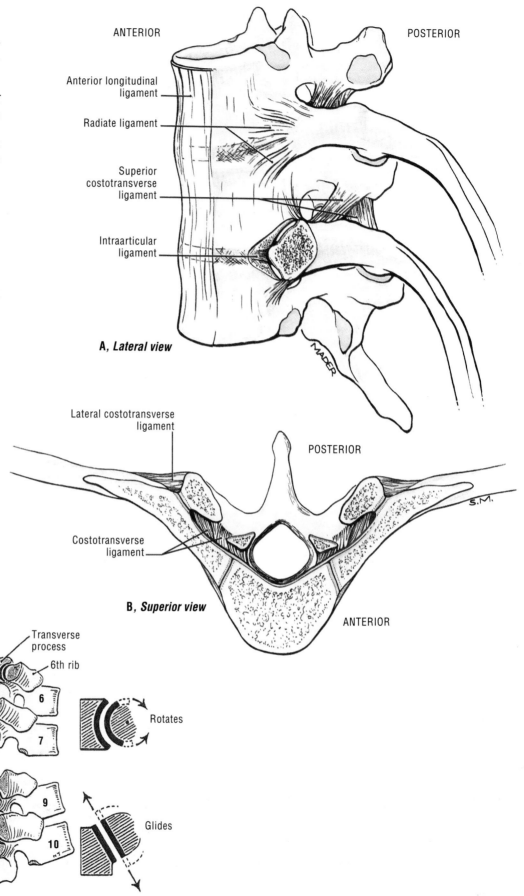

ANTERIOR   POSTERIOR

Anterior longitudinal ligament

Radiate ligament

Superior costotransverse ligament

Intraarticular ligament

A, *Lateral view*

Lateral costotransverse ligament

POSTERIOR

Costotransverse ligament

B, *Superior view*

ANTERIOR

Transverse process

6th rib

6

7

Rotates

9

10

Glides

C

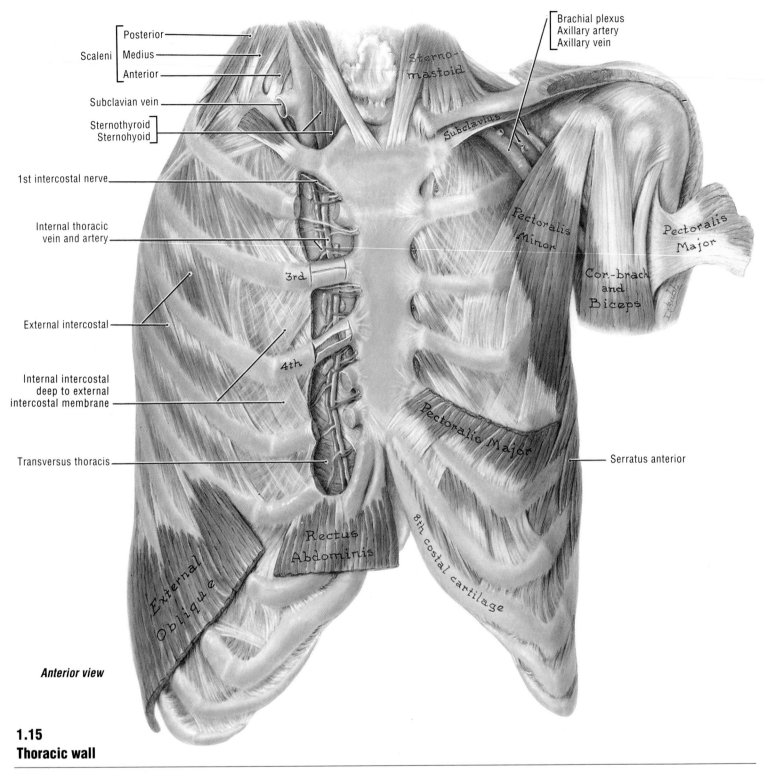

Posterior
Scaleni Medius
Anterior

Subclavian vein

Sternothyroid
Sternohyoid

Sterno-mastoid

Brachial plexus
Axillary artery
Axillary vein

Subclavius

1st intercostal nerve

Internal thoracic
vein and artery

3rd

Pectoralis Minor

Pectoralis Major

Cor-brach
and
Biceps

External intercostal

4th

Internal intercostal
deep to external
intercostal membrane

Pectoralis Major

Transversus thoracis

Serratus anterior

Rectus Abdominis

8th costal cartilage

External Oblique

Anterior view

1.15
Thoracic wall

Observe:

1. The internal thoracic (internal mammary) vessels running inferiorly just lateral to the edge of the sternum and providing intercostal branches;

2. The parasternal lymph nodes (green) that receive lymphatic vessels from the intercostal spaces, from the costal pleura and diaphragm, and from the medial part of the breast; it is by this route that cancer of the breast may spread to the lungs and mediastinum;

3. The subclavian vessels are "sandwiched" between the 1st rib and the clavicle (padded by the subclavius muscle);

4. The H-shaped cut through the perichondrium of the 3rd and 4th cartilages was used to shell out segments of cartilage; similarly, in performing a thoracotomy, the surgeon may shell a segment of rib out of its periosteum; later, bone regenerates from this periosteum.

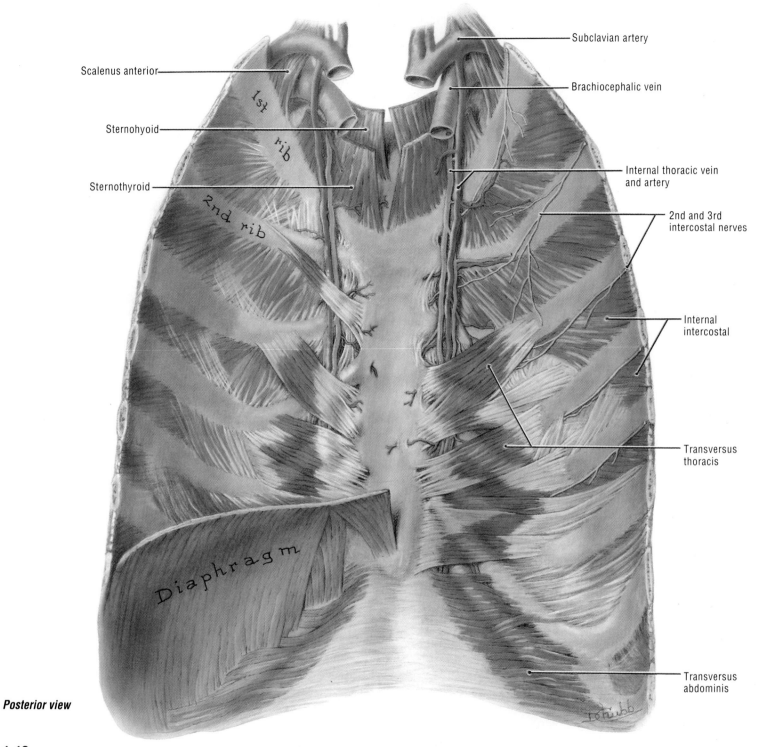

Scalenus anterior

1st rib

Sternohyoid

2nd rib

Sternothyroid

Subclavian artery

Brachiocephalic vein

Internal thoracic vein
and artery

2nd and 3rd
intercostal nerves

Internal
intercostal

Transversus
thoracis

Diaphragm

Transversus
abdominis

Posterior view

1.16
Anterior thoracic wall

Observe:

1. The continuity of the transversus thoracis muscle with the transversus abdominis muscle, these being the innermost layer of the three flat muscles of the thoracoabdominal wall;

2. The internal thoracic (internal mammary) artery, arising from the subclavian artery, accompanied by two veins (venae comitantes) up to the 2nd costal cartilage and superior to this by a single vein

(internal thoracic vein), which drains into the brachiocephalic vein;

3. The inferior portions of the internal thoracic (internal mammary) vessels, covered posteriorly by the transversus thoracis muscle; the superior portions in contact with parietal pleura (removed).

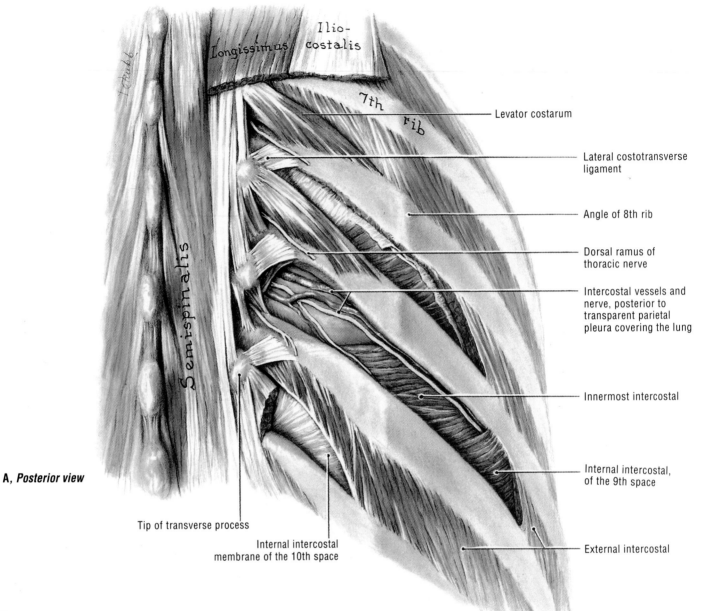

Ilio-
costalis

Longissimus

Levator costarum

Lateral costotransverse
ligament

Angle of 8th rib

Dorsal ramus of
thoracic nerve

Intercostal vessels and
nerve, posterior to
transparent parietal
pleura covering the lung

Innermost intercostal

Semispinalis

7th
rib

A, *Posterior view*

Internal intercostal,
of the 9th space

Tip of transverse process

Internal intercostal
membrane of the 10th space

External intercostal

1.17
Posterior end of an intercostal space

A. The iliocostalis and longissimus muscles have been removed exposing the levator costarum muscle. Of the five intercostal spaces shown:
a) The superior two (6th and 7th) are intact;

b) In the 8th and 10th spaces varying portions of the external intercostal muscle have been removed to reveal the underlying internal intercostal membrane, which is continuous with the internal intercostal muscle; the levator costarum muscle hasbeen removed to show the intercostal vessels and nerve.

Observe:
1. The vessels and nerve appear medially between the superior costotransverse ligament and the transparent parietal pleura covering the lung and disappear laterally between the internal and innermost intercostal muscles;

2. The intercostal nerve is the most inferior of the trio and the least sheltered in the intercostal groove.

B is a diagram of the area shown in **A**. In **A**, the scapula has been removed to reveal the 7th rib posteriorly.

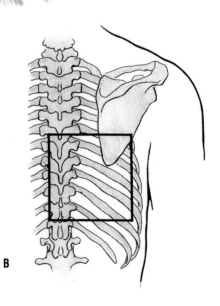

B

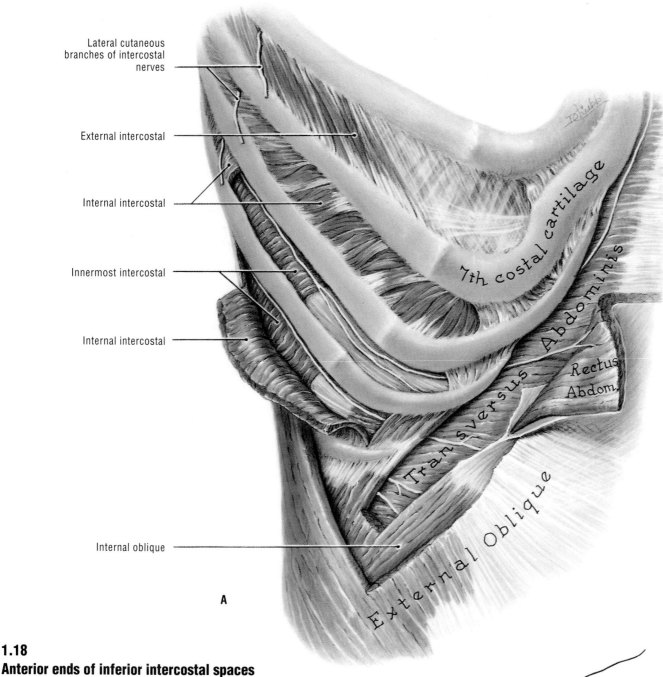

Lateral cutaneous branches of intercostal nerves

External intercostal

Internal intercostal

Innermost intercostal

Internal intercostal

Internal oblique

7th costal cartilage

Transversus Abdominis

Rectus Abdom.

External Oblique

A

1.18
Anterior ends of inferior intercostal spaces

Observe in **A**:

1. The fibers of the external intercostal and external oblique muscles run in the same direction: inferomedially;

2. The internal intercostal and internal oblique muscles are in continuity at the ends of the 9th, 10th, and 11th intercostal spaces;

3. That the intercostal nerves coursing in the intercostal space lie deep to the internal intercostal muscle but superficial to the innermost intercostal muscle; anteriorly these nerves also lie superficial to either the transversus abdominis or transversus thoracis muscles;

4. An intercostal nerve runs parallel to its rib and then to its costal cartilage; thus, on reaching the abdominal wall, nerves T7 and T8 continue superiorly, T9 continues nearly horizontally, and T10 continues inferomedially toward the umbilicus; these nerves provide cutaneous innervation in overlapping segmental bands.

B is a diagram of the area shown in **A**.

B

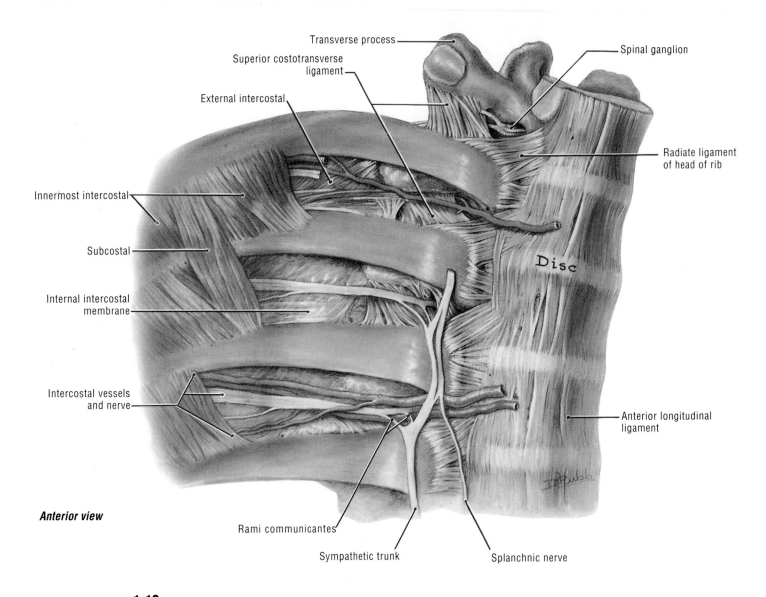

Transverse process

Superior costotransverse ligament

External intercostal

Innermost intercostal

Subcostal

Internal intercostal membrane

Intercostal vessels and nerve

Spinal ganglion

Radiate ligament of head of rib

Disc

Anterior longitudinal ligament

Rami communicantes

Sympathetic trunk

Splanchnic nerve

Anterior view

1.19
Vertebral end of an intercostal space

Observe:

1. Portions of the innermost intercostal muscle that bridge two intercostal spaces are called subcostal muscles;

2. An external intercostal muscle in the superiormost space;

3. An internal intercostal membrane in the middle space, continuous medially with a superior costotransverse ligament;

4. In the most inferior space, the order of the structures: intercostal vein, artery, and nerve; note their collateral branches;

5. Near the top of the illustration, a thoracic nerve; the ventral ramus crosses anterior to the superior costotransverse ligament and the dorsal ramus posterior to it;

6. The attachment of intercostal nerves to the sympathetic trunk by the rami communicantes; the splanchnic nerve is a visceral branch of the trunk.

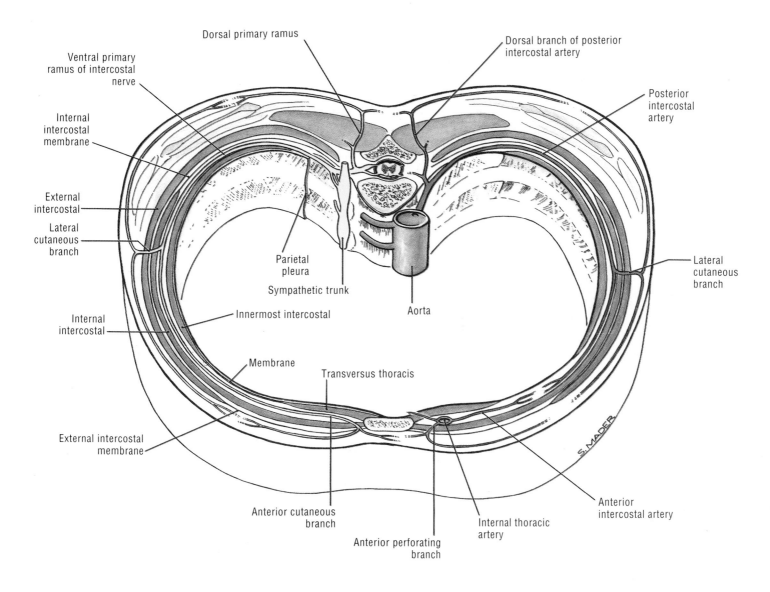

Dorsal primary ramus

Ventral primary
ramus of intercostal
nerve

Internal
intercostal
membrane

External
intercostal

Lateral
cutaneous
branch

Internal
intercostal

Dorsal branch of posterior
intercostal artery

Posterior
intercostal
artery

Parietal
pleura

Sympathetic trunk

Aorta

Lateral
cutaneous
branch

Innermost intercostal

Membrane

Transversus thoracis

External intercostal
membrane

Anterior cutaneous
branch

Anterior perforating
branch

Internal thoracic
artery

Anterior
intercostal artery

S. MADER

1.20
Contents of an intercostal space

This diagram is simplified by showing nerves on the right and arteries on the left.

Observe:

1. Three muscular layers: (a) external intercostal muscle and membrane, (b) internal intercostal muscle and membrane, (c) innermost intercostal and transversus thoracis muscles and the membrane connecting them;

2. The dorsal primary ramus innervating the deep back muscles and the skin adjacent to the vertebral column;

3. The intercostal nerves are the ventral primary rami of spinal nerves T1 to T11; the ventral primary ramus of spinal nerve T12 is the subcostal nerve;

4. The upper intercostal vessels and nerves run in the plane between the middle and innermost layers of muscles; subsequently, the lower intercostal vessels and nerves occupy a corresponding plane in the abdominal wall as shown in Figure 1.18**A**;

5. Posterior intercostal arteries are branches of the aorta (the superior two spaces are supplied from the superior intercostal branch of the costocervical trunk); anterior intercostal arteries are branches of the internal thoracic artery.

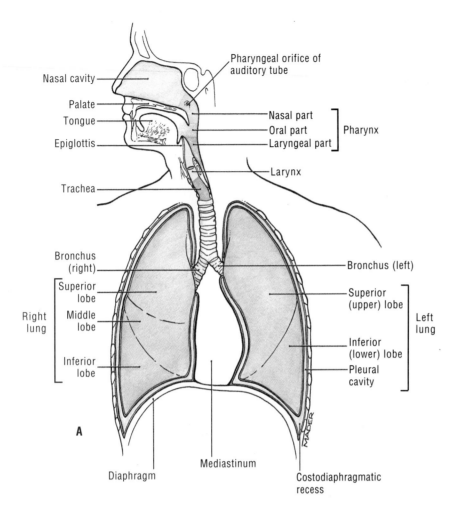

Nasal cavity

Palate

Tongue

Epiglottis

Trachea

Pharyngeal orifice of auditory tube

Nasal part
Oral part ⎤ Pharynx
Laryngeal part ⎦

Larynx

Bronchus (right)

Superior lobe ⎤
Right lung ⎱ Middle lobe
Inferior lobe ⎦

Bronchus (left)

Superior (upper) lobe ⎤
⎰ Inferior (lower) lobe ⎱ Left lung
Pleural cavity ⎦

A

Diaphragm

Mediastinum

Costodiaphragmatic recess

1.21
Diagrams of the respiratory system

Study the three diagrams of the respiratory system: overview (**A**), coronal section through the heart and lungs (**B**), and pleural cavity and pleura (**C**) and observe:

1. The lungs are invaginated by a continuous membranous pleural sac; the part of the membranous sac that covers the lungs is called visceral (pulmonary) pleura and the part that lines the thoracic cavity is called parietal pleura; the visceral and parietal pleurae are continuous at the root of the lung;

2. The pleural cavity is a potential space between the visceral (pulmonary) and parietal pleura, which contains a thin layer of fluid; when the lung collapses, the pleural cavity becomes a "real" space and may contain air, blood, etc. (**C**);

3. The left pleural cavity is smaller than the right pleural cavity due to the projection of the heart to the left side;

4. The parietal pleura can be divided regionally into the costal, diaphragmatic, mediastinal, and cervical pleura; note the costomediastinal recess between the costal and diaphragmatic parietal pleura.

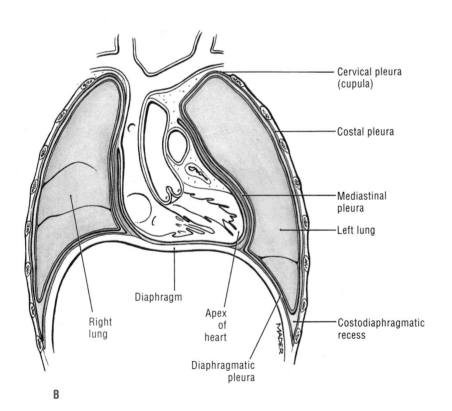

Cervical pleura (cupula)

Costal pleura

Mediastinal pleura

Left lung

Costodiaphragmatic recess

Right lung

Diaphragm

Apex of heart

Diaphragmatic pleura

B

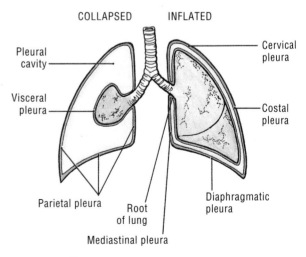

COLLAPSED   INFLATED

Pleural cavity

Visceral pleura

Parietal pleura

Root of lung

Mediastinal pleura

Cervical pleura

Costal pleura

Diaphragmatic pleura

C

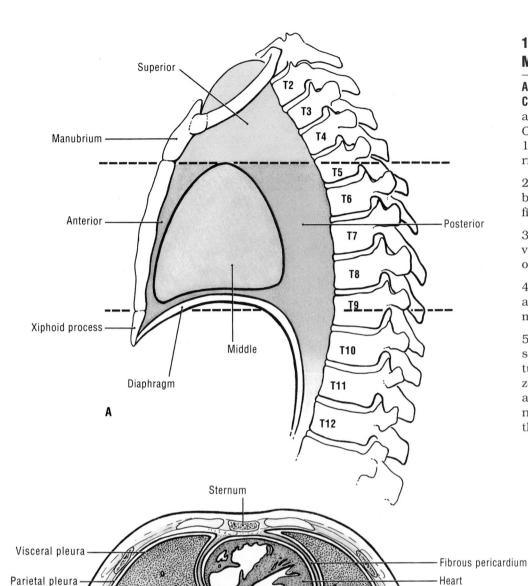

Superior

Manubrium

Anterior

Xiphoid process

Diaphragm

T2
T3
T4
T5
T6
T7
T8
T9
T10
T11
T12

Posterior

Middle

A

A. Subdivisions of the mediastinum. **B** and **C**. Transverse section through the heart and lungs.

Observe:

1. The mediastinum located between the right and left pleural sacs;

2. The anterior mediastinum between the body of the sternum anteriorly and the fibrous pericardium posteriorly;

3. The posterior mediastinum between the vertebral bodies and the posterior surface of the fibrous pericardium;

4. The middle mediastinum between the anterior and posterior subdivisions of the mediastinum;

5. The superior mediastinum is bounded, superiorly, by the superior thoracic aperture (thoracic inlet), inferiorly by a horizontal plane through the sternal angle, anteriorly by the manubrium of the sternum, and posteriorly by the superior four thoracic vertebrae.

Sternum

Visceral pleura

Parietal pleura

Esophagus

B

Fibrous pericardium

Heart

Pleural cavity

Azygos vein, Thoracic duct

Aorta

Vertebral body T7

S.M.

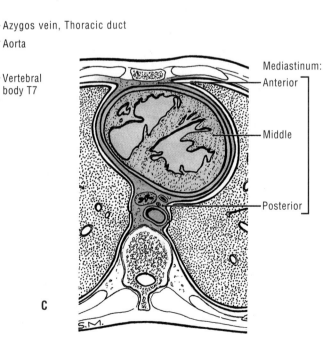

Mediastinum:

Anterior

Middle

Posterior

C

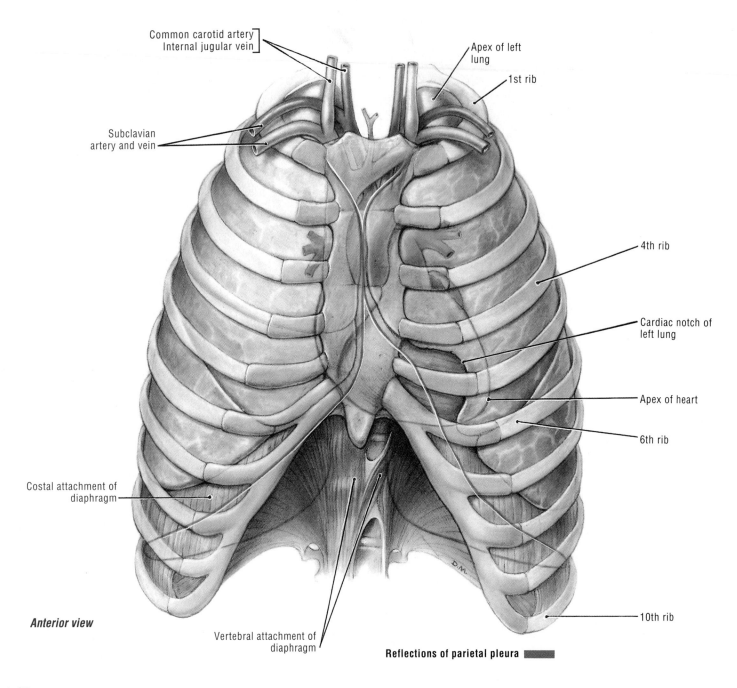

Common carotid artery
Internal jugular vein

Apex of left lung

1st rib

Subclavian artery and vein

4th rib

Cardiac notch of left lung

Apex of heart

6th rib

Costal attachment of diaphragm

10th rib

Anterior view

Vertebral attachment of diaphragm

Reflections of parietal pleura ▬

1.23
Contents of the thorax

Observe:

1. The apex of the lungs at the level of the neck of the 1st rib and the inferior border of the lungs at the 6th costal cartilage/ 6th rib in the midclavicular line and at the 8th rib at the lateral aspect of the bony thorax at the midaxillary line;

2. The cardiac notch of the left lung and the deviation of the parietal pleura away from the median plane toward the left side in the region of the notch;

3. The reflection of parietal pleura inferiorly at the 8th costochondral junction at the midclavicular line and at the 10th rib in the midaxillary line; posterior to the reflection can be seen posterior

to the diaphragm on each side of the vertebral column at the level of the neck of the 12th rib;

4. The apex of the heart in the 5th interspace at the left midclavicular line;

5. The right atrium forming the right border of the heart and extending just beyond the lateral margin of the sternum;

6. The great vessels of the heart and the branches of the great vessels that pass through the superior thoracic aperture (thoracic inlet).

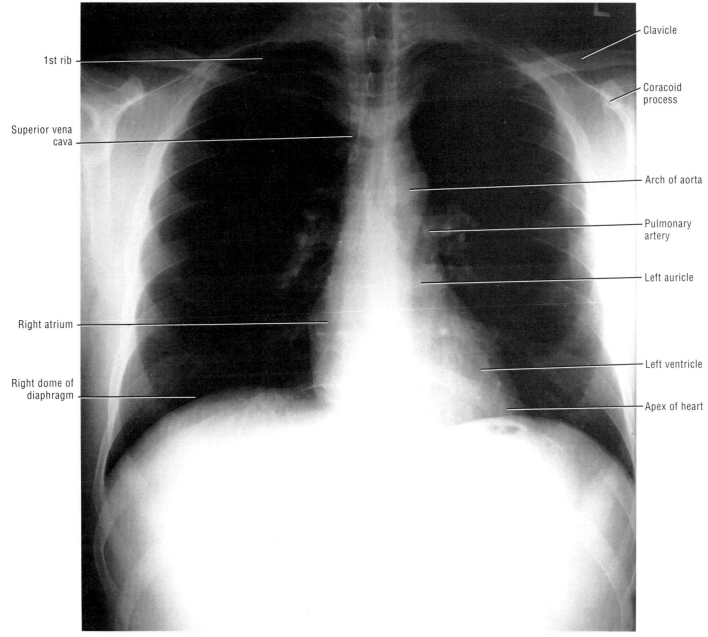

1st rib

Superior vena
cava

Right atrium

Right dome of
diaphragm

Clavicle

Coracoid
process

Arch of aorta

Pulmonary
artery

Left auricle

Left ventricle

Apex of heart

1.24
Radiograph of chest

Using Figure 1.23 for reference, observe in this posteroanterior projection:

1. The body of the 1st thoracic vertebra (T1) and the articulation of the 1st rib with the vertebral body; follow the 1st rib, which curves laterally and then medially crossing the clavicle;

2. The dome of the diaphragm is somewhat higher on the right;

3. The convexity of the right mediastinal border is formed by the right atrium; the lesser convexity above this is produced by the superior vena cava;

4. The left mediastinal border is formed by the arch of the aorta, the pulmonary trunk, the left auricle (not prominent on a normal chest radiograph), and the left ventricle. (Courtesy of Dr. E.L. Lansdown, Professor of Radiology, University of Toronto, Toronto, Ontario, Canada.)

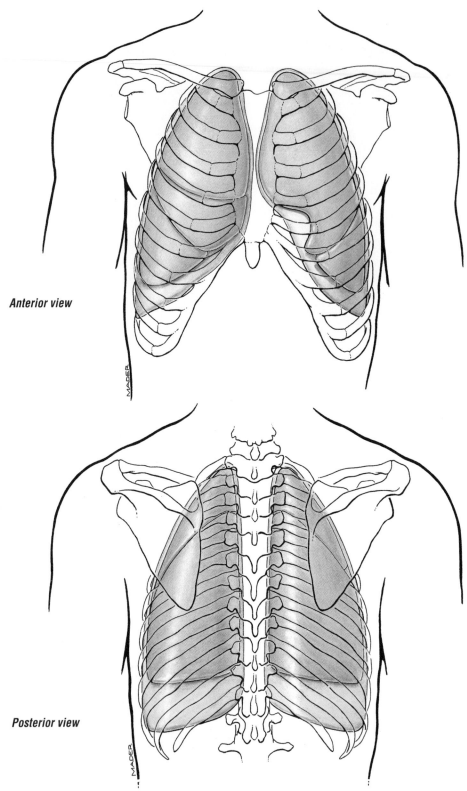

Anterior view

Posterior view

1.25
Outline of the pleura and lungs

Trace the outline of the lung (covered with visceral pleura) and the outline of the parietal pleura as observed in quiet respiration. Note that the apex and anterior border of both lungs lie directly adjacent to the parietal pleura as far as the 4th costal cartilage. At this level, the left lung has a well-defined cardiac notch spanning horizontally along the 4th costal cartilage and rib to the midclavicular line and then curving inferiorly to the 6th rib or costal cartilage. Follow the outline of the inferior border of the lungs and pleura on the anterior, lateral, and posterior aspect of the bony thorax. Note that the apex of the lung and cervical pleura extend to the neck of the 1st rib.

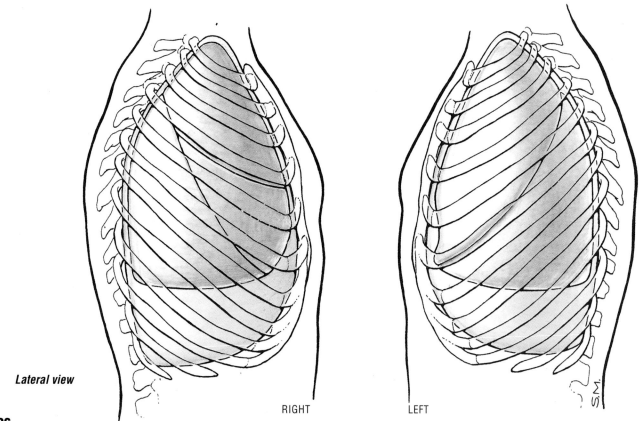

Lateral view

RIGHT   LEFT

1.26
Outline of the pleura and lungs

Follow the outlines of the oblique and horizontal fissures of the right lung and the oblique fissure of the left lung on the anterior, posterior, and lateral views of the bony thorax. Compare the left lateral view of the bony thorax to the MRI (Fig. 1.27).

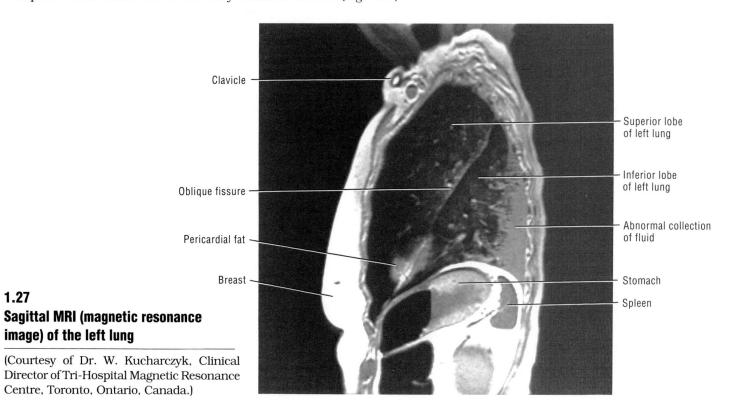

Clavicle

Oblique fissure

Pericardial fat

Breast

Superior lobe
of left lung

Inferior lobe
of left lung

Abnormal collection
of fluid

Stomach

Spleen

1.27
Sagittal MRI (magnetic resonance image) of the left lung

(Courtesy of Dr. W. Kucharczyk, Clinical Director of Tri-Hospital Magnetic Resonance Centre, Toronto, Ontario, Canada.)

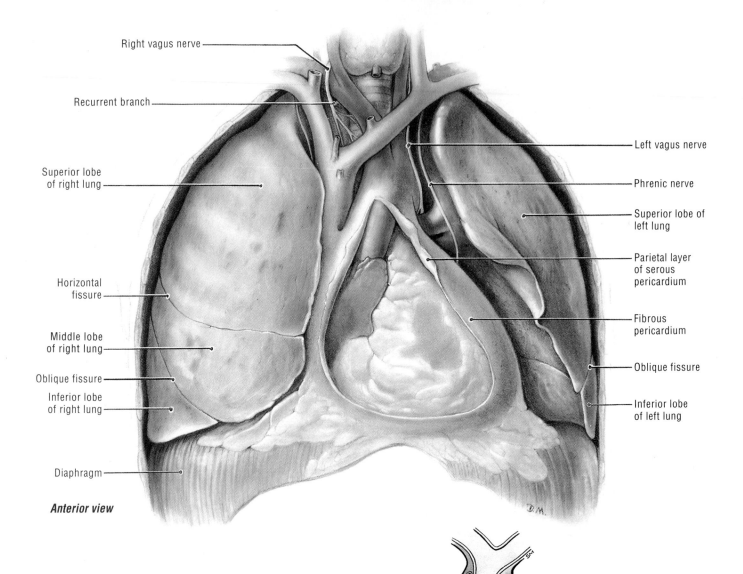

Right vagus nerve

Recurrent branch

Superior lobe
of right lung

Horizontal
fissure

Middle lobe
of right lung

Oblique fissure

Inferior lobe
of right lung

Diaphragm

Anterior view

Left vagus nerve

Phrenic nerve

Superior lobe of
left lung

Parietal layer
of serous
pericardium

Fibrous
pericardium

Oblique fissure

Inferior lobe
of left lung

Fibrous pericardium

Parietal layer ⎤
                 ⎬ Serous
Visceral layer ⎦ pericardium

1.28
Thoracic contents in situ

Observe:

1. The fibrous pericardium is removed anteriorly exposing the heart and great vessels; note the fibrous pericardium is lined by the parietal layer of serous pericardium;

2. The right lung has three lobes; the superior lobe is separated from the middle lobe by the horizontal fissure and the middle lobe is separated from the inferior lobe by the oblique fissure;

3. The left lung has two lobes, superior and inferior, separated by the oblique fissure; the anterior border of the left lung is reflected laterally to enable visualization of the phrenic nerve passing anterior to the root of the lung and the vagus nerve lying anterior to the arch of the aorta and then passing posterior to the root of the lung;

4. The right vagus nerve passing anterior to the right subclavian artery where it gives off the recurrent branch and then divides to contribute fibers to the esophageal, cardiac, and pulmonary plexuses.

1.29
Fibrous and serous pericardia

On the coronal section of the heart, observe that the external layer of the pericardium is fibrous. The fibrous pericardium is lined by a double layered, membranous sac, the serous pericardium. The outer parietal layer lines the fibrous pericardium and is continuous with the inner visceral layer or epicardium that covers the surface of the heart and great vessels. The thin film of fluid between the visceral and parietal layers of serous pericardium allows the heart to move within the sac.

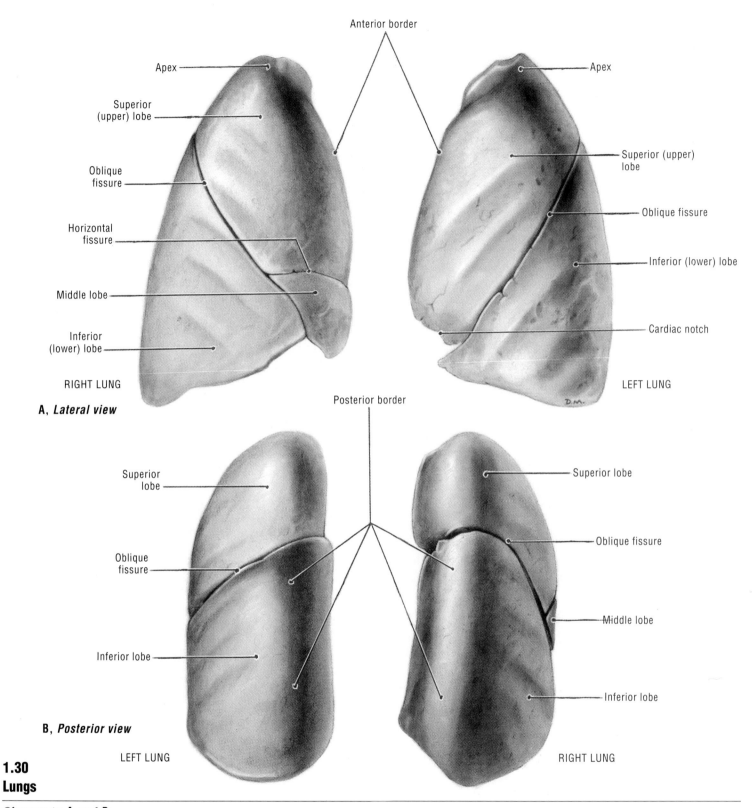

Anterior border

Apex

Superior
(upper) lobe

Oblique
fissure

Horizontal
fissure

Middle lobe

Inferior
(lower) lobe

RIGHT LUNG

A, Lateral view

Apex

Superior (upper)
lobe

Oblique fissure

Inferior (lower) lobe

Cardiac notch

LEFT LUNG

D.M.

Posterior border

Superior
lobe

Oblique
fissure

Inferior lobe

B, Posterior view

LEFT LUNG

Superior lobe

Oblique fissure

Middle lobe

Inferior lobe

RIGHT LUNG

1.30
Lungs

Observe in **A** and **B**:

1. The three lobes of the right lung and the two lobes of the left;

2. The middle lobe (of the right lung) lying anteriorly;

3. The deficiency of the superior (upper) lobe of the left lung, called the cardiac notch;

4. The oblique and horizontal fissures of the right lung and the oblique fissure of the left lung; the fissures may be incomplete or absent on some specimens;

5. The sharp anterior border and the rounded posterior border of the lungs;

6. The impressions of the ribs on the anterior and lateral aspects of the lung.

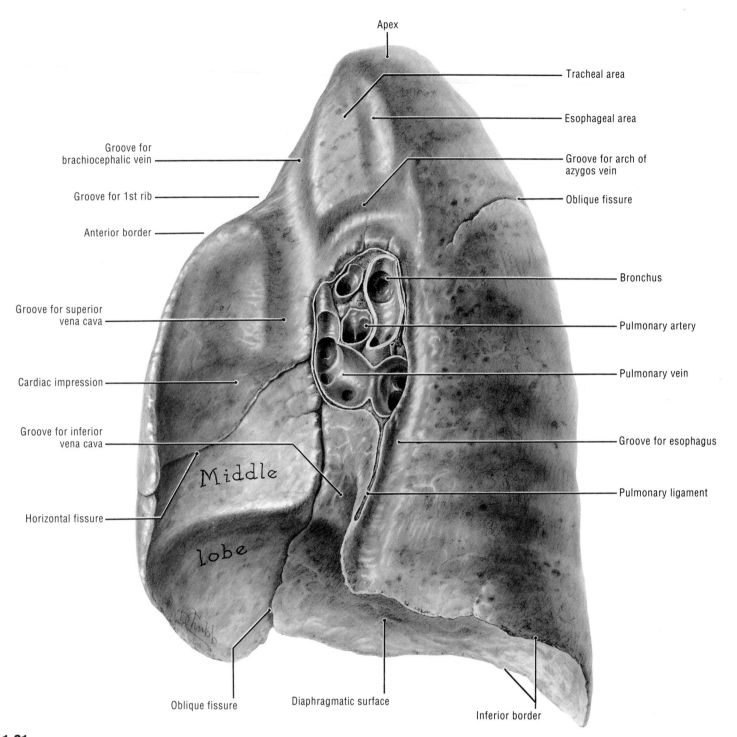

Apex

Tracheal area

Esophageal area

Groove for brachiocephalic vein

Groove for arch of azygos vein

Groove for 1st rib

Oblique fissure

Anterior border

Bronchus

Groove for superior vena cava

Pulmonary artery

Pulmonary vein

Cardiac impression

Groove for inferior vena cava

Groove for esophagus

Pulmonary ligament

Middle

Horizontal fissure

lobe

Oblique fissure

Diaphragmatic surface

Inferior border

1.31
Mediastinal surface of right lung

Observe:

1. The embalmed lungs have impressions of the structures with which they come into contact clearly demarcated as surface features; thus, the base is fashioned by the domes of the diaphragm; the costal surface bears the impressions of the ribs; distended vessels leave their mark; empty vessels and nerves do not;

2. The somewhat "pear"-shaped root of the lung near the center of the mediastinal surface, and the pulmonary ligament descending like a stalk from the root;

3. The groove for (or line of contact with) the esophagus throughout the length of the lung, except where the arch of the azygos vein intervenes; this groove passes posterior to the root and therefore posterior to the pulmonary ligament, which separates it from the groove for the inferior vena cava;

4. The oblique fissure, here incomplete, but complete in Figure 1.32.

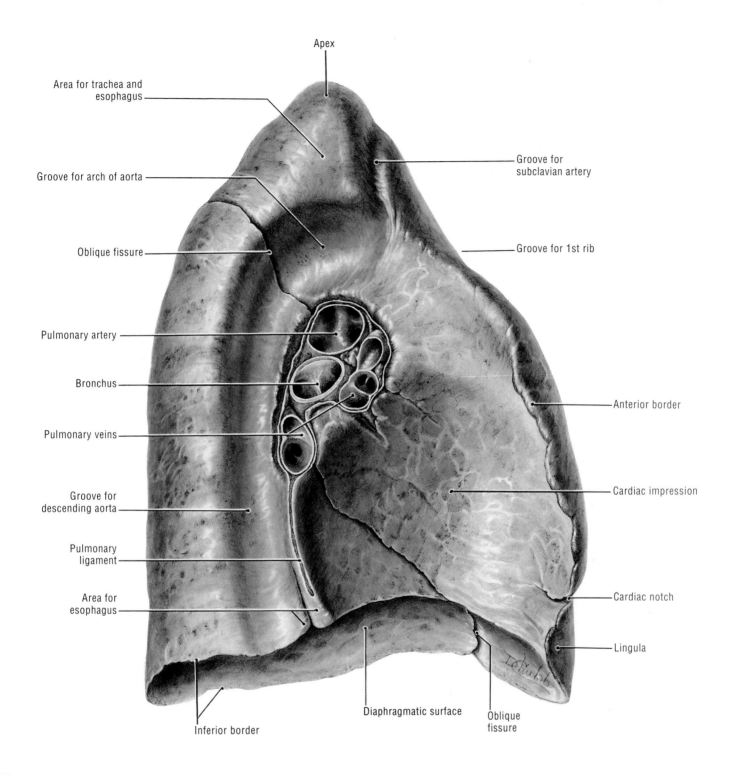

Apex

Area for trachea and
esophagus

Groove for
subclavian artery

Groove for arch of aorta

Oblique fissure

Groove for 1st rib

Pulmonary artery

Bronchus

Anterior border

Pulmonary veins

Groove for
descending aorta

Cardiac impression

Pulmonary
ligament

Area for
esophagus

Cardiac notch

Lingula

Inferior border

Diaphragmatic surface

Oblique
fissure

1.32
Mediastinal surface of left lung

Observe:

1. Near the center, the root and the pulmonary ligament descending from it;

2. The site of contact with the esophagus, between the aorta and the inferior end of the pulmonary ligament;

3. The oblique fissure, cutting completely through the lung substance;

4. In both the right root and the left, the artery is superior, the bronchus is posterior, one vein is anterior, and the other is inferior; in the right root, the bronchus (eparterial) to the superior (upper) lobe is the most superior structure.

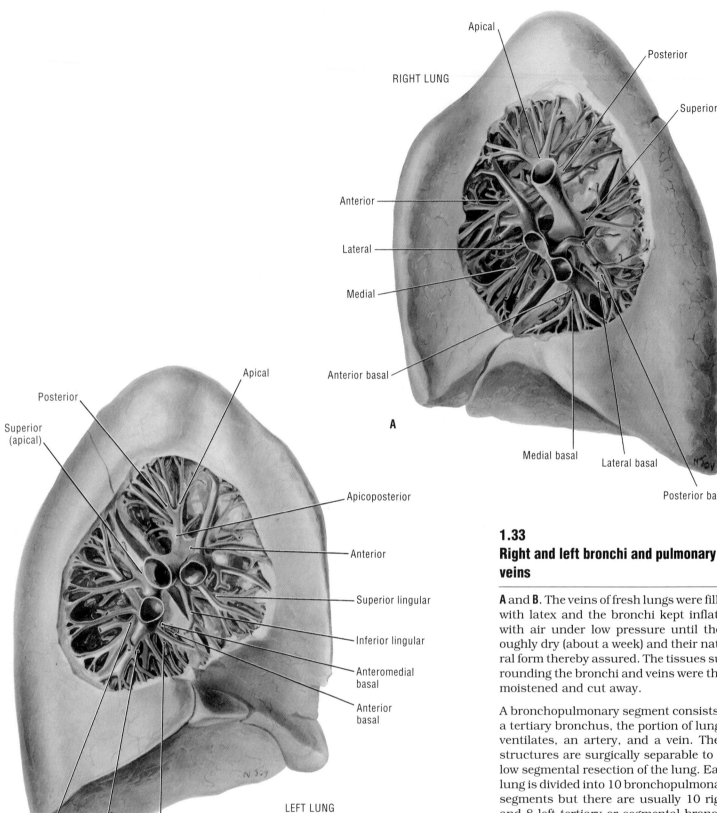

RIGHT LUNG

Apical

Posterior

Superior

Anterior

Lateral

Medial

Anterior basal

Medial basal

Lateral basal

Posterior basal

A

Apical

Posterior

Superior
(apical)

Apicoposterior

Anterior

Superior lingular

Inferior lingular

Anteromedial
basal

Anterior
basal

Posterior
basal

Lateral
basal

Medial
basal

LEFT LUNG

B

1.33
Right and left bronchi and pulmonary veins

A and **B**. The veins of fresh lungs were filled with latex and the bronchi kept inflated with air under low pressure until thoroughly dry (about a week) and their natural form thereby assured. The tissues surrounding the bronchi and veins were then moistened and cut away.

A bronchopulmonary segment consists of a tertiary bronchus, the portion of lung it ventilates, an artery, and a vein. These structures are surgically separable to allow segmental resection of the lung. Each lung is divided into 10 bronchopulmonary segments but there are usually 10 right and 8 left tertiary or segmental bronchi. The reduced number in the left lung is accounted for by the fact that the left apical and posterior bronchi arise from a common stem, as do also the left anterior basal and medial basal.(Terminology is after Jackson and Huber.)

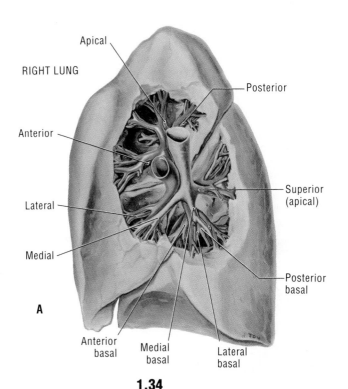

RIGHT LUNG

Apical

Posterior

Anterior

Lateral

Medial

Superior (apical)

Posterior basal

Anterior basal

Medial basal

Lateral basal

A

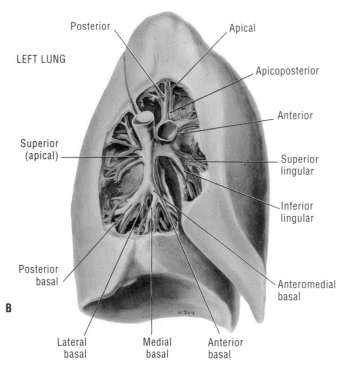

Posterior

Apical

LEFT LUNG

Apicoposterior

Anterior

Superior (apical)

Superior lingular

Inferior lingular

Posterior basal

Anteromedial basal

Lateral basal

Medial basal

Anterior basal

B

1.34
Right (A) and left (B) bronchi and pulmonary arteries

The arteries (blue) of the fresh lungs were filled with red latex and the bronchi (gray) kept inflated and treated as for Figure 1.33.

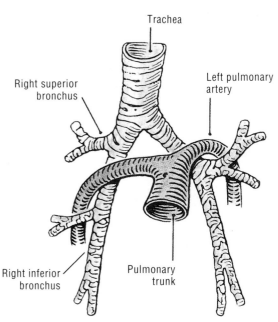

Trachea

Right superior bronchus

Left pulmonary artery

Right inferior bronchus

Pulmonary trunk

1.35

Relationship of the bronchi and the pulmonary artery at the root of the right and left lung

Note that the right pulmonary artery at the root of the lung lies between the secondary bronchi to the superior (upper) and middle lobes and the left pulmonary artery arches anterior to the left primary bronchus.

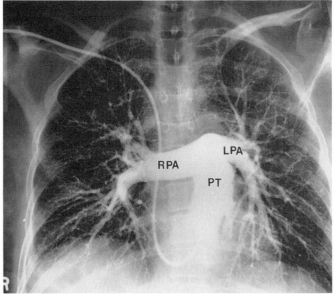

LPA

RPA

PT

R

1.36
Pulmonary angiogram

Observe:

1. The catheter located in the right ventricle and pulmonary trunk *(PT);*

2. The pulmonary trunk *(PT)* dividing into a longer right pulmonary artery *(RPA)* and a shorter left pulmonary artery *(LPA);*

3. The branches of the artery following the corresponding segmental bronchi. (Courtesy of Dr. J. Heslin, Assistant Professor of Anatomy, University of Toronto, Toronto, Ontario, Canada.)

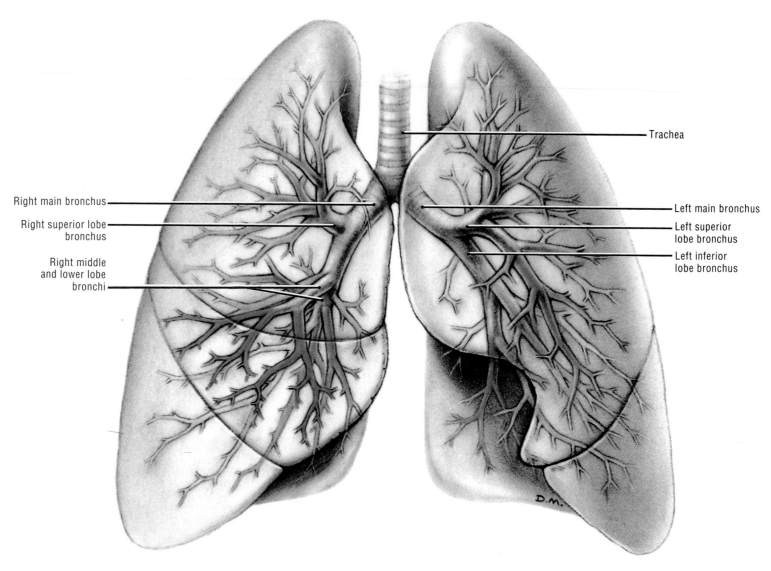

Right main bronchus

Right superior lobe bronchus

Right middle and lower lobe bronchi

Trachea

Left main bronchus

Left superior lobe bronchus

Left inferior lobe bronchus

Anterior view

1.37
Trachea and bronchi in situ

Observe:

1. The bifurcation of the trachea into right and left main (primary) bronchi, at the sternal angle;

2. The right main bronchus is more vertical, has a greater diameter, and is shorter in length than the left main bronchus; therefore, it is more likely that foreign objects will become lodged in the right main bronchus;

3. The right main bronchus gives off the right superior lobe bronchus (eparterial bronchus) before entering the hilum (hilus) of the lung; after entering the hilum, the right middle and inferior lobe bronchi are given off;

4. The left main bronchus divides into the left superior and left inferior lobe bronchi; the left superior lobe bronchus also supplies the lingula;

5. The lobar bronchi further divide into segmental (tertiary) bronchi.

RIGHT LUNG	LEFT LUNG
Superior Lobe	**Superior Lobe**
☐ Apical	☐ Apical
▨ Posterior	▨ Posterior
☐ Anterior	☐ Anterior
	▨ Superior
Middle Lobe	▨ Inferior
▨ Lateral	**Inferior Lobe**
▨ Medial	
	☐ Superior
Inferior Lobe	☐ Anterior basal
	▨ Medial basal
☐ Superior	▨ Lateral basal
☐ Anterior basal	▨ Posterior basal
☐ Medial basal	
▨ Lateral basal	
▨ Posterior basal	

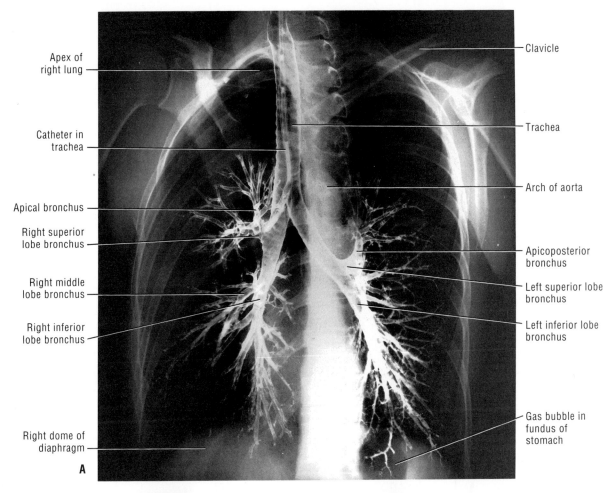

Apex of right lung

Catheter in trachea

Apical bronchus

Right superior lobe bronchus

Right middle lobe bronchus

Right inferior lobe bronchus

Right dome of diaphragm

Clavicle

Trachea

Arch of aorta

Apicoposterior bronchus

Left superior lobe bronchus

Left inferior lobe bronchus

Gas bubble in fundus of stomach

A

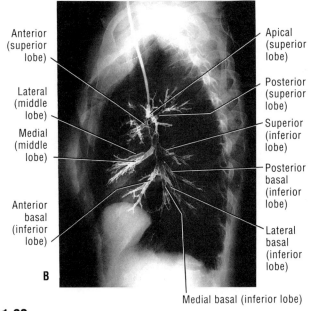

Anterior (superior lobe)

Lateral (middle lobe)

Medial (middle lobe)

Anterior basal (inferior lobe)

Apical (superior lobe)

Posterior (superior lobe)

Superior (inferior lobe)

Posterior basal (inferior lobe)

Lateral basal (inferior lobe)

Medial basal (inferior lobe)

B

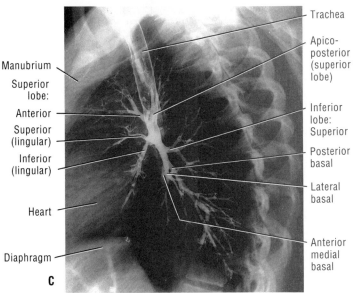

Manubrium

Superior lobe:

Anterior

Superior (lingular)

Inferior (lingular)

Heart

Diaphragm

Trachea

Apico-posterior (superior lobe)

Inferior lobe: Superior

Posterior basal

Lateral basal

Anterior medial basal

C

1.38
Bronchograms

A. Bronchogram of the right and left bronchial tree. This is a slightly oblique, posteroanterior view.

B. Right lateral bronchogram, segmental bronchi.

C. Left lateral bronchogram, segmental bronchi. (Bronchograms courtesy of Dr. D.E. Sanders, Dr. S. Herman, and Dr. E.L. Lansdown, Department of Radiology, University of Toronto, Toronto, Ontario, Canada.)

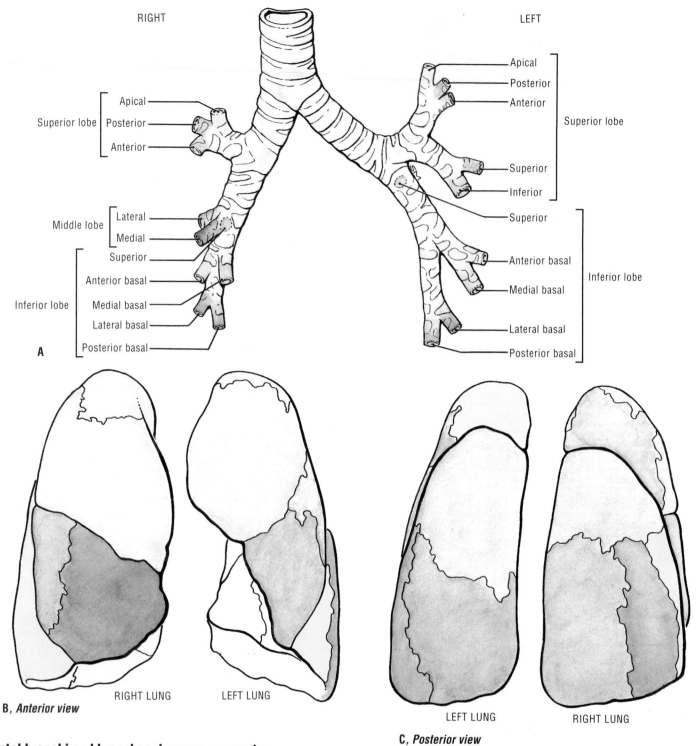

RIGHT

Superior lobe
- Apical
- Posterior
- Anterior

Middle lobe
- Lateral
- Medial

Inferior lobe
- Superior
- Anterior basal
- Medial basal
- Lateral basal
- Posterior basal

LEFT

Superior lobe
- Apical
- Posterior
- Anterior
- Superior
- Inferior

Inferior lobe
- Superior
- Anterior basal
- Medial basal
- Lateral basal
- Posterior basal

A

RIGHT LUNG   LEFT LUNG

B, *Anterior view*

LEFT LUNG   RIGHT LUNG

C, *Posterior view*

1.39
Segmental bronchi and bronchopulmonary segments

A. Segmental bronchi. The right lung has three lobes; the left has two. There are 10 tertiary or segmental bronchi on the right, 8 on the left. Note that on the left, the apical and posterior bronchi arise from a single stem, as do the anterior basal and medial basal.

B and **C**. Bronchopulmonary segments. A bronchopulmonary segment consists of a tertiary bronchus, the portion of lung it ventilates, an artery, and a vein. These are surgically separable. To prepare Figures 1.39**B**, 1.40**A**, and 1.40**B**, the tertiary bronchi of fresh lungs were isolated within the hilus and injected with

latex of various colors. Minor variations in the branching of the bronchi result in variations in the surface patterns.

For detailed information consult Jackson CL, Huber JF. *Correlated applied anatomy of the bronchial tree and lungs with a system of nomenclature.* Dis Chest 1943; 9:319; Boyden EA. *Segmental anatomy of the lungs.* New York: McGraw-Hill Book Company, 1954; Boyden EA. *The nomenclature of the broncho-pulmonary segments and their blood supply.* Dis Chest 1961; 39:1.

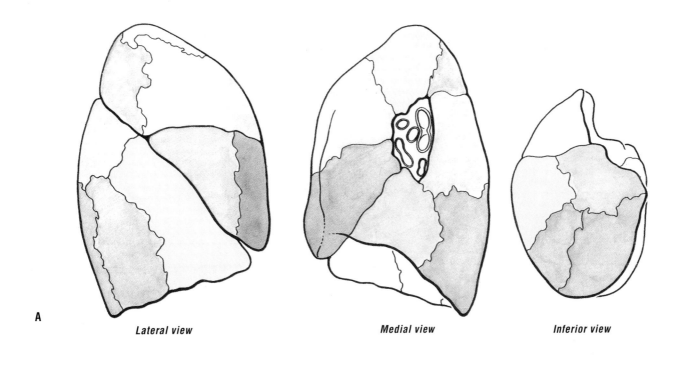

Lateral view   *Medial view*   *Inferior view*

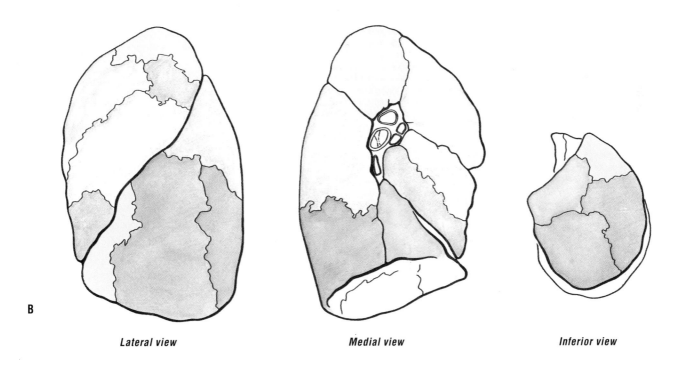

Lateral view   *Medial view*   *Inferior view*

1.40
Bronchopulmonary segments (*continued*)

Right (**A**) and left (**B**) bronchopulmonary segments.

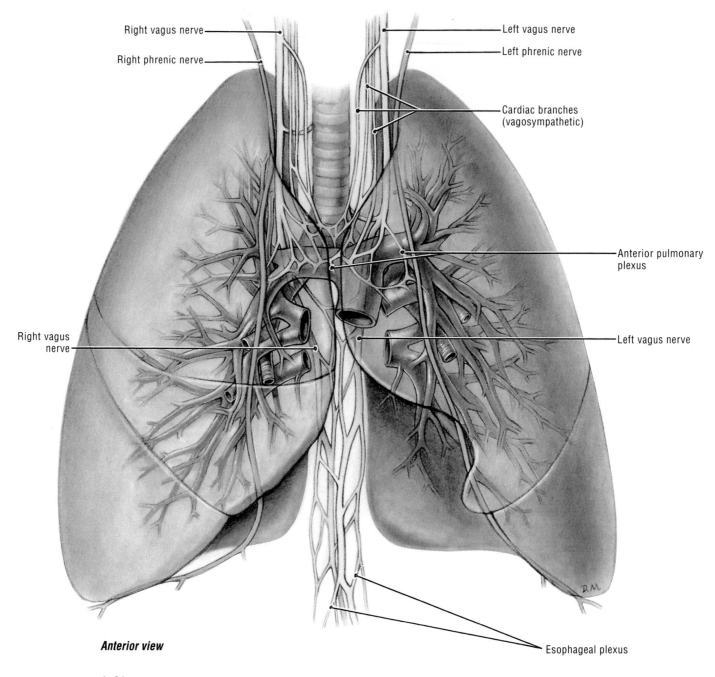

Right vagus nerve

Right phrenic nerve

Left vagus nerve

Left phrenic nerve

Cardiac branches
(vagosympathetic)

Anterior pulmonary
plexus

Right vagus
nerve

Left vagus nerve

Esophageal plexus

Anterior view

1.41
Lungs – innervation

Observe:

1. The anterior and posterior pulmonary plexuses receiving sympathetic contributions from the right and left sympathetic trunks (2nd to 5th thoracic ganglia), not shown, and parasympathetic contributions from the right and left vagus nerves;

2. The right and left vagus nerves passing inferiorly from the posterior pulmonary plexus to contribute fibers to the esophageal plexus;

3. Branches from the pulmonary plexuses continuing along the bronchi and pulmonary vasculature to the lungs;

4. The phrenic nerve passing anterior to the root of the lung to the diaphragm.

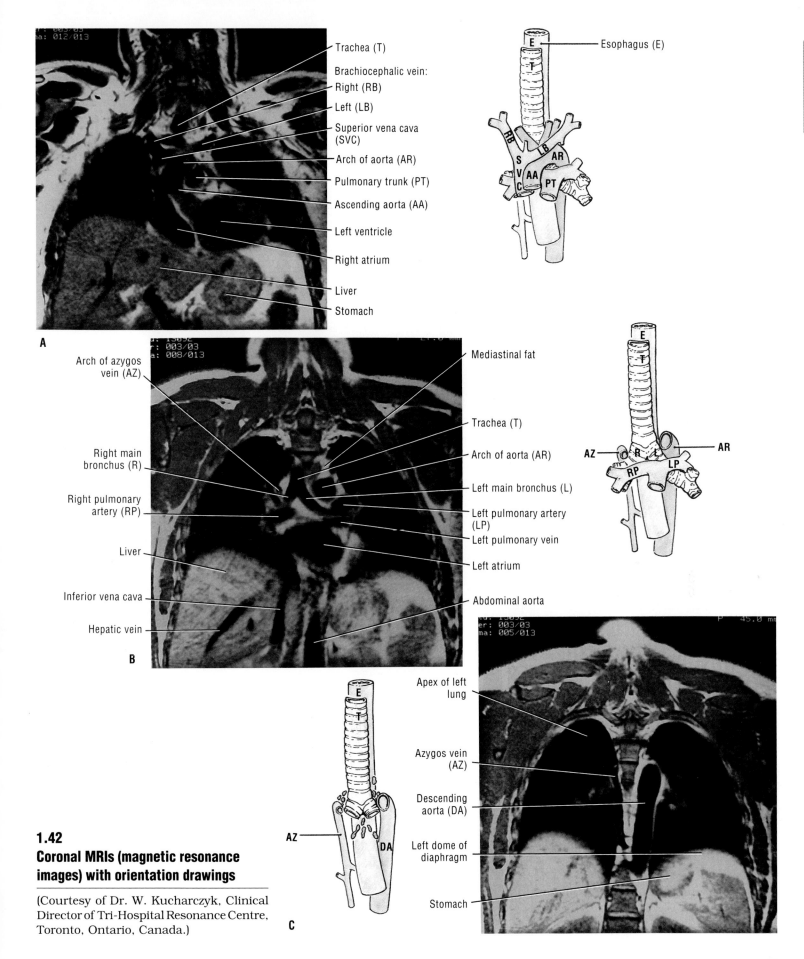

Trachea (T)

Brachiocephalic vein:
Right (RB)
Left (LB)

Superior vena cava
(SVC)

Arch of aorta (AR)

Pulmonary trunk (PT)

Ascending aorta (AA)

Left ventricle

Right atrium

Liver

Stomach

Esophagus (E)

A

Arch of azygos
vein (AZ)

Right main
bronchus (R)

Right pulmonary
artery (RP)

Liver

Inferior vena cava

Hepatic vein

Mediastinal fat

Trachea (T)

Arch of aorta (AR)

Left main bronchus (L)

Left pulmonary artery
(LP)

Left pulmonary vein

Left atrium

Abdominal aorta

B

Apex of left
lung

Azygos vein
(AZ)

Descending
aorta (DA)

Left dome of
diaphragm

Stomach

1.42
Coronal MRIs (magnetic resonance images) with orientation drawings

(Courtesy of Dr. W. Kucharczyk, Clinical
Director of Tri-Hospital Resonance Centre,
Toronto, Ontario, Canada.)

C

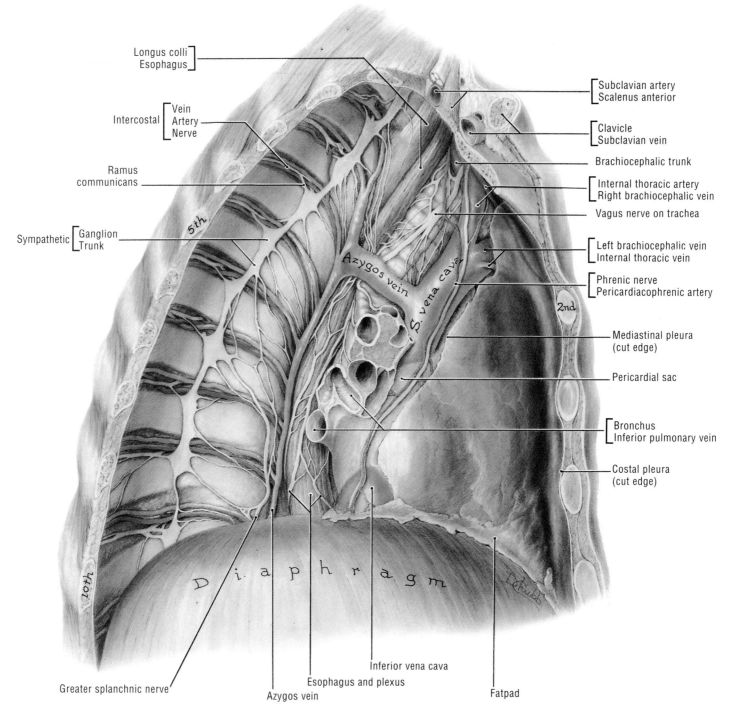

Longus colli
Esophagus

Intercostal
Vein
Artery
Nerve

Ramus
communicans

Sympathetic
Ganglion
Trunk

5th

Azygos vein

S. vena cava

2nd

Subclavian artery
Scalenus anterior

Clavicle
Subclavian vein

Brachiocephalic trunk

Internal thoracic artery
Right brachiocephalic vein

Vagus nerve on trachea

Left brachiocephalic vein
Internal thoracic vein

Phrenic nerve
Pericardiacophrenic artery

Mediastinal pleura
(cut edge)

Pericardial sac

Bronchus
Inferior pulmonary vein

Costal pleura
(cut edge)

Diaphragm

10th

Greater splanchnic nerve

Azygos vein

Esophagus and plexus

Inferior vena cava

Fatpad

1.43
Right side of the mediastinum

The costal and mediastinal pleurae have mostly been removed, exposing the underlying structures. Compare with the mediastinal surface of the right lung in Figure 1.31.

In this important dissection, observe:
1. The right side of the mediastinum is the "blue side," dominated by the arch of the azygos vein, the superior vena cava, and the right atrium;

2. When the mediastinal pleura is removed, the phrenic nerve is free; follow its medial relationships to the diaphragm;

3. The trachea and esophagus are visible;

4. That on entering the mediastinum the right vagus nerve travels on the medial surface of the trachea, passes medial to the arch of the azygos vein and then courses slightly posteriorly to travel along the medial aspect of the esophagus;

5. The sympathetic trunk and its ganglia, the greater splanchnic nerve, and the esophageal plexus.

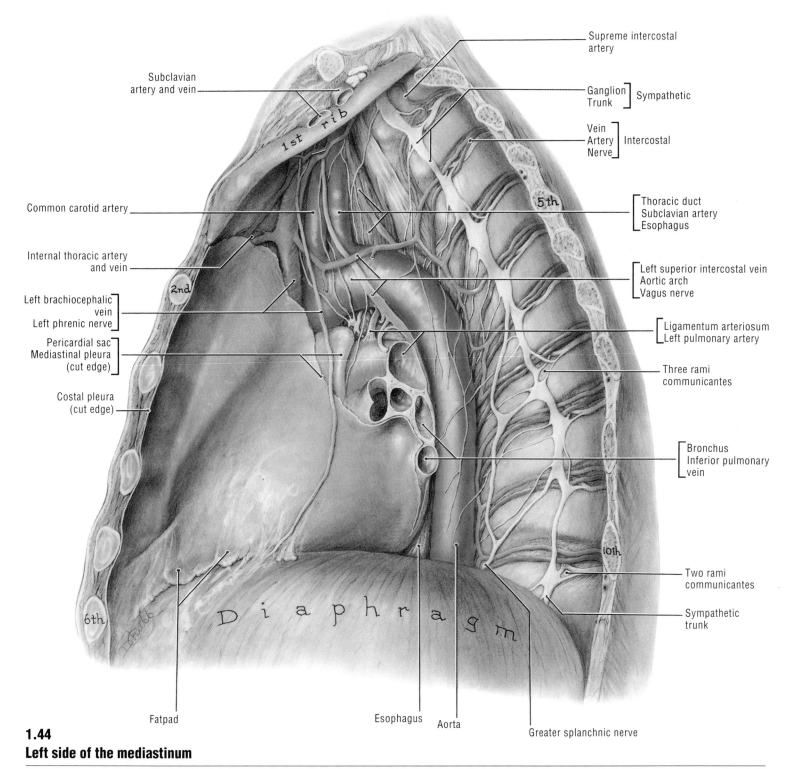

Subclavian artery and vein

1st rib

Common carotid artery

Internal thoracic artery and vein

2nd

Left brachiocephalic vein
Left phrenic nerve

Pericardial sac
Mediastinal pleura (cut edge)

Costal pleura (cut edge)

6th

Diaphragm

Fatpad

Supreme intercostal artery

Ganglion Trunk] Sympathetic

Vein
Artery] Intercostal
Nerve

5th

Thoracic duct
Subclavian artery
Esophagus

Left superior intercostal vein
Aortic arch
Vagus nerve

Ligamentum arteriosum
Left pulmonary artery

Three rami communicantes

Bronchus
Inferior pulmonary vein

10th

Two rami communicantes

Sympathetic trunk

Esophagus   Aorta

Greater splanchnic nerve

1.44
Left side of the mediastinum

The costal and mediastinal pleurae have mostly been removed, exposing the underlying structures. Compare with the mediastinal surface of the left lung in Figure 1.32.

In this important dissection, observe:

1. The left side of the mediastinum is the "red side," dominated by the arch and descending portion of the aorta, the left common carotid and subclavian arteries;

2. The phrenic nerve, freed by removal of pleura, passing anterior to the root of the lung;

3. The thoracic duct on the esophagus;

4. The left vagus nerve passing posterior to the root of the lung, and sending its recurrent laryngeal branch around the ligamentum arteriosum posterior to the arch of the aorta;

5. The sympathetic trunk attached to intercostal nerves by rami communicantes.

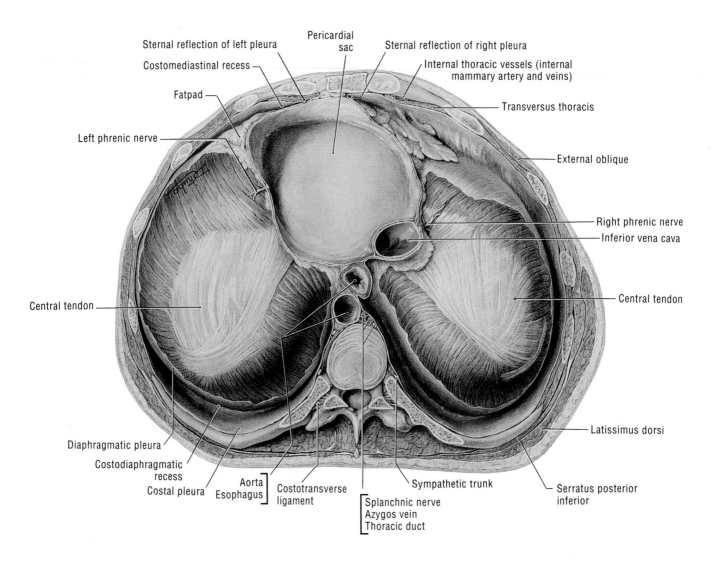

Sternal reflection of left pleura

Pericardial sac

Sternal reflection of right pleura

Costomediastinal recess

Internal thoracic vessels (internal mammary artery and veins)

Fatpad

Transversus thoracis

Left phrenic nerve

External oblique

Right phrenic nerve

Inferior vena cava

Central tendon

Central tendon

Latissimus dorsi

Diaphragmatic pleura

Costodiaphragmatic recess

Costal pleura

Aorta
Esophagus

Costotransverse ligament

Splanchnic nerve
Azygos vein
Thoracic duct

Sympathetic trunk

Serratus posterior inferior

1.45
Diaphragm and pericardial sac

In this superior view, the diaphragmatic pleura is mostly removed. Observe:

1. The pericardial sac, situated on the anterior half of the diaphragm; one-third being to the right of the median plane and two-thirds being to the left; the most caudal point being anteriorly and to the left, like the apex of the heart;

2. The openings of the large hepatic veins into the inferior vena cava;

3. The sternal reflection of the left pleural sac, failing to meet that of the right sac in the median plane, anterior to the pericardium;

4. The right and left pleural sacs almost meeting between the esophagus and aorta to form a mesoesophagus;

5. The costodiaphragmatic and costomediastinal recesses;

6. The costal pleura, on reaching the vertebral column imperceptibly becoming the mediastinal pleura.

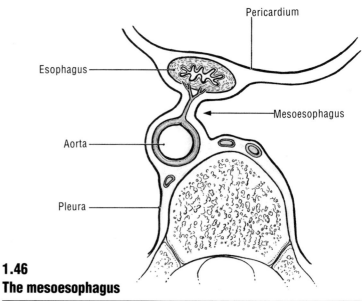

Pericardium

Esophagus

Mesoesophagus

Aorta

Pleura

1.46
The mesoesophagus

Between the inferior part of the esophagus and the aorta, the right and left layers of mediastinal pleura form a dorsal mesoesophagus.

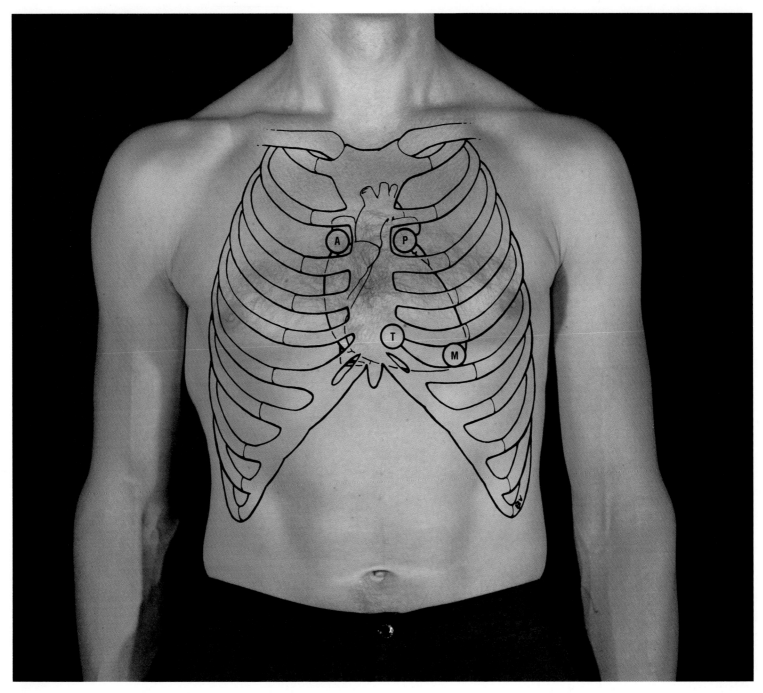

1.47

Surface markings of the heart and points of auscultation

Observe:

1. The superior border of the heart represented by a slightly oblique line joining the right and left 3rd costal cartilages, the convex right side of the heart projecting lateral to the sternum and inferiorly lying at the 6th or 7th costochondral junction, the inferior border of the heart lying, superior to the central tendon of the diaphragm, and sloping slightly inferiorly to the apex at the 5th interspace in the midclavicular line;

2. Auscultation points are the areas where sounds from each of the heart's valves may be heard most distinctly through a stethoscope; aortic and mitral valves are deep in the chest and their sounds are heard best at the points where the direction of blood flow is closer to the chest wall; aortic *(A)* and pulmonary *(P)* areas are in the 2nd interspace to the right and left of the sternal border; the tricuspid area *(T)* is near the left sternal border in the 5th or 6th interspace; the mitral valve *(M)* is heard best near the apex of the heart in the 5th intercostal space in the midclavicular line.

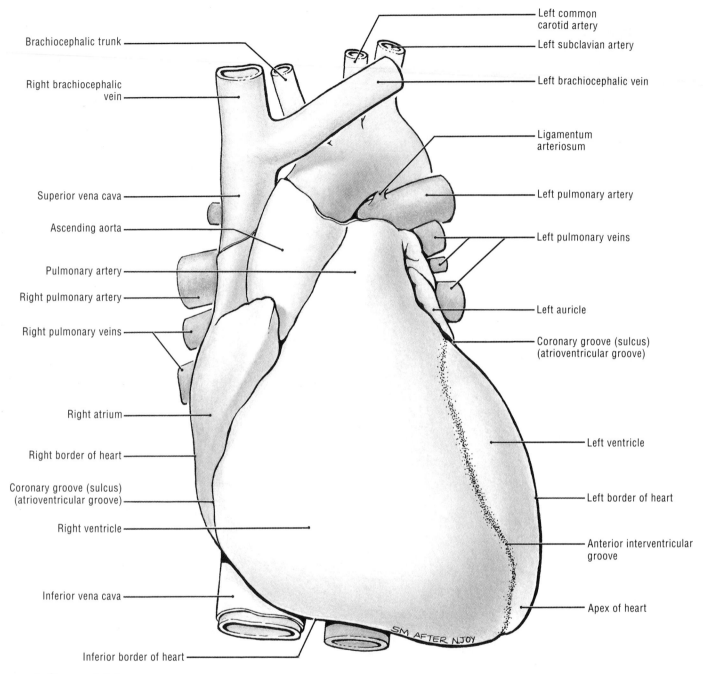

Brachiocephalic trunk

Right brachiocephalic vein

Superior vena cava

Ascending aorta

Pulmonary artery

Right pulmonary artery

Right pulmonary veins

Right atrium

Right border of heart

Coronary groove (sulcus) (atrioventricular groove)

Right ventricle

Inferior vena cava

Inferior border of heart

Left common carotid artery

Left subclavian artery

Left brachiocephalic vein

Ligamentum arteriosum

Left pulmonary artery

Left pulmonary veins

Left auricle

Coronary groove (sulcus) (atrioventricular groove)

Left ventricle

Left border of heart

Anterior interventricular groove

Apex of heart

SM AFTER N.JOY

A, *Sternocostal view*

1.48
Heart and great vessels, hardened in situ and removed en masse

Observe in **A**:

1. The right border, formed by the right atrium, slightly convex and almost in line with the superior vena cava and the inferior vena cava; enlargement of the right atrium shows as a bulging of the right border of the heart;

2. The inferior border is formed primarily by the right ventricle and a small part of the left ventricle; dilation of the right ventricle is directed toward the pulmonary artery and causes the heart to rotate so that more of the right ventricle forms the left border of the heart;

3. The left border is formed primarily by the left ventricle and a small portion by the left auricle; when the left ventricle is dilated, the apex of the heart extends further to the left;

4. The pulmonary artery bifurcating inferior to the arch of the aorta into the right and left pulmonary arteries;

5. The ligamentum arteriosum passing from the root of the left pulmonary artery to the arch of the aorta.

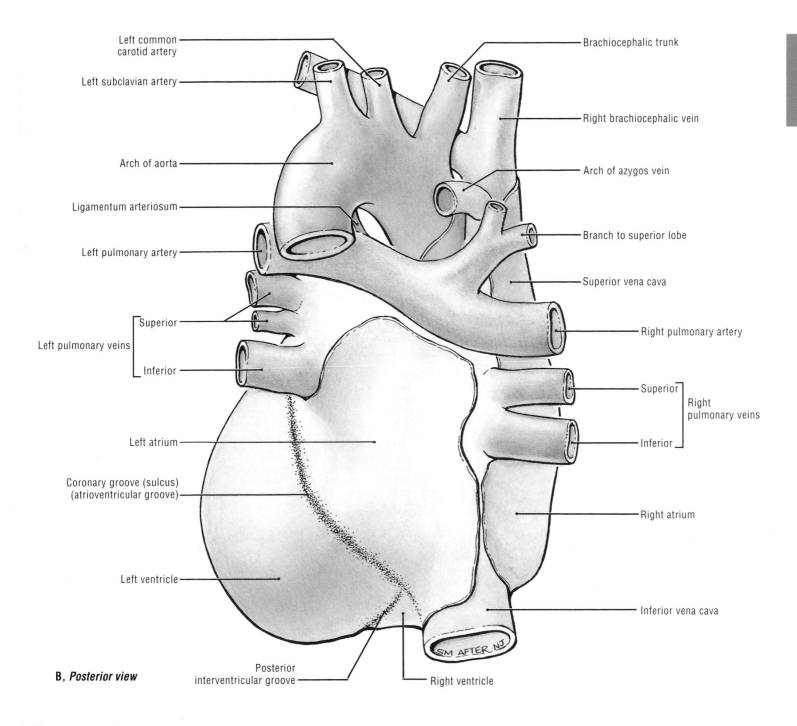

Left common carotid artery

Left subclavian artery

Arch of aorta

Ligamentum arteriosum

Left pulmonary artery

Left pulmonary veins {Superior / Inferior}

Left atrium

Coronary groove (sulcus) (atrioventricular groove)

Left ventricle

Posterior interventricular groove

Brachiocephalic trunk

Right brachiocephalic vein

Arch of azygos vein

Branch to superior lobe

Superior vena cava

Right pulmonary artery

Right pulmonary veins {Superior / Inferior}

Right atrium

Inferior vena cava

Right ventricle

SM AFTER NJ

B, *Posterior view*

1.48

Heart and great vessels, hardened in situ and removed en masse *(continued)*

Observe in **B**:

1. Visible from the posterior: most of the left atrium, much of the left ventricle, a little of the right atrium, and almost none of the right ventricle;

2. The right and left pulmonary veins, converging to open into the left atrium;

3. The right and left pulmonary arteries, just superior and parallel to the pulmonary veins and inclining from the left side inferiorly and to the right; hence, the root of the right lung is more inferior than that of the left;

4. The aorta, arching over the left pulmonary vessels (and bronchus); the azygos vein arching over the right pulmonary vessels (and bronchus);

5. The arch of the aorta, arched in two planes: (a) superiorly and (b) to the left; the convexity to the left is molded on the esophagus and trachea;

6. The atrioventricular groove or coronary groove (sulcus) between the left atrium and left ventricle.

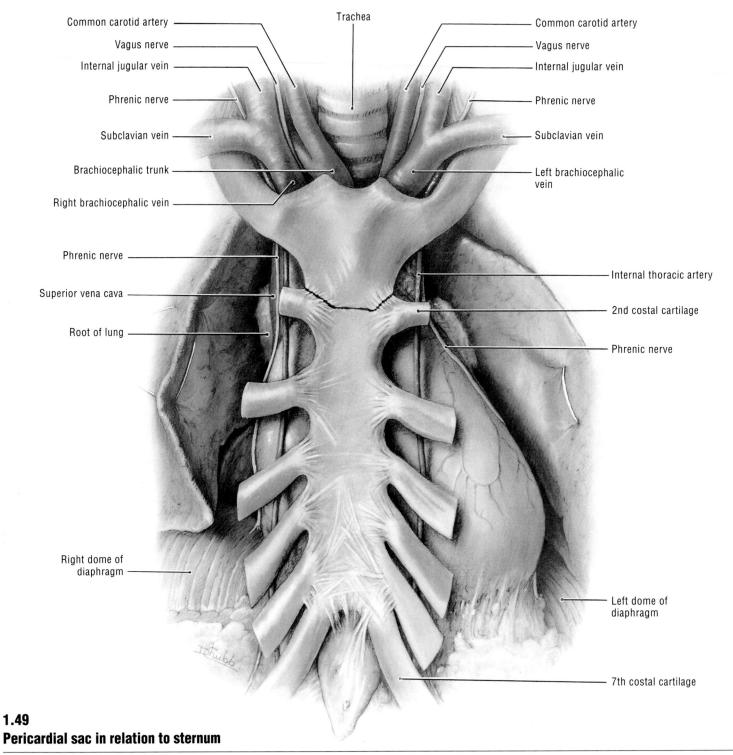

Common carotid artery

Vagus nerve

Internal jugular vein

Phrenic nerve

Subclavian vein

Brachiocephalic trunk

Right brachiocephalic vein

Phrenic nerve

Superior vena cava

Root of lung

Right dome of diaphragm

Trachea

Common carotid artery

Vagus nerve

Internal jugular vein

Phrenic nerve

Subclavian vein

Left brachiocephalic vein

Internal thoracic artery

2nd costal cartilage

Phrenic nerve

Left dome of diaphragm

7th costal cartilage

1.49
Pericardial sac in relation to sternum

Observe:

1. The pericardial sac lies posterior to the body of the sternum from just superior to the sternomanubrial joint (sternal angle) to the level of the xiphisternal joint; about one-third lies to the right of the median plane and two-thirds to the left;

2. The heart thus lies between the sternum and the anterior mediastinum anteriorly and the vertebral column and the posterior mediastinum posteriorly; in cardiac compression, the sternum is depressed 4 to 5 cm, forcing blood out of the heart and into the great vessels;

3. The internal thoracic arteries lateral to the borders of the sternum;

4. The right and left phrenic nerves applied to the pericardial sac;

5. The relationship of the nerves and vessels at the superior thoracic aperture (thoracic inlet).

Note that in order to complete this dissection the manubriosternal (sternomanubrial) joint was divided to enable the body of the sternum to be turned inferiorly.

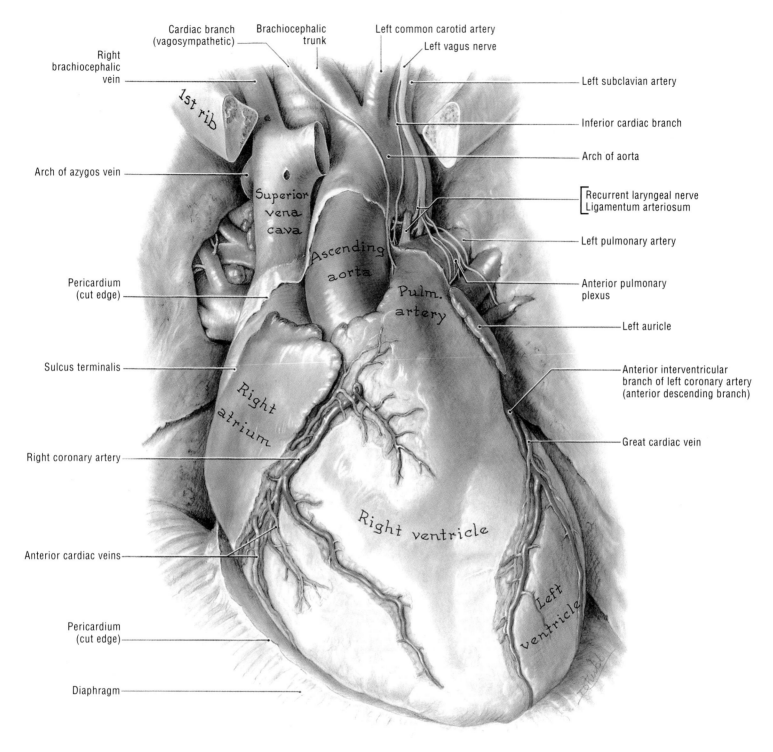

Right brachiocephalic vein

Cardiac branch (vagosympathetic)

Brachiocephalic trunk

Left common carotid artery

Left vagus nerve

Left subclavian artery

1st rib

Inferior cardiac branch

Arch of azygos vein

Arch of aorta

Superior vena cava

Recurrent laryngeal nerve
Ligamentum arteriosum

Left pulmonary artery

Pericardium (cut edge)

Ascending aorta

Anterior pulmonary plexus

Pulm. artery

Left auricle

Sulcus terminalis

Right atrium

Anterior interventricular branch of left coronary artery (anterior descending branch)

Right coronary artery

Great cardiac vein

Right ventricle

Anterior cardiac veins

Left ventricle

Pericardium (cut edge)

Diaphragm

1.50
Sternocostal surface of the heart and great vessels, in situ

Observe:

1. The entire right auricle and much of the right atrium are visible anteriorly, but only a small portion of the left auricle is visible; the auricles, like two closing claws, grasp the pulmonary artery and ascending aorta from the posterior;

2. The ligamentum arteriosum, passing from the root of the left pulmonary artery to the arch of the aorta beyond the site of origin of the left subclavian artery;

3. The right coronary artery in the anterior atrioventricular groove and the anterior interventricular (anterior descending) artery in the anterior interventricular groove;

4. The left vagus nerve passing anterior to the arch of the aorta and then posterior to the root of the lung; the recurrent branch passing inferior to the arch of the aorta just lateral to the ligamentum arteriosum.

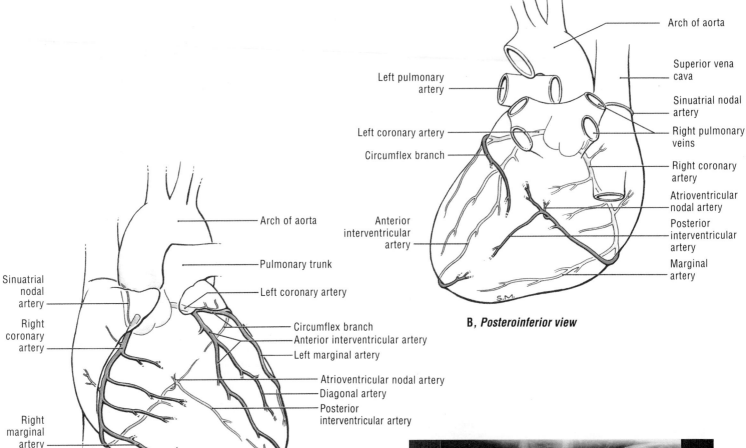

A, Anterior view

1.51
Coronary arteries

Observe in **A** and **B**:

1. The right coronary artery travels in the coronary groove (sulcus) to reach the posterior surface of the heart where it will anastomose with the circumflex branch of the left coronary artery; early in its course it gives off the sinuatrial (SA) nodal artery that supplies the right atrium and reaches the SA node; major branches are a marginal branch supplying much of the anterior wall of the right ventricle, an atrioventricular (AV) nodal artery given off near the posterior border of the interventricular septum, and a posterior interventricular artery in the interventricular groove that anastomoses with the anterior interventricular artery a branch of the left coronary artery.

2. The left coronary artery divides into a circumflex branch that passes posteriorly to anastomose with the right coronary on the posterior aspect of the heart, and an anterior descending branch in the interventricular groove; the origin of the SA nodal artery is variable and it may also be a branch of the left coronary artery;

3. The interventricular septum receives its blood supply from septal branches of the two descending branches: the anterior two-thirds from the left coronary, the posterior one-third from the right.

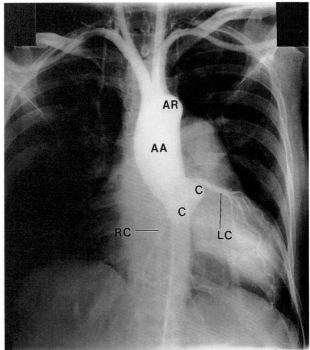

1.52
Aortic root angiogram

AR - Arch of aorta, *AA* - Ascending aorta, *C* - Cusp of aortic valve, *LC* - Left coronary artery, *RC* - Right coronary artery. (Courtesy of Dr. J. Heslin, Assistant Professor of Anatomy, University of Toronto, Toronto, Ontario, Canada.)

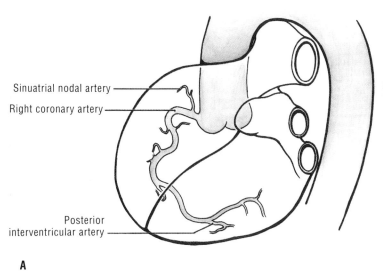

Sinuatrial nodal artery

Right coronary artery

Posterior interventricular artery

A

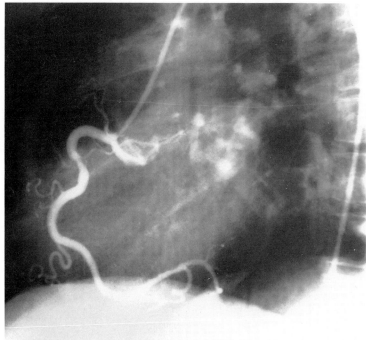

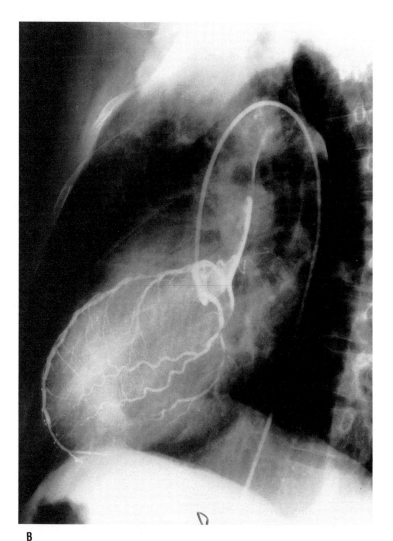

B

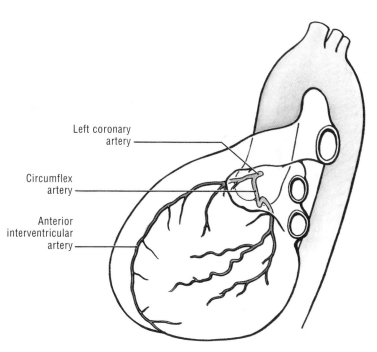

Left coronary artery

Circumflex artery

Anterior interventricular artery

1.53
Coronary arteriograms with orientation drawings

The right (**A**) and left (**B**) coronary arteriograms are from a left anterior oblique, almost lateral view. (Arteriograms courtesy of Dr. I. Morrow, Department of Radiology, Health Sciences Centre, University of Manitoba, Winnipeg, Manitoba, Canada.)

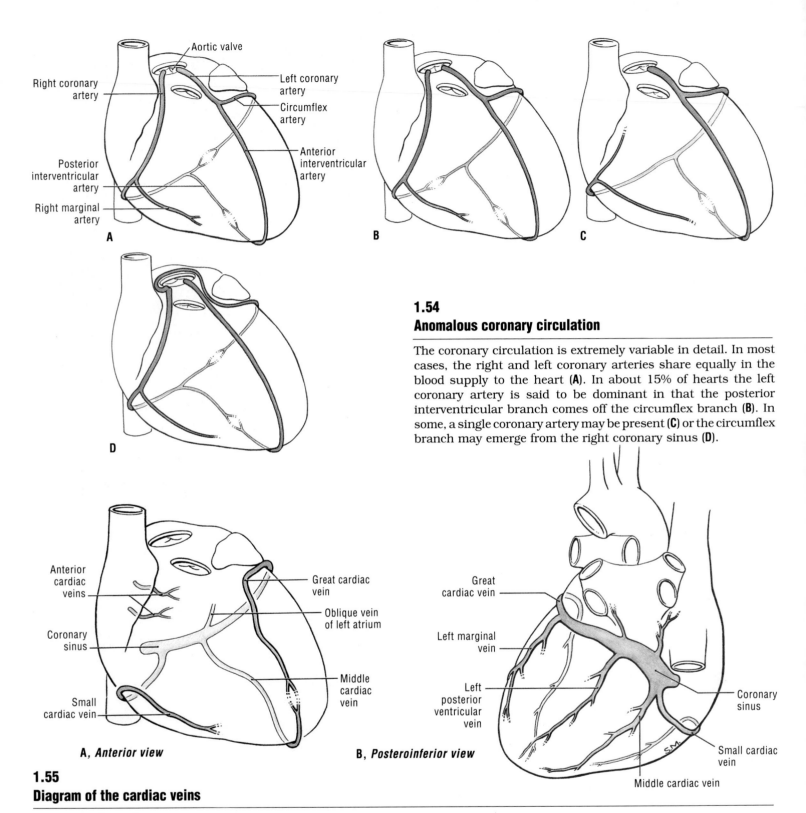

A

- Aortic valve
- Right coronary artery
- Left coronary artery
- Circumflex artery
- Posterior interventricular artery
- Anterior interventricular artery
- Right marginal artery

B

C

D

1.54
Anomalous coronary circulation

The coronary circulation is extremely variable in detail. In most cases, the right and left coronary arteries share equally in the blood supply to the heart (**A**). In about 15% of hearts the left coronary artery is said to be dominant in that the posterior interventricular branch comes off the circumflex branch (**B**). In some, a single coronary artery may be present (**C**) or the circumflex branch may emerge from the right coronary sinus (**D**).

- Anterior cardiac veins
- Coronary sinus
- Small cardiac vein
- Great cardiac vein
- Oblique vein of left atrium
- Middle cardiac vein

A, Anterior view

- Great cardiac vein
- Left marginal vein
- Left posterior ventricular vein
- Coronary sinus
- Small cardiac vein
- Middle cardiac vein

B, Posteroinferior view

1.55
Diagram of the cardiac veins

Observe in **A** and **B**:

1. The coronary sinus is the major venous drainage vessel of the heart, which empties into the right atrium and is located posteriorly in the coronary sulcus;

2. The great, middle, and small cardiac veins, the oblique vein of the left atrium, and the posterior vein of the left ventricle are the principal vessels draining into the coronary sinus; the anterior cardiac veins drain directly into the right atrium;

3. The cardiac veins accompany the coronary arteries and their branches – great cardiac vein and the anterior interventricular artery, middle cardiac vein and the posterior interventricular artery, etc.;

4. The smallest vessels, the venae cordis minimae, drain the myocardium directly into the atria and ventricles.

1.56
Aortic angiogram

Observe the ascending aorta *(AA)*, the arch of the aorta *(AR)*, the descending aorta *(DA)*, the brachiocephalic *(BT)* trunk (artery) branching into the right subclavian *(RS)* and right common carotid *(RC)* arteries, the left subclavian *(LS)* and left common carotid *(LC)* arteries arising directly from the aorta. (Courtesy of Dr. E.L. Lansdown, Professor of Radiology, University of Toronto, Ontario, Canada.)

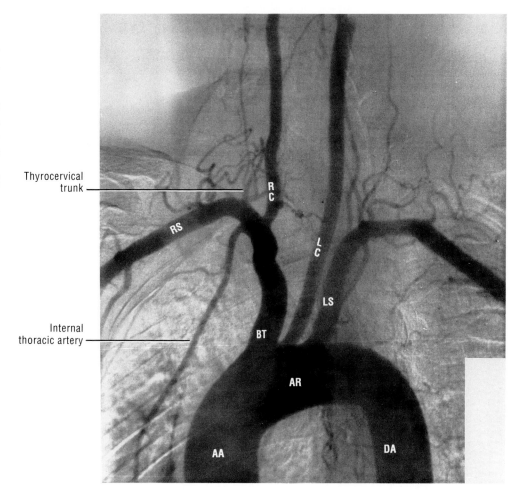

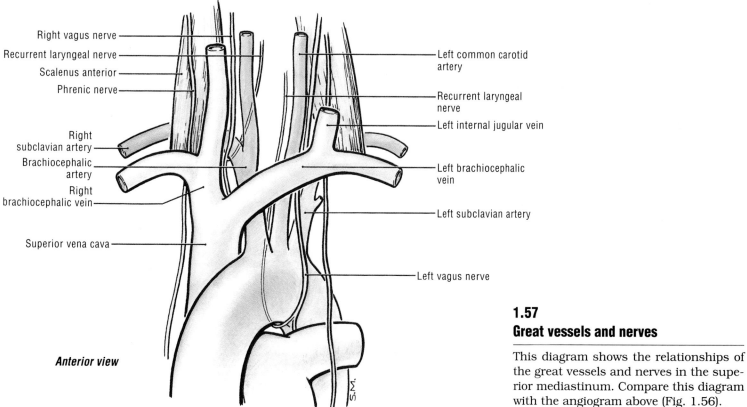

Anterior view

1.57
Great vessels and nerves

This diagram shows the relationships of the great vessels and nerves in the superior mediastinum. Compare this diagram with the angiogram above (Fig. 1.56).

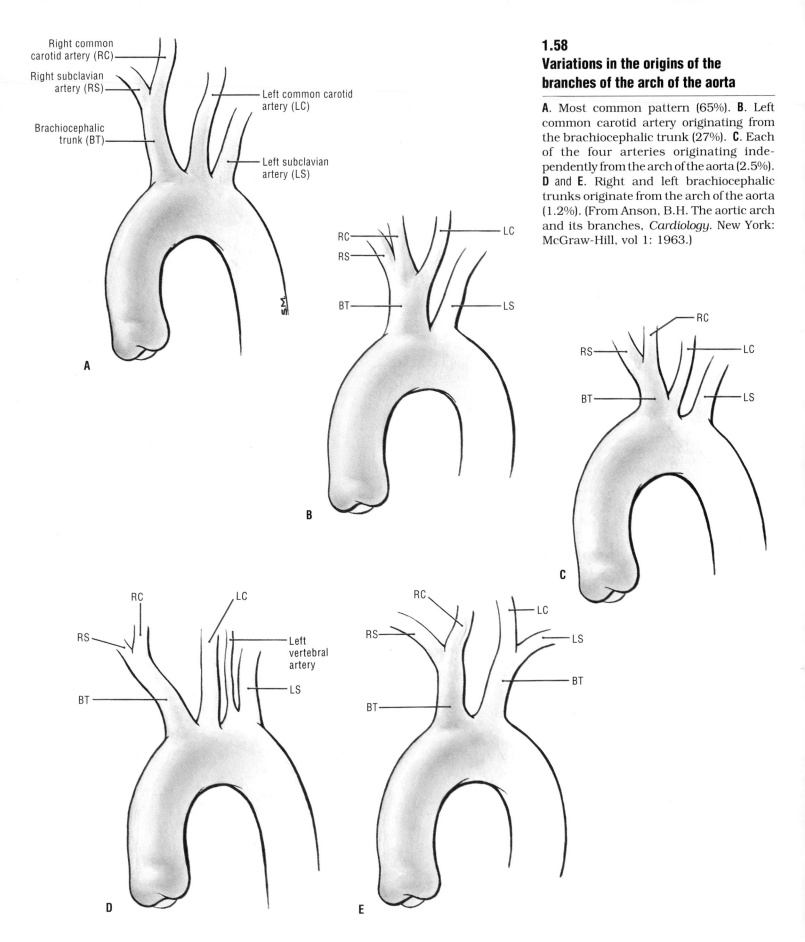

Right common carotid artery (RC)

Right subclavian artery (RS)

Brachiocephalic trunk (BT)

Left common carotid artery (LC)

Left subclavian artery (LS)

A

RC

RS

BT

LC

LS

B

RC

RS

BT

LC

LS

C

RC

RS

BT

LC

Left vertebral artery

LS

D

RC

RS

BT

LC

LS

BT

E

1.58

Variations in the origins of the branches of the arch of the aorta

A. Most common pattern (65%). **B**. Left common carotid artery originating from the brachiocephalic trunk (27%). **C**. Each of the four arteries originating independently from the arch of the aorta (2.5%). **D** and **E**. Right and left brachiocephalic trunks originate from the arch of the aorta (1.2%). (From Anson, B.H. The aortic arch and its branches, *Cardiology*. New York: McGraw-Hill, vol 1: 1963.)

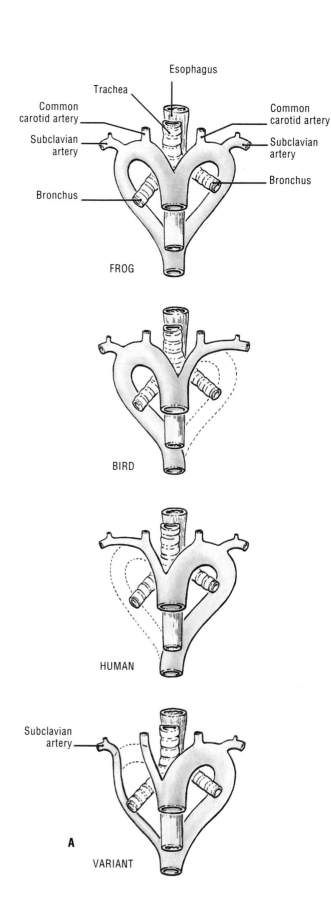

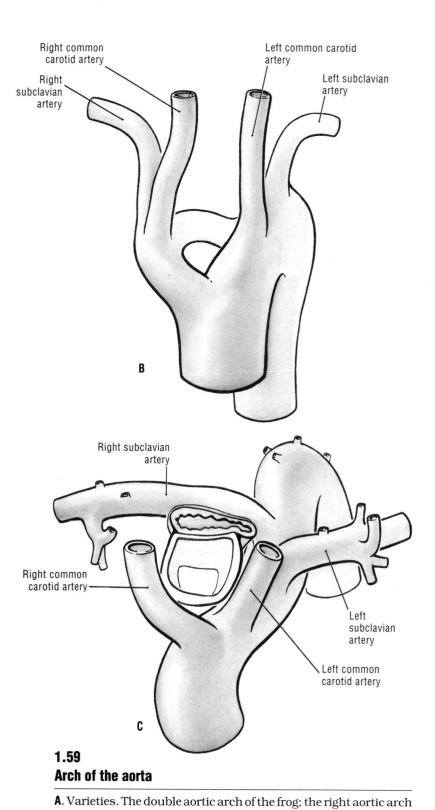

1.59

Arch of the aorta

A. Varieties. The double aortic arch of the frog; the right aortic arch of the bird; the left aortic arch of the mammal, including man and a variant. **B**. Double aortic arch. Both the right and left aortic arches persist completely, as in the frog. In this rare condition, the esophagus and trachea pass through the so-formed "aortic ring." **C**. Retroesophageal right subclavian artery. The artery arises as the last branch of the arch of the aorta. It passes posterior to the esophagus and trachea. The right recurrent laryngeal nerve, having no vessel around which to recur, takes a direct course to the larynx.

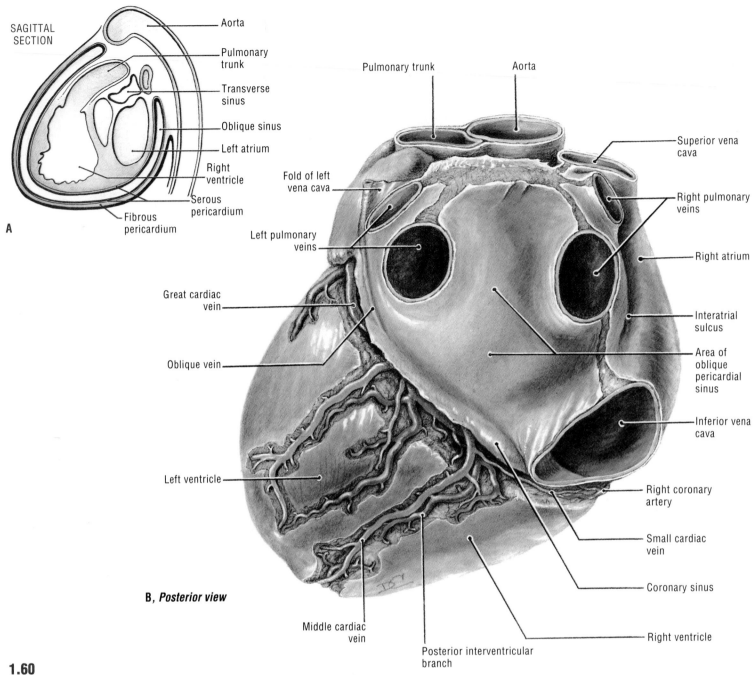

SAGITTAL
SECTION

Aorta

Pulmonary trunk

Transverse sinus

Oblique sinus

Left atrium

Right ventricle

Serous pericardium

Fibrous pericardium

A

Pulmonary trunk

Aorta

Superior vena cava

Fold of left vena cava

Right pulmonary veins

Left pulmonary veins

Right atrium

Great cardiac vein

Interatrial sulcus

Area of oblique pericardial sinus

Oblique vein

Inferior vena cava

Left ventricle

Right coronary artery

Small cardiac vein

B, *Posterior view*

Coronary sinus

Middle cardiac vein

Right ventricle

Posterior interventricular branch

1.60
Heart

This heart was removed from the specimen in Figure 1.61. Observe in **A** and **B**:

1. The entire base, or posterior surface, and part of the diaphragmatic surface are in view;

2. The superior vena cava and the much larger inferior vena cava joining the upper and lower limits of the right atrium;

3. The left atrium, forming the greater part of the posterior surface;

4. The coronary arteries, here irregular in that the left one supplies the posterior interventricular branch;

5. Branches of the cardiac veins, when crossing branches of the coronary arteries, mostly do so superficially;

6. The visceral layer of serous pericardium covering the heart and reflecting onto the great vessels of the heart; from around the great vessels of the heart the serous pericardium reflects to line the fibrous pericardium, as the parietal layer of serous pericardium (Fig. 1.61);

7. The cut edge of the reflections of serous pericardia around the arterial vessels (the pulmonary trunk and aorta) and the venous vessels (the superior and inferior vena cava and the pulmonary veins);

8. The right pulmonary artery (removed) lay on the bare strip at the superior border of the atria, and intervened between the oblique sinus and the transverse sinus (not labeled).

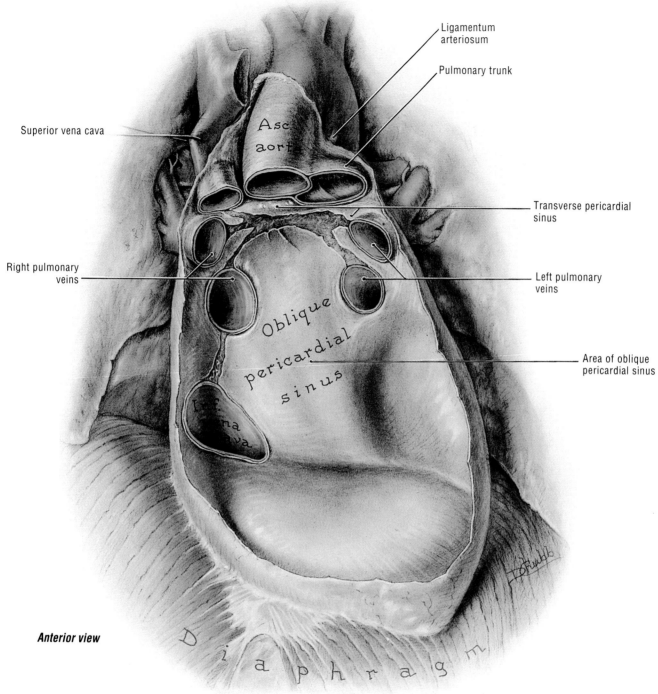

Ligamentum
arteriosum

Pulmonary trunk

Superior vena cava

Asc. aorta

Transverse pericardial
sinus

Right pulmonary
veins

Left pulmonary
veins

Oblique pericardial sinus

Area of oblique
pericardial sinus

Inferior vena cava

Anterior view

Diaphragm

1.61
Interior of the pericardial sac

Observe:

1. The eight vessels severed on excising the heart: two caval veins (superior and inferior venae cavae), four pulmonary veins, and two pulmonary arteries;

2. The oblique sinus bounded anteriorly by the visceral layer of serous pericardium covering the left atrium (Fig. 1.60B), posteriorly by the parietal layer of serous pericardium lining the fibrous pericardium, and superiorly and laterally by the reflection of serous pericardium around the four pulmonary veins and the superior and inferior venae cavae;

3. The oblique sinus, circumscribed by five veins, opens inferiorly and to the left;

4. The transverse sinus bounded anteriorly by the serous pericardium covering the posterior aspect of pulmonary trunk and aorta and posteriorly by the visceral pericardium covering the atria (Figs. 1.60**A** and 1.67);

5. The peak of the pericardial sac, near the junction of the ascending aorta and arch of the aorta;

6. The superior vena cava, partly inside and partly outside the pericardium, and the ligamentum arteriosum entirely outside.

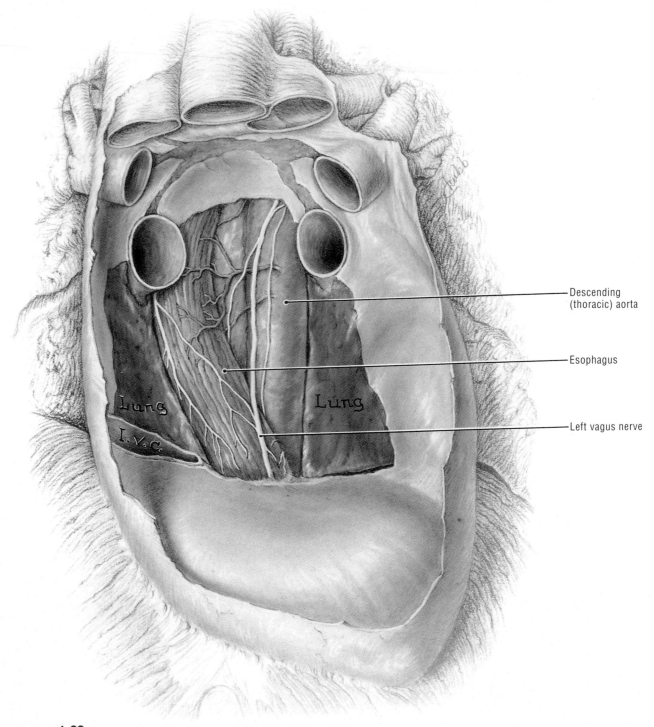

Descending (thoracic) aorta

Esophagus

Left vagus nerve

Lung

Lung

I.V.C.

1.62
Posterior relations of heart and pericardium

The fibrous and parietal layers of serous pericardium have been removed from posterior and lateral to the oblique sinus.

Observe:

1. The posterior relations: part of the right lung and the esophagus grooving it; part of the left lung and the aorta grooving it; and the vagus nerves forming a plexus on the esophagus;

2. The esophagus is here unduly deflected to the right; it usually lies in contact with the aorta.

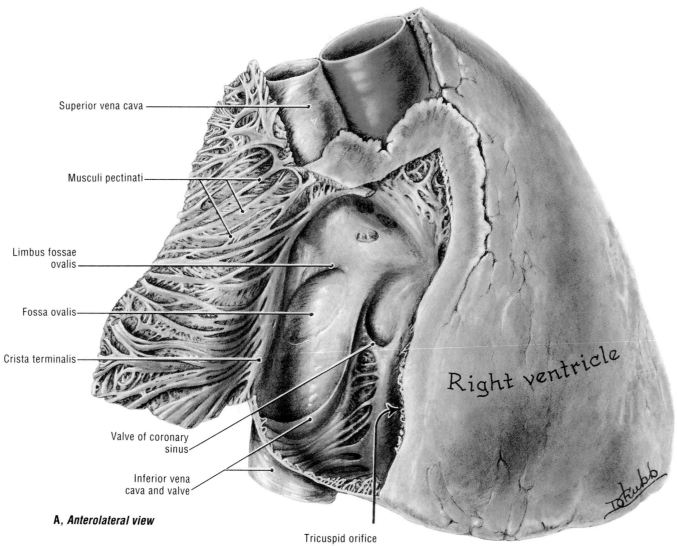

Superior vena cava

Musculi pectinati

Limbus fossae ovalis

Fossa ovalis

Crista terminalis

Valve of coronary sinus

Inferior vena cava and valve

A, Anterolateral view

Right ventricle

Tricuspid orifice

1.63
Right atrium

A. Interior. Observe:

1. The smooth part of the atrial wall formed by the absorption of the right horn of the sinus venosus and the rough part formed from the primitive atrium;

2. Crista terminalis, the valve of the inferior vena cava, and the valve of the coronary sinus, separating the smooth part from the rough part;

3. The musculi pectinati, passing anterior from the crista terminalis like teeth from the back of a comb; the crista underlies the sulcus terminalis, which is a groove visible externally on the posterolateral surface of the right atrium between the superior and inferior vena cavae;

4. The superior and inferior vena cavae and the coronary sinus opening onto the smooth part (sinus venarum) of the right atrium, the anterior cardiac veins and the venae cordis minimae, not visible, also open into the atrium;

6. The right atrioventricular or tricuspid orifice, situated at the anterior aspect of the atrium;

B. Inflow. The inflow from the superior vena cava is directed toward the tricuspid orifice, while blood from the inferior vena cava is directed toward the fossa ovalis.

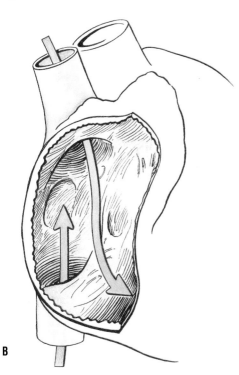

B

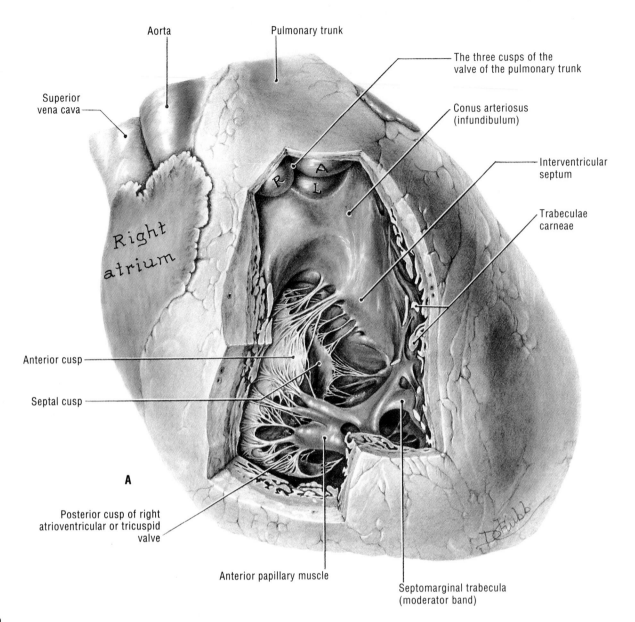

Aorta

Pulmonary trunk

The three cusps of the
valve of the pulmonary trunk

Superior
vena cava

Conus arteriosus
(infundibulum)

R A
L

Interventricular
septum

Right
atrium

Trabeculae
carneae

Anterior cusp

Septal cusp

A

Posterior cusp of right
atrioventricular or tricuspid
valve

Anterior papillary muscle

Septomarginal trabecula
(moderator band)

1.64
Right ventricle

A. Interior. Observe:

1. The entrance to this chamber (right atrioventricular or tricuspid orifice) situated posteriorly; the exit (orifice of the pulmonary trunk) situated superiorly;

2. The smooth funnel-shaped wall (conus arteriosus) inferior to the pulmonary orifice; the remainder of the ventricle, rough with fleshy trabeculae;

3. Three types of trabeculae: (a) mere ridges, (b) bridges, attached only at each end, and (c) finger-like projections called papillary muscles; the anterior papillary muscle rising from the anterior wall; the posterior (not labeled) from the posterior wall; and a series of small septal papillae from the septal wall;

4. The septomarginal trabecula, here very thick, extending from the septum to the base of the anterior papillary muscle;

5. The chordae tendineae, passing from the tips of the papillary muscles to the free margins and ventricular surfaces of the three cusps of the tricuspid valve;

6. Each papillary muscle controlling the adjacent sides of two cusps.

B. Diagram of the right atrioventricular valve, spread out.

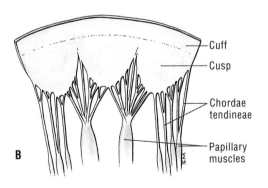

Cuff

Cusp

Chordae
tendineae

B

Papillary
muscles

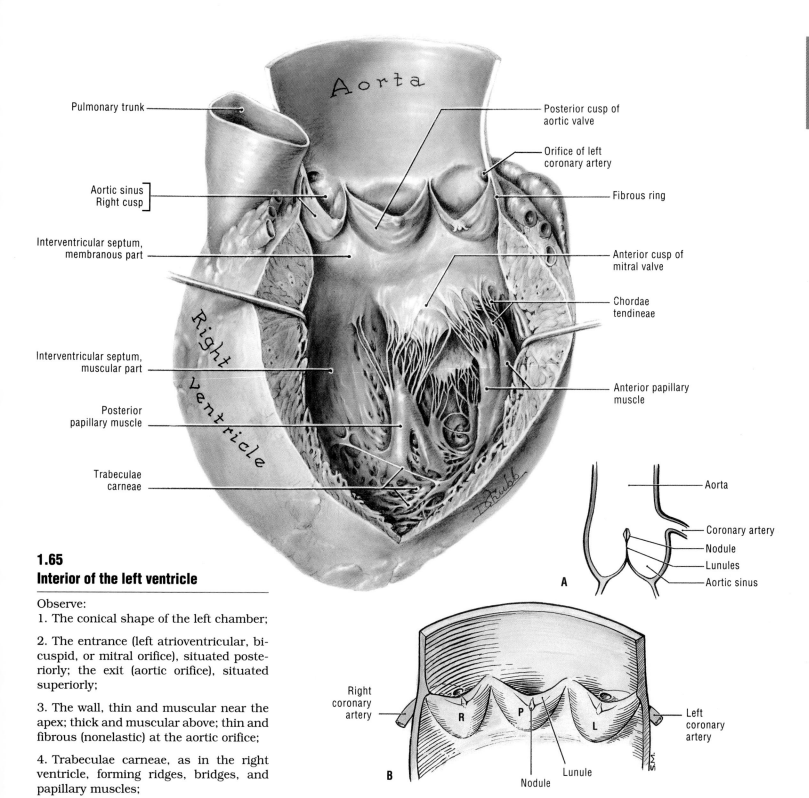

Pulmonary trunk

Aortic sinus
Right cusp

Interventricular septum,
membranous part

Interventricular septum,
muscular part

Posterior
papillary muscle

Trabeculae
carneae

Aorta

Right Ventricle

Posterior cusp of
aortic valve

Orifice of left
coronary artery

Fibrous ring

Anterior cusp of
mitral valve

Chordae
tendineae

Anterior papillary
muscle

1.65
Interior of the left ventricle

Observe:

1. The conical shape of the left chamber;

2. The entrance (left atrioventricular, bicuspid, or mitral orifice), situated posteriorly; the exit (aortic orifice), situated superiorly;

3. The wall, thin and muscular near the apex; thick and muscular above; thin and fibrous (nonelastic) at the aortic orifice;

4. Trabeculae carneae, as in the right ventricle, forming ridges, bridges, and papillary muscles;

5. Two large papillary muscles: the anterior from the anterior wall and the posterior from the posterior wall each controlling, via chordae tendineae, the adjacent halves of two cusps of the mitral valve;

6. The anterior cusp of the mitral valve intervening between the inlet (mitral orifice) and the outlet (aortic orifice).

Aorta

Coronary artery
Nodule
Lunules
Aortic sinus

A

Right
coronary
artery

R   P   L

Left
coronary
artery

Lunule
Nodule

B

1.66
Diagram of the aortic valve

This, like the valve of the pulmonary trunk, has three semilunar cusps (right (R), posterior (P), left (L)), each with a fibrous nodule at the midpoint of its free edge and a thin connective tissue area, the lunula, to each side of the nodule. When the valve is closed, the nodules and lunulae meet in the center. **A**. Longitudinal section, closed valve. **B**. Spread out valve.

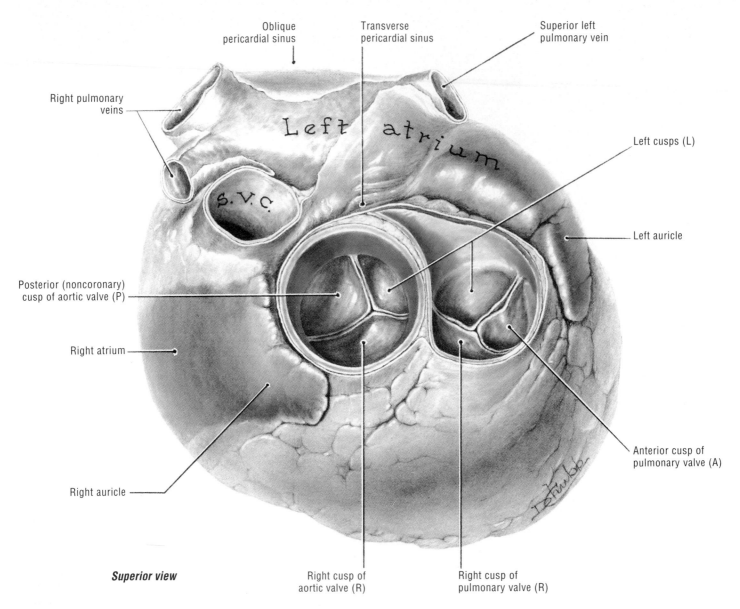

Oblique pericardial sinus

Transverse pericardial sinus

Superior left pulmonary vein

Right pulmonary veins

Left atrium

Left cusps (L)

S.V.C.

Posterior (noncoronary) cusp of aortic valve (P)

Left auricle

Right atrium

Right auricle

Anterior cusp of pulmonary valve (A)

Superior view

Right cusp of aortic valve (R)

Right cusp of pulmonary valve (R)

1.67
Excised heart

Observe:

1. The anterior position of the ventricles; the posterior position of the atria;

2. The stems of the aorta and pulmonary artery, which conduct blood from the ventricles, accordingly placed anterior to the atria and their incoming blood vessels (the superior vena cava and the pulmonary veins);

3. The aorta and pulmonary artery, enclosed within a common tube of serous pericardium and partly embraced by the auricles of the atria;

4. The transverse pericardial sinus, curving posterior to the enclosed stems of the aorta and pulmonary trunk, and anterior to the superior vena cava and upper limits of the atria;

5. The three cusps of the aortic valve and of the pulmonary valve; the names of the cusps of the aortic and pulmonary valves have a developmental origin, as explained in Figure 1.68.

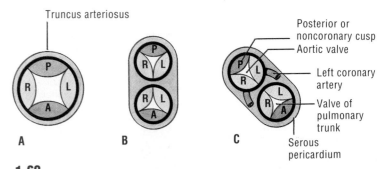

Truncus arteriosus

Posterior or noncoronary cusp

Aortic valve

Left coronary artery

Valve of pulmonary trunk

Serous pericardium

A   **B**   **C**

1.68
Pulmonary and aortic valve names

The names applied to these cusps are explained on a developmental basis: The truncus arteriosus with four cusps (**A**) splits to form two valves, each with three cusps (**B**). The heart undergoes partial rotation to the left on its axis resulting in the arrangement of cusps shown in **C**. Inability of the valve to close completely is called insufficiency and results in regurgitation. Fusion of the cusps to each other produces stenosis.

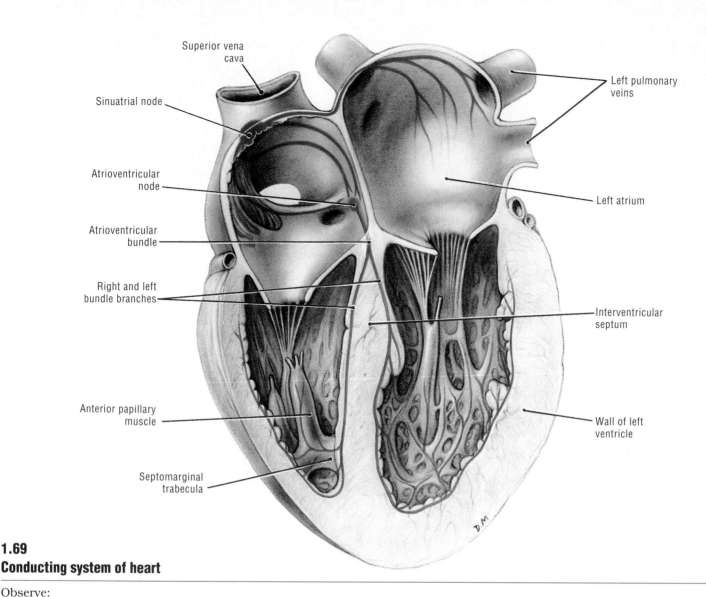

Superior vena cava

Sinuatrial node

Atrioventricular node

Atrioventricular bundle

Right and left bundle branches

Anterior papillary muscle

Septomarginal trabecula

Left pulmonary veins

Left atrium

Interventricular septum

Wall of left ventricle

1.69
Conducting system of heart

Observe:

1. The sinuatrial (SA) node in the wall of the right atrium near the superior end of the sulcus terminalis and extending over the anterior aspect of the opening of the superior vena cava; the SA node is the "pacemaker" of the heart because it initiates cardiac muscle contraction and determines the heart rate; it is supplied by the sinuatrial nodal artery, usually a branch of the right coronary artery, but may also be a branch of the left coronary artery (From Hudson REB. *Cardiovascular pathology*. London: Arnold, 1965);

2. Contraction spreads through the atrial wall until it reaches the atrioventricular (AV) node in the interatrial septum just superior to the opening of the coronary sinus; the AV node is supplied by the atrioventricular nodal artery arising, usually, from the right coronary artery posteriorly at the inferior margin of the interatrial septum;

3. The atrioventricular bundle (AV) bundle, usually supplied by the right coronary artery, passes from the AV node in the membranous part of the interventricular septum and divides into right and left bundle branches on either side of the muscular part of the septum;

4. The right bundle branch travels inferiorly in the interventricu-

lar septum to the anterior wall of the ventricle, then via the septomarginal trabecula to the anterior papillary muscle; excitation spreads throughout the right ventricular wall via a network of branches from the right bundle (Purkinje fibers);

5. The left bundle branch lies beneath the endocardium on the left side of the interventricular septum and branches to enter the anterior and posterior papillary muscles and the wall of the left ventricle; further branching into a plexus of Purkinje fibers allows the impulses to be conveyed throughout the left ventricular wall; the bundle branches are usually supplied by the left coronary except for the posterior limb of the left bundle branch, which receives supply from both coronary arteries;

6. Damage to the conducting system (often by compromised blood supply as in coronary artery disease) leads to disturbances of cardiac muscle contraction; damage to the AV node results in "heart block" as the atrial excitation wave does not reach the ventricles that begin to contract independently at their own rate which is slower than that of the atria; damage to one of the branches results in "bundle branch block" in which excitation goes down the unaffected branch to cause systole of that ventricle; the impulse then spreads to the other ventricle producing later asynchronous contraction.

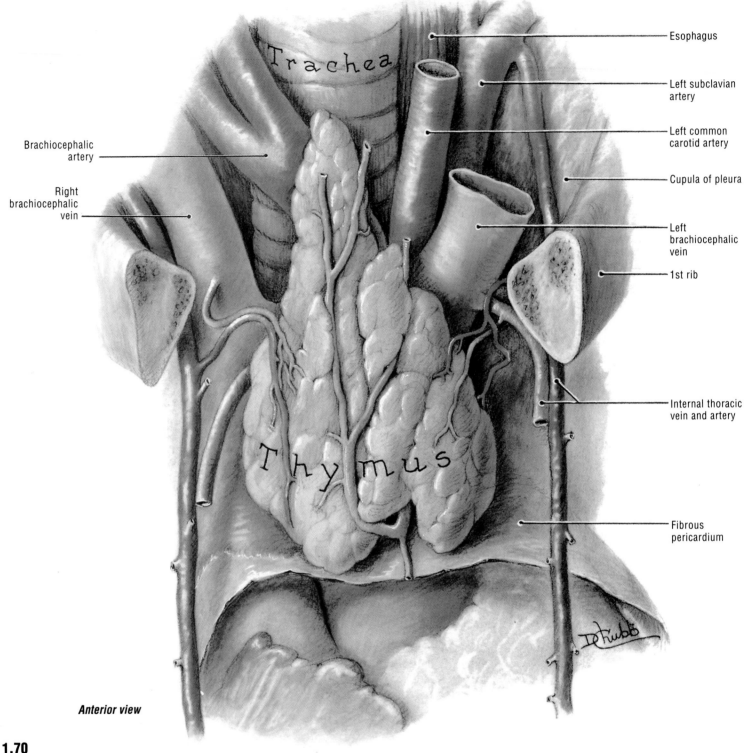

Esophagus

Left subclavian artery

Left common carotid artery

Cupula of pleura

Left brachiocephalic vein

1st rib

Internal thoracic vein and artery

Fibrous pericardium

Brachiocephalic artery

Right brachiocephalic vein

Trachea

Thymus

Anterior view

1.70
Superior mediastinum–I: superficial dissection

The sternum and ribs have been excised and the pleurae removed. It is unusual in an adult to see so discrete a thymus, which is impressive during puberty but subsequently regresses and becomes largely replaced by fat and fibrous tissue.

Observe:

1. The thymus lying in the superior mediastinum; overlapping the pericardial sac inferiorly; and extending superiorly into the neck farther than usual;

2. The longitudinal fissure that divides the thymus into two asymmetrical lobes, a larger right and a smaller left; these two developmentally separate parts are easily separated from each other by blunt dissection;

3. The blood supply to the thymus: arteries from the internal thoracic arteries; veins to the brachiocephalic and internal thoracic veins and communicating superiorly with the inferior thyroid veins.

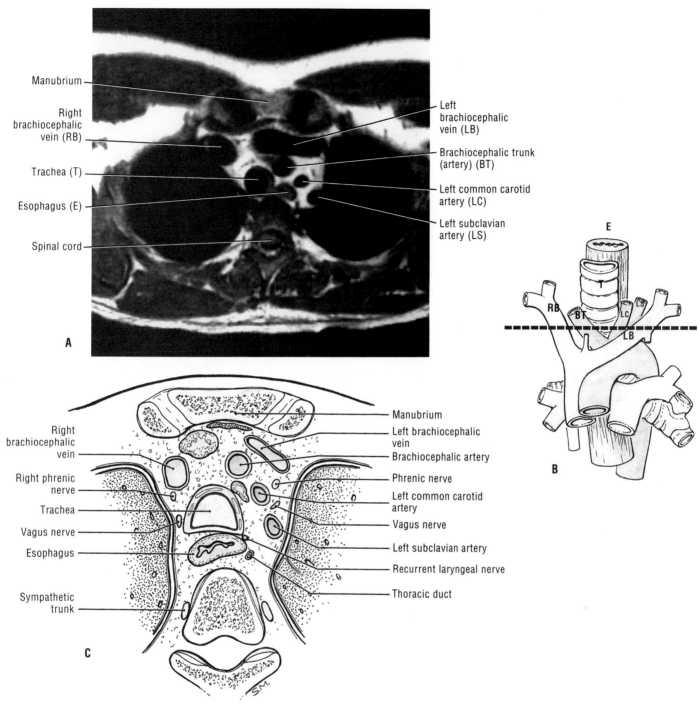

Manubrium

Right
brachiocephalic
vein (RB)

Trachea (T)

Esophagus (E)

Spinal cord

Left
brachiocephalic
vein (LB)

Brachiocephalic trunk
(artery) (BT)

Left common carotid
artery (LC)

Left subclavian
artery (LS)

A

E

B

Right
brachiocephalic
vein

Right phrenic
nerve

Trachea

Vagus nerve

Esophagus

Sympathetic
trunk

Manubrium

Left brachiocephalic
vein

Brachiocephalic artery

Phrenic nerve

Left common carotid
artery

Vagus nerve

Left subclavian artery

Recurrent laryngeal nerve

Thoracic duct

C

1.71
Superior mediastinum

A. Transverse MRI (magnetic resonance image) of the superior mediastinum superior to the arch of the aorta. (Courtesy of Dr. W. Kucharczyk, Clinical Director of Tri-Hospital Magnetic Resonance Centre, Toronto, Ontario, Canada.) **B**. Diagram showing the level of the MRI (magnetic resonance image). **C**. Diagram of transverse section of superior mediastinum at same level as the scan (**A**) above.

Observe:
1. The left brachiocephalic vein is sectioned as it is crossing the mediastinum from left to right to join the right brachiocephalic

vein; the right and left brachiocephalic veins join to form the superior vena cava;

2. The brachiocephalic, left common carotid and left subclavian arteries are sectioned, indicating the level of section is superior to the arch of the aorta;

3. The esophagus lies posterior to the trachea;

4. The phrenic nerves lie anterior to the vagus nerves.

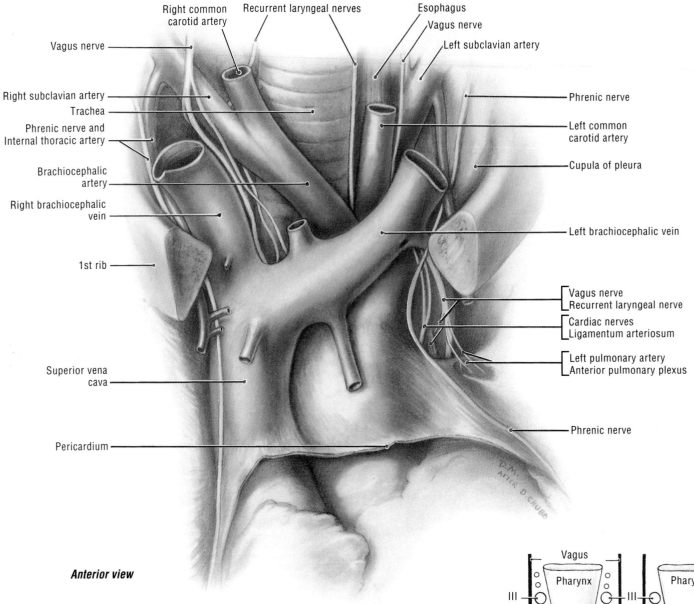

Right common carotid artery — Recurrent laryngeal nerves — Esophagus

Vagus nerve

Vagus nerve

Left subclavian artery

Right subclavian artery

Trachea

Phrenic nerve and Internal thoracic artery

Brachiocephalic artery

Right brachiocephalic vein

1st rib

Superior vena cava

Pericardium

Phrenic nerve

Left common carotid artery

Cupula of pleura

Left brachiocephalic vein

Vagus nerve
Recurrent laryngeal nerve

Cardiac nerves
Ligamentum arteriosum

Left pulmonary artery
Anterior pulmonary plexus

Phrenic nerve

Anterior view

1.72
Superior mediastinum–II: root of the neck, thymus gland removed

Observe:

1. The great veins, anterior to the great arteries;

2. The posterior direction of the arch of the aorta and the nerves crossing its left side;

3. The ligamentum arteriosum, outside the pericardial sac and having the left recurrent nerve on its left side and the vagal and sympathetic branches to the superficial cardiac plexus on its right;

4. The right vagus nerve, crossing anterior to the right subclavian artery, there giving off its recurrent branch, and passing medially to reach the trachea and esophagus;

5. The left vagus nerve, crossing anterior to the arch of the aorta, there giving off its recurrent branch that passes posterior to the arch of the aorta and then ascends between the trachea and esophagus to the larynx; the left vagus nerve then passes posterior to the root of the lung;

6. The left phrenic nerve, crossing the path of the vagus nerve, but 1 cm anterior to it.

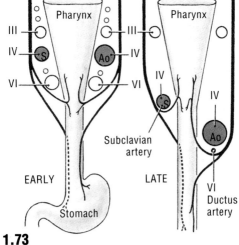

1.73
Recurrent laryngeal nerves

Scheme to explain the asymmetrical courses of the right and left recurrent laryngeal nerves. (*III, IV,* and *VI* are embryonic aortic arches.)

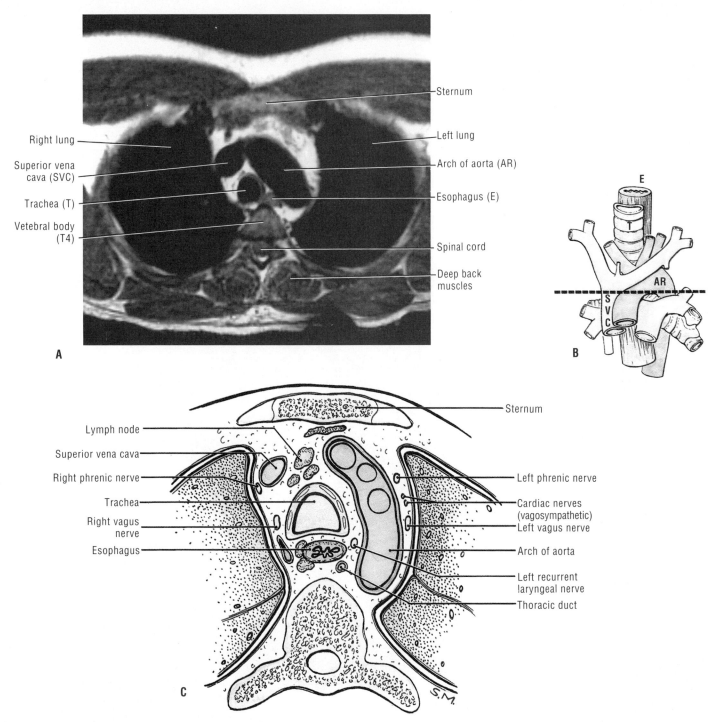

A. Transverse MRI (magnetic resonance image) of the superior mediastinum at the level of the arch of the aorta. Labels: Right lung, Superior vena cava (SVC), Trachea (T), Vetebral body (T4), Sternum, Left lung, Arch of aorta (AR), Esophagus (E), Spinal cord, Deep back muscles.

B. Diagram showing the level of the MRI. Labels: E, T, AR, SVC.

C. Diagram of transverse section of superior mediastinum. Labels: Lymph node, Superior vena cava, Right phrenic nerve, Trachea, Right vagus nerve, Esophagus, Sternum, Left phrenic nerve, Cardiac nerves (vagosympathetic), Left vagus nerve, Arch of aorta, Left recurrent laryngeal nerve, Thoracic duct. S.M.

1.74
Superior mediastinum

A. Transverse MRI (magnetic resonance image) of the superior mediastinum at the level of the arch of the aorta. (Courtesy of Dr. W. Kucharczyk, Clinical Director of TriHospital Magnetic Resonance Centre, Toronto, Ontario, Canada.) **B.** Diagram showing the level of the MRI (magnetic resonance image). **C.** Diagram of transverse section of superior mediastinum at same level as the scan (**A**).

Observe:

1. The posterior direction of the arch of the aorta and the left vagus, phrenic, and vagosympathetic (autonomic) nerves passing to the left of the arch of the aorta;

2. The left recurrent laryngeal nerve between the trachea and esophagus; the absence of the right recurrent laryngeal nerve, which would be found in more cranial sections superior to the right subclavian artery;

3. The relationship of the thoracic duct and right vagus nerve to the trachea and esophagus.

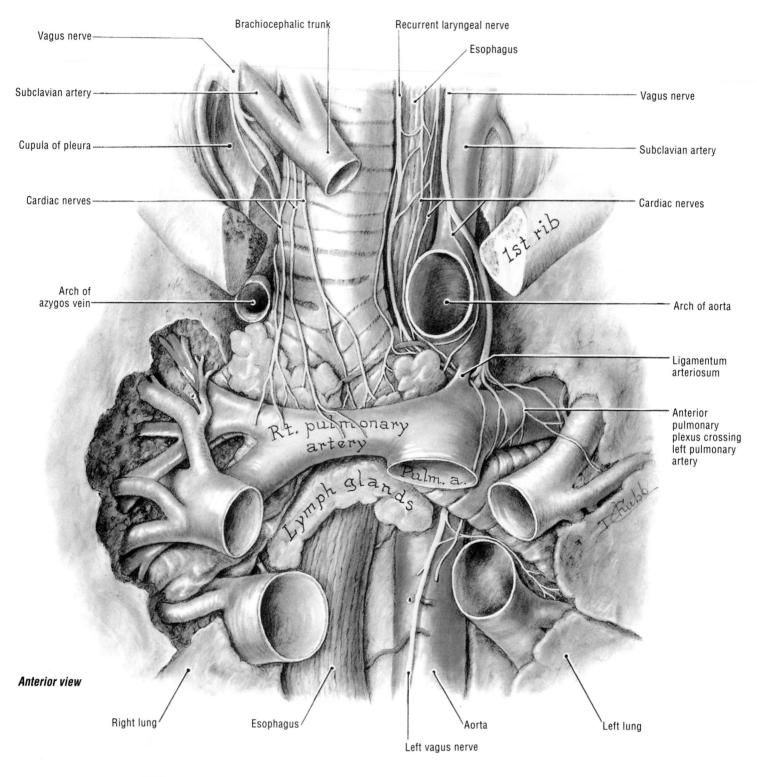

Vagus nerve

Brachiocephalic trunk

Recurrent laryngeal nerve

Esophagus

Vagus nerve

Subclavian artery

Cupula of pleura

Cardiac nerves

1st rib

Subclavian artery

Cardiac nerves

Arch of
azygos vein

Arch of aorta

Ligamentum
arteriosum

Rt. pulmonary
artery

Pulm. a.

Lymph glands

Anterior
pulmonary
plexus crossing
left pulmonary
artery

Anterior view

Right lung

Esophagus

Left vagus nerve

Aorta

Left lung

1.75
Superior mediastinum–III: pulmonary arteries

Observe:

1. The pulmonary trunk, dividing into right and left pulmonary arteries, the right pulmonary artery crossing inferior to the bifurcation of the trachea and separated from the esophagus by lymph nodes (green);

2. Cardiac branches of the vagus and sympathetic nerves, streaming down the sides of the trachea and forming the cardiac plexuses.

1.76
Superior mediastinum–IV: tracheal bifurcation and bronchi

Observe:

1. Four parallel structures: the trachea, esophagus, left recurrent laryngeal nerve, and thoracic duct; the esophagus bulges to the left of the trachea, the recurrent nerve lies in the angle between the trachea and esophagus, and the duct is at the left side of the esophagus;

2. The arch of the aorta passes posteriorly to the left of these four structures, and the arch of the azygos vein passes anteriorly to the right of the four structures;

3. The trachea inclining slightly to the right with the result that the right bronchus is more vertical than the left and its stem is shorter and wider; the first right branch arises about 2.5 cm from the bifurcation, whereas the first left branch arises about 5 cm from the bifurcation;

4. The U-shaped rings of the trachea, commonly bifurcated; the ring at the bifurcation of the trachea being V-shaped;

5. The bronchial arteries that supply the trachea and follow the bronchial tree to supply the bronchi, lung tissue, and lymph nodes.

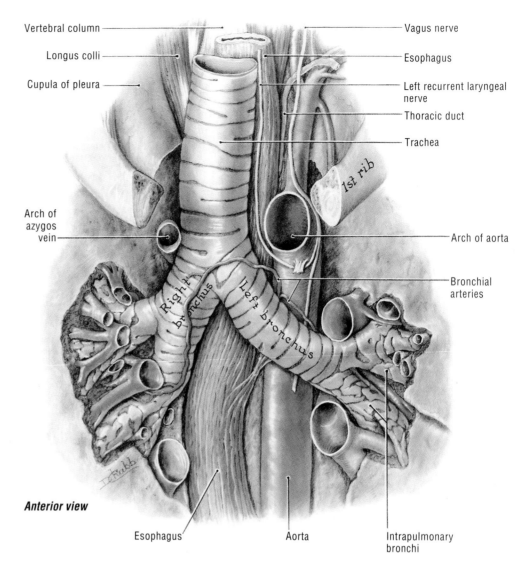

Vertebral column — — Vagus nerve
Longus colli — — Esophagus
Cupula of pleura — — Left recurrent laryngeal nerve
— Thoracic duct
— Trachea
1st rib
Arch of azygos vein — — Arch of aorta
— Bronchial arteries
Right bronchus Left bronchus
Intrapulmonary bronchi

Anterior view

Esophagus Aorta Intrapulmonary bronchi

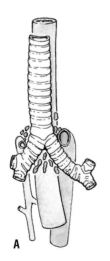
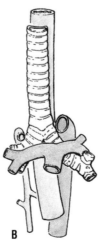
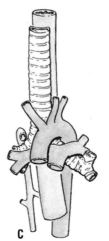
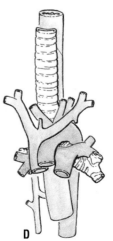

A B C D

1.77
Relations at bifurcation of trachea built up sequentially from deep to superficial

A. Lymph nodes at the tracheal bifurcation.

B. Pulmonary arteries.

C. Ascending aorta and arch of the aorta.

D. Brachiocephalic veins forming the superior vena cava and the arch of the azygos vein entering it posteriorly.

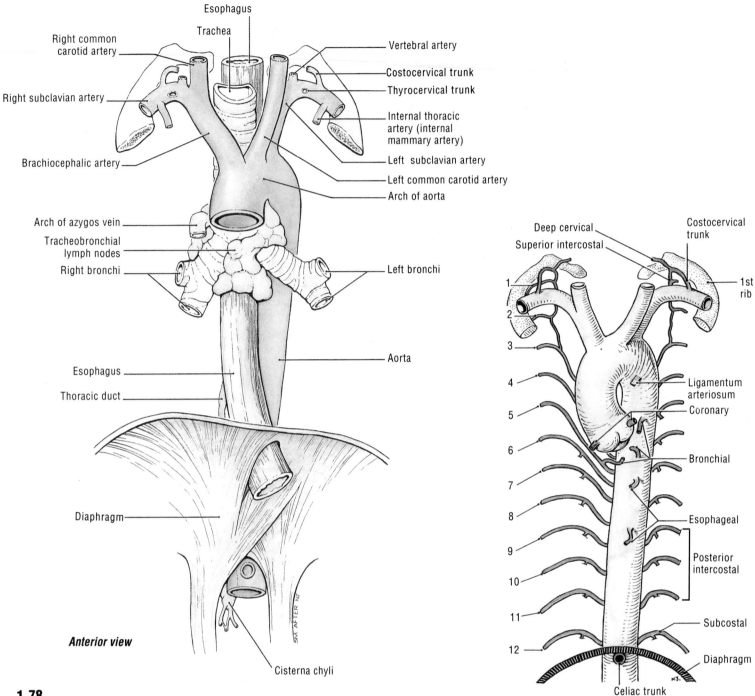

Esophagus

Trachea

Right common
carotid artery

Right subclavian artery

Brachiocephalic artery

Vertebral artery

Costocervical trunk

Thyrocervical trunk

Internal thoracic
artery (internal
mammary artery)

Left subclavian artery

Left common carotid artery

Arch of aorta

Arch of azygos vein

Tracheobronchial
lymph nodes

Right bronchi

Left bronchi

Aorta

Esophagus

Thoracic duct

Diaphragm

Anterior view

Cisterna chyli

Deep cervical

Superior intercostal

Costocervical
trunk

1st
rib

Ligamentum
arteriosum

Coronary

Bronchial

Esophageal

Posterior
intercostal

Subcostal

Diaphragm

Celiac trunk

1.78
Esophagus, trachea, and aorta

Observe:

1. The arch of the aorta, arching posteriorly to the left of the trachea and esophagus, and the arch of the azygos vein arching anteriorly to the right of these structures; each arches superior to the root of a lung;

2. The posterior relation of the trachea is the esophagus;

3. The anterior relations of the thoracic part of the esophagus from superior to inferior are the: trachea (throughout its entire length), right and left bronchi, inferior tracheobronchial lymph nodes, pericardium (removed) and, finally, diaphragm;

4. Superior to the level of the arch of the aorta, the esophagus bulges to the left beyond the trachea; the left recurrent laryngeal nerve lies anterior to the esophagus in this area.

1.79
Branches of the thoracic aorta

The superior phrenic branches arising from the inferior part of the thoracic aorta are not shown. These small vessels supply the posterosuperior aspect of the diaphragm. Note that the right bronchial artery usually arises from either the upper left bronchial or 3rd right posterior intercostal artery (here the 5th) or the aorta directly.

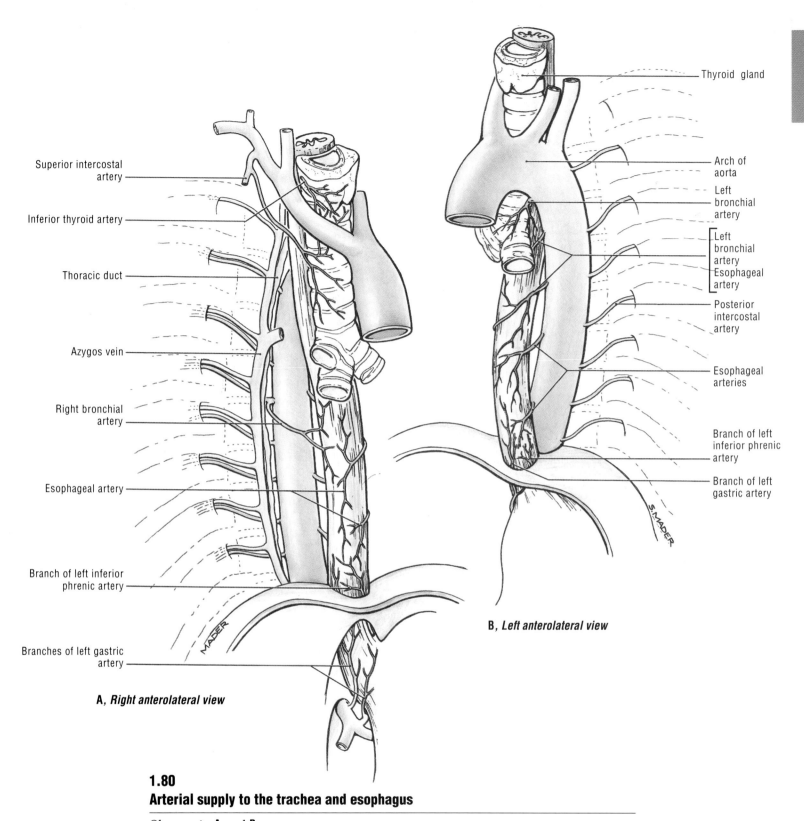

Superior intercostal artery

Inferior thyroid artery

Thoracic duct

Azygos vein

Right bronchial artery

Esophageal artery

Branch of left inferior phrenic artery

Branches of left gastric artery

A, *Right anterolateral view*

Thyroid gland

Arch of aorta

Left bronchial artery

[Left bronchial artery Esophageal artery]

Posterior intercostal artery

Esophageal arteries

Branch of left inferior phrenic artery

Branch of left gastric artery

B, *Left anterolateral view*

1.80
Arterial supply to the trachea and esophagus

Observe in **A** and **B**:

1. The unpaired median bronchial and esophageal branches of the descending thoracic aorta, which supply the trachea, bronchi, and esophagus;

2. The continuous anastomotic chain of arteries on the esophagus formed: (a) by branches of the right and left inferior thyroid and right superior thoracic arteries superiorly; (b) by the unpaired median aortic branches; and (c) by branches of the left gastric and left inferior phrenic arteries inferiorly.

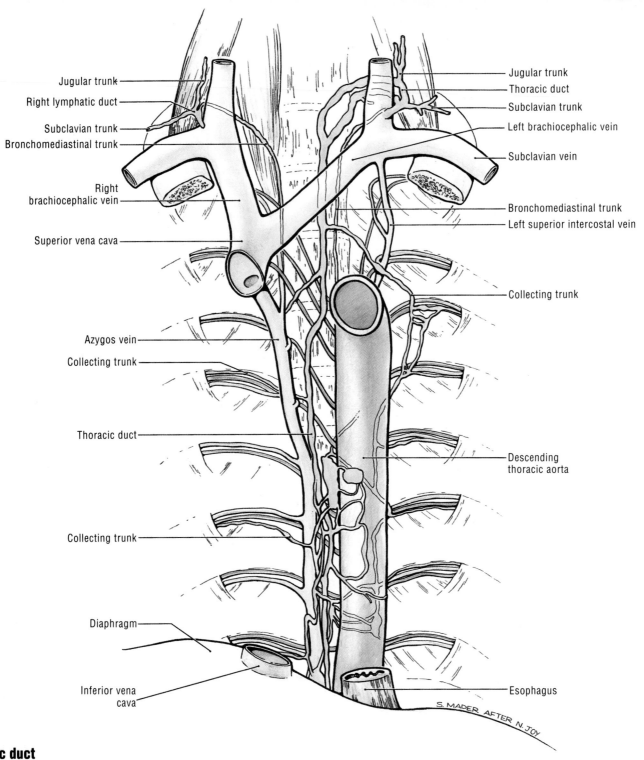

Jugular trunk
Right lymphatic duct
Subclavian trunk
Bronchomediastinal trunk
Right brachiocephalic vein
Superior vena cava
Azygos vein
Collecting trunk
Thoracic duct
Collecting trunk
Diaphragm
Inferior vena cava

Jugular trunk
Thoracic duct
Subclavian trunk
Left brachiocephalic vein
Subclavian vein
Bronchomediastinal trunk
Left superior intercostal vein
Collecting trunk
Descending thoracic aorta
Esophagus

S. MADER AFTER N. JOY

1.81
Thoracic duct

The descending aorta is pulled slightly to the left and the azygos vein slightly to the right. Observe:

1. The thoracic duct (a) ascending on the vertebral column between the azygos vein and the descending aorta and (b) at the junction of the posterior and superior mediastina, passing to the left and continuing its ascent to the neck where (c) it arches laterally to open near, or at, the angle of union of the internal jugular and subclavian veins;

2. The duct, here, as commonly (a) plexiform in the posterior mediastinum and (b) splitting and reuniting in the neck;

3. The duct receiving branches from the intercostal spaces of both sides via several collecting trunks and also branches from posterior mediastinal structures;

4. The duct finally receiving the jugular, subclavian, and bronchomediastinal trunks;

5. The right lymph duct, very short and formed by the union of the right jugular, subclavian, and bronchomediastinal trunks.

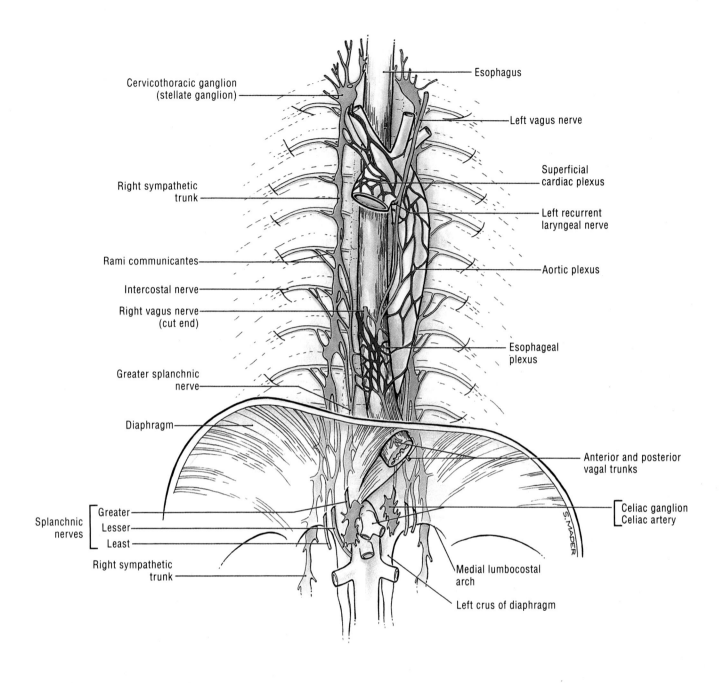

Cervicothoracic ganglion (stellate ganglion)

Esophagus

Left vagus nerve

Right sympathetic trunk

Superficial cardiac plexus

Left recurrent laryngeal nerve

Rami communicantes

Aortic plexus

Intercostal nerve

Right vagus nerve (cut end)

Esophageal plexus

Greater splanchnic nerve

Diaphragm

Anterior and posterior vagal trunks

Celiac ganglion
Celiac artery

Splanchnic nerves
[Greater
Lesser
Least]

Right sympathetic trunk

Medial lumbocostal arch

Left crus of diaphragm

S. MADER

1.82
Autonomic nerves of the posterior and superior mediastinum

Observe:

1. The right and left thoracic sympathetic trunks entering the abdomen by passing deep to the medial lumbocostal arch of the diaphragm;

2. The large cervicothoracic ganglion formed by the fusion of the inferior cervical ganglion and the 1st thoracic ganglion;

3. The sympathetic nerve cell bodies are located in the lateral horn of gray matter of the spinal cord in segments T1– L2 or L3; the fibers are conveyed through the ventral roots, spinal nerves, and rami communicantes to the sympathetic trunk; from the thoracic sympathetic trunk fibers are distributed (a) superiorly to the cervical sympathetic trunk, (b) inferiorly to the lumbar

sympathetic trunk, (c) to thoracic viscera by contributions to the plexes (e.g., cardiac, esophageal), (d) to abdominal ganglia (e.g., celiac, superior mesenteric) by the greater, lesser, and least splanchnic nerves, (e) to the intercostal nerves by the rami communicantes;

4. The left vagus and recurrent laryngeal nerves contributing parasympathetic fibers to the pulmonary, cardiac, and esophageal plexuses; the cut end of the right vagus nerve, which also contributes fibers to these plexuses;

5. The vagus nerves passing through the esophageal opening of the diaphragm to become the anterior and posterior vagal trunks.

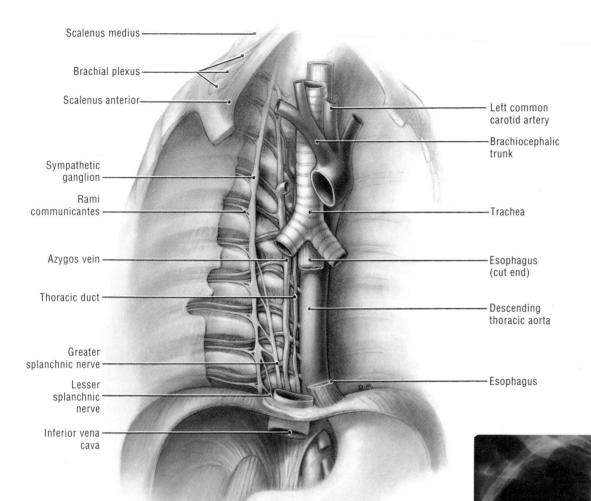

Scalenus medius

Brachial plexus

Scalenus anterior

Sympathetic ganglion

Rami communicantes

Azygos vein

Thoracic duct

Greater splanchnic nerve

Lesser splanchnic nerve

Inferior vena cava

Left common carotid artery

Brachiocephalic trunk

Trachea

Esophagus (cut end)

Descending thoracic aorta

Esophagus

1.83
Posterior mediastinum viewed from the right

Observe:

1. The parietal pleura is intact on the left side and partially removed on the right side;

2. A portion of the esophagus, between the bifurcation of the trachea and the diaphragm, is removed;

3. The thoracic sympathetic trunk lying against the heads of the ribs, the sympathetic ganglia, and the rami communicantes connecting to each intercostal nerve;

4. The greater splanchnic nerve formed by fibers from the 5th to the 10th thoracic ganglia and the lesser splanchnic nerve receiving fibers from the 10th and 11th thoracic ganglia; both nerves contain preganglionic and visceral afferent fibers and enter the abdomen by piercing the crus of the diaphragm;

5. The azygos vein passing anterior to the intercostal vessels and to the right of the thoracic duct and thoracic aorta.

1.84
Azygogram

I – Posterior intercostal vein, *AR* – Arch of azygos vein, *A* – Azygos vein, *T* – Trachea, *L* – Left bronchus. (Courtesy of Dr. J. Heslin, Assistant Professor of Anatomy, University of Toronto, Toronto, Ontario, Canada.)

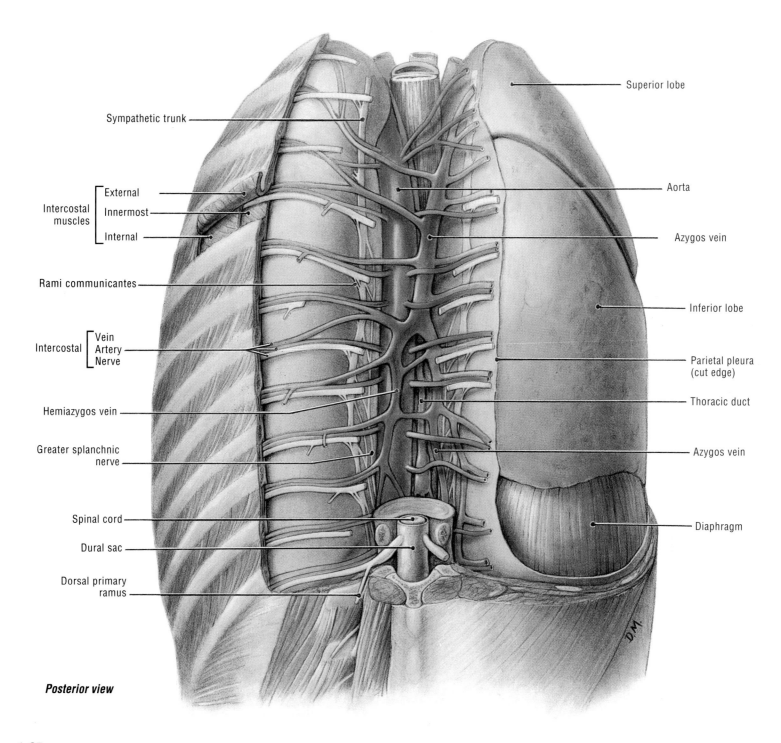

Superior lobe

Sympathetic trunk

Intercostal muscles
- External
- Innermost
- Internal

Rami communicantes

Intercostal
- Vein
- Artery
- Nerve

Hemiazygos vein

Greater splanchnic nerve

Spinal cord

Dural sac

Dorsal primary ramus

Aorta

Azygos vein

Inferior lobe

Parietal pleura (cut edge)

Thoracic duct

Azygos vein

Diaphragm

Posterior view

D.M.

1.85
Mediastinum and lungs

Observe:

1. The thoracic vertebral column and thoracic cage is removed on the right; on the left, the ribs and intercostal musculature is removed posteriorly as far laterally as the angles of the ribs;

2. The parietal pleura is intact on the left side, but is partially removed on the right to reveal the visceral pleura covering the left lung;

3. The azygos vein on the right side; the hemiazygos vein on the left side crossing the midline, usually at T9 but higher in this specimen, to join the azygos vein; the absence of the accessory hemiazygos vein, instead three posterior intercostal veins draining directly into the azygos vein;

4. The thoracic aorta lying against the left lung and partially embedded in the parietal pleura.

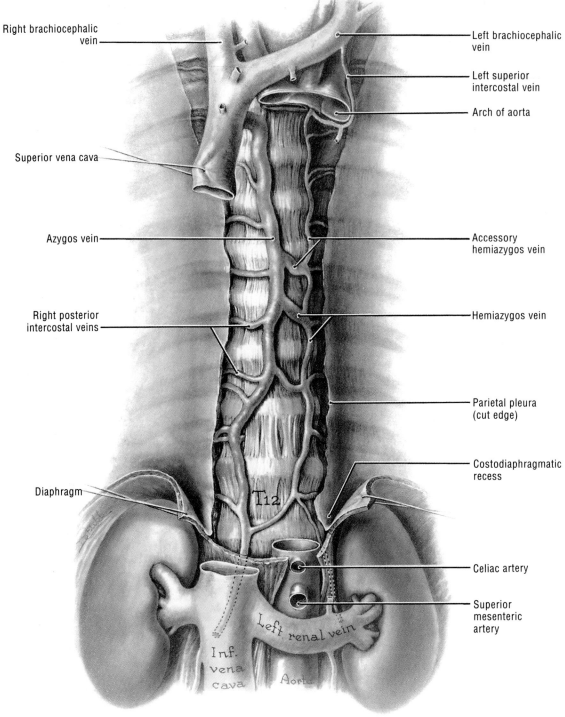

Right brachiocephalic vein

Left brachiocephalic vein

Left superior intercostal vein

Arch of aorta

Superior vena cava

Azygos vein

Accessory hemiazygos vein

Right posterior intercostal veins

Hemiazygos vein

Parietal pleura (cut edge)

Costodiaphragmatic recess

Diaphragm

T12

Celiac artery

Superior mesenteric artery

Inf. vena cava

Left renal vein

Aorta

1.86
Azygos system of veins

While consulting Figure 1.87 on the facing page, observe:
1. The left renal vein anterior to the aorta; the left brachiocephalic vein anterior to the three branches of the arch of the aorta; these two cross-channels conduct blood from the left side of the body to the right side and so to the right atrium;

2. The paired and approximately symmetrical longitudinal veins anterior to the vertebral column; the azygos vein, on the right side, communicating inferiorly with the inferior vena cava; the hemiazygos vein, on the left side, communicating with the left renal vein; and each receiving the respective right and left posterior intercostal veins;

3. In this specimen, the hemiazygos, accessory hemiazygos, and left superior intercostal veins are continuous, but commonly they are discontinuous as in Figure 1.87;

4. The hemiazygos vein crossing the vertebral column at approximately T9 and the accessory hemiazygos vein at T8 to enter the azygos vein; in this specimen, note the presence of four cross connecting channels between the azygos and hemiazygos systems;

5. The azygos vein arches superior to the root of the right lung, at T4, to drain into the superior vena cava.

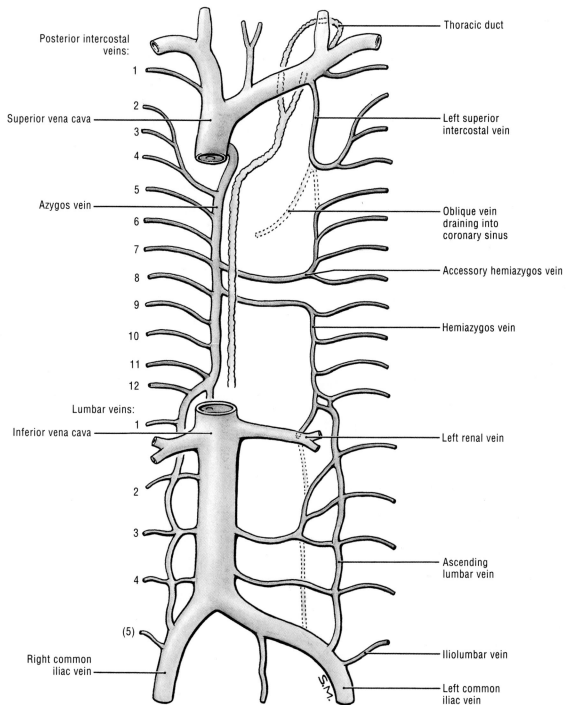

Posterior intercostal veins:

1
2
3
4
5
6
7
8
9
10
11
12

Superior vena cava

Azygos vein

Lumbar veins:
1

Inferior vena cava

2

3

4

(5)

Right common iliac vein

Thoracic duct

Left superior intercostal vein

Oblique vein draining into coronary sinus

Accessory hemiazygos vein

Hemiazygos vein

Left renal vein

Ascending lumbar vein

Iliolumbar vein

Left common iliac vein

S.M.

1.87
Azygos, hemiazygos, and lumbar veins

Observe:

1. That this system is of great importance, in continued venous return to the heart, if there is an obstruction of the venae cavae;

2. The lumbar veins lie directly anterior to the vertebral bodies and drain blood from the posterior abdominal wall and from vertebral structures (vertebral column, spinal cord, meninges, etc.) into the inferior vena cava; branches of the lumbar veins also anastomose with the vertebral venous plexes;

3. The ascending lumbar veins connect the common iliac veins to the lumbar veins and join the subcostal veins to become the lateral root of the azygos or hemiazygos veins;

4. The medial roots of the azygos and hemiazygos veins are usually from the inferior vena cava and left renal vein, if present;

5. The right posterior intercostal veins draining into the azygos and right superior intercostal veins; the left posterior intercostal veins draining into the hemiazygos, accessory hemiazygos, and left superior intercostal veins;

6. The hemiazygos vein (at T9) and accessory hemiazygos vein (at T8) crossing the vertebral column to drain into the azygos vein; the azygos vein arching anteriorly superior to the root of the lung, at T4, to enter the superior vena cava.

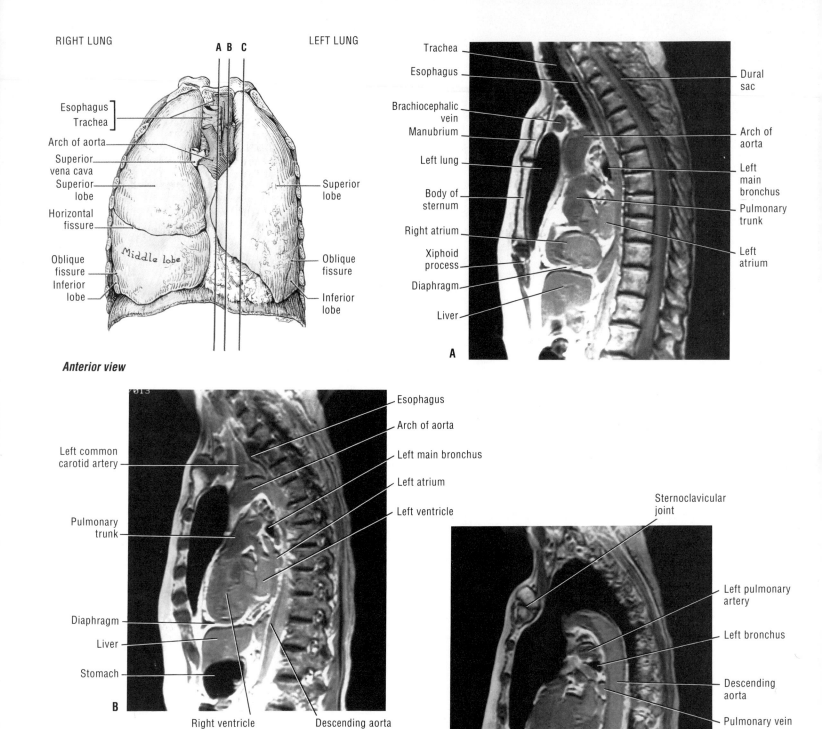

RIGHT LUNG   A B C   LEFT LUNG

Esophagus
Trachea

Arch of aorta

Superior vena cava

Superior lobe

Horizontal fissure

Middle lobe

Oblique fissure

Inferior lobe

Superior lobe

Oblique fissure

Inferior lobe

Anterior view

Trachea

Esophagus

Brachiocephalic vein

Manubrium

Left lung

Body of sternum

Right atrium

Xiphoid process

Diaphragm

Liver

Dural sac

Arch of aorta

Left main bronchus

Pulmonary trunk

Left atrium

A

Esophagus

Arch of aorta

Left main bronchus

Left atrium

Left ventricle

Left common carotid artery

Pulmonary trunk

Diaphragm

Liver

Stomach

B

Right ventricle

Descending aorta

Sternoclavicular joint

Left pulmonary artery

Left bronchus

Descending aorta

Pulmonary vein

Left ventricle

Stomach

C

1.88
Sagittal MRIs (magnetic resonance images) of the thorax

The line diagram indicates the location of the section (**A**, **B**, and **C**) of the MRIs. (Courtesy of Dr. W. Kucharczyk, Clinical Director of Tri-Hospital Magnetic Resonance Centre, Toronto, Ontario, Canada.)

2   The Abdomen

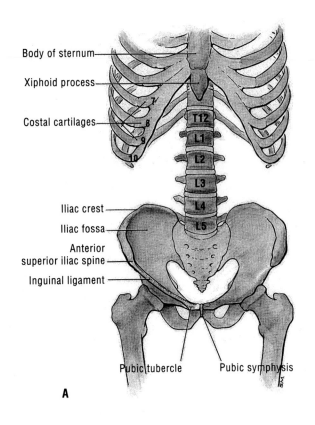

Body of sternum

Xiphoid process

Costal cartilages

7
8
9
10

T12
L1
L2
L3
L4
L5

Iliac crest

Iliac fossa

Anterior
superior iliac spine

Inguinal ligament

Pubic tubercle

Pubic symphysis

A

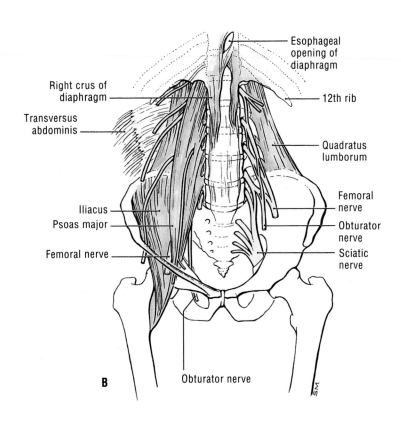

Right crus of
diaphragm

Transversus
abdominis

Iliacus

Psoas major

Femoral nerve

Obturator nerve

Esophageal
opening of
diaphragm

12th rib

Quadratus
lumborum

Femoral
nerve

Obturator
nerve

Sciatic
nerve

B

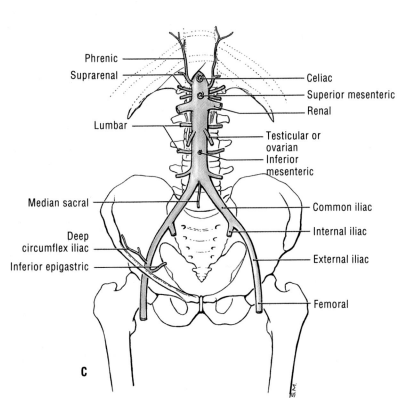

Phrenic

Suprarenal

Lumbar

Median sacral

Deep
circumflex iliac

Inferior epigastric

Celiac

Superior mesenteric

Renal

Testicular or
ovarian

Inferior
mesenteric

Common iliac

Internal iliac

External iliac

Femoral

C

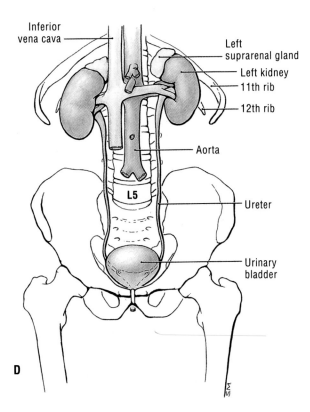

Inferior
vena cava

Left
suprarenal gland

Left kidney

11th rib

12th rib

Aorta

L5

Ureter

Urinary
bladder

D

2.1
Overview diagrams of the abdomen and pelvis

A. Skeleton of abdomen and pelvis. **B**. Posterior wall, musculature and lumbosacral
plexus. **C**. Abdominal aorta. **D**. Urinary apparatus.

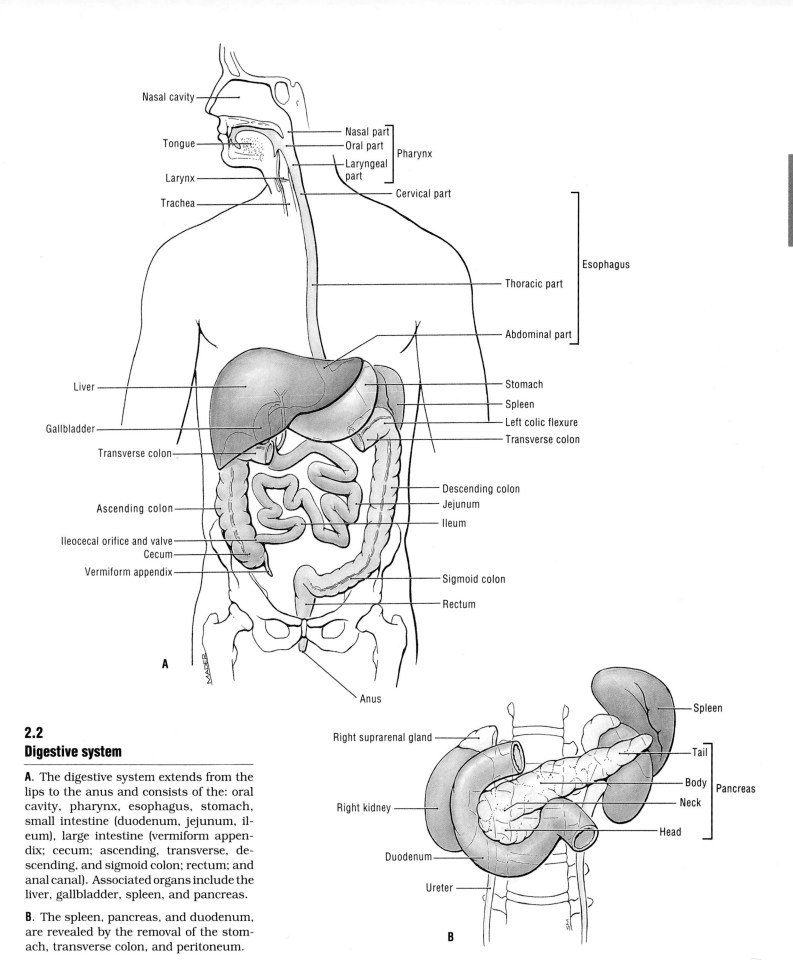

Nasal cavity

Tongue

Larynx

Trachea

Nasal part ⎤
Oral part ⎬ Pharynx
Laryngeal part ⎦

Cervical part

Esophagus

Thoracic part

Abdominal part

Liver

Gallbladder

Transverse colon

Ascending colon

Ileocecal orifice and valve

Cecum

Vermiform appendix

Stomach

Spleen

Left colic flexure

Transverse colon

Descending colon

Jejunum

Ileum

Sigmoid colon

Rectum

A

Anus

Spleen

Right suprarenal gland

Tail ⎤
Body ⎬ Pancreas
Neck
Head ⎦

Right kidney

Duodenum

Ureter

B

2.2
Digestive system

A. The digestive system extends from the lips to the anus and consists of the: oral cavity, pharynx, esophagus, stomach, small intestine (duodenum, jejunum, ileum), large intestine (vermiform appendix; cecum; ascending, transverse, descending, and sigmoid colon; rectum; and anal canal). Associated organs include the liver, gallbladder, spleen, and pancreas.

B. The spleen, pancreas, and duodenum, are revealed by the removal of the stomach, transverse colon, and peritoneum.

2.3
Surface anatomy of the anterior abdominal wall
(at right and lower right)

Observe:

1. The linea alba extending the full length of the anterior abdominal wall, from the xiphoid process to the symphysis pubis; the linea alba is formed by the interweaving of the aponeurotic fibers of the external, internal, and transversus abdominis muscles (**B**);

2. The right and left rectus abdominis muscles spanning from the pubic bone to the xiphoid process and costal cartilages of the 5th, 6th, and 7th ribs; the linea semilunaris located at the lateral border of the rectus abdominis muscle;

3. The transversely oriented tendinous intersections that interrupt the continuity of the rectus abdominis muscle; the tendinous intersections are adherent to the anterior rectus sheath and seldom penetrate through the full thickness of the muscle belly (Fig. 2.5);

4. The inguinal ligament lying between the anterior superior iliac spine and the pubic tubercle; the inguinal ligament is formed by the inferior margin of the aponeurosis of the external oblique muscle (Fig. 2.10).

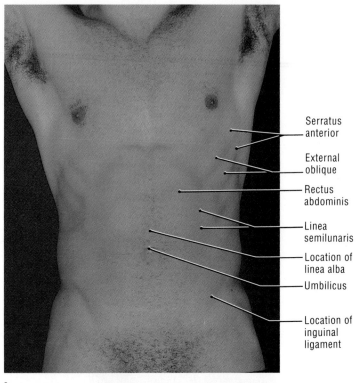

Serratus anterior

External oblique

Rectus abdominis

Linea semilunaris

Location of linea alba

Umbilicus

Location of inguinal ligament

A

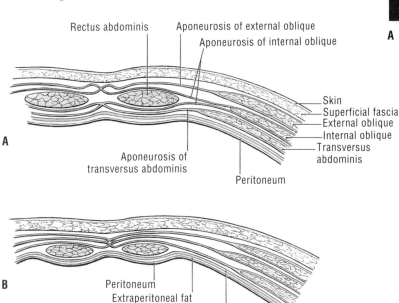

Rectus abdominis

Aponeurosis of external oblique

Aponeurosis of internal oblique

Skin
Superficial fascia
External oblique
Internal oblique
Transversus abdominis

A

Aponeurosis of transversus abdominis

Peritoneum

Peritoneum
Extraperitoneal fat
Transversalis fascia

B

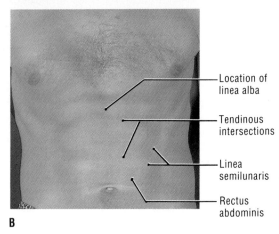

Location of linea alba

Tendinous intersections

Linea semilunaris

Rectus abdominis

B

2.4
Rectus sheath *(above)*

Transverse section of the anterior abdominal wall superior to the umbilicus (**A**) and inferior to the umbilicus (**B**).

Observe in **A** and **B**:

1. The aponeuroses of the external oblique, internal oblique, and transversus abdominis muscles are each bilaminar;

2. The decussation and interweaving of the aponeuroses, occurring at the linea alba, is not only from side to side but also from superficial to deep;

3. Superior to the umbilicus, both anterior and posterior rectus sheaths are trilaminar: anteriorly, the two layers of the aponeurosis of the external oblique muscle and the superficial layer of the aponeurosis of the internal oblique muscle; posteriorly, the deep layer of the aponeurosis of the internal oblique muscle and the two layers of the aponeurosis of the transversus abdominis muscle;

4. Approximately midway between the umbilicus and the symphysis pubis, all the aponeuroses pass anterior to the rectus abdominis muscle; the posterior rectus sheath gradually ends as the arcuate line and the transversalis fascia comes to lie in contact with the posterior aspect of the rectus abdominis muscle. (From Rizk NN. *A new description of the anterior abdominal wall in man and mammals.* J Anat 1980; 131:373-385.)

2.5
Anterior abdominal wall

A. Superficial dissection. Anterior layer of rectus sheath is reflected, on the left side.

Observe:

1. The anterior cutaneous nerves (T7 to T12) piercing the rectus abdominis muscle and the anterior layer of its sheath; T10 supplies the region of the umbilicus;

2. In the fatty superficial layer of superficial fascia, the three superficial inguinal branches of the femoral artery and the great (long) saphenous vein;

3. The membranous deep layer of the superficial fascia: (a) blending with the fascia lata of the thigh, a finger's breadth inferior to the inguinal ligament and thereby forming a gutter that empties into the superficial perineal region; (b) following along the penis and the spermatic cord to the scrotum, and from here continuing posteriorly to blend with the deep layer of superficial fascia of the perineum;

4. The spermatic cord and the ilioinguinal nerve passing through the superficial inguinal ring.

B. Membranous deep layer of superficial fascia of the abdomen.

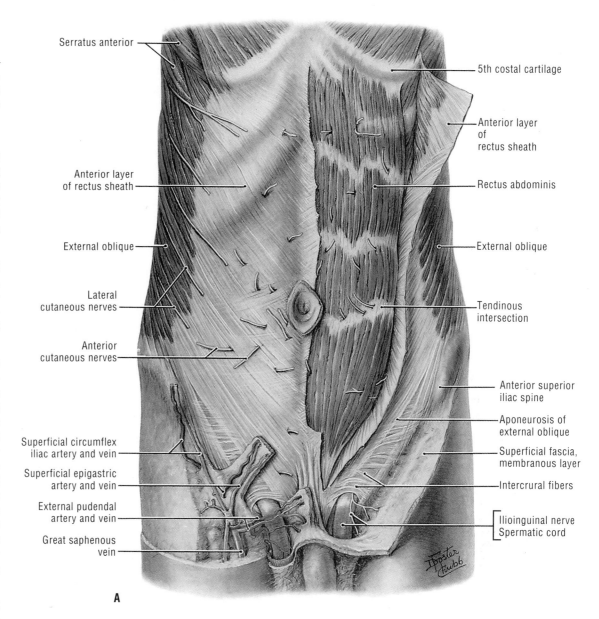

Serratus anterior

5th costal cartilage

Anterior layer of rectus sheath

Anterior layer of rectus sheath

Rectus abdominis

External oblique

External oblique

Lateral cutaneous nerves

Tendinous intersection

Anterior cutaneous nerves

Anterior superior iliac spine

Superficial circumflex iliac artery and vein

Aponeurosis of external oblique

Superficial epigastric artery and vein

Superficial fascia, membranous layer

External pudendal artery and vein

Intercrural fibers

Great saphenous vein

Ilioinguinal nerve
Spermatic cord

A

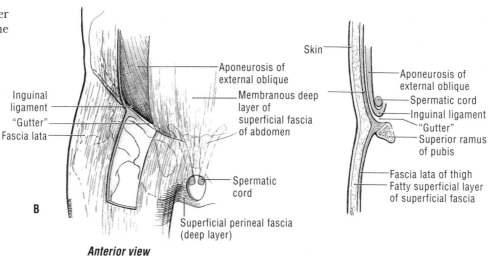

Inguinal ligament

Aponeurosis of external oblique

Skin

"Gutter"

Membranous deep layer of superficial fascia of abdomen

Aponeurosis of external oblique

Fascia lata

Spermatic cord

Inguinal ligament

"Gutter"

Superior ramus of pubis

Spermatic cord

Fascia lata of thigh

Fatty superficial layer of superficial fascia

Superficial perineal fascia (deep layer)

B

Anterior view

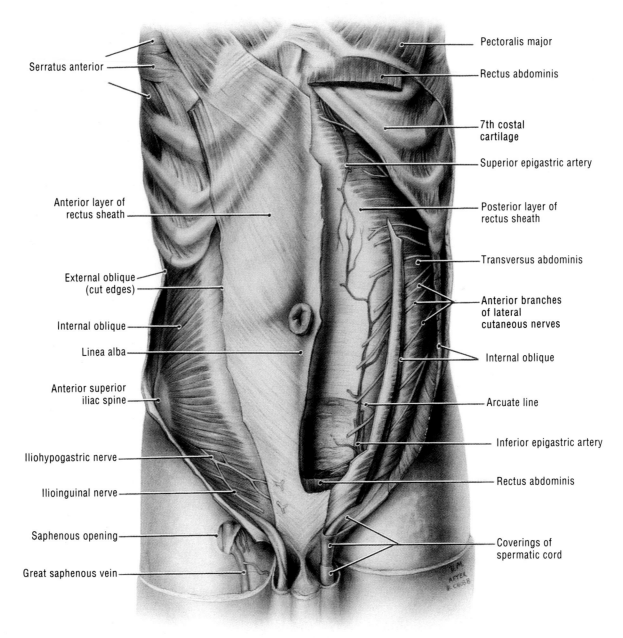

Serratus anterior

Anterior layer of
rectus sheath

External oblique
(cut edges)

Internal oblique

Linea alba

Anterior superior
iliac spine

Iliohypogastric nerve

Ilioinguinal nerve

Saphenous opening

Great saphenous vein

Pectoralis major

Rectus abdominis

7th costal
cartilage

Superior epigastric artery

Posterior layer of
rectus sheath

Transversus abdominis

Anterior branches
of lateral
cutaneous nerves

Internal oblique

Arcuate line

Inferior epigastric artery

Rectus abdominis

Coverings of
spermatic cord

2.6
Anterior abdominal wall, deep dissection

On the right side, most of the external oblique muscle is excised.

On the left, the rectus abdominis muscle is excised and the internal oblique muscle divided.

Observe:

1. The fibers of the internal oblique muscle running horizontally at the level of the anterior superior iliac spine; running obliquely upward superior to this level, and obliquely downward inferior to it;

2. The arcuate line at the level of the anterior superior iliac spine;

3. The anastomosis between the superior and inferior epigastric arteries that indirectly unites the arteries of the upper limb to those of the lower limb (subclavian to external iliac);

4. The linea alba is not an unyielding ligament uniting the sternum to the symphysis pubis, but an extendible line across which fibers decussate in bias.

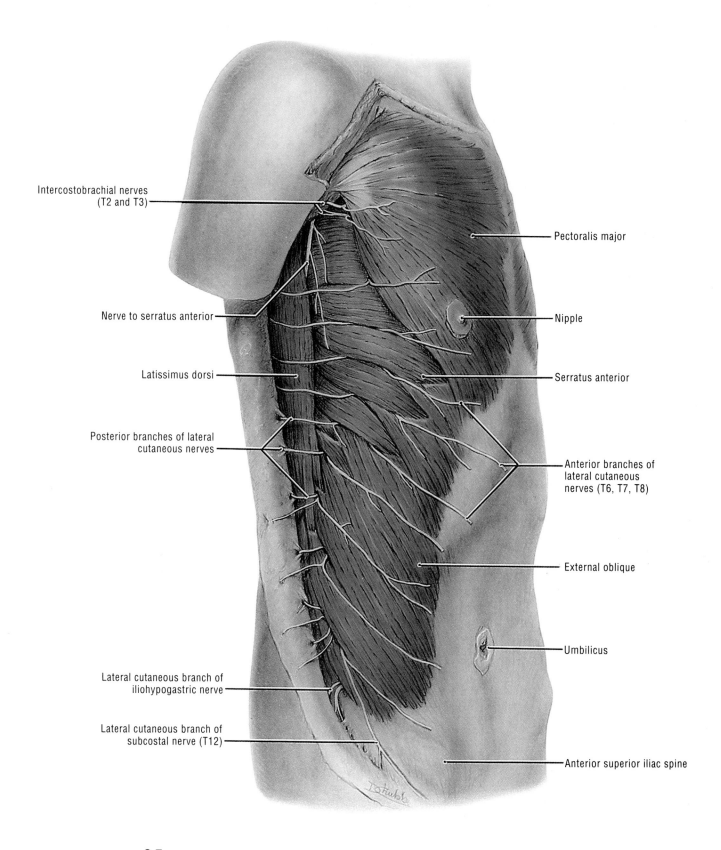

Intercostobrachial nerves (T2 and T3)

Nerve to serratus anterior

Latissimus dorsi

Posterior branches of lateral cutaneous nerves

Lateral cutaneous branch of iliohypogastric nerve

Lateral cutaneous branch of subcostal nerve (T12)

Pectoralis major

Nipple

Serratus anterior

Anterior branches of lateral cutaneous nerves (T6, T7, T8)

External oblique

Umbilicus

Anterior superior iliac spine

2.7
Lateral view of the trunk

This superficial dissection shows the external oblique muscle and the lateral cutaneous nerves. Observe the interdigitations of the fibers of the serratus anterior muscle with the external oblique muscle.

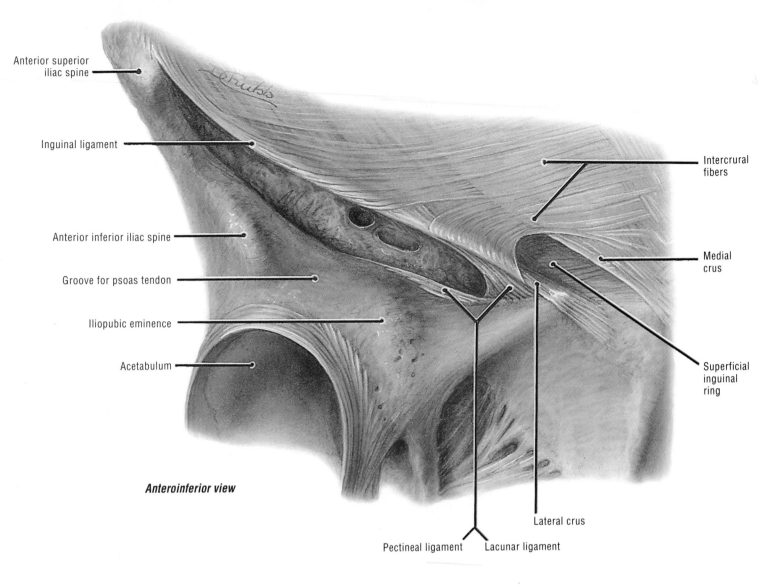

Anterior superior iliac spine

Inguinal ligament

Anterior inferior iliac spine

Groove for psoas tendon

Iliopubic eminence

Acetabulum

Anteroinferior view

Intercrural fibers

Medial crus

Superficial inguinal ring

Lateral crus

Pectineal ligament   Lacunar ligament

2.8
Inguinal ligament

Observe:

1. The inguinal ligament formed by the inferior, underturned fibers of the aponeurosis of the external oblique muscle;

2. The intercrural fibers, well developed in this specimen, preventing the crura of the inguinal ring from spreading;

3. The superficial inguinal ring is triangular, its central point being superior to the pubic tubercle, its base being the lateral half of the pubic crest, its lateral crus being the inguinal ligament, and its medial crus being fibers of the aponeurosis of the external oblique muscle that cross the pubic crest at its midpoint;

4. The fibers of the inguinal ligament, that falling short of the pubic tubercle, find attachment to the pectineal line as the lacunar ligament; this ligament forms the medial boundary of the femoral ring, through which a femoral hernia may descend;

5. The pectineal ligament whose fibers run horizontally along the pectineal line.

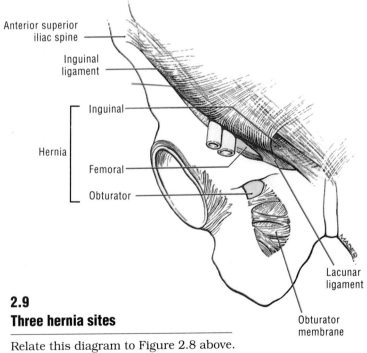

Anterior superior iliac spine

Inguinal ligament

Inguinal

Hernia

Femoral

Obturator

Lacunar ligament

Obturator membrane

2.9
Three hernia sites

Relate this diagram to Figure 2.8 above.

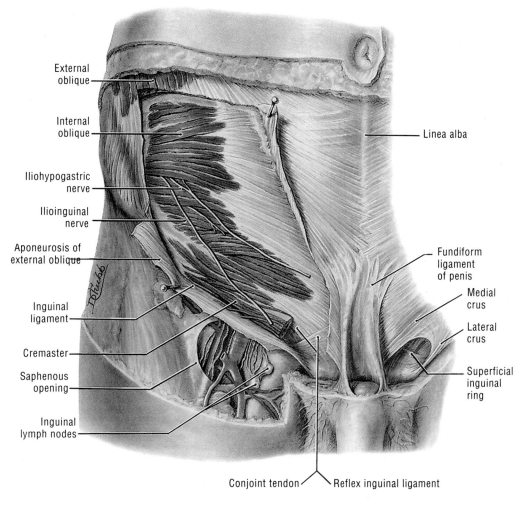

External
oblique

Internal
oblique

Iliohypogastric
nerve

Ilioinguinal
nerve

Aponeurosis of
external oblique

Inguinal
ligament

Cremaster

Saphenous
opening

Inguinal
lymph nodes

Linea alba

Fundiform
ligament
of penis

Medial
crus

Lateral
crus

Superficial
inguinal
ring

Conjoint tendon — Reflex inguinal ligament

2.10
Inguinal region of the male–I

The aponeurosis of the external oblique muscle is partly cut away and the spermatic cord is cut short.

Observe:
1. The laminated, fundiform ligament of the penis descending to the junction of the fixed and mobile parts of the organ;

2. The reflex inguinal ligament, which represents aponeurotic fibers of the external oblique muscle, lying anterior to the conjoint tendon; the conjoint tendon is formed by the aponeurosis of the internal oblique and transversus abdominis muscles;

3. The only two structures that course between external and internal obliques, namely, the iliohypogastric and ilioinguinal branches of the 1st lumbar nerve; they are sensory from this point to their terminations;

4. The fleshy fibers of internal oblique muscle at the level of the anterior superior iliac spine running horizontally; those from the iliac crest passing superomedially; and those from the inguinal ligament arching inferomedially;

5. The cremaster muscle covering the spermatic cord and filling the arched space between conjoint tendon and inguinal ligament;

6. At the level of the umbilicus, the aponeurosis of external oblique muscle blending with the aponeurosis of the internal oblique muscle near the lateral border of the rectus abdominis muscle, but in the suprapubic region free as far as the median plane.

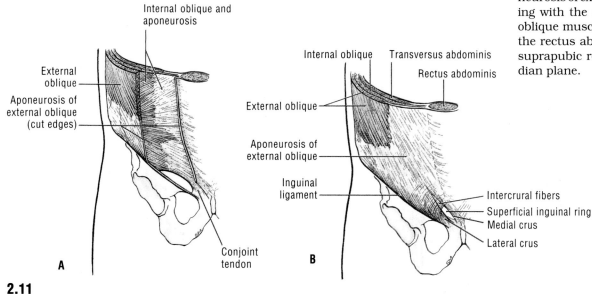

Internal oblique and
aponeurosis

External
oblique

Aponeurosis of
external oblique
(cut edges)

Conjoint
tendon

Internal oblique   Transversus abdominis

Rectus abdominis

External oblique

Aponeurosis of
external oblique

Inguinal
ligament

Intercrural fibers

Superficial inguinal ring

Medial crus

Lateral crus

A   B

2.11
Diagrams of the inguinal region

A. Internal oblique and conjoint tendon. **B.** Superficial inguinal ring.

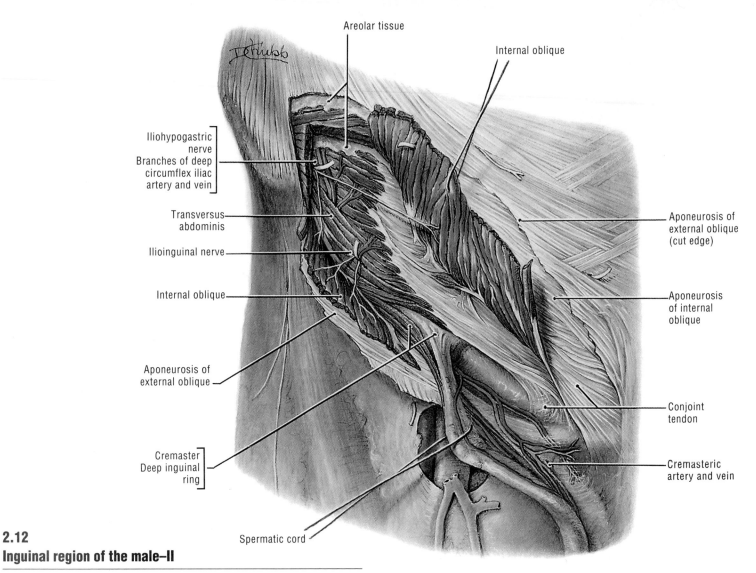

Areolar tissue

Internal oblique

Iliohypogastric nerve

Branches of deep circumflex iliac artery and vein

Transversus abdominis

Ilioinguinal nerve

Internal oblique

Aponeurosis of external oblique

Cremaster
Deep inguinal ring

Spermatic cord

Aponeurosis of external oblique (cut edge)

Aponeurosis of internal oblique

Conjoint tendon

Cremasteric artery and vein

2.12

Inguinal region of the male–II

The internal oblique muscle is reflected and the spermatic cord is retracted.

Observe:

1. The transversus abdominis muscle taking, in this region, the same common inferomedial direction as the fibers of external oblique aponeurosis and internal oblique muscle;

2. The internal oblique portion of the conjoint tendon attached to the pubic crest; transversus portion extending laterally along the pectineal line;

3. The conjoint tendon not sharply defined from fascia transversalis, but blending with it;

4. The iliohypogastric and ilioinguinal nerves, supplying the fibers of internal oblique and transversus abdominis muscles that control the conjoint tendon;

5. Fascia transversalis evaginated to form the tubular internal spermatic fascia; the mouth of the tube, called the deep inguinal ring, situated lateral to the inferior epigastric vessels;

6. The cremasteric artery (a branch of the inferior epigastric artery) that supplies the testes along with the testicular artery and the artery of the deferent duct;

7. The cremaster muscle arising from the inguinal ligament.

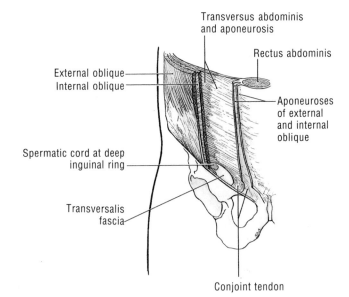

Transversus abdominis and aponeurosis

Rectus abdominis

External oblique
Internal oblique

Aponeuroses of external and internal oblique

Spermatic cord at deep inguinal ring

Transversalis fascia

Conjoint tendon

2.13

Diagram of the inguinal region – transversus abdominis, conjoint tendon, and transversalis fascia

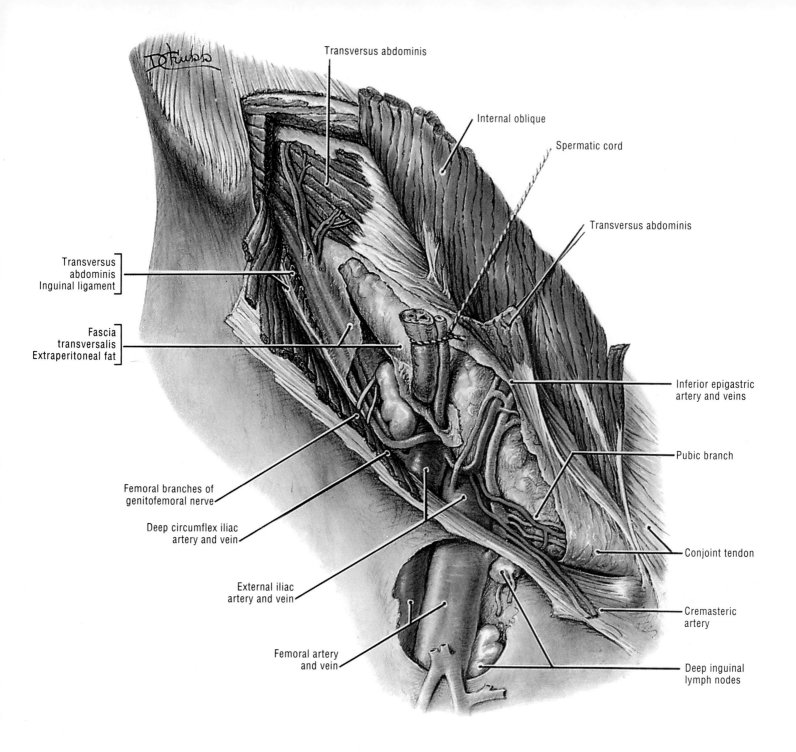

Transversus abdominis

Internal oblique

Spermatic cord

Transversus abdominis

Transversus
abdominis
Inguinal ligament

Fascia
transversalis
Extraperitoneal fat

Inferior epigastric
artery and veins

Pubic branch

Femoral branches of
genitofemoral nerve

Deep circumflex iliac
artery and vein

Conjoint tendon

External iliac
artery and vein

Cremasteric
artery

Femoral artery
and vein

Deep inguinal
lymph nodes

2.14

Inguinal region of the male–III

The inguinal part of transversus abdominis muscle and fascia transversalis is partly cut away and the spermatic cord is excised.

Observe:

1. The inferior limit of the peritoneal sac; it lies some distance superior to the inguinal ligament laterally but close to it medially;

2. The location of the deep inguinal ring, a finger's breadth superior to the inguinal ligament at the midpoint between the anterior superior iliac spine and the pubic tubercle;

3. The testicular vessels and the deferent duct (retracted) starting to part company at the deep inguinal ring;

4. The proximity of the external iliac artery and vein to the inguinal canal;

5. The only two branches of the external iliac artery, the deep circumflex iliac and inferior epigastric arteries; note also the cremasteric and pubic branches of the latter.

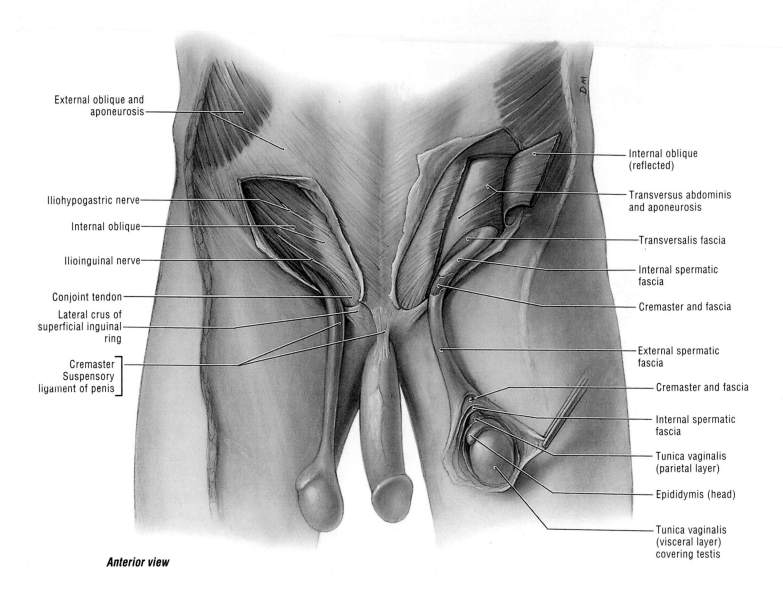

External oblique and aponeurosis

Iliohypogastric nerve

Internal oblique

Ilioinguinal nerve

Conjoint tendon

Lateral crus of superficial inguinal ring

Cremaster
Suspensory ligament of penis

Internal oblique (reflected)

Transversus abdominis and aponeurosis

Transversalis fascia

Internal spermatic fascia

Cremaster and fascia

External spermatic fascia

Cremaster and fascia

Internal spermatic fascia

Tunica vaginalis (parietal layer)

Epididymis (head)

Tunica vaginalis (visceral layer) covering testis

Anterior view

2.15
Inguinal region, spermatic cord, and testis

Observe on the right side:

1. The aponeurosis of the external oblique muscle is incised and reflected to reveal the more deeply located internal oblique muscle and aponeurosis;

2. Inferiorly, the aponeuroses of internal oblique and transversus abdominis muscles forming the conjoint tendon; the internal oblique portion of the conjoint tendon attaching to the pubic crest; the transversus portion extending laterally along the pectineal line;

3. The cremaster muscle arising from the internal oblique muscle to form a covering for the spermatic cord and testes;

4. The iliohypogastric and ilioinguinal branches of the 1st lumbar nerve; both are motor to the internal oblique and transversus abdominis muscles and terminate as sensory nerves supplying the skin in the area of the superficial inguinal ring and the medial aspect of the thigh and scrotum, respectively.

Observe on the left side:

1. A window has been made by cutting and reflecting the internal oblique muscle laterally to expose the deeply located transversus abdominis muscle and aponeurosis; also visible is the fascia transversalis evaginated to form the tubular internal spermatic fascia; the mouth of the tube is called the deep inguinal ring;

2. The inguinal arch of the transversus abdominis muscle and aponeurosis, laterally, arching superior to the spermatic cord and, medially terminating posterior to it; the oblique course of the spermatic cord in the inguinal canal, i.e., from the deep to the superficial inguinal ring;

3. All of the layers covering the right testis have been cut open sequentially: the external spermatic fascia, the cremaster muscle and fascia, the internal spermatic fascia, and the tunica vaginalis of the testis consisting of visceral and parietal layers.

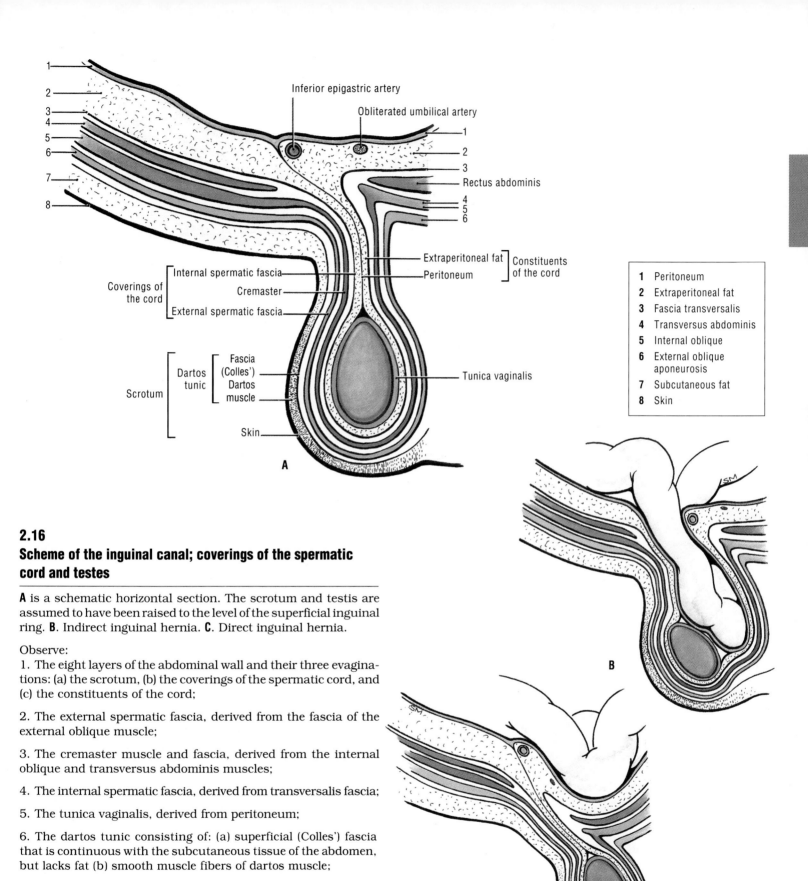

Inferior epigastric artery

Obliterated umbilical artery

Rectus abdominis

Extraperitoneal fat ⎤ Constituents
Peritoneum ⎦ of the cord

Coverings of the cord
Internal spermatic fascia
Cremaster
External spermatic fascia

Scrotum
Dartos tunic
Fascia (Colles')
Dartos muscle

Skin

Tunica vaginalis

A

1	Peritoneum
2	Extraperitoneal fat
3	Fascia transversalis
4	Transversus abdominis
5	Internal oblique
6	External oblique aponeurosis
7	Subcutaneous fat
8	Skin

B

C

2.16
Scheme of the inguinal canal; coverings of the spermatic cord and testes

A is a schematic horizontal section. The scrotum and testis are assumed to have been raised to the level of the superficial inguinal ring. **B**. Indirect inguinal hernia. **C**. Direct inguinal hernia.

Observe:

1. The eight layers of the abdominal wall and their three evaginations: (a) the scrotum, (b) the coverings of the spermatic cord, and (c) the constituents of the cord;

2. The external spermatic fascia, derived from the fascia of the external oblique muscle;

3. The cremaster muscle and fascia, derived from the internal oblique and transversus abdominis muscles;

4. The internal spermatic fascia, derived from transversalis fascia;

5. The tunica vaginalis, derived from peritoneum;

6. The dartos tunic consisting of: (a) superficial (Colles') fascia that is continuous with the subcutaneous tissue of the abdomen, but lacks fat (b) smooth muscle fibers of dartos muscle;

7. The deep inguinal ring is lateral to the inferior epigastric artery; indirect inguinal hernias pass through this ring, the sac following the course of the spermatic cord (**B**); direct inguinal hernias bulge directly through the abdominal wall medial to the inferior epigastric artery (**C**).

2.17
Transverse section of right testis

Observe:

1. The cavity of the tunica vaginalis testis surrounding the testis anteriorly and laterally and extending between testis and epididymis as the sinus of the epididymis;

2. The epididymis lying posterolateral to the testis; it indicates to which side a testis belongs, for it is on the right side of a right testis and on the left side of a left testis;

3. The ductus deferens with its fine lumen and thick wall lying posteromedial to the testis;

4. The three groups of longitudinal veins (a) around the testicular artery, (b) medial to the duct with the artery of the duct, and (c) lateral to the duct;

5. The pyramidal compartments of the seminiferous tubules, shown semidiagrammatically; each of the 250 compartments contains two or three hair-like seminiferous tubules that join in the mediastinum testis to form a rete.

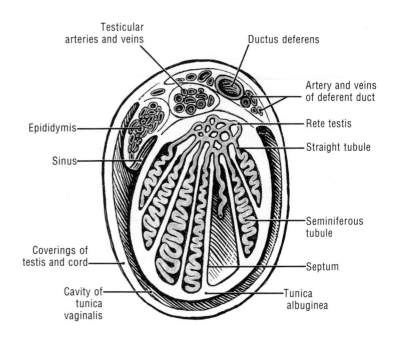

2.18
Lymphatic drainage of the testis and scrotum

Note the lymphatic drainage of the testis into the lateral and preaortic lymph nodes. The lymph vessels originate just deep to the tunica vaginalis and deeply within the testis, and then follow the spermatic cord and testicular vessels to the aorta. The scrotal lymphatics drain into the superficial inguinal nodes.

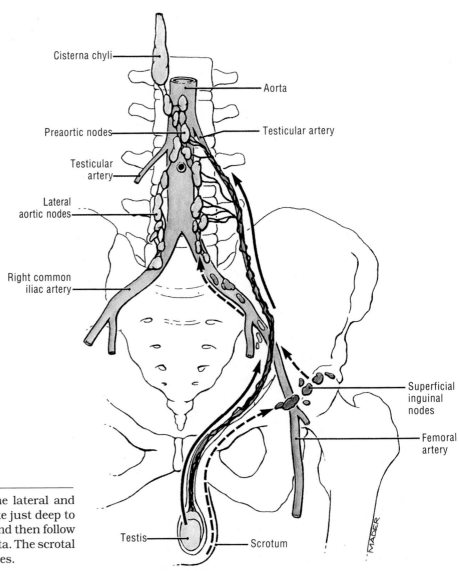

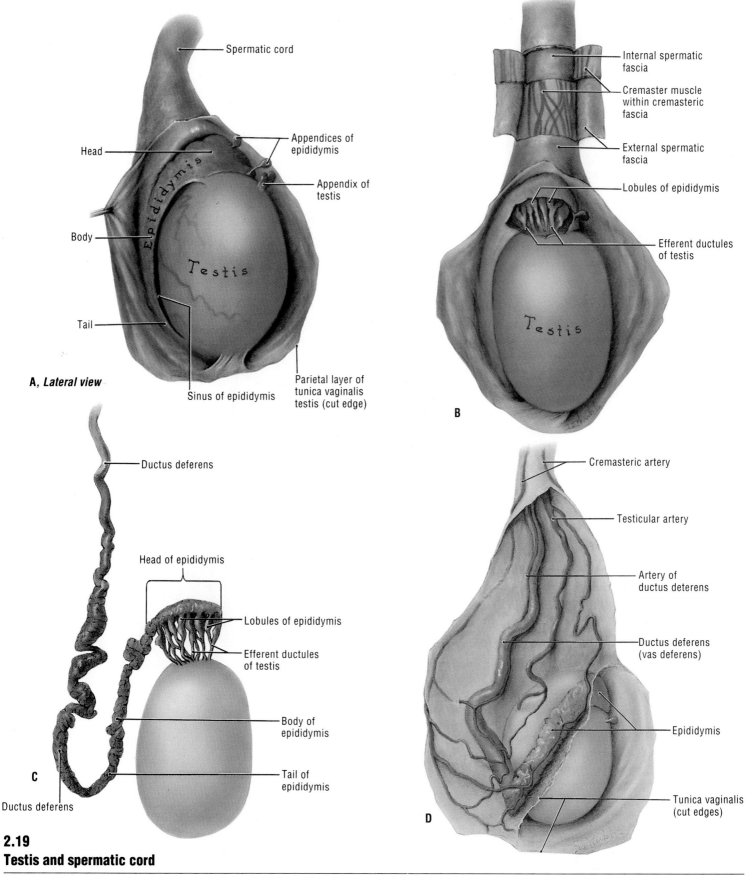

A, *Lateral view*

- Spermatic cord
- Head
- Appendices of epididymis
- Appendix of testis
- Body
- Tail
- Sinus of epididymis
- Parietal layer of tunica vaginalis testis (cut edge)
- Epididymis
- Testis

- Internal spermatic fascia
- Cremaster muscle within cremasteric fascia
- External spermatic fascia
- Lobules of epididymis
- Efferent ductules of testis
- Testis

B

- Ductus deferens
- Head of epididymis
- Lobules of epididymis
- Efferent ductules of testis
- Body of epididymis
- Tail of epididymis
- Ductus deferens

C

- Cremasteric artery
- Testicular artery
- Artery of ductus deterens
- Ductus deferens (vas deferens)
- Epididymis
- Tunica vaginalis (cut edges)

D

2.19
Testis and spermatic cord

A. Testis. The tunica vaginalis testis has been incised longitudinally. **B**. Coverings of the cord. **C**. Epididymis. Note the eight efferent ductules uniting the epididymis to the superior pole of the testis. **D**. Blood supply of the testis. The epididymis is displaced slightly to the lateral side. Note the anastomosis between the three arteries.

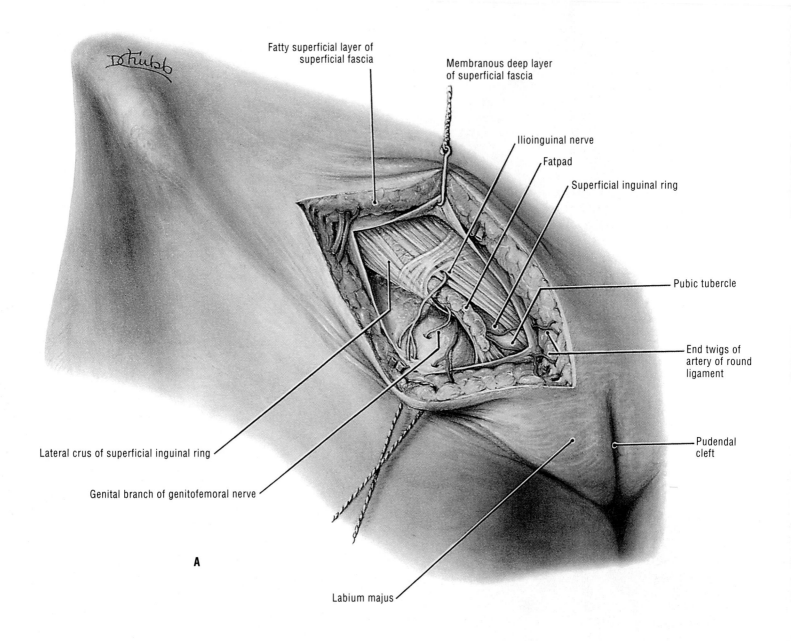

Fatty superficial layer of
superficial fascia

Membranous deep layer
of superficial fascia

Ilioinguinal nerve

Fatpad

Superficial inguinal ring

Pubic tubercle

End twigs of
artery of round
ligament

Pudendal
cleft

Lateral crus of superficial inguinal ring

Genital branch of genitofemoral nerve

A

Labium majus

2.20
Female inguinal canal–I

Progressive dissections of the female inguinal canal.

Observe:

1. In **A**, the superficial inguinal ring, which is small, and its crura are prevented from spreading by the intercrural fibers;

2. Passing through the superficial inguinal ring: (a) the round ligament of the uterus, (b) a closely applied pad of fat, (c) the genital branch of the genitofemoral nerve, and (d) the artery of the round ligament of the uterus;

3. The ilioinguinal nerve, here perforating the medial crus of the superficial inguinal ring.

4. In **B**, the cremaster muscle, not extending beyond the ring;

5. In **C**, the round ligament breaking up into strands as it leaves the inguinal canal and approaches the labium majus;

6. In **D**, the close relationship of the external iliac artery and vein to the inguinal canal.

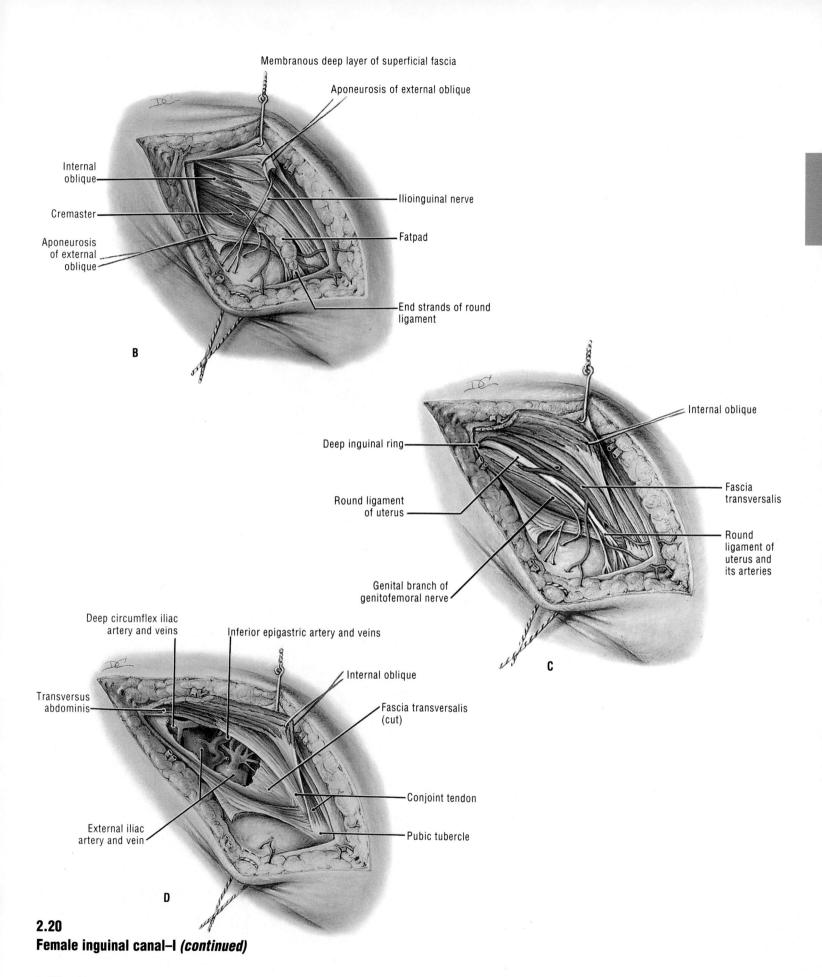

Membranous deep layer of superficial fascia

Aponeurosis of external oblique

Internal oblique

Cremaster

Aponeurosis of external oblique

Ilioinguinal nerve

Fatpad

End strands of round ligament

B

Deep inguinal ring

Round ligament of uterus

Genital branch of genitofemoral nerve

Internal oblique

Fascia transversalis

Round ligament of uterus and its arteries

C

Deep circumflex iliac artery and veins

Inferior epigastric artery and veins

Internal oblique

Transversus abdominis

Fascia transversalis (cut)

External iliac artery and vein

Conjoint tendon

Pubic tubercle

D

2.20

Female inguinal canal–I (continued)

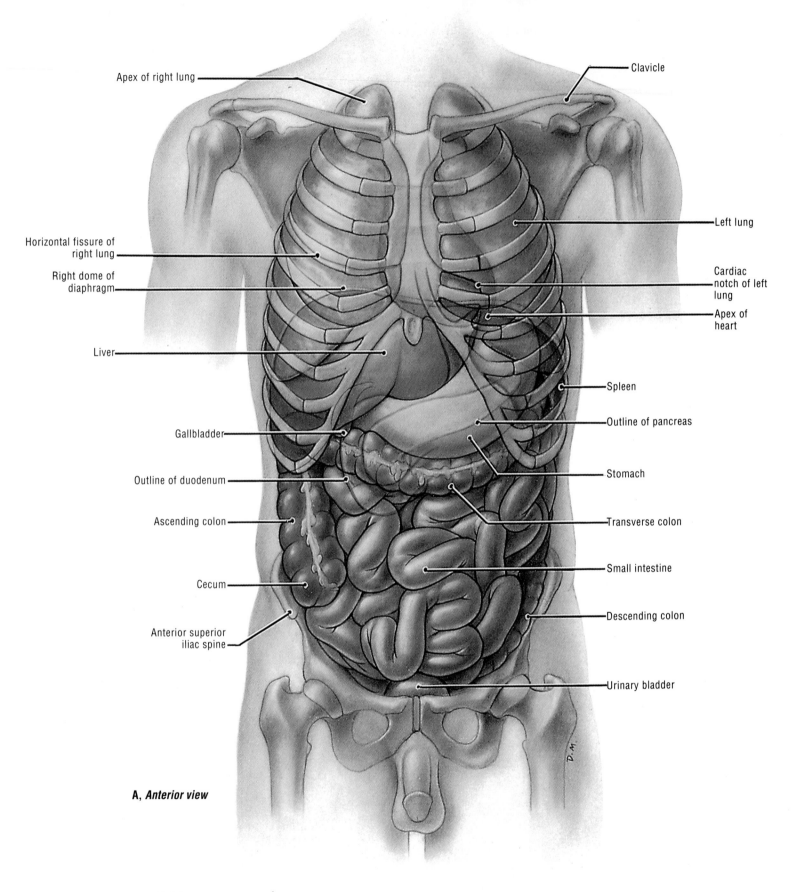

Apex of right lung

Clavicle

Horizontal fissure of right lung

Right dome of diaphragm

Liver

Left lung

Cardiac notch of left lung

Apex of heart

Spleen

Outline of pancreas

Gallbladder

Outline of duodenum

Ascending colon

Cecum

Anterior superior iliac spine

Stomach

Transverse colon

Small intestine

Descending colon

Urinary bladder

D.M.

A, *Anterior view*

2.21
Overview of the viscera of the thorax and abdomen

Grant's Atlas of Anatomy

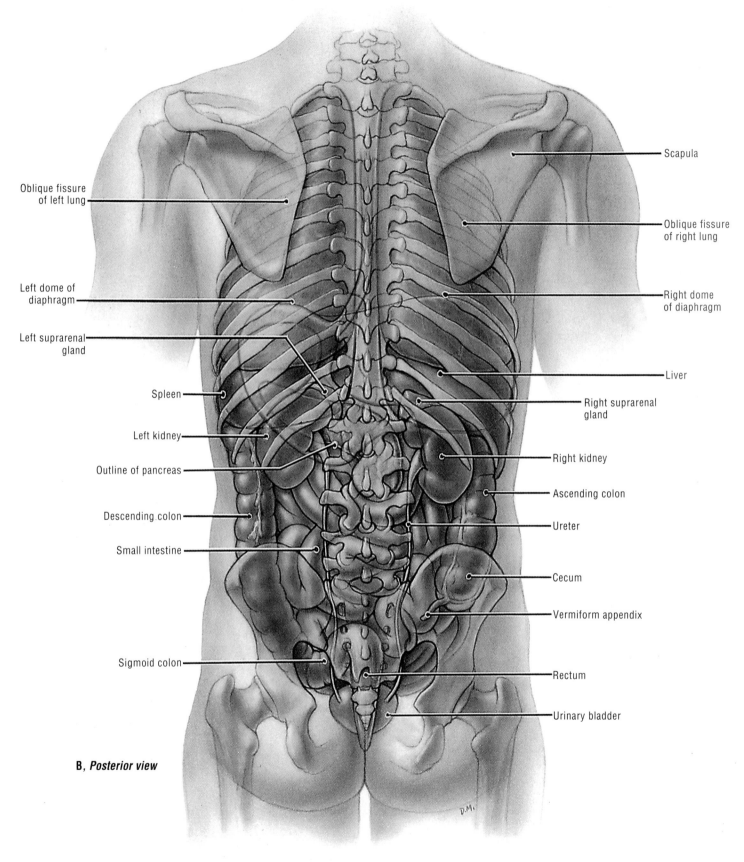

Oblique fissure of left lung

Oblique fissure of right lung

Scapula

Left dome of diaphragm

Right dome of diaphragm

Left suprarenal gland

Spleen

Liver

Left kidney

Right suprarenal gland

Outline of pancreas

Right kidney

Descending colon

Ascending colon

Small intestine

Ureter

Cecum

Vermiform appendix

Sigmoid colon

Rectum

Urinary bladder

B, *Posterior view*

2.21
Overview of the viscera of the thorax and abdomen *(continued)*

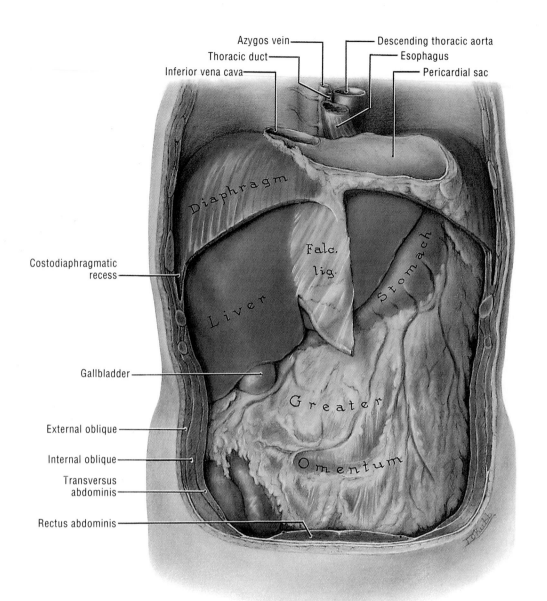

Azygos vein — Descending thoracic aorta
Thoracic duct — Esophagus
Inferior vena cava — Pericardial sac

Diaphragm

Costodiaphragmatic
recess —

Falc.
lig.

Stomach

Liver

Gallbladder —

Greater

External oblique —

Internal oblique —

Transversus
abdominis —

Omentum

Rectus abdominis —

2.22
Abdominal contents, undisturbed

The anterior abdominal and thoracic walls are cut away.

Observe:

1. The falciform ligament, with the ligamentum teres in its free edge, severed at its attachment to the abdominal wall and diaphragm in the median plane; its attachment to the liver is its own width to the right of the median plane; it resists displacement of the liver to the right;

2. The gallbladder projecting inferior to the sharp, inferior border of the liver;

3. The internal oblique muscle, the thickest of the three flat abdominal muscles;

4. The pleural cavities separating the diaphragm and the superior abdominal viscera from the body wall;

5. Two-thirds of the pericardial sac lying to the left of the median plane; its apex, i.e., the lowest and leftmost point, overlying the stomach.

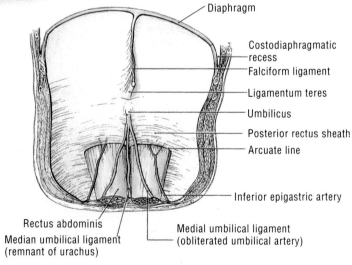

Diaphragm

Costodiaphragmatic
recess
Falciform ligament

Ligamentum teres

Umbilicus

Posterior rectus sheath

Arcuate line

Inferior epigastric artery

Rectus abdominis

Median umbilical ligament
(remnant of urachus)

Medial umbilical ligament
(obliterated umbilical artery)

2.23
Diagram of the posterior aspect of the anterior abdominal wall

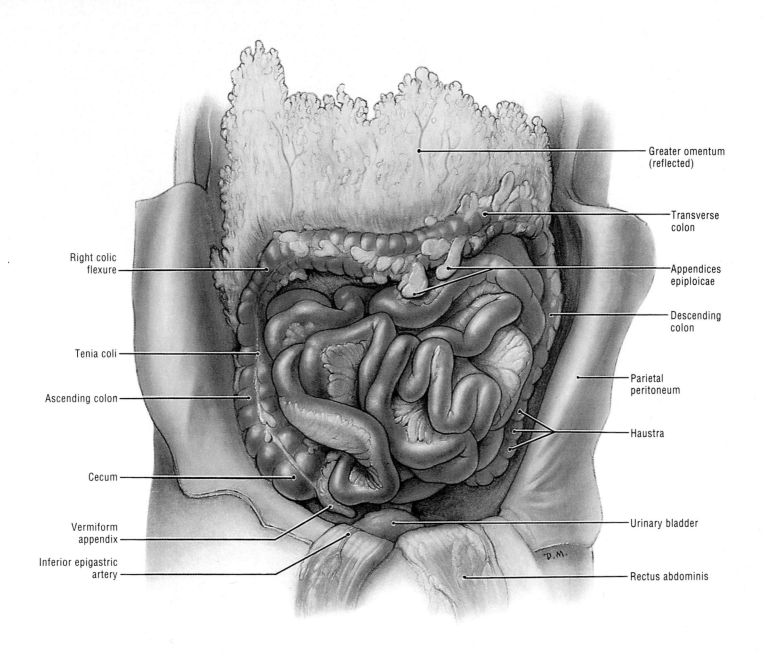

Greater omentum (reflected)

Transverse colon

Right colic flexure

Appendices epiploicae

Descending colon

Tenia coli

Parietal peritoneum

Ascending colon

Haustra

Cecum

Vermiform appendix

Urinary bladder

Inferior epigastric artery

Rectus abdominis

D. M.

2.24
Abdominal contents, greater omentum reflected superiorly

Observe:

1. The extensive coiling of the jejunum and ileum of the small intestine (together about 6 m in length);

2. The small intestine continuous with the large intestine at the cecum;

3. That the ileum is reflected to reveal the vermiform appendix, in the lower right quadrant; the vermiform appendix usually lies posterior to the cecum (retrocecal) or, as in this case, it may project over the pelvic brim;

4. The large intestine forming 3 1/2 sides of a square picture frame around the jejunum and ileum; on the right side, the cecum and ascending colon; the transverse colon superiorly; on the left, the descending colon and the sigmoid colon (not fully seen);

5. The right colic flexure, which lies inferior to the liver, placed at a lower level than the left colic flexure, which lies inferior to the spleen;

6. The distinguishing features of the large intestine: (a) its position around the small intestine, (b) the teniae coli or longitudinal muscle bands, (c) the sacculations or haustra, and (d) the appendices epiploicae.

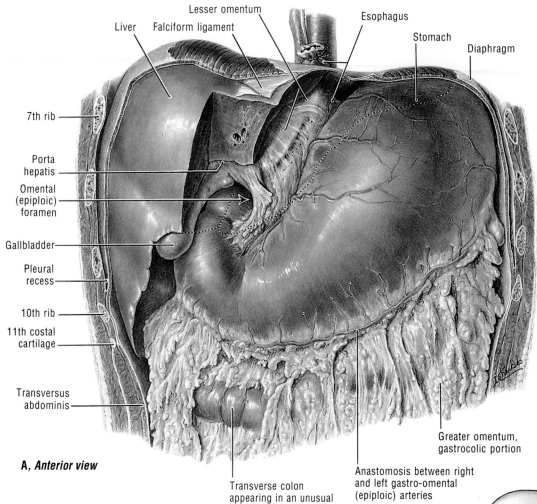

Lesser omentum
Liver Falciform ligament Esophagus
  Stomach
  Diaphragm
7th rib
Porta
hepatis
Omental
(epiploic)
foramen
Gallbladder
Pleural
recess
10th rib
11th costal
cartilage

Transversus
abdominis

Greater omentum,
gastrocolic portion

A, *Anterior view*

Transverse colon
appearing in an unusual
gap in the greater
omentum

Anastomosis between right
and left gastro-omental
(epiploic) arteries

2.25
Stomach and the omenta

A. The lesser and greater omenta. The stomach is inflated with air; the left part of the liver is cut away.

Observe:
1. The pyloric end of the stomach that, during development, had moved to the right and has come to lie inferoposterior to the gallbladder; the first or superior part of the duodenum placed posterior to the arrowhead almost occluding the omental (epiploic) foramen (mouth of the lesser sac);

2. The gallbladder, followed superiorly, leading to the free margin of the lesser omentum, and hence acting as a guide to the epiploic foramen, which lies posterior to that free margin;

3. The lesser omentum passing from the lesser curvature of the stomach and first inch of the duodenum to the fissure for the ligamentum venosum and porta hepatis; this omentum, thickened at its free margin but elsewhere thin, much perforated, and the caudate lobe of the liver visible through it;

4. The greater omentum hanging from the greater curvature of the stomach;

5. The right dome of the diaphragm rising higher than the left dome.

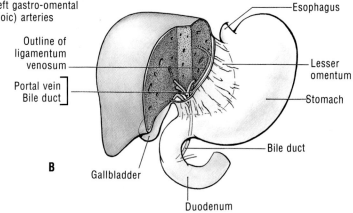

Esophagus

Outline of
ligamentum
venosum

Lesser
omentum

Portal vein
Bile duct

Stomach

Bile duct

B

Gallbladder

Duodenum

B. The lesser omentum. Two sagittal cuts have been made through the liver: one at the fissure for the ligamentum venosum; the other at the right limit of the porta hepatis. These two cuts have been joined by a coronal cut.

Observe:
1. The lesser omentum may be regarded as the "mesentery" of the bile passages, seeing they occupy its free edge;

2. The lesser omentum extends from the lesser curvature of the stomach and first inch of the duodenum to the fissure for the ligamentum venosum and to the porta hepatis; the part attached to the body of the stomach passes to the fissure; the part attached to the pyloric part of the stomach and duodenum passes to the porta hepatis.

2.26
Median section to show the vertical extent of omental bursa (lesser sac)

The *arrow* passes from the greater sac of peritoneum through the omental (epiploic) foramen into the omental bursa (lesser sac).

Observe:

1. The superior recess of the omental bursa between the liver and the posterior attachment of the diaphragm;

2. The inferior recess of the omental bursa between the two double layers of the greater omentum; the inferior recess in the adult usually only extends inferiorly as far as the transverse colon due to the fusion of the two double peritoneal layers at birth.

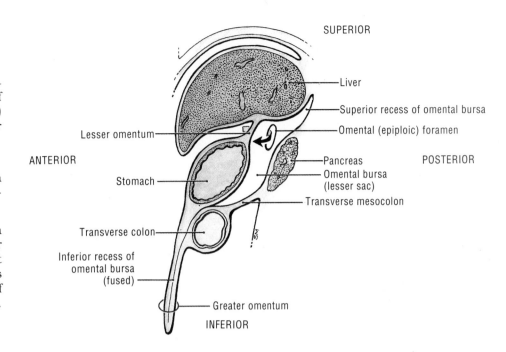

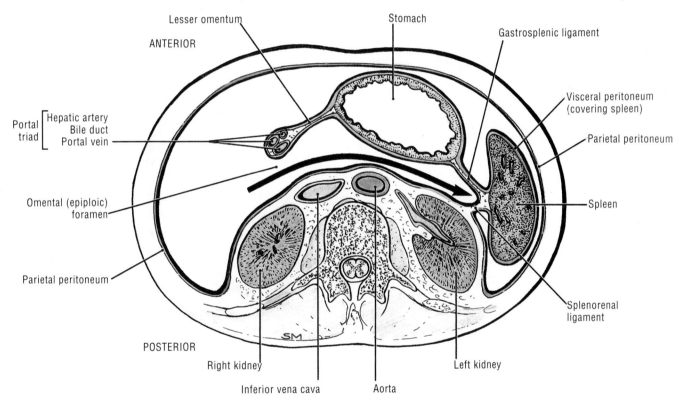

2.27
Transverse section at the level of the omental (epiploic) foramen to show the horizontal extent of omental bursa

The *arrow* passes from the greater sac through the omental foramen into the omental bursa (lesser sac).

Observe:

1. The gastrosplenic and splenorenal ligaments suspending the spleen between the kidney and the stomach; the ligaments forming a pedicle (stalk) that conveys blood vessels to and from the hilum of the spleen;

2. The gastrosplenic and splenorenal ligaments are double layers of peritoneum forming the left boundary of the omental bursa (lesser sac); the inner layers consisting of peritoneum lining the omental bursa (lesser sac); the outer layers consisting of peritoneum lining the peritoneal cavity (greater sac).

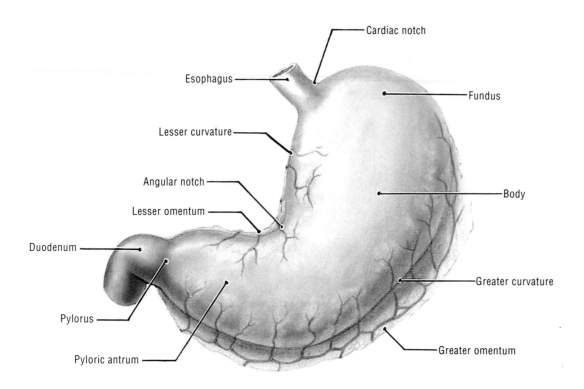

Cardiac notch

Esophagus

Fundus

Lesser curvature

Angular notch

Body

Lesser omentum

Duodenum

Greater curvature

Pylorus

Pyloric antrum

Greater omentum

A, *Anterior view*

2.28
Stomach

A. External surface. B. Internal surface (mucous membrane).

Observe in **B**:

1. The esophagogastric junction usually located to the left of the midline, at the 11th thoracic vertebra; the pylorus usually located at L1 vertebral level to the right of the midline at the transpyloric plane;

2. The angular notch separating the body from the pyloric region of the stomach; the pyloric sphincter, a ring of circular muscle, at the junction of the stomach and duodenum;

3. The lesser omentum attaching to the lesser curvature of the stomach; the continuous greater omentum and gastrosplenic ligament attaching to the greater curvature of the stomach;

4. Along the lesser curvature, several longitudinal ridges extending from the esophagus to the pylorus; elsewhere the mucous membrane is rugose when the stomach is empty.

C. Pylorus. The pylorus pouts into the 1st (superior) part of the duodenum. The first 4 cm of the duodenum have no plicae circulares, but the mucous membrane may be rugose.

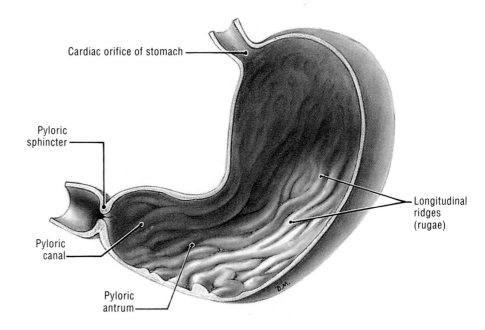

Cardiac orifice of stomach

Pyloric sphincter

Longitudinal ridges (rugae)

Pyloric canal

Pyloric antrum

B

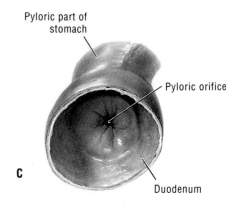

Pyloric part of stomach

Pyloric orifice

Duodenum

C

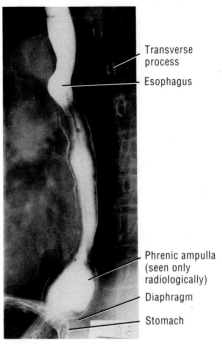

Transverse process

Esophagus

Phrenic ampulla (seen only radiologically)

Diaphragm

Stomach

Lateral view

2.29
Radiograph of esophagus

This is a radiograph of the esophagus after swallowing barium. The esophageal ampulla is the distensible portion of the esophagus seen only radiologically. (Courtesy of Dr. E.L. Lansdown, Professor of Radiology, University of Toronto, Toronto, Ontario, Canada.)

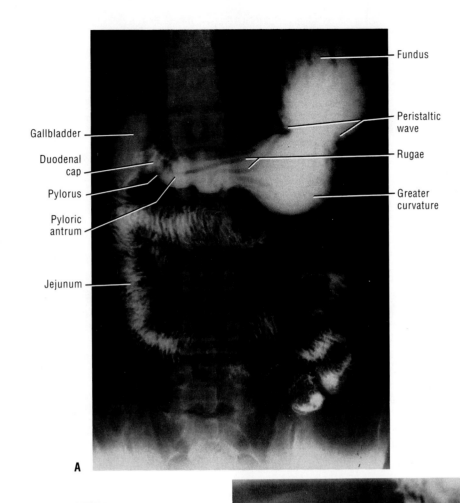

Fundus

Gallbladder

Duodenal cap

Pylorus

Pyloric antrum

Jejunum

Peristaltic wave

Rugae

Greater curvature

A

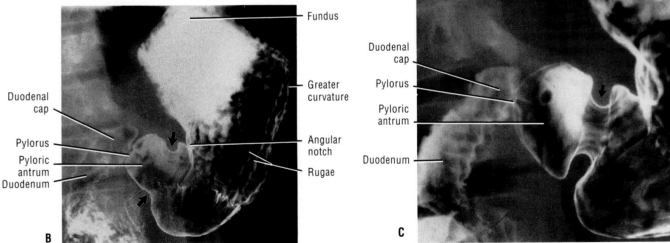

Fundus

Duodenal cap

Pylorus

Pyloric antrum

Duodenum

Greater curvature

Angular notch

Rugae

B

Duodenal cap

Pylorus

Pyloric antrum

Duodenum

C

2.30
Radiographs of stomach, small intestine, and gallbladder

A. The stomach, small intestine, and gallbladder are shown. **B.** In the radiograph of the stomach and small intestine following a barium meal, observe: longitudinal ridges of mucous membrane (rugae); the angular notch: a peristaltic wave *(arrowheads)*; pylorus; duodenal "cap"; the feathery appearance of barium in the small intestine; the relationship of the gallbladder to the first part of the duodenum. **C.** Radiograph of the pyloric region of the stomach and the proximal duodenum. (**A** Courtesy of Dr. J. Heslin, Assistant Professor of Anatomy, University of Toronto, Toronto, Ontario, Canada; **B** and **C** courtesy of Dr. E.L. Lansdown, Professor of Radiology, University of Toronto, Toronto, Ontario, Canada.)

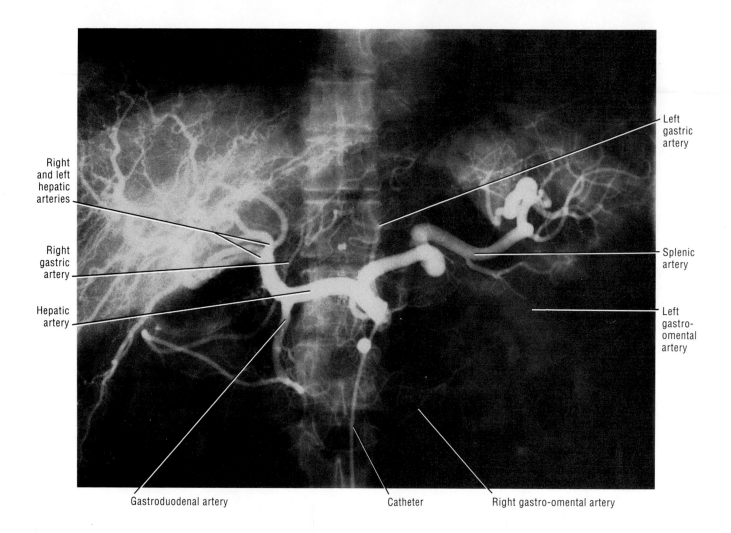

Right and left hepatic arteries

Right gastric artery

Hepatic artery

Left gastric artery

Splenic artery

Left gastro-omental artery

Gastroduodenal artery

Catheter

Right gastro-omental artery

2.31
Celiac arteriogram

Observe:
The hepatic artery; the right gastro-omental (gastroepiploic) artery following the greater curvature of the stomach; the tortuous splenic artery and the left gastric artery.

Consult Figures 2.32 and 2.33. (Courtesy of Dr. J. Heslin, Assistant Professor of Anatomy, University of Toronto, Toronto, Ontario, Canada.)

2.32
Diagram of the branches of the celiac trunk

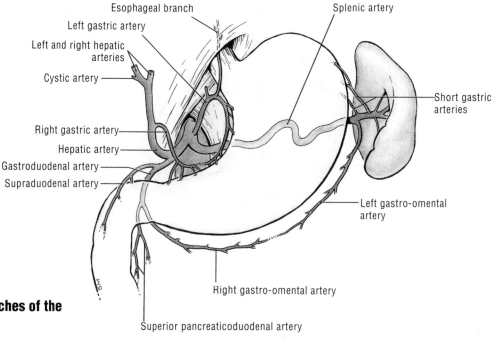

Esophageal branch

Left gastric artery

Left and right hepatic arteries

Cystic artery

Splenic artery

Short gastric arteries

Right gastric artery

Hepatic artery

Gastroduodenal artery

Supraduodenal artery

Left gastro-omental artery

Right gastro-omental artery

Superior pancreaticoduodenal artery

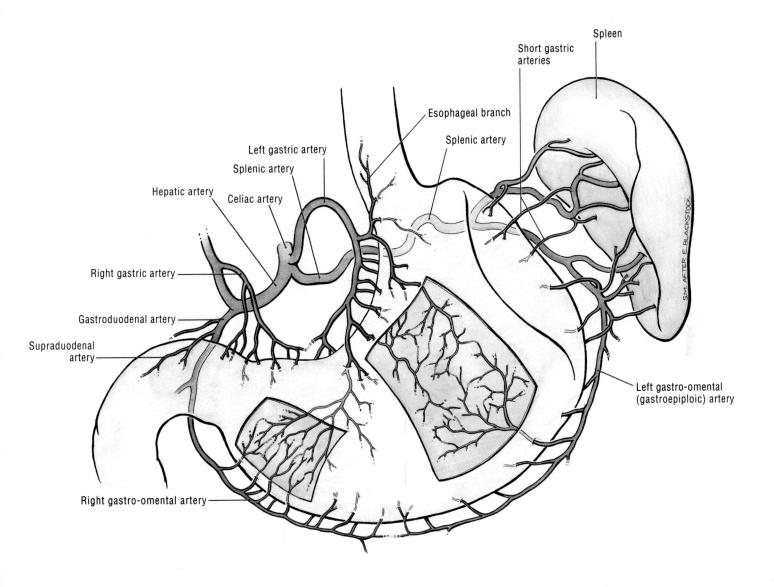

Spleen

Short gastric
arteries

Esophageal branch

Splenic artery

Left gastric artery

Splenic artery

Hepatic artery

Celiac artery

Right gastric artery

Gastroduodenal artery

Supraduodenal
artery

Left gastro-omental
(gastroepiploic) artery

Right gastro-omental artery

S.M. AFTER E. BLACKSTOCK

2.33
Arteries of the stomach and spleen

The serous and muscular coats are removed from two areas of the stomach, thereby revealing the anastomotic networks in the submucous coat.

Observe:

1. The arterial arch on the lesser curvature formed by the larger left gastric artery and the much smaller right gastric artery;

2. The arterial arch on the greater curvature formed equally by the right and the left gastro-omental (gastroepiploic) arteries; the anastomoses between their two trunks is attentuated; commonly it is absent;

3. The anastomoses between the branches of the two foregoing arterial arches taking place in the submucous coat two-thirds of the distance from lesser to greater curvature;

4. Four or five tenuous short gastric arteries leaving the terminal branches of the splenic artery close to the spleen; and the left gastroepiploic artery, belonging to the short gastric artery series, arising within 2.5 cm of the hilum of the spleen.

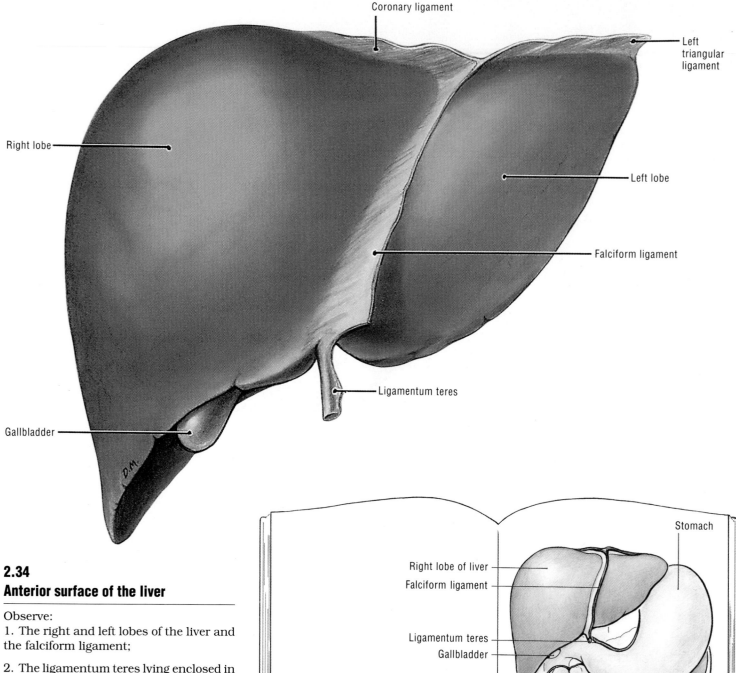

Coronary ligament

Left triangular ligament

Right lobe

Left lobe

Falciform ligament

Ligamentum teres

Gallbladder

D.M.

2.34
Anterior surface of the liver

Observe:

1. The right and left lobes of the liver and the falciform ligament;

2. The ligamentum teres lying enclosed in the free edge of the falciform ligament; the ligamentum teres is the obliterated umbilical vein that carried oxygenated blood from the placenta to the liver before birth;

3. The falciform ligament has been severed from its attachment to the diaphragm and anterior abdominal wall; the two layers of peritoneum forming the falciform ligament separate over the superior aspect of the liver to form the superior layer of the coronary ligament on the right, and on the left, the left triangular ligament;

4. The fundus of the gallbladder visible at the inferior border of the liver.

Stomach

Right lobe of liver

Falciform ligament

Ligamentum teres

Gallbladder

Transverse mesocolon (cut edge)

Site where ascending colon removed

Mesentery of small intestine (cut edge)

Anterior view

MADER AFTER N.JOY

Site where descending colon removed

1

2.35
Diagram of the peritoneal ligaments of the liver

Note that the jejunum, ileum, as well as the ascending, transverse, and descending colon have been removed.

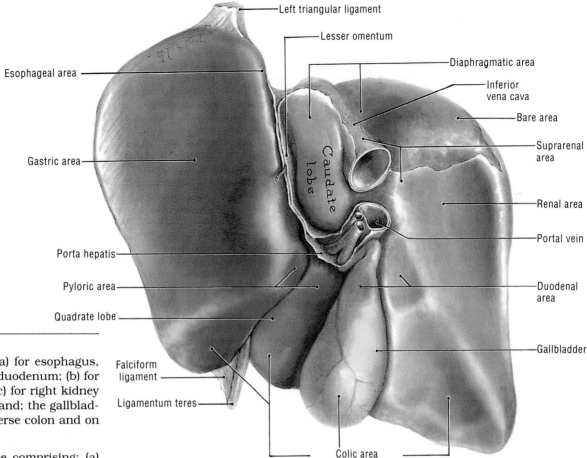

Left triangular ligament

Lesser omentum

Esophageal area

Diaphragmatic area

Inferior vena cava

Bare area

Gastric area

Suprarenal area

Renal area

Caudate lobe

Porta hepatis

Portal vein

2.36
Inferior and posterior surfaces of the liver

Pyloric area

Quadrate lobe

Duodenal area

Gallbladder

Falciform ligament

Ligamentum teres

Colic area

Observe:

1. The visceral areas: (a) for esophagus, stomach, pylorus, and duodenum; (b) for transverse colon; and (c) for right kidney and right suprarenal gland; the gallbladder rests on the transverse colon and on the duodenum;

2. The posterior surface comprising: (a) the bare area, occupied on its left by the inferior vena cava, (b) the caudate lobe, and (c) the groove for the esophagus;

3. The caudate lobe separated from the quadrate lobe by the porta hepatis, and joined to the right lobe by the caudate process;

4. The bare area is triangular; hence, the coronary ligament which surrounds it is three-sided; its left side or base is between the inferior vena cava and the caudate lobe; its apex is at the right triangular ligament, where the superior and inferior layers of the coronary ligament meet;

5. The inferior layer of the coronary ligament is reflected from the liver onto: the diaphragm, right kidney, and right suprarenal gland; it is called the hepatorenal ligament by the surgeon; followed medially, this layer crosses the inferior vena cava at the omental (epiploic) foramen, and turning superiorly it becomes the left layer of the coronary ligament; followed to the left, this layer of peritoneum forms the superior limit of the superior recess of the omental bursa and then turns inferiorly as the posterior layer of the lesser omentum.

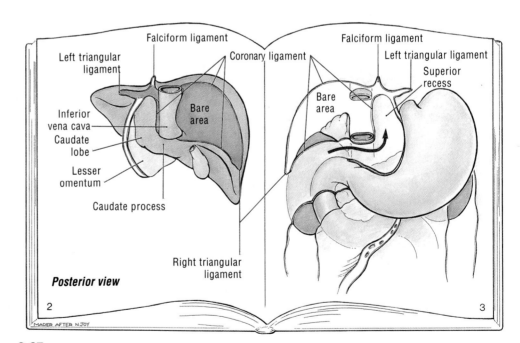

Falciform ligament

Left triangular ligament

Coronary ligament

Falciform ligament

Left triangular ligament

Superior recess

Bare area

Inferior vena cava

Caudate lobe

Bare area

Lesser omentum

Caudate process

Right triangular ligament

Posterior view

2

MADER AFTER N.JOY

3

2.37
Diagram of the peritoneal ligaments of the liver

The attachments of the liver are cut through and the liver is turned to the right side of the cadaver, as you would turn the page of a book; the posterior aspect of the liver is shown on page **2** and its posterior relations on page **3** of the diagram above. The *arrow* indicates the site of the omental foramen.

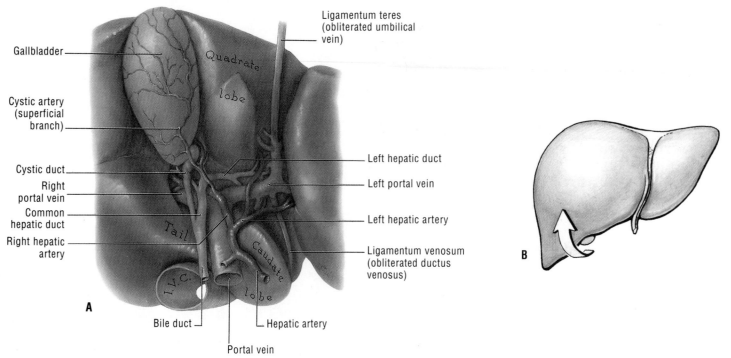

Gallbladder

Cystic artery
(superficial
branch)

Cystic duct

Right
portal vein

Common
hepatic duct

Right hepatic
artery

Ligamentum teres
(obliterated umbilical
vein)

Quadrate
lobe

Tail

I.V.C.

Caudate
lobe

A

Bile duct

Portal vein

Hepatic artery

Left hepatic duct

Left portal vein

Left hepatic artery

Ligamentum venosum
(obliterated ductus
venosus)

B

2.38
Porta hepatis and the cystic artery

You are standing on the right side of the cadaver and facing the head. The attachments of the liver are severed and the inferior border of the liver is raised as in **B**, the orientation drawing.

Observe in **A**:
1. The caudate lobe forming the superior boundary of the omental (epiploic) foramen, and lying between the portal vein and the inferior vena cava;

2. The relation of structures as they ascend to the porta hepatis–duct to the right, artery to the left, vein posterior;

3. The order of structures at the porta hepatis–duct, artery, and vein from anterior to posterior;

4. The left portal vein and left hepatic artery supplying the quadrate and caudate lobes en route to the left lobe, and accompanied by tributaries of the left hepatic duct;

5. The ligamentum teres passing to the left portal vein, and the ligamentum venosum arising opposite it and ascending to the inferior vena cava (Fig. 2.37);

6. The cystic artery springing from the right hepatic artery and dividing into a superficial and a deep branch that arborize on the respective surfaces of the gallbladder;

7. The cystic duct, sinuous at its origin.

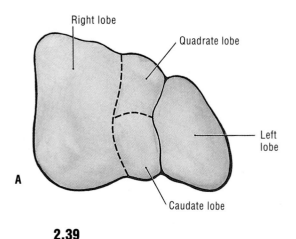

Right lobe

Quadrate lobe

Left
lobe

A

Caudate lobe

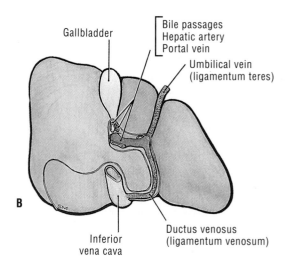

Gallbladder

Bile passages
Hepatic artery
Portal vein

Umbilical vein
(ligamentum teres)

B

Inferior
vena cava

Ductus venosus
(ligamentum venosum)

2.39
Diagrams of the liver

A. The four lobes of the liver. **B**. The occupants of the posterior and inferior aspects of the liver.

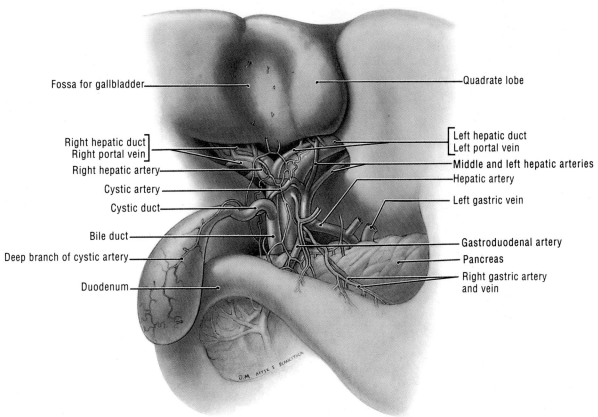

Fossa for gallbladder

Quadrate lobe

Right hepatic duct
Right portal vein

Left hepatic duct
Left portal vein

Right hepatic artery

Middle and left hepatic arteries

Cystic artery

Hepatic artery

Cystic duct

Left gastric vein

Bile duct

Gastroduodenal artery

Deep branch of cystic artery

Pancreas

Duodenum

Right gastric artery
and vein

2.40
Vessels in the porta hepatis, on the deep surface of the gallbladder, and in the fossa for the gallbladder

The gallbladder is freed from its bed or fossa and turned inferiorly and to the right. Observe:

1. The anastomoses seen in the porta hepatis, here involving various branches of the right hepatic artery;

2. The deep branch of the cystic artery, ramifying on the deep or attached surface of the gallbladder, anastomosing with twigs of the superficial branch of the cystic artery, and sending twigs into the bed of the gallbladder (the cut ends of the arterial and venous twigs can be seen);

3. The network of arteries on the gallbladder; most of the smaller arteries lying on a deeper plane than the larger arteries.

4. Many fine sinuous arterial twigs supplying the bile passages and springing from nearby arteries;

5. Several anastomotic arteries capable of bringing blood from various gastric and pancreatic arteries to the porta hepatis;

6. Veins (not all shown), accompanying faithfully most arteries.

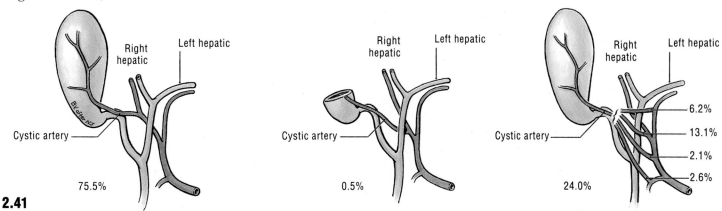

Right hepatic   Left hepatic

Cystic artery

75.5%

Right hepatic   Left hepatic

Cystic artery

0.5%

Right hepatic   Left hepatic

Cystic artery

6.2%

13.1%

2.1%

2.6%

24.0%

2.41
Variations in the origin and course of the cystic artery

The cystic artery usually arises from the right hepatic artery in the angle between the common hepatic duct and the cystic duct, and has no occasion to cross the common hepatic duct. When, however, it arises on the left of the bile passages, it almost always crosses anterior to the passages.

Diagrams are based on 580 cases. (From Daseler EH, Anson BJ, Hambley WC, Reimann AF. *The cystic artery and constituents of the hepatic pedicle.* Surg Gynecol Obstet 1947; 85:47.)

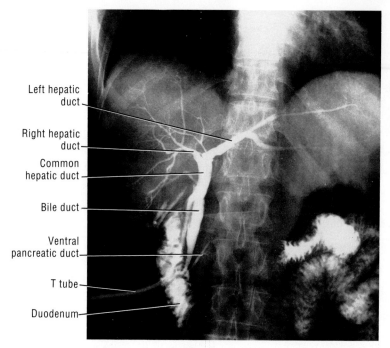

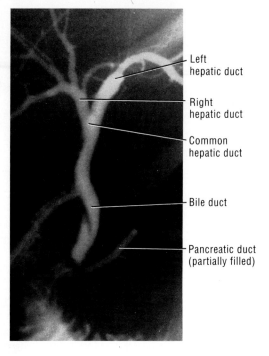

Left hepatic duct

Right hepatic duct

Common hepatic duct

Bile duct

Ventral pancreatic duct

T tube

Duodenum

Left hepatic duct

Right hepatic duct

Common hepatic duct

Bile duct

Pancreatic duct (partially filled)

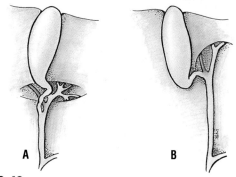

A   **B**

2.42
Radiographs of the biliary passages *(above)*

Following a cholecystectomy (removal of the gallbladder), contrast medium has been injected via a T tube inserted into the bile passages. (Courtesy of Dr. J. Heslin, Assistant Professor of Anatomy, University of Toronto, Toronto, Ontario, Canada.)

2.43
Accessory hepatic ducts *(above)*

"Accessory" hepatic ducts are segmental ducts that arise early. They are common and in positions of surgical danger. Of 95 gallbladders and bile passages studied, seven had accessory ducts. Of these: **A.** Four joined the common hepatic duct near the cystic ducts. **B.** Two joined the cystic duct; and one was an anastomosing duct connecting the cystic with the common hepatic duct.

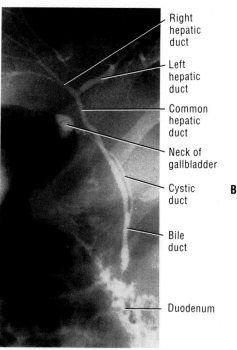

Right hepatic duct

Left hepatic duct

Common hepatic duct

Neck of gallbladder

Cystic duct

Bile duct

Duodenum

A

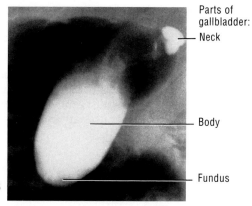

Parts of gallbladder:
— Neck

Body

Fundus

B

2.44
Endoscopic retrograde
cholangiography of the gallbladder and biliary passages *(above)*

The cystic duct usually lies on the right of the common hepatic duct and joins it just superior to the first part of the duodenum. The course and length of the cystic duct is variable. (Courtesy of Dr. G.B. Haber, Assistant Professor of Medicine, University of Toronto, Toronto, Ontario, Canada.)

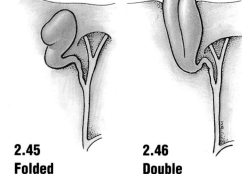

2.45
Folded
gallbladder

2.46
Double
gallbladder

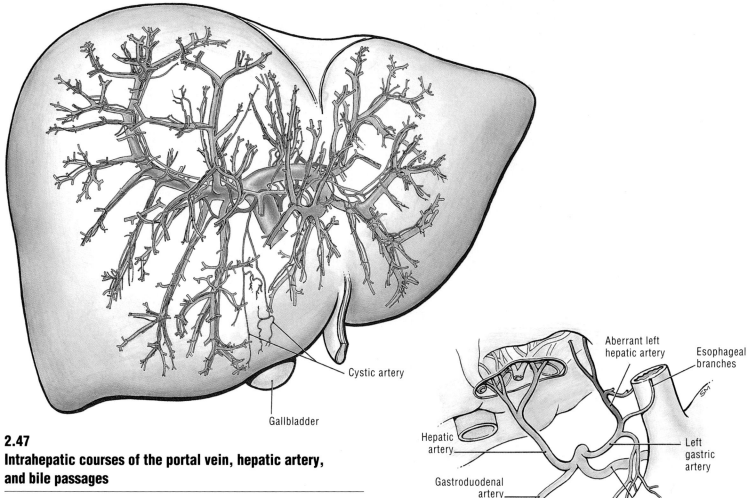

Cystic artery

Gallbladder

2.47

Intrahepatic courses of the portal vein, hepatic artery, and bile passages

This figure was traced from a projected Kodachrome of a corrosion specimen. It is simplest to regard the portal vein, hepatic artery, and bile passages as branching and rebranching dichotomously, although the left portal vein differs slightly in branching pattern from the left hepatic artery and left bile duct. Note the segmental distribution of these vessels.

Aberrant left
hepatic artery

Esophageal
branches

Hepatic
artery

Left
gastric
artery

Gastroduodenal
artery

Splenic artery

Right gastric artery

2.48
Aberrant left hepatic artery

The left hepatic artery was entirely replaced by a branch of the left gastric artery, as in this specimen, in 11.5% of 200 cadavers; and in another 11.5%, it was partially replaced. (From Michels NA. *Newer anatomy of the liver and its variant blood supply and collateral circulation*, Am J Surg 1966; 112:337.)

Left hepatic
artery

Right
hepatic
artery

Left hepatic
artery

Right
hepatic
artery

Left hepatic
artery

Right
hepatic
artery

24%

64%

12%

A

Hepatic artery

Hepatic artery

Hepatic artery

2.49
Variations in the hepatic arteries

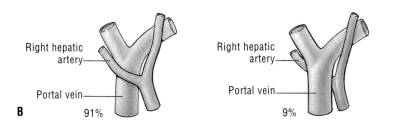

Right hepatic
artery

Portal vein

91%

Right hepatic
artery

Portal vein

9%

B

In a study of 165 cadavers, (**A**) three patterns were seen: right hepatic artery crossed ventral to bile passages, 24%; right hepatic artery crossed dorsal to bile passages, 64%; aberrant artery arising from the superior mesenteric artery, 12%. **B**. The artery crossed ventral to the portal vein in 91% and dorsal in 9%.

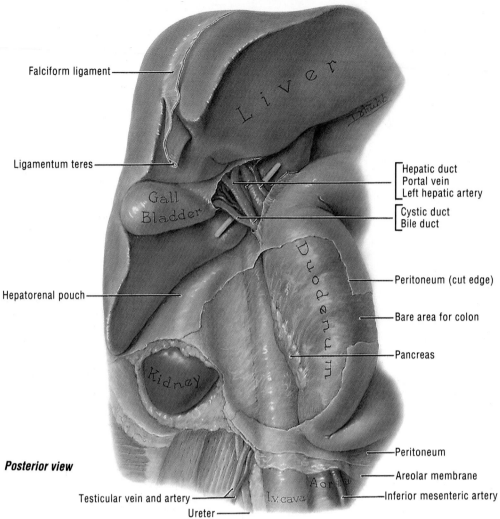

Falciform ligament

Liver

Ligamentum teres

Hepatic duct
Portal vein
Left hepatic artery

Cystic duct
Bile duct

Hepatorenal pouch

Gall Bladder

Duodenum

Peritoneum (cut edge)

Bare area for colon

Pancreas

Kidney

Peritoneum

Posterior view

Areolar membrane

Testicular vein and artery

Aorta

I.v. cava

Inferior mesenteric artery

Ureter

2.50
Exposure of the bile duct–I

A white rod is passed through the omental (epiploic) foramen; the lesser omentum and transverse colon are removed; the peritoneum is cut along the right border of the duodenum, and this part of the duodenum is swung anteriorly like a door on a hinge.

Observe:

1. The space opened up reveals two smooth areolar membranes applied to each other; here one membrane covers the posterior aspect of the second part of the duodenum and the head of the pancreas; the other covers the aorta, inferior vena cava, renal vessels, and perirenal fat;

2. To find the omental foramen either: (a) follow the liver at the superior limit of the hepatorenal pouch, medially to the caudate process, forming the superior wall of the foramen, and the inferior vena cava forming the posterior wall; or (b) follow the gallbladder to the cystic duct, which occupies the free edge of the lesser omentum, and forms the anterior wall of the foramen;

3. Of the three main structures in the anterior wall, the portal vein is posterior, the hepatic artery ascends from the left, and the bile passages descend to the right;

4. In this specimen the right hepatic artery springs from the superior mesenteric artery, a common variant (Fig. 2.48).

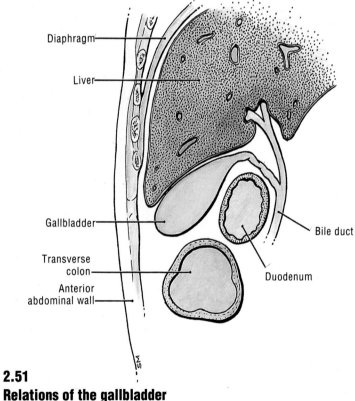

Diaphragm

Liver

Gallbladder

Transverse colon

Anterior abdominal wall

Bile duct

Duodenum

2.51
Relations of the gallbladder

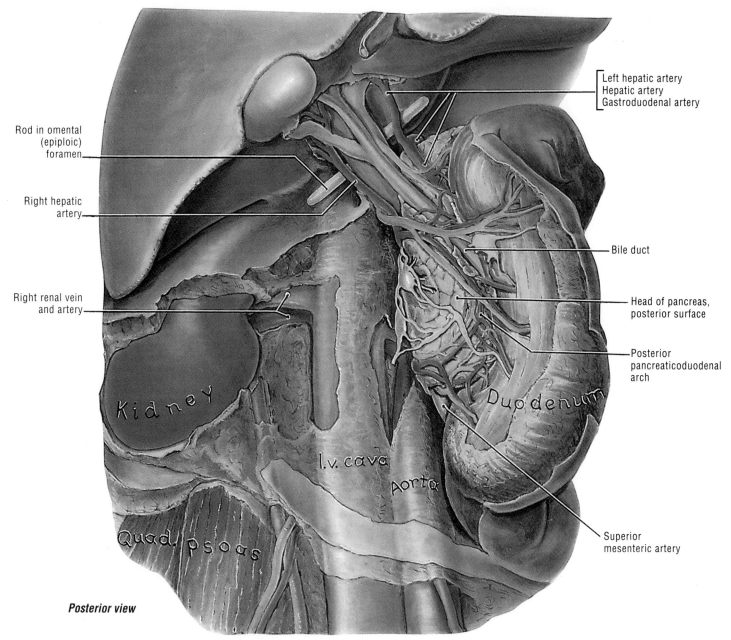

Rod in omental
(epiploic)
foramen

Right hepatic
artery

Right renal vein
and artery

Kidney

I.v. cava

Aorta

Quad. psoas

Left hepatic artery
Hepatic artery
Gastroduodenal artery

Bile duct

Head of pancreas,
posterior surface

Posterior
pancreaticoduodenal
arch

Duodenum

Superior
mesenteric artery

Posterior view

2.52
Exposure of the bile duct–II

In this further dissection of Figure 2.50, the duodenum is swung still further anteriorly and to the left, taking the head of the pancreas with it. In effect, the omental foramen has been enlarged inferiorly; the areolar membrane covering the pancreas and duodenum is largely removed; that covering the great vessels is in part removed.

Observe:
1. The bile duct descending in a groove on the posterior aspect of the head of the pancreas;

2. The bile duct ending at the level of the hilum of the kidney;

3. The very close relationship of the inferior vena cava to the portal vein; they are separated by the omental foramen; a portacaval shunt to divert the portal circulation into the caval system may be done here by an end-to-side anastomosis;

4. Vasa recta, accompanied by veins and lymph vessels, passing from the posterior pancreaticoduodenal arch to the duodenum;

5. Of the two posterior pancreaticoduodenal arteries that form the posterior arch, the inferior arises from the superior mesenteric artery, and the superior here from the right hepatic artery, but usually from the gastroduodenal artery;

6. The posterior superior pancreaticoduodenal vein ending in the portal vein;

7. The right renal vein is short; the right renal artery is long and passes posterior to the inferior vena cava to the hilus of the kidney.

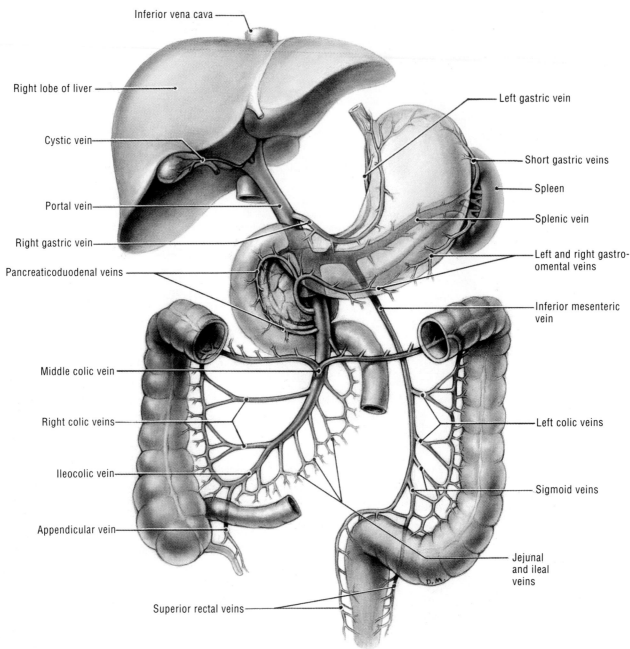

Inferior vena cava

Right lobe of liver

Cystic vein

Portal vein

Right gastric vein

Pancreaticoduodenal veins

Middle colic vein

Right colic veins

Ileocolic vein

Appendicular vein

Superior rectal veins

Left gastric vein

Short gastric veins

Spleen

Splenic vein

Left and right gastro-
omental veins

Inferior mesenteric
vein

Left colic veins

Sigmoid veins

Jejunal
and ileal
veins

D. M.

2.53
Portal venous system

Observe:

1. The portal vein draining venous blood from the gastrointestinal tract, spleen, pancreas, and gallbladder to the sinusoids of the liver; from the sinusoids of the liver the blood is conveyed to the systemic venous system by the hepatic veins that drain directly into the inferior vena cava;

2. The portal vein forming posterior to the neck of the pancreas by the union of the superior mesenteric and splenic veins, with the inferior mesenteric vein joining at or near the angle of union; here, the left gastric vein joins the portal vein; usually, it is also joined by the right gastric vein, cystic vein, and one or two small duodenal or pancreatic veins;

3. The splenic vein drains blood from the inferior mesenteric, left gastro-omental (epiploic), short gastric, and pancreatic veins;

4. The superior mesenteric vein to be joined by the right gastro-omental (epiploic), pancreaticoduodenal, jejunal, ileal, right and middle colic veins;

5. The inferior mesenteric vein commences, in the rectal plexus, as the superior rectal vein and, after crossing the common iliac vessels, becomes the inferior mesenteric vein; branches include the sigmoid and left colic veins;

6. The portal vein dividing into right and left branches at the porta hepatis; the left hepatic vein carries mainly, but not exclusively, blood from the inferior mesenteric, gastric, and splenic veins and the right hepatic vein carries blood from the superior mesenteric vein.

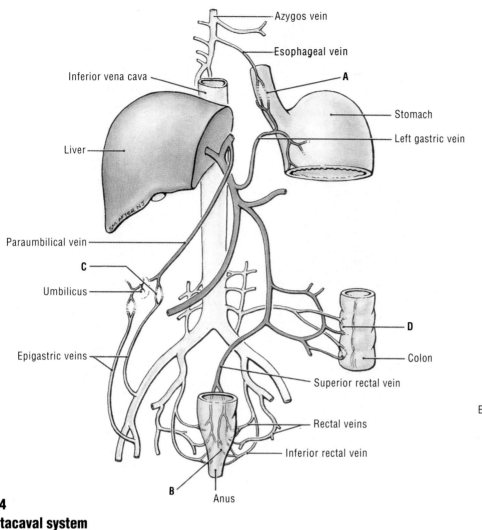

2.54
Portacaval system

In this diagram, portal tributaries are a darker blue, systemic tributeries and communicating veins are a lighter blue. In portal hypertension (as in hepatic cirrhosis) the portal blood cannot drain freely into the liver and the tiny anastomotic veins become engorged, dilated, and varicose and, as a consequence, may rupture. The sites of the anastomosis shown are:

A, Between esophageal veins draining into either the azygos vein (systemic) or the left gastric vein (portal); when dilated these are esophageal varices;

B, Between rectal veins, the inferior and middle draining into the inferior vena cava (systemic) and the superior rectal vein continuing as the inferior mesenteric vein (portal); when dilated these are hemorrhoids;

C, Paraumbilical veins (portal) anastomosing with small epigastric veins of the anterior abdominal wall (systemic); may produce the "caput medusae";

D, Twigs of colic veins (portal) anastomosing with systemic retroperitoneal veins.

Note also the proximity to each other of the splenic vein and the left renal vein, a relationship used in the surgical relief of portal hypertension through a splenorenal shunt (see Figs. 2.60 and 2.85).

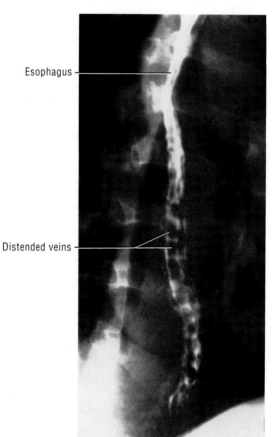

2.55
Esophageal varices

Note how the barium outlines the distended veins (esophageal varices) encroaching on the lumen. (Courtesy of Dr. E.L. Lansdown, Professor of Radiology, University of Toronto, Toronto, Ontario, Canada.)

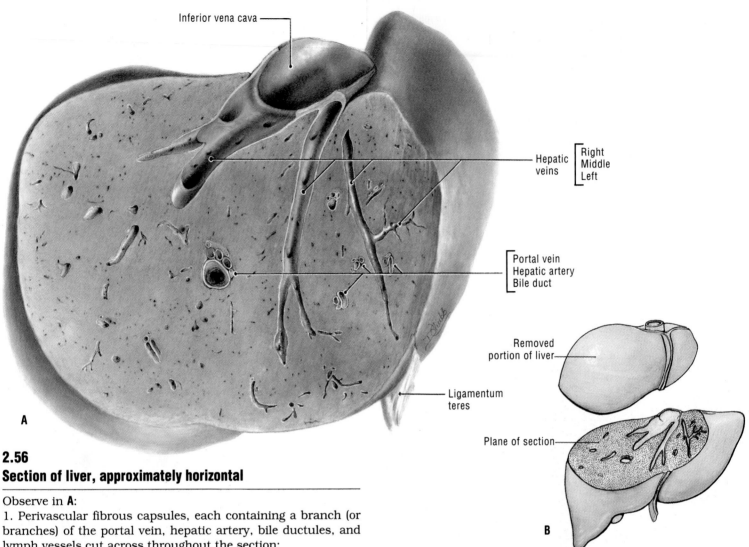

Inferior vena cava

Hepatic veins — Right Middle Left

Portal vein Hepatic artery Bile duct

Removed portion of liver

Plane of section

Ligamentum teres

A

B

2.56
Section of liver, approximately horizontal

Observe in **A**:

1. Perivascular fibrous capsules, each containing a branch (or branches) of the portal vein, hepatic artery, bile ductules, and lymph vessels cut across throughout the section;

2. Interdigitating with these are branches of the three main hepatic veins which, unaccompanied and having no capsules, converge fanwise on the inferior vena cava.

B. Orientation drawing.

2.57
Ultrasound scan of hepatic veins

Compare the scan to the drawing of the section of the liver (Fig. 2.56). The transducer was placed under the costal margin, angled toward the diaphragm. (Courtesy of Dr. A.M. Arenson, Assistant Professor of Radiology, University of Toronto, Toronto, Ontario, Canada.)

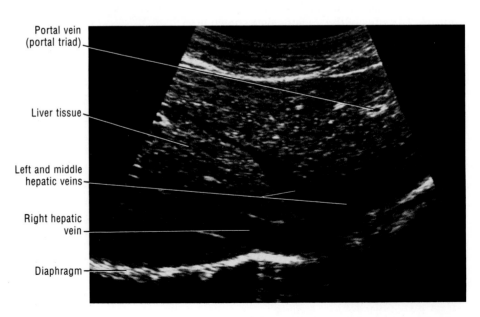

Portal vein (portal triad)

Liver tissue

Left and middle hepatic veins

Right hepatic vein

Diaphragm

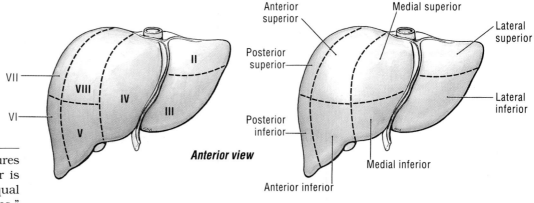

Anterior view

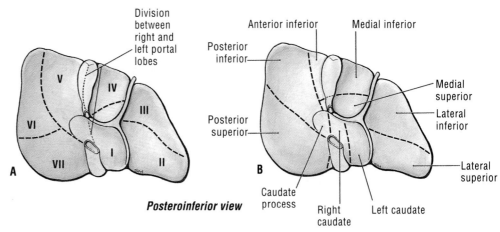

Posteroinferior view

2.58
Segments of the liver

Corrosion specimen of the portal structures (Fig. 2.47) have shown that the liver is divisible functionally into almost equal halves, "the right and left portal lobes," served by right and left portal veins, hepatic arteries, and bile passages. The two lobes are demarcated by a plane passing through the gallbladder fossa and the fossa for the inferior vena cava. Each of the lobes is further subdivided into segments that can be numerically identified, as in **A**, or named, as in **B**. (**A** from Couinaud C. *Lobes et segments hepatiques: Note sur l'architecture anatomique et chirurgicale du foie.* Presse Med 1954; 62:709. **B** from Healy JE, Schroy PC. *Anatomy of the biliary ducts within the human liver: Analysis of the prevailing pattern of branchings and the major variations of the biliary ducts.* Arch Surg 1953; 66:599.)

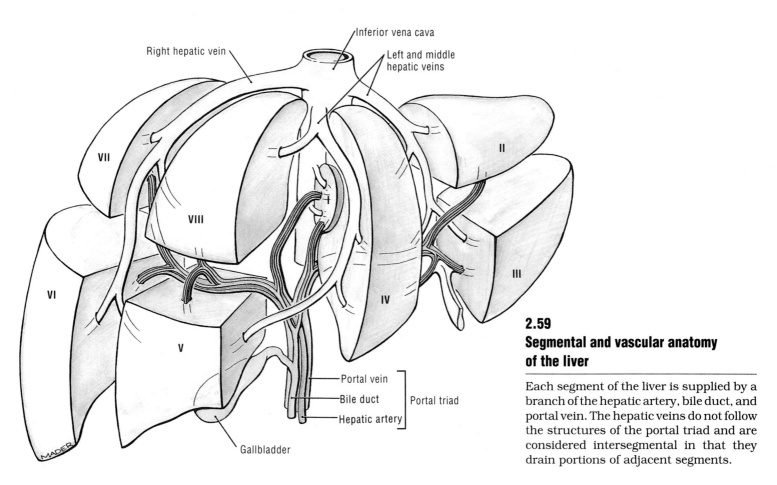

2.59
Segmental and vascular anatomy of the liver

Each segment of the liver is supplied by a branch of the hepatic artery, bile duct, and portal vein. The hepatic veins do not follow the structures of the portal triad and are considered intersegmental in that they drain portions of adjacent segments.

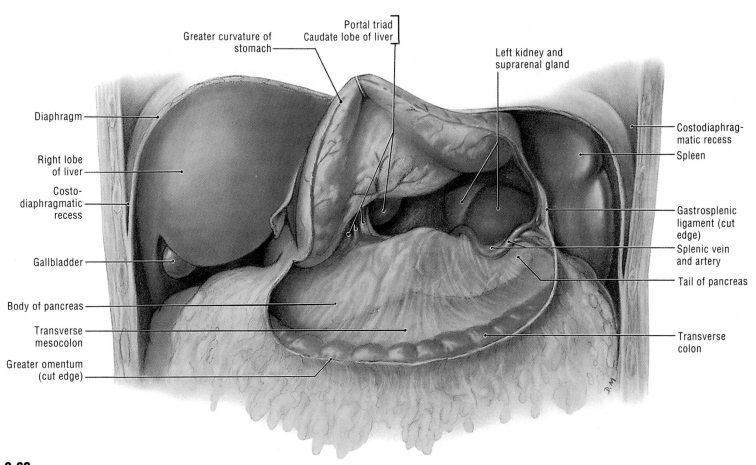

Greater curvature of stomach

Portal triad
Caudate lobe of liver

Left kidney and suprarenal gland

Diaphragm

Right lobe of liver

Costo-diaphragmatic recess

Gallbladder

Body of pancreas

Transverse mesocolon

Greater omentum (cut edge)

Costodiaphrag-matic recess

Spleen

Gastrosplenic ligament (cut edge)

Splenic vein and artery

Tail of pancreas

Transverse colon

2.60
Posterior relationships of the omental bursa

Observe:

1. The greater omentum and gastrosplenic ligament have been cut along the greater curvature of the stomach and the stomach reflected superiorly;

2. The lesser omentum is removed to reveal the portal triad (bile duct, hepatic artery, and portal vein) situated anterior to the opening of the omental (epiploic) foramen; the caudate lobe of the liver forming the superior boundary of the omental foramen;

3. The transverse mesocolon and the visceral peritoneum covering the spleen, the left kidney, and the left suprarenal gland;

4. The splenic artery and vein entering the hilum of the spleen; the tail of the pancreas extending to the spleen; the relationship of the spleen to the costodiaphragmatic recess.

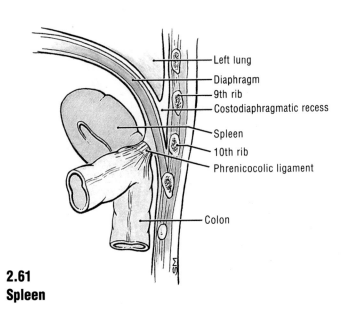

Left lung

Diaphragm

9th rib

Costodiaphragmatic recess

Spleen

10th rib

Phrenicocolic ligament

Colon

2.61
Spleen

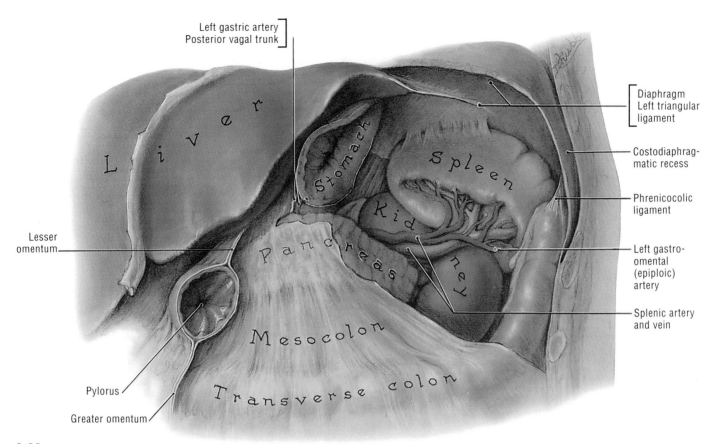

2.62
Stomach bed

The stomach is excised. The peritoneum of the omental bursa, or lesser sac, covering the stomach bed is largely removed; so is the peritoneum of the greater sac covering the inferior part of the kidney and pancreas; the pancreas is unusually short; the adhesions binding the spleen to diaphragm are pathological but not unusual.

2.63
Spleen, visceral surface

For orientation see Figure 2.61. Observe:

1. A "circumferential border" comprising the inferior, superior, and anterior borders, and separating the visceral surface from the diaphramatic surface;

2. The notches characteristic of the superior border;

3. The left limit of the omental bursa at the hilum of the spleen, between the splenorenal and gastrosplenic ligaments;

4. The spleen taking the impressions of the structures in contact with it;

5. The long axis of the spleen lying parallel to the 9th, 10th, and 11th ribs; it is not usually palpable inferior to the costal margin, unless it is enlarged (Figs. 2.21**A** and **B**).

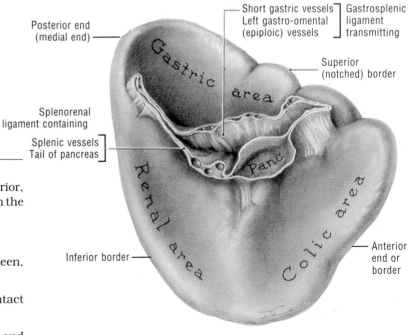

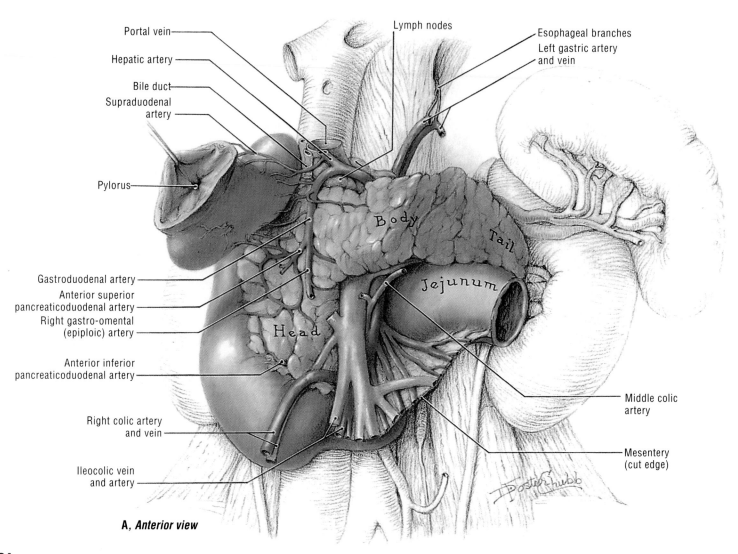

Portal vein
Hepatic artery
Bile duct
Supraduodenal artery
Pylorus
Gastroduodenal artery
Anterior superior pancreaticoduodenal artery
Right gastro-omental (epiploic) artery
Anterior inferior pancreaticoduodenal artery
Right colic artery and vein
Ileocolic vein and artery

Lymph nodes
Esophageal branches
Left gastric artery and vein
Body
Tail
Jejunum
Head
Middle colic artery
Mesentery (cut edge)

A, _Anterior view_

2.64
Duodenum and pancreas

Observe in **A** and **B**:

1. The duodenum molded around the head of the pancreas; its 1st or superior part (retracted) passing posteriorly, superiorly, and to the right; the remaining parts (2nd, 3rd, and 4th) overlapped by the pancreas; near the junction of its 3rd and 4th parts, the duodenum is crossed by the superior mesenteric vessels, which descend anterior to the uncinate process, and enter the root of the mesentery; they may, by constricting the duodenum, cause its 1st, 2nd, and 3rd parts to be dilated;

2. The tail of the pancreas, here very short, usually abuts on the spleen;

3. The celiac trunk, which lies posterior to the superior border of the pancreas, sending (a) the left gastric artery superiorly toward the cardiac orifice of the stomach to enter the lesser omentum; (b) the splenic artery to the left; and (c) the hepatic artery to the right, giving off the gastroduodenal artery;

4. In **B**, the posterior view of the specimen depicted in **A**, only the end of the 1st part of the duodenum is in view; the bile duct is descending in a fissure (opened up) in the posterior part of the head of the pancreas.

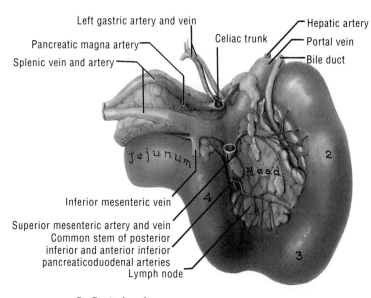

Left gastric artery and vein
Pancreatic magna artery
Splenic vein and artery
Celiac trunk
Hepatic artery
Portal vein
Bile duct
Jejunum
Head
2
Inferior mesenteric vein
Superior mesenteric artery and vein
Common stem of posterior inferior and anterior inferior pancreaticoduodenal arteries
Lymph node
4
3

B, _Posterior view_

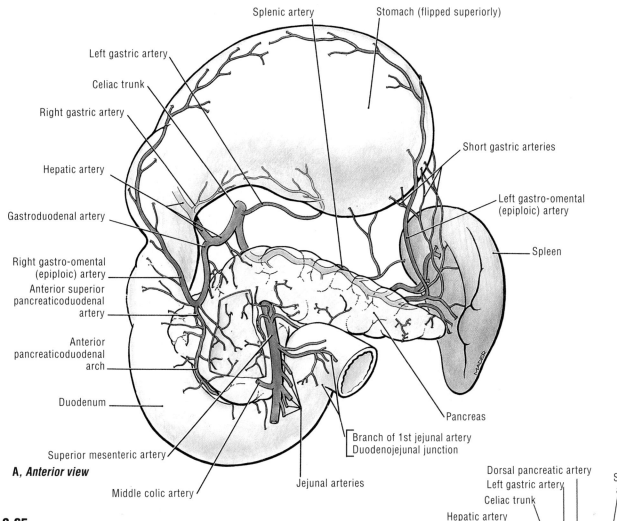

A, *Anterior view*

Labels in figure A:
- Splenic artery
- Stomach (flipped superiorly)
- Left gastric artery
- Celiac trunk
- Right gastric artery
- Short gastric arteries
- Hepatic artery
- Left gastro-omental (epiploic) artery
- Gastroduodenal artery
- Spleen
- Right gastro-omental (epiploic) artery
- Anterior superior pancreaticoduodenal artery
- Anterior pancreaticoduodenal arch
- Duodenum
- Pancreas
- Branch of 1st jejunal artery
- Duodenojejunal junction
- Superior mesenteric artery
- Middle colic artery
- Jejunal arteries

2.65
Blood supply to the pancreas, duodenum, and spleen

Observe:

1. This territory is supplied by the hepatic, splenic, and superior mesenteric arteries;

2. Several retroduodenal branches from the right gastro-omental (epiploic) artery;

3. The anterior superior pancreaticoduodenal branch of the gastroduodenal artery and the anterior inferior pancreatico–duodenal branch of the superior mesenteric artery form an arch anterior to the head of the pancreas; the posterior superior and posterior inferior branches of the same two arteries form another arch posterior to the pancreas; the anterior and posterior inferior arteries here, as usual, spring from a common stem; from each arch thus formed straight vessels, called vasa recta duodeni, pass to the anterior and posterior surfaces, respectively, of the 2nd, 3rd, and 4th parts of the duodenum;

4. The fine network of arteries supplying the pancreas are derived from: the common hepatic artery, the gastroduodenal artery, the pancreaticoduodenal arches, the splenic artery, and the superior mesenteric artery. (For more details, consult Michels NA. *The anatomic variations of the arterial pancreaticoduodenal arcades, etc.* J Int Coll Surgeons 1962; 37:13; and Woodbourne RT, Olsen LL. *The arteries of the pancreas.* Anat Rec 1951; 111:255.)

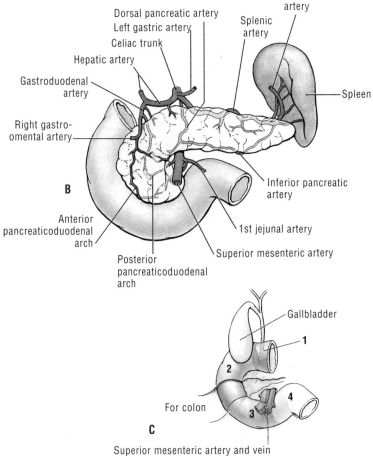

Labels in figure B:
- Dorsal pancreatic artery
- Left gastric artery
- Splenic artery
- Celiac trunk
- Left gastro-omental artery
- Hepatic artery
- Gastroduodenal artery
- Spleen
- Right gastro-omental artery
- Inferior pancreatic artery
- Anterior pancreaticoduodenal arch
- 1st jejunal artery
- Posterior pancreaticoduodenal arch
- Superior mesenteric artery

B

Labels in figure C:
- Gallbladder
- 1
- 2
- For colon
- 4
- 3
- Superior mesenteric artery and vein

C

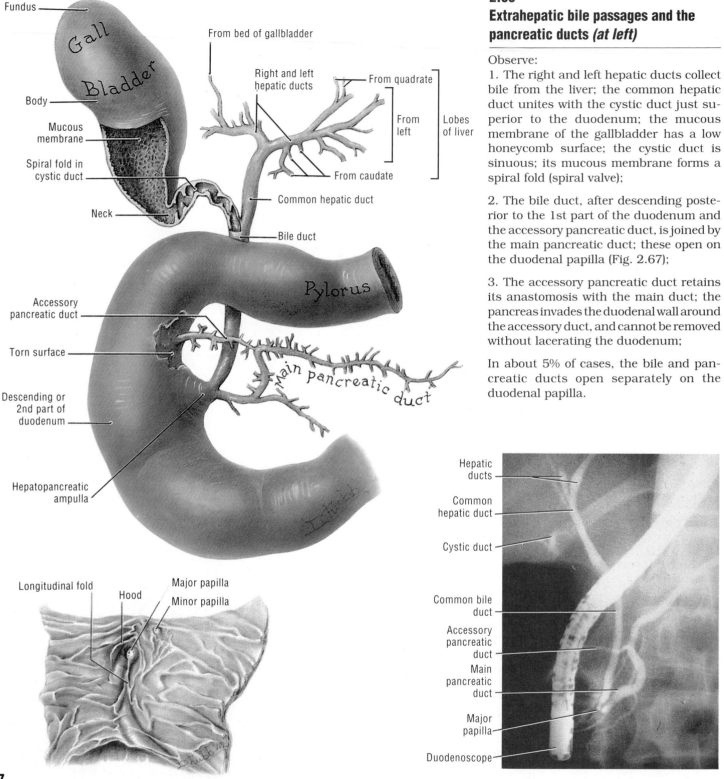

Fundus

Gall Bladder

Body

Mucous membrane

Spiral fold in cystic duct

Neck

From bed of gallbladder

Right and left hepatic ducts

From quadrate

From left — Lobes of liver

From caudate

Common hepatic duct

Bile duct

Pylorus

Accessory pancreatic duct

Torn surface

Descending or 2nd part of duodenum

Hepatopancreatic ampulla

main pancreatic duct

2.66
Extrahepatic bile passages and the pancreatic ducts (*at left*)

Observe:

1. The right and left hepatic ducts collect bile from the liver; the common hepatic duct unites with the cystic duct just superior to the duodenum; the mucous membrane of the gallbladder has a low honeycomb surface; the cystic duct is sinuous; its mucous membrane forms a spiral fold (spiral valve);

2. The bile duct, after descending posterior to the 1st part of the duodenum and the accessory pancreatic duct, is joined by the main pancreatic duct; these open on the duodenal papilla (Fig. 2.67);

3. The accessory pancreatic duct retains its anastomosis with the main duct; the pancreas invades the duodenal wall around the accessory duct, and cannot be removed without lacerating the duodenum;

In about 5% of cases, the bile and pancreatic ducts open separately on the duodenal papilla.

Longitudinal fold

Hood

Major papilla

Minor papilla

Hepatic ducts

Common hepatic duct

Cystic duct

Common bile duct

Accessory pancreatic duct

Main pancreatic duct

Major papilla

Duodenoscope

2.67
Interior of the 2nd part of the duodenum (*above*)

Observe the larger duodenal papilla projecting into the duodenum about 9 cm from the pylorus; a hood is thrown over the larger papilla, a longitudinal fold descends from it, and the small duodenal papilla, of the accessory pancreatic duct, lies just anterosuperior to it; the plicae circulares are pronounced.

2.68
Endoscopic retrograde cholangiography and pancreatography (ERCP) of the bile and pancreatic ducts

(Courtesy of Dr. G.B. Haber, Assistant Professor of Medicine, University of Toronto, Toronto, Ontario, Canada.)

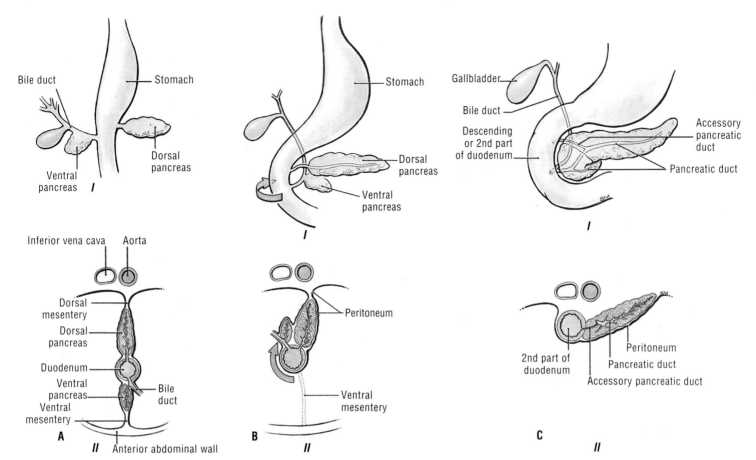

2.69
Development of the pancreatic ducts

In seeking a developmental explanation for variability of pancreatic ducts, examine the anterior views *(I)* and transverse sections *(II)* of the stages in the development of the pancreas.

A *(I* and *II).* A smaller primitive ventral bud arises in common with the bile duct, and a larger primitive dorsal bud arises independently from the duodenum, cranial to this.

B *(I* and *II).* The 2nd or descending part of the duodenum rotates on its long axis, which brings the ventral bud and the bile duct posterior to the dorsal bud.

C *(I* and *II).* A connecting segment unites the dorsal duct to the ventral duct, whereupon the duodenal end of the dorsal duct tends to atrophy and the direction of flow within it is reversed.

2.70
Variability of pancreatic ducts

Millbourn's radiographic study of 200 cases showed the following: in 44%, the accessory duct has lost its connection with the duodenum; in 10%, the accessory duct is large enough to relieve an obstructed main duct; in 20%, the accessory duct could probably substitute for the main duct; in 9%, the primitive dorsal duct persists quite unconnected with the primitive ventral duct, pancreas divisum (shown in the adjacent radiograph). (See Millbourn E. *On the excretory ducts of the pancreas in man, with special reference to their relations to each other, to the common bile duct and to the duodenum: radiological and anatomical study.* Acta Anat 1950; 9:1, and Dawson W, Langman J. *An anatomical-radiological study on the pancreatic duct pattern in man.* Anat Rec 1961; 139:59.) (Courtesy of Dr. G.B. Haber, Assistant Professor of Medicine, University of Toronto, Toronto, Ontario, Canada.)

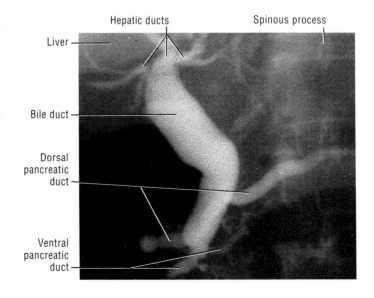

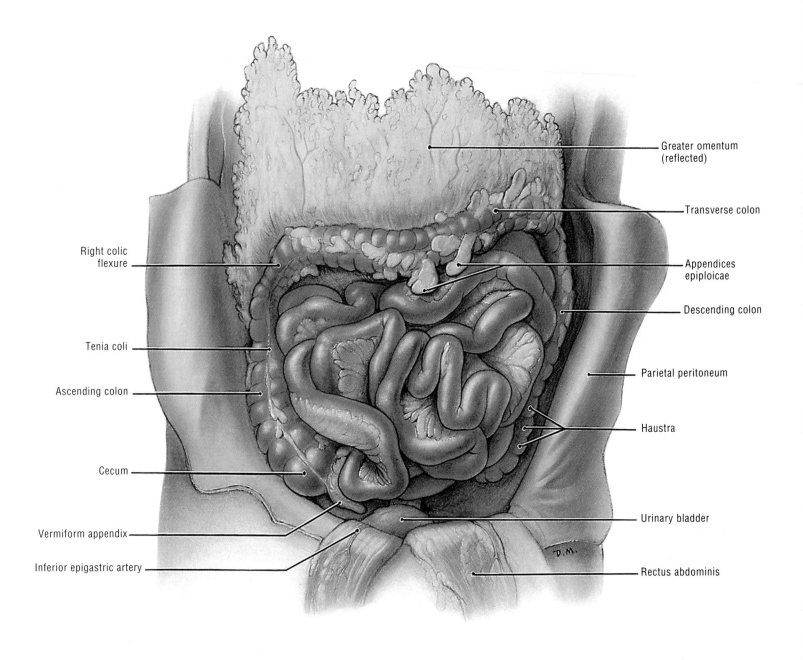

Greater omentum (reflected)

Transverse colon

Right colic flexure

Appendices epiploicae

Descending colon

Tenia coli

Parietal peritoneum

Ascending colon

Haustra

Cecum

Urinary bladder

Vermiform appendix

Rectus abdominis

Inferior epigastric artery

2.71
Small and large intestine in situ–I

Observe:

1. The extensive coiling of the jejunum and ileum of the small intestine (together about 6 m in length);

2. The small intestine continuous with the large intestine at the cecum;

3. The ileum is reflected to reveal the vermiform appendix, in the lower right quadrant; the vermiform appendix usually lies posterior to the cecum (retrocecal) or, as in this case, it may project over the pelvic brim;

4. The large intestine forming 3 1/2 sides of a square picture frame around the jejunum and ileum; on the right side, the cecum and ascending colon; the transverse colon superiorly; on the left, the descending colon and the sigmoid colon (not fully seen).

2.72
Interior of a dried cecum and diverticulum ilei (Meckel's diverticulum)

This cecum was filled with air until dry, opened, and varnished.

Observe:

1. The ileocecal valve guarding the ileocecal orifice; its pouting upper lip overhanging the lower lip; and the folds running horizontally from the corners of the lips;

2. The slight fold closing the superior part of the orifice of the appendix;

3. Meckel's diverticulum, found in 2% of persons, is the remains of the prenatal yolk stalk (vitellointestinal duct); it projects from the side of the ileum and is attached to it by a short peritoneal fold; usually less than 5 cm in length, it may attain 25 cm; about 72% of diverticula are located within 100 cm of the ileocecal orifice and 25% from 100 to 160 cm. (See Jay GD III, Margulis RR, McGraw AB, Northrip RR. *Meckel's diverticulum: survey of 103 cases.* Arch Surg 1950; 61:158.)

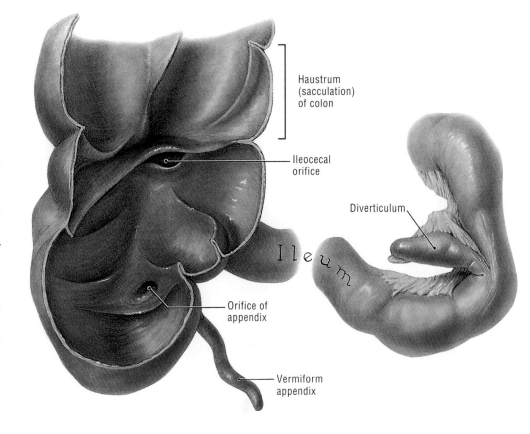

Haustrum (sacculation) of colon

Ileocecal orifice

Diverticulum

Ileum

Orifice of appendix

Vermiform appendix

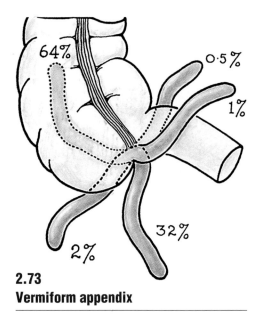

2.73
Vermiform appendix

This diagram shows the approximate incidence of various locations of the appendix. Like the hands of a clock, the appendix may be long or short, and it may occupy any position consistent with its length. (See Wakeley CPG. *The position of the vermiform appendix as ascertained by the analysis of 10,000 cases.* J Anat 1933; 67:277; Maisel H. *The position of the human vermiform appendix in fetal and adult age groups.* Anat Rec 1960; 136:385.)

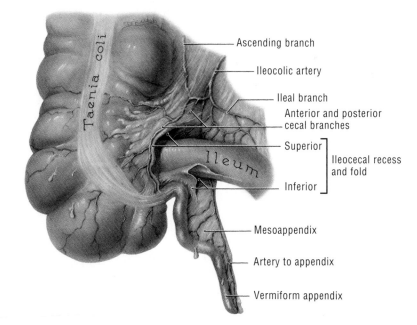

Ascending branch

Ileocolic artery

Ileal branch

Anterior and posterior cecal branches

Superior

Ileocecal recess and fold

Inferior

Mesoappendix

Artery to appendix

Vermiform appendix

Taenia coli

Ileum

2.74
Blood supply of ileocecal region

Observe:

1. The appendix in one free border of the mesoappendix and the artery in the other;

2. The anterior tenia coli leading to the appendix; this is a guide to the surgeon;

3. The inferior ileocecal (bloodless) fold extending from ileum to mesoappendix;

4. The vascular cecal fold is the official name for the superior ileocecal fold.

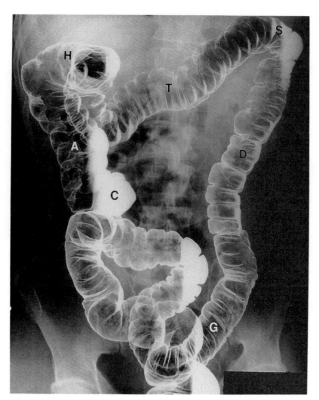

A, *Anteroposterior view*

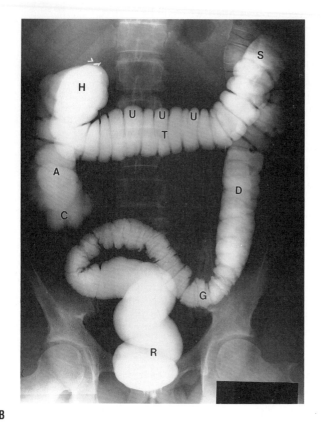

B

2.75
Barium enema examination of the colon

A. Double contrast. Barium can be seen coating the walls of the colon distended with air, giving a vivid view of the mucosal relief and haustra. (Courtesy of Dr. C.S. Ho, Professor of Radiology, University of Toronto, Toronto, Ontario Canada.)

B. Single contrast. A barium enema has filled the colon. Observe the relative levels of the hepatic and splenic flexures. (Courtesy of Dr. E.L. Lansdown, Professor of Radiology, University of Toronto, Toronto, Ontario, Canada.) *C* - Cecum, *A* - Ascending colon, *H* - Hepatic (right colic) flexure, *T* - Transverse colon, *S* - Splenic (left colic) flexure, *D* - Descending colon, *G* - Sigmoid colon, *R* - Rectum, *U* - Haustra.

C. Coronal MRI (magnetic resonance image) of the abdomen. (Courtesy of Dr. W. Kucharczyk, Clinical Director of Tri-Hospital Resonance Centre, Toronto, Ontario, Canada.)

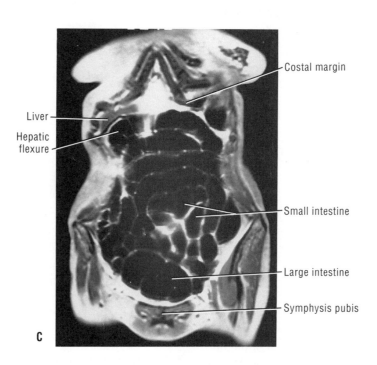

Liver

Hepatic flexure

Costal margin

Small intestine

Large intestine

Symphysis pubis

C

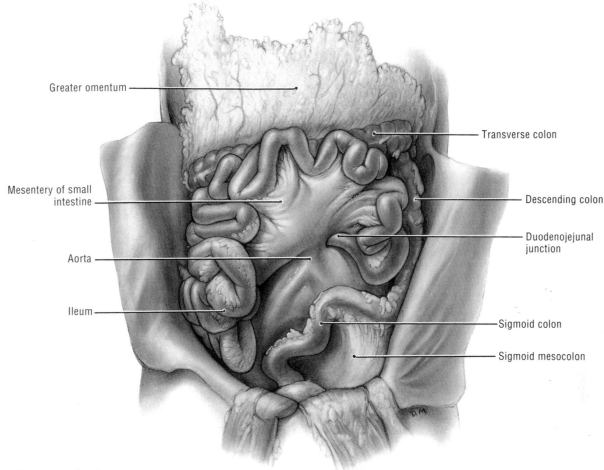

Greater omentum

Mesentery of small intestine

Aorta

Ileum

Transverse colon

Descending colon

Duodenojejunal junction

Sigmoid colon

Sigmoid mesocolon

2.76
Small and large intestine in situ

The greater omentum, and together with it the transverse colon, is lifted superiorly. The small intestine has been pushed aside to the right to expose the mesentery of the small intestine, the sigmoid colon, and rectum.

Observe:

1. The duodenojejunal junction, situated to the left of the median plane; the first few centimeters of the jejunum descending inferiorly and to the left, anterior to the left kidney;

2. The root of the mesentery of the small intestine, about 15 to 20 cm in length, extending between the duodenojejunal junction and the ileocecal junction; the mesentery fanning extensively to accommodate the jejunum and ileum, about 6 m in length;

3. The descending colon, the narrowest part of the large intestine, spannning from the left colic flexure to the pelvic brim where it is continuous with the sigmoid colon;

4. The descending colon is retroperitoneal, but the sigmoid colon has a mesentery, the sigmoid mesocolon; the sigmoid colon is continuous with the rectum at the point at which the sigmoid mesocolon is no longer present;

5. The aorta, covered with peritoneum, bifurcating into the common iliac arteries at vertebral level L4.

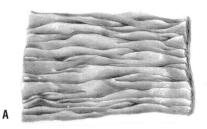

A

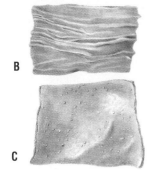

B

C

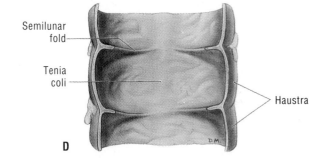

Semilunar fold

Tenia coli

Haustra

D

2.77
Interior of the intestine

A. Jejunum, proximal part: the plicae circulares are tall, closely packed, and commonly branched.

B. Ileum, proximal part: the plicae circulares are low and becoming sparse. The caliber of the gut is reduced and the wall is thinner.

C. Ileum, distal part: plicae are now absent. Solitary lymph nodules stud the wall.

D. Transverse colon: the semilunar folds and teniae coli form prominent features on the smooth-surfaced wall.

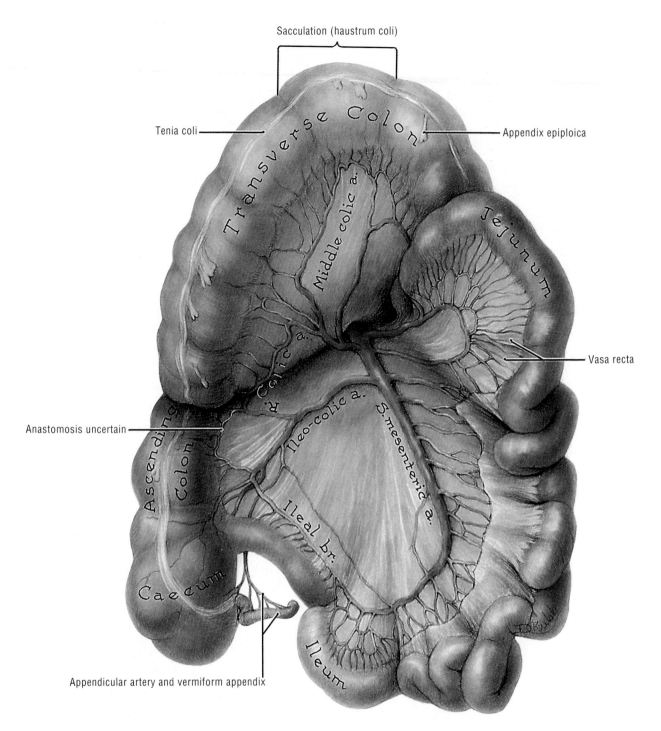

Sacculation (haustrum coli)

Tenia coli

Transverse Colon

Appendix epiploica

Middle colic a.

Jejunum

R. Colic a.

Colic a.

Vasa recta

Anastomosis uncertain

Ileo-colic a.

S. mesenteric a.

Ascending Colon

Ileal br.

Caecum

Ileum

Appendicular artery and vermiform appendix

2.78
Superior mesenteric artery

The peritoneum is, in part, stripped off.

Observe:

1. The superior mesenteric artery ending by anastomosing with one of its own branches, the ileal branch of the ileocolic artery;

2. Its branches: (a) from its left side, 12 or more jejunal and ileal branches; these anastomose to form arcades from which vasta recta pass to the small intestine; (b) from its right side, the middle colic, the ileocolic, and commonly, but not here, an independent right colic artery; these anastomose to form a marginal artery

from which vasa recta pass to the large intestine; (c) the two inferior pancreaticoduodenal arteries arise from the main artery either directly or in conjunction with the first jejunal branch;

3. Teniae coli, sacculations, and appendices epiploicae that distinguish the large intestine from the smooth-walled small intestine. (For details, consult Basmajian JV. *The marginal anastomoses of the arteries to the large intestine.* Surg Gynecol Obstet 1954; 99:614; Basmajian JV. *The main arteries of the large intestine.* Surg Gynecol Obstet 1955; 101:585.)

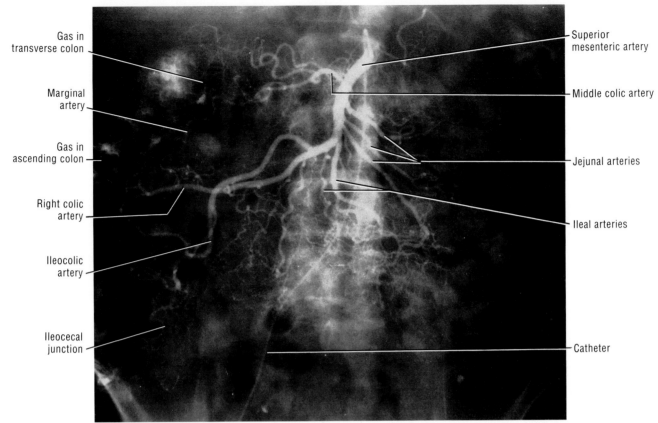

Gas in transverse colon

Marginal artery

Gas in ascending colon

Right colic artery

Ileocolic artery

Ileocecal junction

Superior mesenteric artery

Middle colic artery

Jejunal arteries

Ileal arteries

Catheter

2.79
Superior mesenteric arteriogram

Consult Figure 2.78 to identify the branches of the superior mesenteric artery. Observe, in particular, examples of anasto-motic loops. (Courtesy of Dr. E.L. Lansdown, Professor of Radiology, University of Toronto, Toronto, Ontario, Canada.)

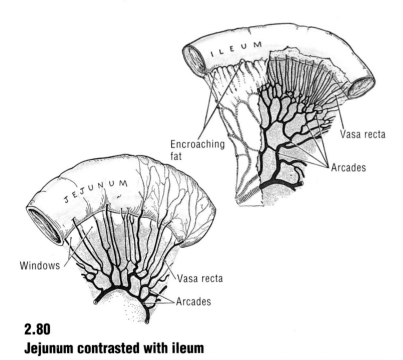

ILEUM

Encroaching fat

Vasa recta

Arcades

JEJUNUM

Windows

Vasa recta

Arcades

2.80
Jejunum contrasted with ileum

Compare diameter, thickness of wall, number of arterial arcades, long or short vasa recta, presence of translucent (fat free) areas at the mesenteric border, and fat encroaching on the wall of the gut.

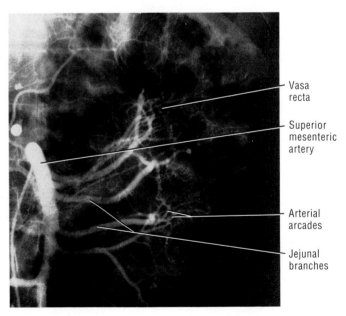

Vasa recta

Superior mesenteric artery

Arterial arcades

Jejunal branches

2.81
Superior mesenteric arteriogram, jejunal branches, and arterial arcades

(Courtesy of Dr. J. Heslin, Assistant Professor of Anatomy, University of Toronto, Toronto, Ontario, Canada.)

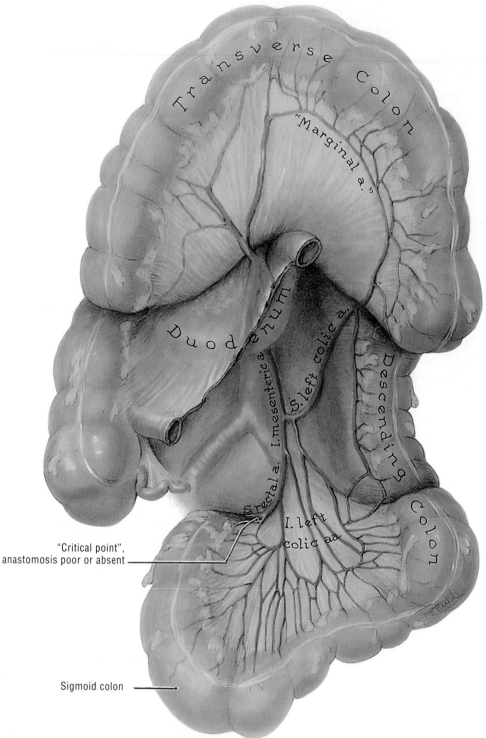

Transverse Colon

"Marginal a."

Duodenum

S. left colic a.

Descending Colon

S. rectal a. I. mesenteric a.

I. left colic aa.

"Critical point", anastomosis poor or absent

Sigmoid colon

2.82
Inferior mesenteric artery

The mesentery has been cut at its root and discarded with the jejunum and ileum.

Observe:

1. The inferior mesenteric artery arising posterior to the duodenum, 4 cm superior to the bifurcation of the aorta; on crossing the left common iliac artery, it becomes the superior rectal artery;

2. Its branches: (a) a single left colic artery, and (b) several sigmoid arteries (inferior left colic arteries) springing from its left side; in

this specimen the two inferior sigmoid arteries from the superior rectal artery; the point at which the last artery to the colon leaves the artery to the rectum is known as the "critical point of Sudeck." (For details, see Michels NA, Siddharth P, Kornblith PL, Parke WW. *The variant blood supply to the small and large intestine based on four hundred dissections, etc.* J Int Coll Surg 1963; 39:127; also *The variant blood supply to the descending colon, rectosigmoid and rectum.* Dis Colon Rectum 1965; 8:251.

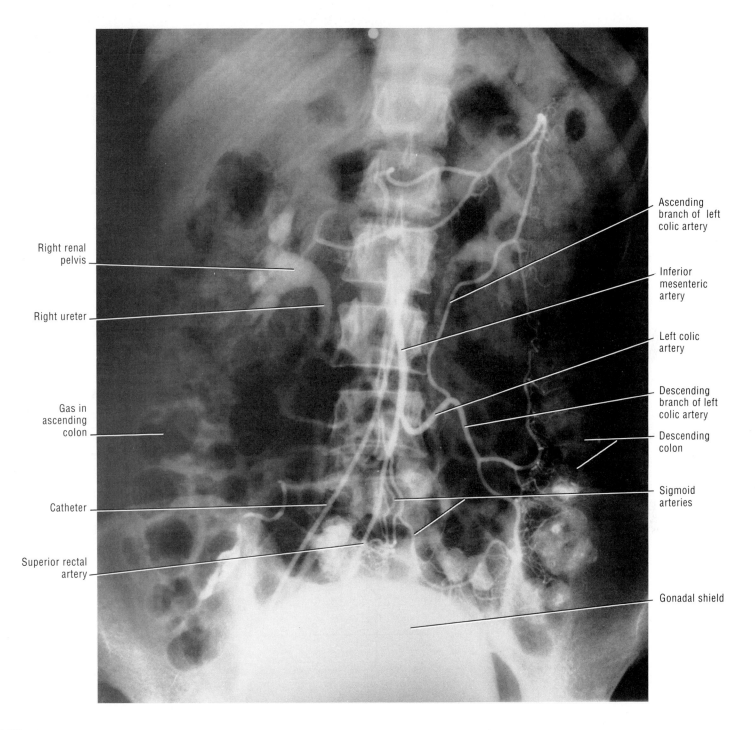

Right renal pelvis

Right ureter

Gas in ascending colon

Catheter

Superior rectal artery

Ascending branch of left colic artery

Inferior mesenteric artery

Left colic artery

Descending branch of left colic artery

Descending colon

Sigmoid arteries

Gonadal shield

2.83
Inferior mesenteric arteriogram

Consult Figure 2.82.

Observe:

1. The left colic artery, coursing to the left toward the descending colon and splitting into an ascending and a descending branch;

2. The sigmoid arteries, two to four in number, supplying the sigmoid colon;

3. The superior rectal artery, the continuation of the inferior mesenteric artery, supplying the rectum; it anastomoses with branches of the middle and inferior rectal arteries (from the internal iliac artery). (Courtesy of Dr. K. Sniderman, Associate Professor of Radiology, University of Toronto, Toronto, Ontario, Canada.)

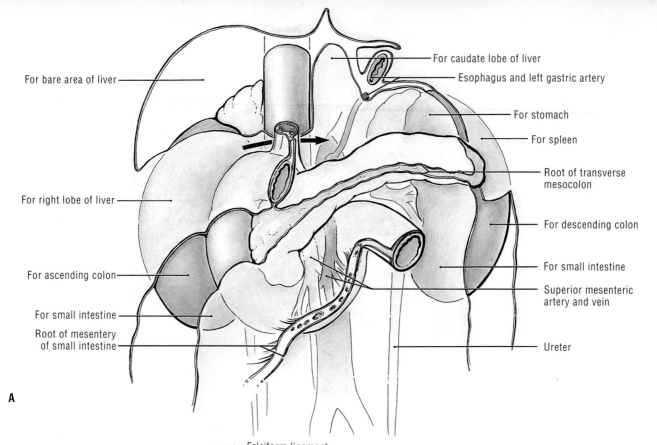

For bare area of liver

For caudate lobe of liver

Esophagus and left gastric artery

For stomach

For spleen

Root of transverse mesocolon

For right lobe of liver

For descending colon

For small intestine

For ascending colon

Superior mesenteric artery and vein

For small intestine

Root of mesentery of small intestine

Ureter

A

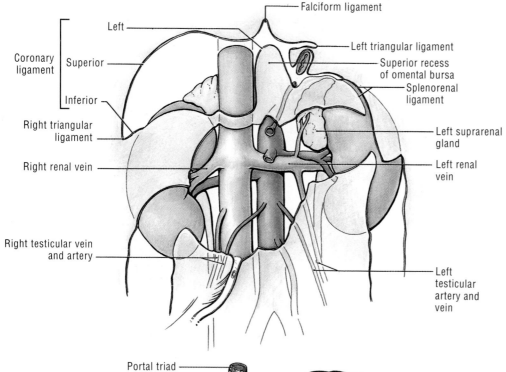

Falciform ligament

Left

Left triangular ligament

Coronary ligament

Superior

Superior recess of omental bursa

Splenorenal ligament

Inferior

Right triangular ligament

Left suprarenal gland

Right renal vein

Left renal vein

Right testicular vein and artery

Left testicular artery and vein

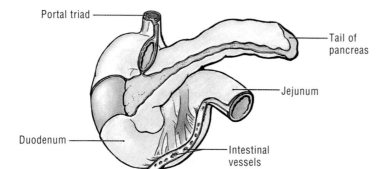

Portal triad

Tail of pancreas

Jejunum

B

Duodenum

Intestinal vessels

2.84
Relationships of the pancreas and duodenum

A. Duodenum and pancreas in situ. **B.** Duodenum and pancreas removed.

Observe in **A** and **B**:

1. The peritoneal covering of the pancreas and duodenum;

2. The colic area of right kidney, descending or 2nd part of duodenum, and head of pancreas; the line of attachment of the transverse mesocolon to the body and tail of the pancreas and the colic area of the left kidney;

3. (a) The intestinal vessels lying on a plane anterior to (b) that of the testicular vessels, and these, in turn, lying (c) anterior to the plane of the kidney, its vessels, and the ureter;

4. The right suprarenal gland at the omental (epiploic) foramen, indicated by an *arrow*;

5. The three parts of the coronary ligament attached to the diaphragm except where the inferior vena cava, suprarenal gland, and kidney intervene;

6. The relationships of the two kidneys to the suprarenal glands, the liver, the colon, the duodenum, the stomach, the pancreas, and the spleen.

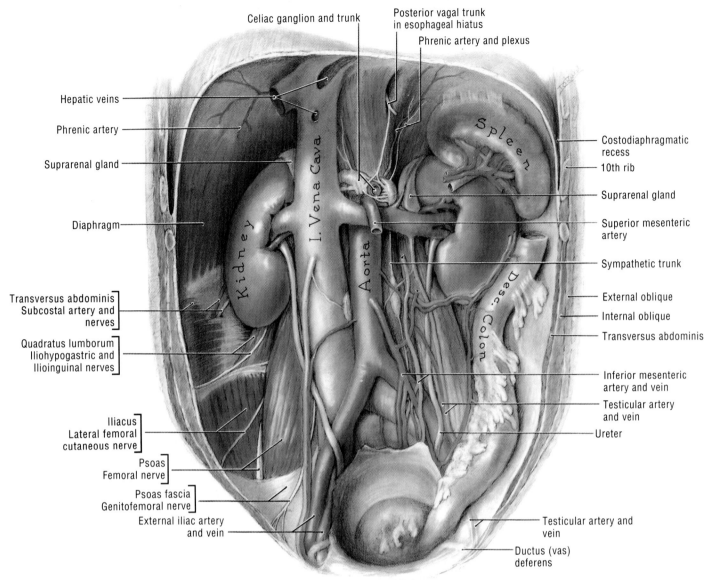

Celiac ganglion and trunk

Posterior vagal trunk in esophageal hiatus

Phrenic artery and plexus

Hepatic veins

Phrenic artery

Suprarenal gland

Diaphragm

Transversus abdominis
Subcostal artery and nerves

Quadratus lumborum
Iliohypogastric and Ilioinguinal nerves

Iliacus
Lateral femoral cutaneous nerve

Psoas
Femoral nerve

Psoas fascia
Genitofemoral nerve

External iliac artery and vein

Kidney

I. Vena Cava

Aorta

Spleen

Desc. Colon

Costodiaphragmatic recess

10th rib

Suprarenal gland

Superior mesenteric artery

Sympathetic trunk

External oblique

Internal oblique

Transversus abdominis

Inferior mesenteric artery and vein

Testicular artery and vein

Ureter

Testicular artery and vein

Ductus (vas) deferens

2.85
Great vessels: kidneys: suprarenal glands

Observe that:

1. The abdominal aorta is shorter and of smaller caliber than the inferior vena cava;

2. The celiac trunk is surrounded by the celiac plexus and celiac ganglia; the ganglia receive a branch of the posterior gastric nerve;

3. The superior mesenteric artery arises just inferior to the celiac trunk, and in the angle it makes with the aorta runs the left renal vein (Fig. 2.86);

4. The inferior mesenteric artery arises 4 cm superior to the aortic bifurcation and crosses the left common iliac vessels to become the superior rectal artery.

5. The kidneys lie anterior to the diaphragm, transversus abdominis aponeurosis, quadratus lumborum, and psoas muscles; the left renal vein drains the left testis, left suprarenal gland, and left kidney; the renal arteries are posterior to the renal veins;

6. The ureter crosses the external iliac artery just beyond the common iliac bifurcation; the blood supply to the ureter comes from three main sources, (a) from the renal artery superiorly, (b) from a vesical artery inferiorly, and (c) from either the common iliac artery or the aorta;

7. The testicular vessels cross anterior to the ureter and join the ductus deferens at the deep inguinal ring.

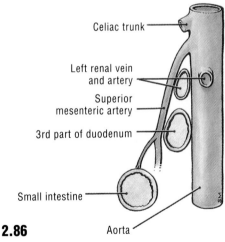

Celiac trunk

Left renal vein and artery

Superior mesenteric artery

3rd part of duodenum

Small intestine

Aorta

2.86
Nutcrackers

Diagram illustrating that the left renal vein and duodenum are compressed between the aorta posteriorly and the superior mesenteric artery suspending the weight of the intestine anteriorly.

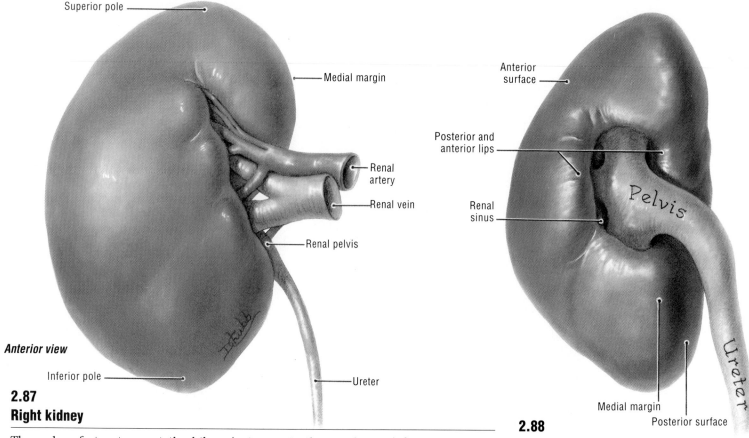

Superior pole

Medial margin

Renal
artery

Renal vein

Renal pelvis

Anterior view

Inferior pole

Ureter

2.87
Right kidney

The order of structures at the hilum (entrance to the renal sinus) from anterior to posterior is vein, artery, renal pelvis, or ureter; often a branch of the artery passes posterior to the renal pelvis; the superior pole of the kidney is usually wider than the inferior pole and is closer to the median plane.

Anterior
surface

Posterior and
anterior lips

Renal
sinus

Pelvis

Ureter

Medial margin

Posterior surface

2.88
Sinus of the kidney

The renal sinus is a vertical "pocket" on the medial side of the kidney. Tucked into the pocket are the renal pelvis and the renal vessels.

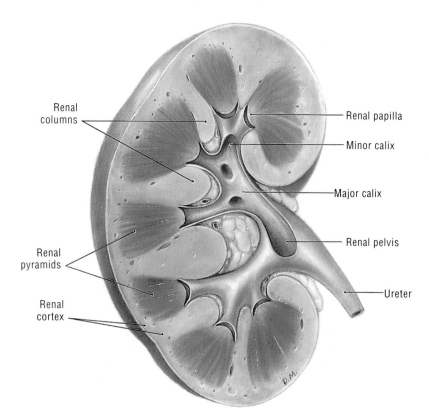

Renal
columns

Renal papilla

Minor calix

Major calix

Renal pelvis

Renal
pyramids

Ureter

Renal
cortex

2.89
Coronal section of kidney,
internal structure

Observe:
1. The conical renal pyramids radiating from the renal sinus toward the surface of the kidney; their blunted apex, the renal papilla, pouts into a minor calix into which it discharges urine from the openings of its collecting tubules; the pyramids, which appear striated, form the medulla of the kidney and contain loops of Henle and collecting tubules;

2. The renal cortex forming the outer one-third of the renal substance, extending between pyramids as renal columns, appears rather granular, and contains glomeruli and convoluted tubules; interlobar arteries travel in the renal columns;

3. The ureter draining the renal pelvis that receives two or three major calices; each kidney has seven to fourteen minor calices.

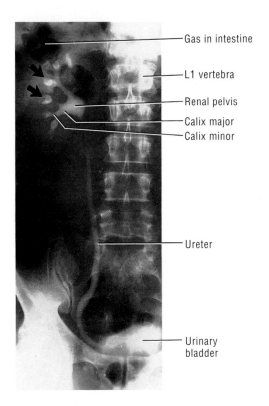

- Gas in intestine
- L1 vertebra
- Renal pelvis
- Calix major
- Calix minor
- Ureter
- Urinary bladder

2.90
Pyelogram

Radiopaque material outlines the cavities conducting urine. Note the papillae (indicated with *arrows*) bulging into the minor calices that empty into a major calix, which, in turn, opens into the renal pelvis, which drains into the ureter. The ureter travels inferiorly, toward the urinary bladder, along the transverse processes of the lumbar vertebrae. (Courtesy of Dr. E.L. Lansdown, Professor of Radiology, University of Toronto, Toronto, Ontario, Canada.)

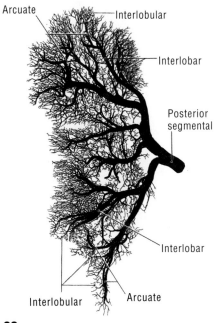

- Arcuate
- Interlobular
- Interlobar
- Posterior segmental
- Interlobar
- Interlobular
- Arcuate

2.92
Corrosion cast of the posterior segmental artery of the kidney

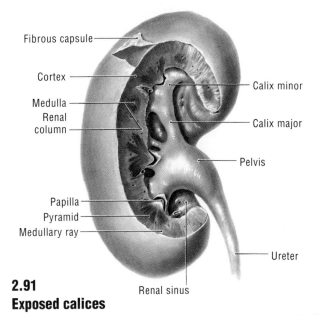

- Fibrous capsule
- Cortex
- Medulla
- Renal column
- Papilla
- Pyramid
- Medullary ray
- Renal sinus
- Calix minor
- Calix major
- Pelvis
- Ureter

2.91
Exposed calices

The anterior lip of the sinus has been cut away to expose the renal pelvis and the calices. This gives a three dimensional view to assist in interpreting coronal sections of the kidney (Fig. 2.55).

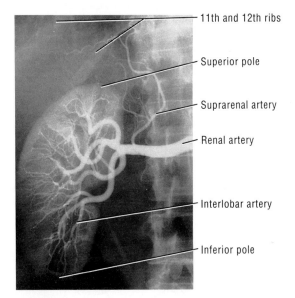

- 11th and 12th ribs
- Superior pole
- Suprarenal artery
- Renal artery
- Interlobar artery
- Inferior pole

2.93
Renal arteriogram

Typically, the renal artery divides into five branches, each supplying a segment of the kidney; a segmental artery provides a lobar artery to each pyramid; these divide to provide two or three interlobar arteries that travel between pyramids; near the junction of the medulla and cortex, arcuate arteries are given off at right angles to the parent stem, these do not anastomose; from the arcuate arteries (and some from the interlobar arteries), interlobular arteries pass into the cortex; the arterioles supplying the glomeruli are mainly from these interlobular arteries; although the veins of the kidney anastomose freely, segmental arteries are end arteries. (See Graves FT. *The arterial anatomy of the kidney.* Bristol: John Wright & Sons, Ltd., 1971.) (Courtesy of Dr. E.L. Lansdown, Professor of Radiology, University of Toronto, Toronto, Ontario, Canada.)

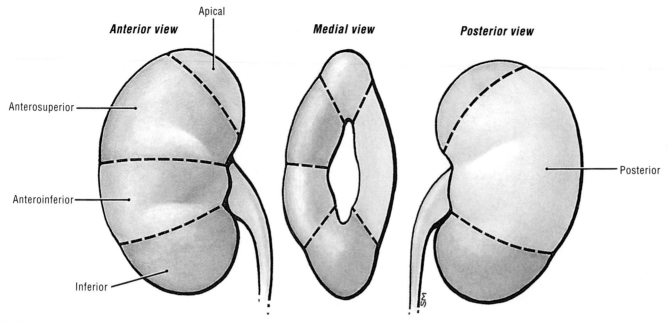

Anterior view   Medial view   Posterior view

Apical

Anterosuperior

Anteroinferior

Inferior

Posterior

2.94
Segments of the kidney

According to its arterial supply the kidney has five segments: (a) apical; (b) anterosuperior (upper anterior); (c) anteroinferior (middle anterior); (d) inferior (lower); and (e) posterior.

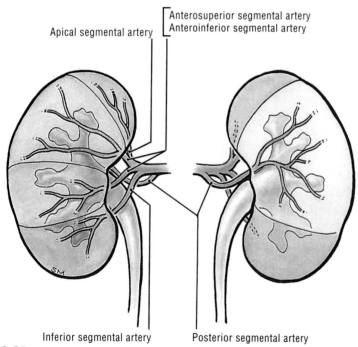

Apical segmental artery

Anterosuperior segmental artery
Anteroinferior segmental artery

Inferior segmental artery   Posterior segmental artery

2.95
Segmental arteries

Only the apical and inferior arteries supply the whole thickness of the kidney. The posterior artery crosses superior to the renal pelvis to reach its segment.

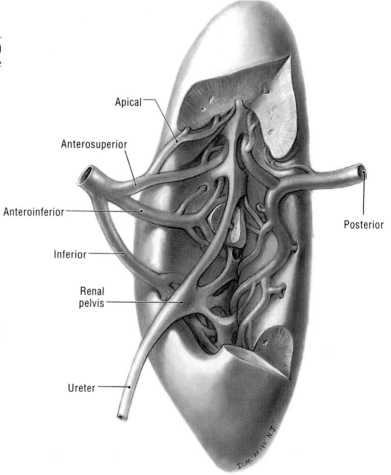

Apical

Anterosuperior

Anteroinferior

Posterior

Inferior

Renal pelvis

Ureter

2.96
Branches of the renal artery within the sinus

About 25% of kidneys receive directly 2nd, 3rd, and even 4th branches from the aorta. These enter either through the renal sinus or at the superior or inferior pole.

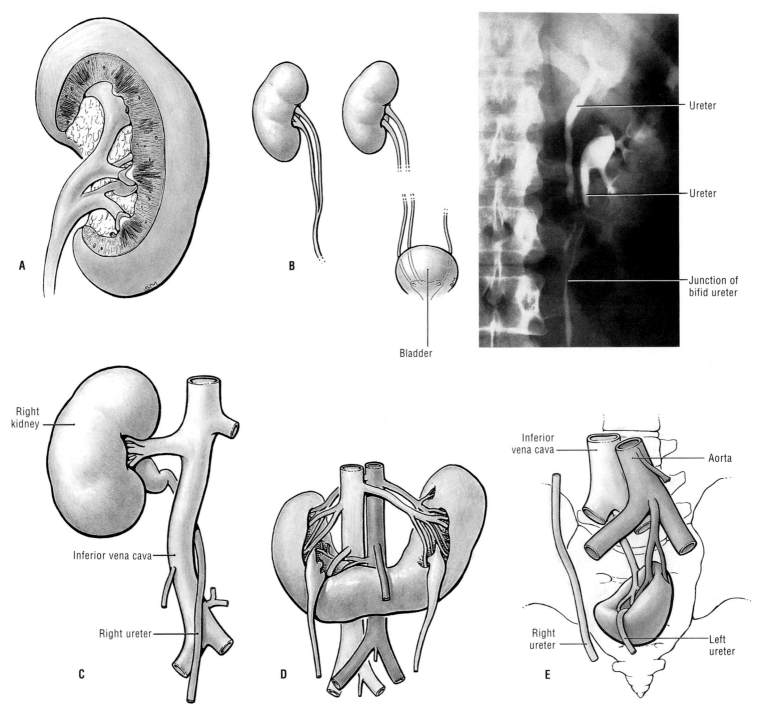

2.97
Anomalies of the kidney and ureter

A. Bifid pelves. The pelves are almost replaced by two long major calices, which lie partly within and partly outside the sinus.

B. Duplicated or bifid ureters. These may be either unilateral or bilateral, and either complete or incomplete. The incidence is less than 1%. (See Campbell M. *Ureteral reduplication (double ureter).* Urology, Vol. 1 Philadelphia: WB Saunders, 1954: 309.) (Pyelogram courtesy of Dr. E.L. Lansdown, Professor of Radiology, University of Toronto, Toronto, Ontario, Canada.)

C. Retrocaval ureter. (See Pick JW, Anson BJ. *Retrocaval ureter.* J Urol 1940; 43:672; Lowsley OS. *Postcaval ureter-operation for its*

correction. Surg Gynecol Obstet 1946; 82:549.)

D. Horseshoe kidney. This occurs in 0.25% of cases. (See Yamaguchi B. *A dissection-case of horseshoe kidney.* Sapporo Med J 1964; 25:141.)

E. Ectopic pelvic kidney. Pelvic kidneys have no fatty capsule and may be unilateral or bilateral. During childbirth, they may both cause obstruction and suffer injury. (See Anderson GA, Rice GG, Harris BA. *Pregnancy and labor complicated by pelvic ectopic kidney anomalies; a review.* Obstet Gynecol Surv 1949; 4:737.)

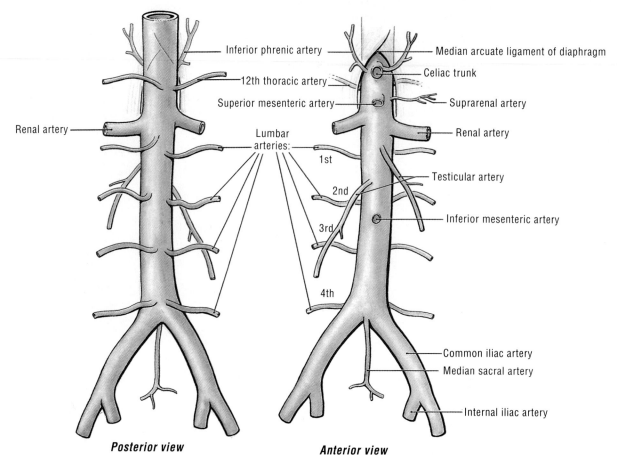

Inferior phrenic artery

Median arcuate ligament of diaphragm

12th thoracic artery

Celiac trunk

Superior mesenteric artery

Suprarenal artery

Renal artery

Renal artery

Lumbar
arteries:

1st

Testicular artery

2nd

3rd

Inferior mesenteric artery

4th

Common iliac artery

Median sacral artery

Internal iliac artery

Posterior view

Anterior view

2.98
Abdominal aorta and its branches

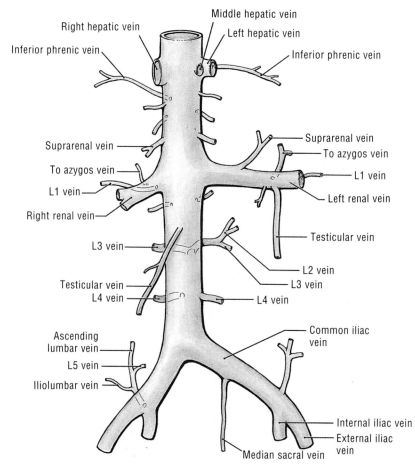

Middle hepatic vein

Right hepatic vein

Left hepatic vein

Inferior phrenic vein

Inferior phrenic vein

Suprarenal vein

Suprarenal vein

To azygos vein

To azygos vein

L1 vein

L1 vein

Left renal vein

Right renal vein

Testicular vein

L3 vein

L2 vein

L3 vein

Testicular vein

L4 vein

L4 vein

Ascending
lumbar vein

Common iliac
vein

L5 vein

Iliolumbar vein

Internal iliac vein

External iliac
vein

Median sacral vein

2.99
Inferior vena cava and its tributaries

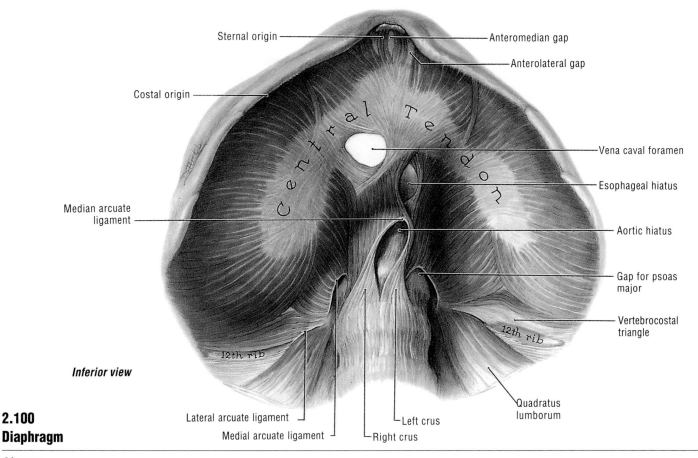

Sternal origin —————— ———— Anteromedian gap

———— Anterolateral gap

Costal origin ——————

Central Tendon

———— Vena caval foramen

———— Esophageal hiatus

Median arcuate
ligament ——————

———— Aortic hiatus

———— Gap for psoas
major

———— Vertebrocostal
triangle

12th rib

12th rib

Quadratus
lumborum

Inferior view

2.100
Diaphragm

Lateral arcuate ligament ⌐

Medial arcuate ligament ⌐

⌐ Left crus

⌐ Right crus

Observe:

1. The trefoil-shaped central tendon, which is the aponeurotic insertion of the muscle;

2. The fleshy origins: anteriorly from the inner surface of the xiphoid process, circumferentially from the lower six costal cartilages, and posteriorly from the superior three lumbar vertebral bodies via right and left crura that unite anterior to the aortic hiatus to form the median arcuate ligament; thickenings of the psoas and quadratus lumborum fascia (the medial and lateral arcuate ligaments) also afford origin to the diaphragm;

3. The diaphragm, in this specimen, failing to arise from the left lateral arcuate ligament, hence the vertebrocostal triangle through which a herniation of abdominal contents into the pleural cavity may occur.

Nerve supply: Each phrenic nerve (C3, C4, C5) is the sole motor nerve to its own half of the diaphragm; it is also sensory to its own half, including the pleura superiorly and the peritoneum inferiorly, but the lower intercostal nerves are sensory to the peripheral edge of the diaphragm.

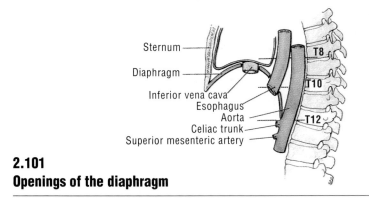

Sternum ————
Diaphragm ————
Inferior vena cava ————
Esophagus ————
Aorta ————
Celiac trunk ————
Superior mesenteric artery ————

T8

T10

T12

2.101
Openings of the diaphragm

There are three large openings in the diaphragm for major structures to pass from the thorax into the abdomen: (a) the opening for the inferior vena cava, most anterior, at the T8 level and to the right of the midline; (b) the esophageal opening, intermediate, at T10, and to the left; (c) the aorta passes posterior to the vertebral attachment of the diaphragm in the midline, at T12.

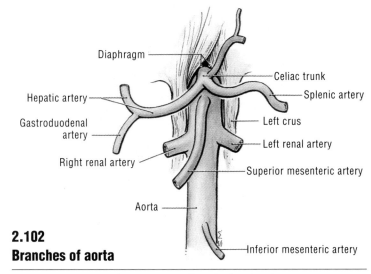

Diaphragm ————
———— Celiac trunk
Hepatic artery ————
———— Splenic artery
Gastroduodenal artery ————
———— Left crus
Right renal artery ————
———— Left renal artery
———— Superior mesenteric artery
Aorta ————
———— Inferior mesenteric artery

2.102
Branches of aorta

Autonomic nerve plexuses travel with these arteries to viscera.

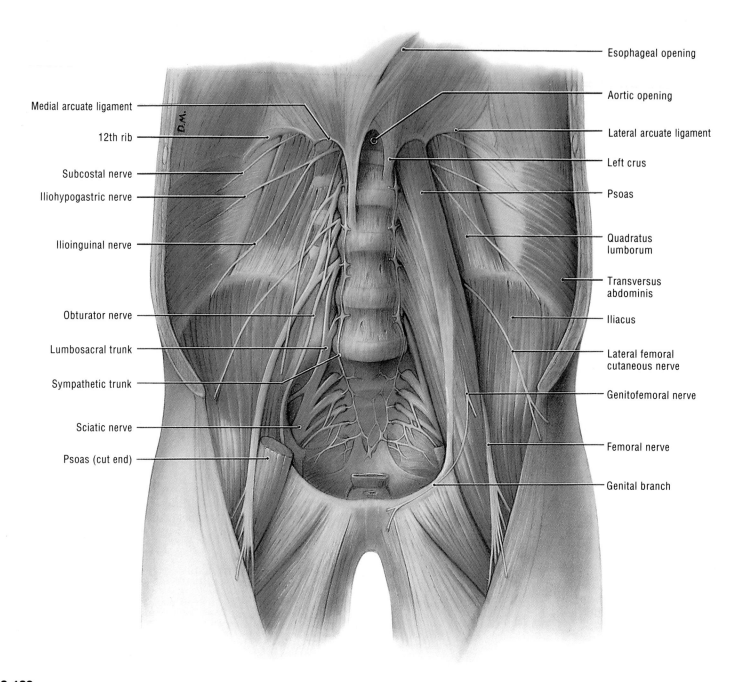

Esophageal opening

Aortic opening

Medial arcuate ligament

12th rib

Lateral arcuate ligament

Subcostal nerve

Left crus

Iliohypogastric nerve

Psoas

Ilioinguinal nerve

Quadratus lumborum

Transversus abdominis

Obturator nerve

Iliacus

Lumbosacral trunk

Lateral femoral cutaneous nerve

Sympathetic trunk

Genitofemoral nerve

Sciatic nerve

Femoral nerve

Psoas (cut end)

Genital branch

2.103
Posterior abdominal wall: lumbar plexus

Muscles. Transversus abdominis becomes aponeurotic on a line dropped from the tip of the 12th rib. Quadratus lumborum has an oblique lateral border; its fascia is thickened to form the lateral arcuate ligament superiorly and the iliolumbar ligament inferiorly. Iliacus lies inferior to the iliac crest. Psoas major rises superior to the crest and extends superior to the medial arcuate ligament, which is thickened psoas fascia.

Nerves. The subcostal nerve (T12) passes posterior to the lateral arcuate ligament and runs at some distance inferior to the 12th rib (with its artery). The next four nerves appear at the lateral border of psoas. Of these, the iliohypogastric (T12, L1) takes the characteristic course shown here; the ilioinguinal (L1) and the lateral femoral cutaneous nerve (lateral cutaneous of the thigh)

(L2, L3) are variable; the femoral (L2, L3, L4) descends in the angle between iliacus and psoas. The genitofemoral nerve (L1, L2) pierces the psoas and its fascia anteriorly. The obturator nerve (L2, L3, L4) and a branch of L4 that joins with L5 to form the lumbosacral trunk appear at the medial border of psoas, and, crossing the ala of the sacrum, enter the pelvis.

The sympathetic trunk enters the abdomen with psoas major posterior to the medial arcuate ligament. It descends on vertebral bodies and intervertebral discs, following closely the attached border of psoas to enter the pelvis. Its rami communicantes run dorsally with, or near, the lumbar arteries to join the lumbar nerves.

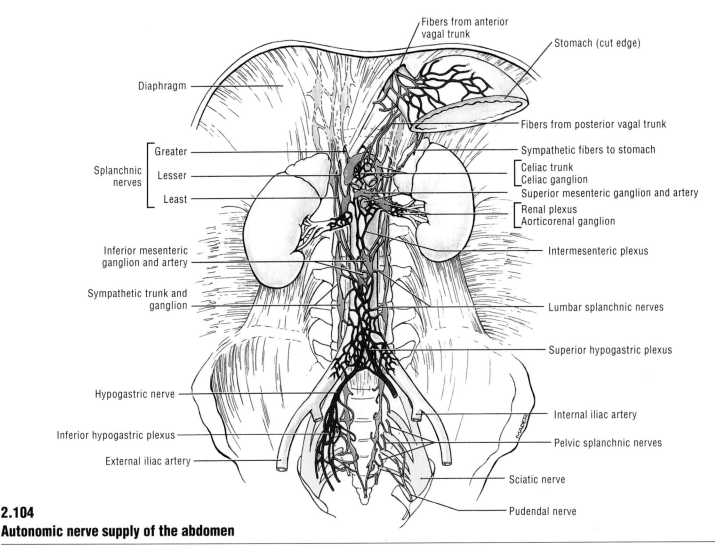

Diaphragm

Splanchnic nerves
Greater
Lesser
Least

Inferior mesenteric ganglion and artery

Sympathetic trunk and ganglion

Hypogastric nerve

Inferior hypogastric plexus

External iliac artery

Fibers from anterior vagal trunk

Stomach (cut edge)

Fibers from posterior vagal trunk

Sympathetic fibers to stomach

Celiac trunk
Celiac ganglion
Superior mesenteric ganglion and artery

Renal plexus
Aorticorenal ganglion

Intermesenteric plexus

Lumbar splanchnic nerves

Superior hypogastric plexus

Internal iliac artery

Pelvic splanchnic nerves

Sciatic nerve

Pudendal nerve

2.104
Autonomic nerve supply of the abdomen

Sympathetic and parasympathetic nerves mingle in the rich tangle of nerve plexuses anterior to the aorta; both kinds of fibers are distributed by "hitchhiking" on the walls of branches of the abdominal aorta to their destinations; this network is variable and difficult to dissect.

The above, somewhat simplified diagram is useful for general orientation. Observe:

1. The interconnected plexuses on abdominal aorta; the stems of the celiac, superior mesenteric, and inferior mesenteric arteries and the areas between these vessels are surrounded by networks of nerve fibers, e.g., the celiac, superior mesenteric, intermesenteric, and inferior mesenteric plexuses; the plexuses follow the branches of these arteries to the viscera and are named according to which vessels they follow, e.g., renal, testicular, ovarian, gastric, cystic plexuses; the superior hypogastric plexus, at the bifurcation of the aorta, is connected via the hypogastric nerves to the inferior hypogastric plexus;

2. Sympathetic input is via preganglionic fibers (splanchnic nerves) from right and left sympathetic trunks: greater, lesser, and least splanchnic nerves from the thorax and lumbar splanchnic nerves from the abdomen; the greater splanchnic nerve is from thoracic ganglia 5 to 9; the lesser from thoracic ganglia 10 and 11; the least from thoracic ganglion 12, the lumbar splanchnics from the four lumbar ganglia.

3. The sympathetic splanchnic nerves synapse in preaortic ganglia, e.g., the greater splanchnic nerve ending in the celiac ganglion; the lesser splanchnic nerve ending in the renal plexus (aorticorenal ganglion); the lumbar splanchnics in the intermesenteric and superior hypogastric plexuses; usually, the greater splanchnic nerve pierces the crus at the level of the celiac trunk; the lesser nerve inferolateral to this; and the sympathetic trunk enters with the psoas major;

4. The sympathetic trunk lying on the bodies of the vertebrae and descending along the anterior border of the psoas major; the trunk is slender where it enters the abdomen; its ganglia are ill defined; about six lumbar splanchnic nerves leave it anteromedially;

5. Parasympathetic fibers via the posterior and anterior vagal trunks (formerly right and left vagus nerves) are distributed to the foregut and midgut; pelvic splanchnic nerves from branches of the anterior primary rami of sacral spinal nerves 2, 3, and 4 supply parasympathetic fibers to the hindgut and pelvic viscera;

6. The posterior and anterior vagal trunks entering the abdomen on the esophagus and supplying gastric branches; the celiac branch of the posterior vagal trunk leaving to make its contribution to the preaortic plexuses; hepatic branches of the anterior vagal trunk joined by sympathetic fibers from the celiac plexus.

2.105
Lymphatic drainage of the abdomen

A. Stomach and small intestine. **B**. Spleen and pancreas.

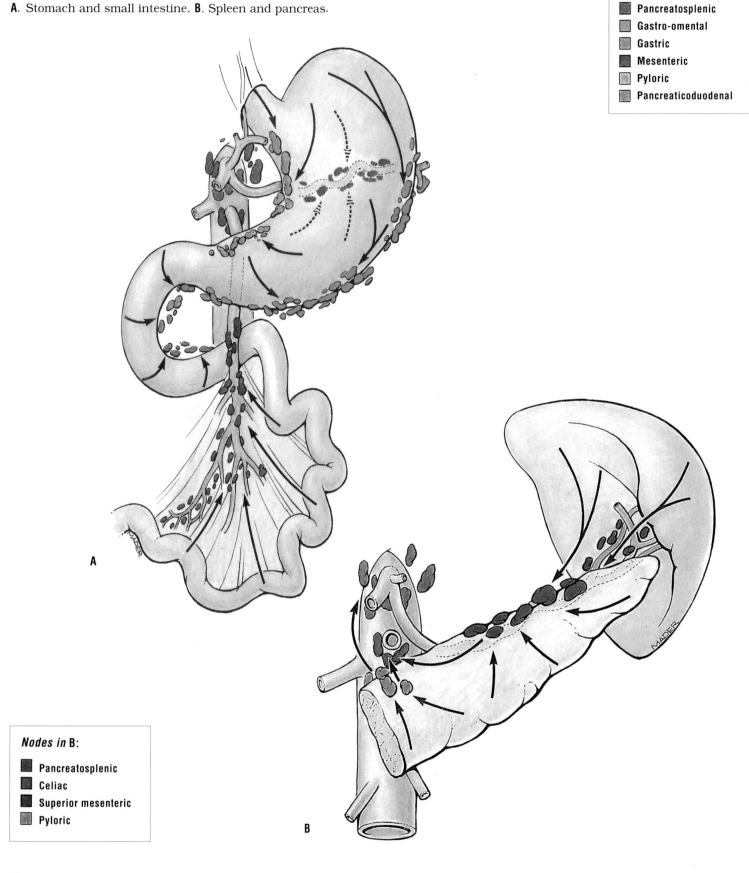

Nodes in A:

- Celiac
- Pancreatosplenic
- Gastro-omental
- Gastric
- Mesenteric
- Pyloric
- Pancreaticoduodenal

Nodes in B:

- Pancreatosplenic
- Celiac
- Superior mesenteric
- Pyloric

Lymphatic drainage of the abdomen *(continued)*

A. Large intestine. **B.** Liver and kidney.

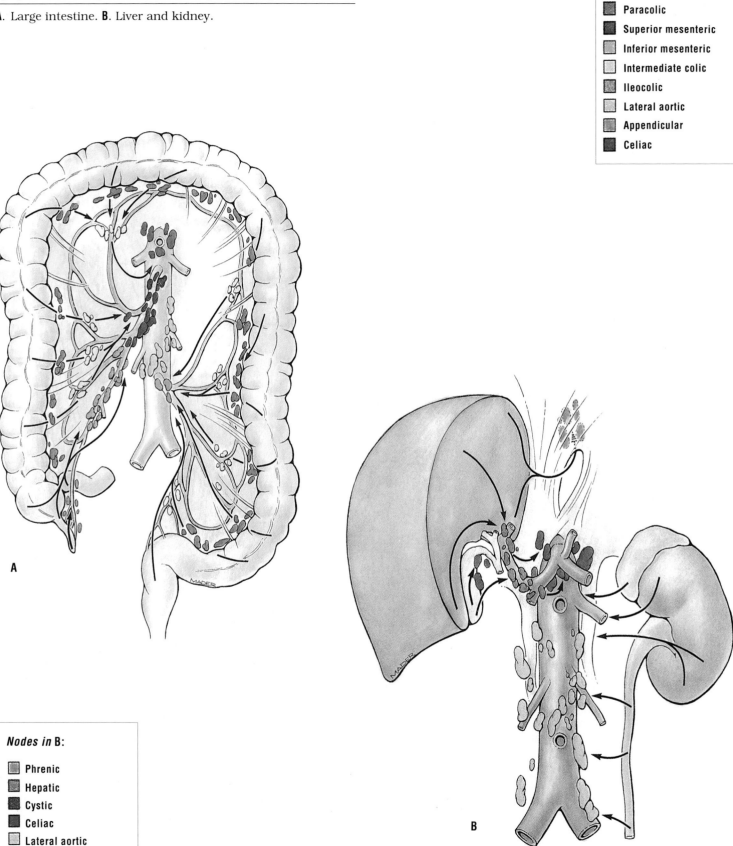

Nodes in A:

- ■ Paracolic
- ■ Superior mesenteric
- ■ Inferior mesenteric
- □ Intermediate colic
- ■ Ileocolic
- ■ Lateral aortic
- ■ Appendicular
- ■ Celiac

Nodes in B:

- ■ Phrenic
- ■ Hepatic
- ■ Cystic
- ■ Celiac
- ■ Lateral aortic

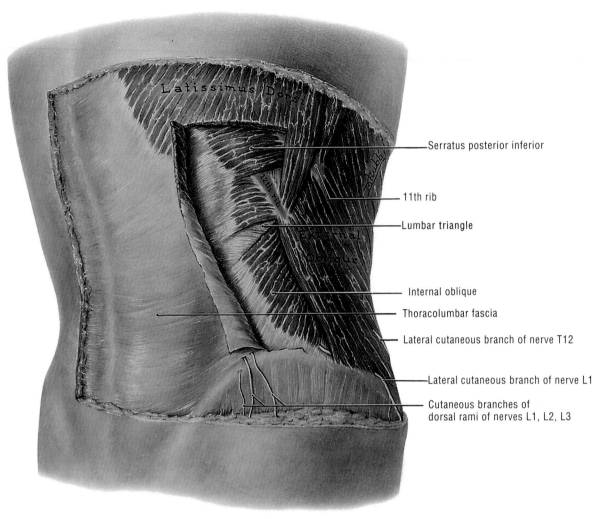

Posterolateral view

2.107
Posterior abdominal wall–I

Latissimus dorsi is, in part, reflected.

Observe:

1. External oblique muscle having an oblique, free, posterior border that extends from the tip of the 12th rib to the midpoint of the iliac crest;

2. Internal oblique muscle extending posterior to the external oblique muscle; it forms the floor of the lumbar triangle, creeps up on to the lumbar fascia, and has a triangle between it and serratus posterior inferior; this is the "superior lumbar triangle."

Labels for figure 2.107:
- Serratus posterior inferior
- 11th rib
- Lumbar triangle
- Internal oblique
- Thoracolumbar fascia
- Lateral cutaneous branch of nerve T12
- Lateral cutaneous branch of nerve L1
- Cutaneous branches of dorsal rami of nerves L1, L2, L3
- Latissimus Dorsi
- External oblique

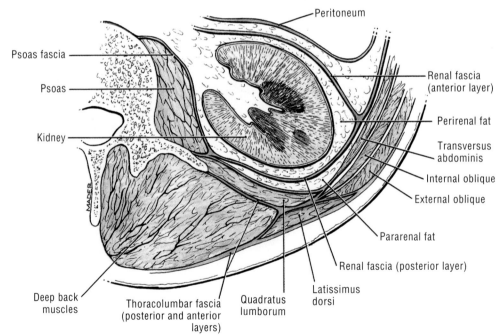

Labels for figure 2.108:
- Peritoneum
- Psoas fascia
- Psoas
- Kidney
- MADER
- Deep back muscles
- Thoracolumbar fascia (posterior and anterior layers)
- Quadratus lumborum
- Latissimus dorsi
- Renal fascia (posterior layer)
- Pararenal fat
- External oblique
- Internal oblique
- Transversus abdominis
- Perirenal fat
- Renal fascia (anterior layer)

2.108
Transverse section of the kidney: relationships of muscle and fascia

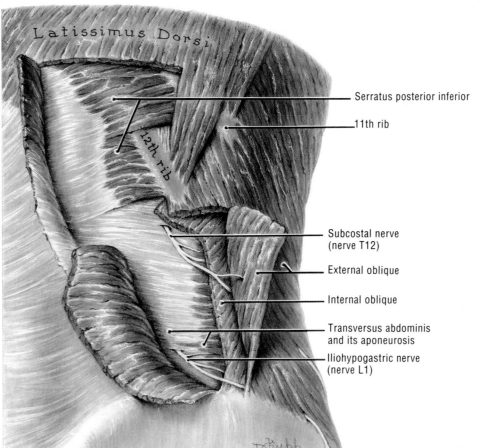

Serratus posterior inferior

11th rib

Subcostal nerve
(nerve T12)

External oblique

Internal oblique

Transversus abdominis
and its aponeurosis

Iliohypogastric nerve
(nerve L1)

2.109
Posterior abdominal wall–II

When the external oblique muscle has been incised and turned laterally and the internal oblique muscle incised and turned medially, transversus abdominis muscle and its posterior aponeurosis are exposed where pierced by the subcostal (T12) and iliohypogastric (L1) nerves; these nerves give off motor twigs and lateral cutaneous branches, and continue anteriorly between internal oblique and transversus abdominis muscles.

2.110
Posterior abdominal wall–III

On dividing the posterior aponeurosis of transversus abdominis between the subcostal and iliohypogastric nerves, and lateral to the oblique lateral border of quadratus lumborum muscle, the retroperitoneal fat surrounding the kidney is exposed; the renal fascia is within this fat; the portion of fat inside the renal fascia is termed fatty renal capsule (perirenal fat); the fat outside is pararenal fat.

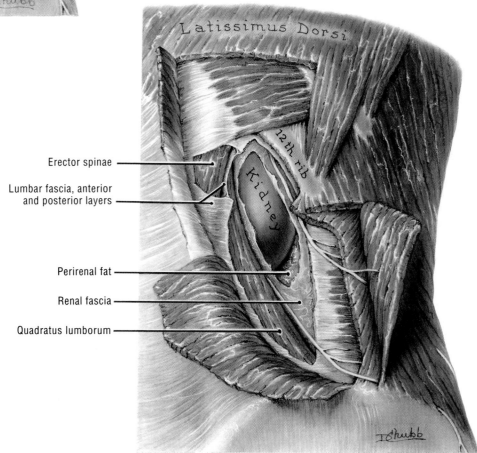

Erector spinae

Lumbar fascia, anterior
and posterior layers

Perirenal fat

Renal fascia

Quadratus lumborum

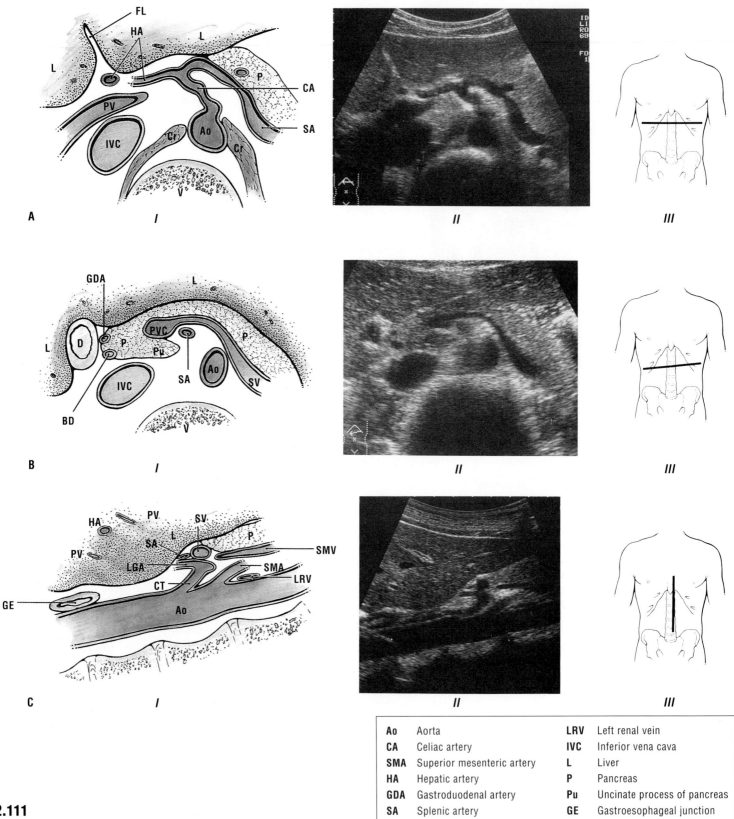

2.111
Ultrasound scans of the abdomen

A. Transverse scan through the celiac trunk. **B**. Transverse scan through the pancreas. **C**. Sagittal scan through the aorta. (Courtesy of Dr. A.M. Arenson, Assistant Professor of Radiology, University of Toronto, Toronto, Ontario, Canada.)

Ao	Aorta	**LRV**	Left renal vein
CA	Celiac artery	**IVC**	Inferior vena cava
SMA	Superior mesenteric artery	**L**	Liver
HA	Hepatic artery	**P**	Pancreas
GDA	Gastroduodenal artery	**Pu**	Uncinate process of pancreas
SA	Splenic artery	**GE**	Gastroesophageal junction
LGA	Left gastric artery	**D**	Duodenum
PVC	Portal venous confluence	**Cr**	Crus of diaphragm
SMV	Superior mesenteric vein	**FL**	Falciform ligament
SV	Splenic vein	**BD**	Bile duct
PV	Portal vein	**V**	Vertebra

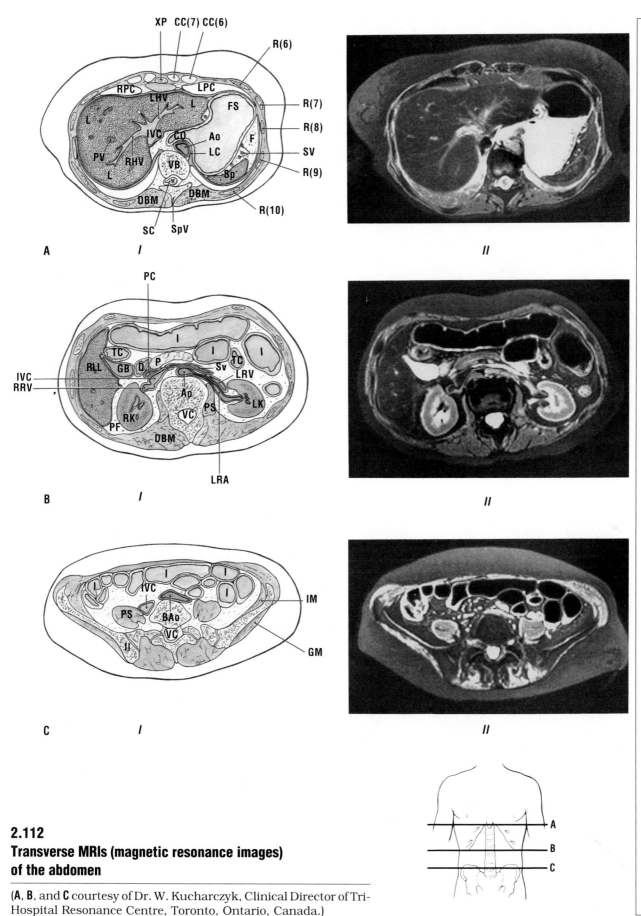

Ao — Aorta
BAo — Bifurcation of aorta
LRA — Left renal artery
IVC — Inferior vena cava
LHV — Left hepatic vein
RHV — Right hepatic vein
PV — Portal vein (triad)
PC — Portal confluence
SV — Splenic vessels
Sv — Splenic vein
LRV — Left renal vein
RRV — Right renal vein
L — Liver
RLL — Right lobe of liver
GB — Gallbladder
P — Pancreas
FS — Fundus of stomach
CO — Cardiac orifice of stomach
D — Duodenum
TC — Transverse colon
DC — Descending colon
I — Intestine
RK — Right kidney
LK — Left kidney
Sp — Spleen
PF — Perirenal fat
F — Fat
XP — Xiphoid process
CC — Costal cartilage
R — Rib
RPC — Right pleural cavity
LPC — Left pleural cavity
VB — Vertebral body
SpV — Spinous process of vertebra
VC — Vertebral canal
SC — Spinal cord
II — Ilium
PS — Psoas muscle
IM — Iliacus muscle
GM — Gluteus medius muscle
DBM — Deep back muscles
LC — Left crus

2.112

Transverse MRIs (magnetic resonance images) of the abdomen

(**A**, **B**, and **C** courtesy of Dr. W. Kucharczyk, Clinical Director of Tri-Hospital Resonance Centre, Toronto, Ontario, Canada.)

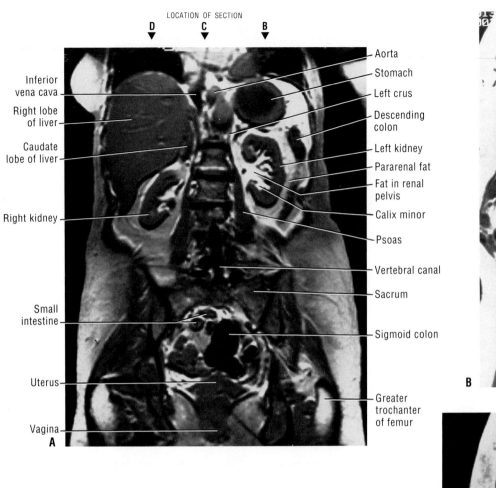

LOCATION OF SECTION
D   C   B

Inferior vena cava
Right lobe of liver
Caudate lobe of liver
Right kidney
Small intestine
Uterus
Vagina

A

Aorta
Stomach
Left crus
Descending colon
Left kidney
Pararenal fat
Fat in renal pelvis
Calix minor
Psoas
Vertebral canal
Sacrum
Sigmoid colon
Greater trochanter of femur

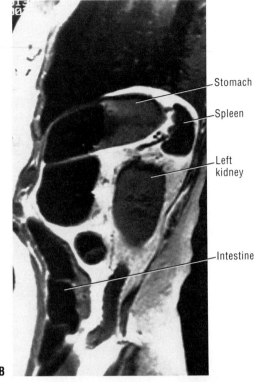

Stomach
Spleen
Left kidney
Intestine

B

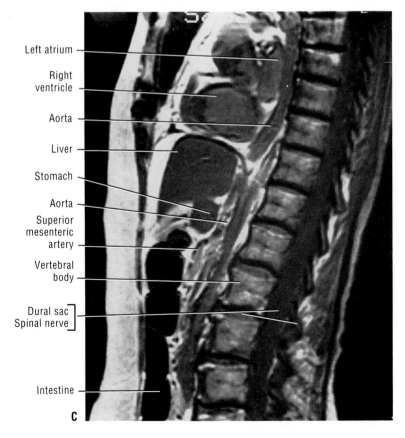

Left atrium
Right ventricle
Aorta
Liver
Stomach
Aorta
Superior mesenteric artery
Vertebral body
Dural sac
Spinal nerve
Intestine

C

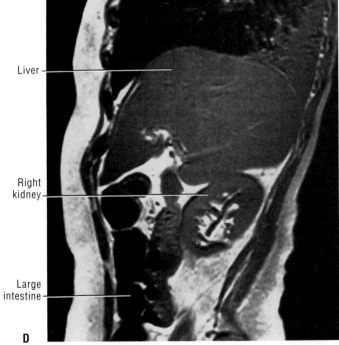

Liver
Right kidney
Large intestine

D

2.113
MRIs (magnetic resonance images) of the abdomen and pelvis

Note that the location of the plane of section for each image is shown on **A**. **A** is a coronal scan. **B**, **C**, and **D** are sagittal scans. (Courtesy of Dr. W. Kucharczyk, Clinical Director of Tri-Hospital Resonance Centre, Toronto, Ontario, Canada.)

3   The Perineum and Pelvis

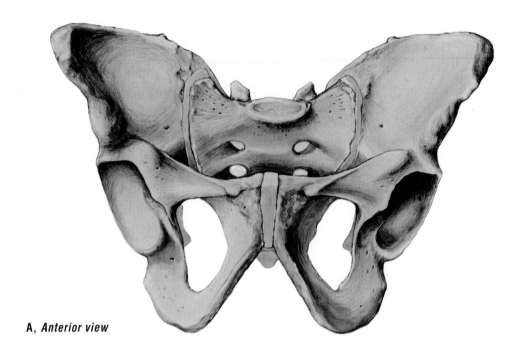

A, *Anterior view*

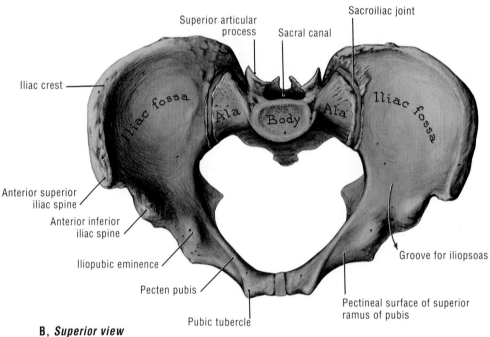

Superior articular
process

Sacral canal

Sacroiliac joint

Iliac crest

Iliac fossa

Ala

Body

Ala

Iliac fossa

Anterior superior
iliac spine

Anterior inferior
iliac spine

Iliopubic eminence

Groove for iliopsoas

Pecten pubis

Pectineal surface of superior
ramus of pubis

Pubic tubercle

B, *Superior view*

3.1
Male pelvis

A and **B.** The pelvis major (false pelvis) is formed by the iliac fossae and the alae of the sacrum. The pelvis minor (true pelvis) is formed by the inner surface of ischium, pubis, some ilium, sacrum, and coccyx. The groove between the anterior inferior iliac spine and the iliopubic eminence conducts the iliopsoas muscle from the pelvis major to the thigh. **C.** Orientation of the pelvis. When the subject is standing in the anatomical position, note that the anterior superior iliac spines and the anterior aspect of the pubic symphysis lie in the same vertical plane.

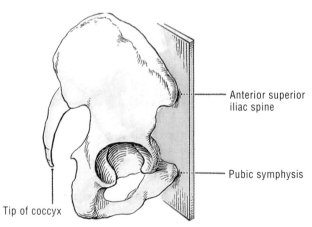

Anterior superior
iliac spine

Pubic symphysis

Tip of coccyx

C, *Lateral view*

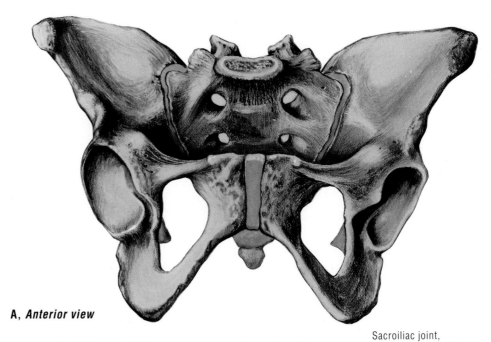

A, *Anterior view*

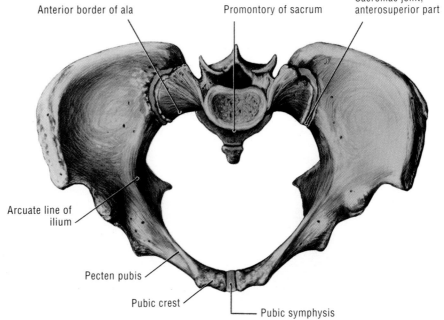

Anterior border of ala

Promontory of sacrum

Sacroiliac joint, anterosuperior part

Arcuate line of ilium

Pecten pubis

Pubic crest

Pubic symphysis

B, *Superior view*

3.2
Female pelvis

A and **B.** The pelvic brim, surrounding the superior pelvic aperture (pelvic inlet), is formed by three bones and three joints. The bones are: two hip bones (os coxae) and the sacrum. The joints are: the symphysis pubis and the two sacroiliac joints. The component parts of the pelvic brim are labeled on Figure 3.3. Compare the following features of the male and female pelvis: (a) the angle of the pubic arch; (b) the relative breadth of alae to body of sacrum; (c) the shape and dimensions of the pelvic brim.

3.3
Superior and inferior pelvic apertures, median section

In the anatomical position, the pelvis is tilted anteriorly so that the plane of the superior pelvic aperture (pelvic inlet) forms an angle of 50°-60° with the horizontal plane. Similarly, the inferior pelvic aperature (pelvic outlet) forms an angle of about 15° to the horizontal plane.

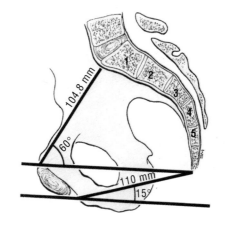

104.8 mm

60°

110 mm

15°

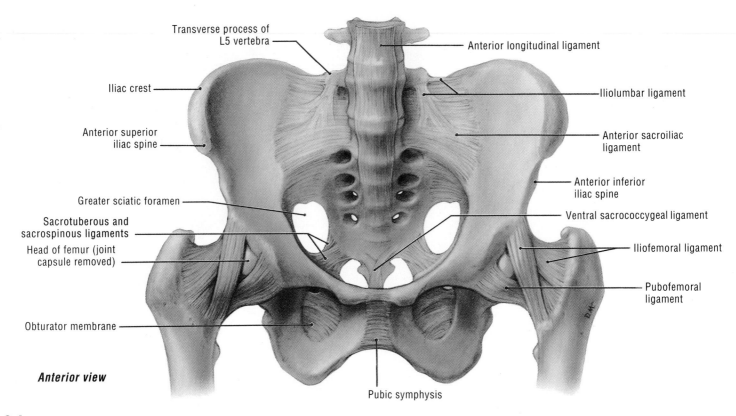

Transverse process of L5 vertebra

Iliac crest

Anterior superior iliac spine

Greater sciatic foramen

Sacrotuberous and sacrospinous ligaments

Head of femur (joint capsule removed)

Obturator membrane

Anterior view

Anterior longitudinal ligament

Iliolumbar ligament

Anterior sacroiliac ligament

Anterior inferior iliac spine

Ventral sacrococcygeal ligament

Iliofemoral ligament

Pubofemoral ligament

Pubic symphysis

3.4
Ligaments of the pelvis

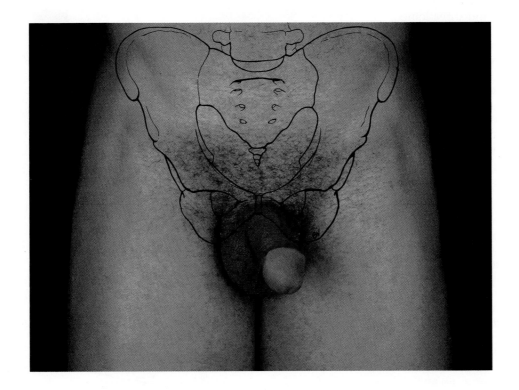

Anterior view

3.5
Pelvis in situ

Grant's Atlas of Anatomy

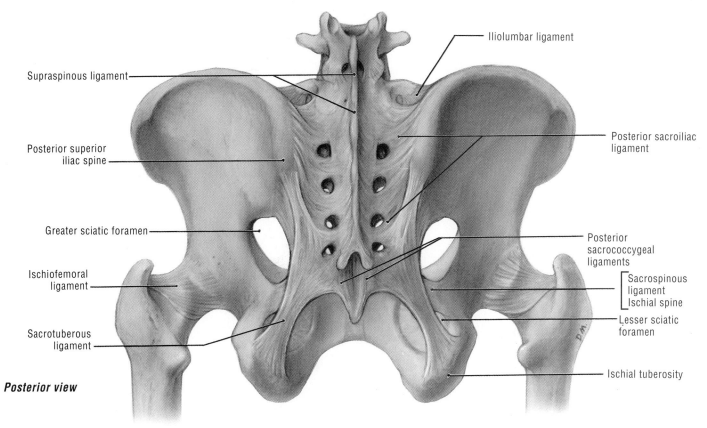

Supraspinous ligament

Iliolumbar ligament

Posterior superior
iliac spine

Posterior sacroiliac
ligament

Greater sciatic foramen

Posterior
sacrococcygeal
ligaments

Ischiofemoral
ligament

Sacrospinous
ligament
Ischial spine

Sacrotuberous
ligament

Lesser sciatic
foramen

Ischial tuberosity

Posterior view

3.6
Ligaments of the pelvis

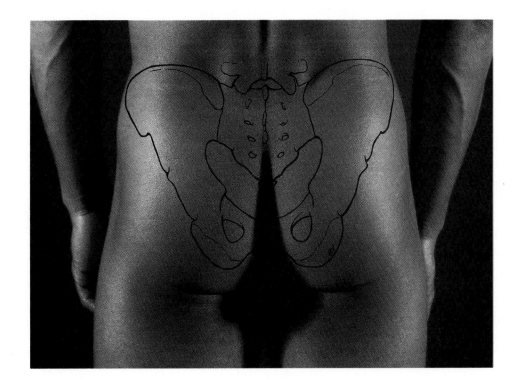

Posterior view

3.7
Pelvis in situ

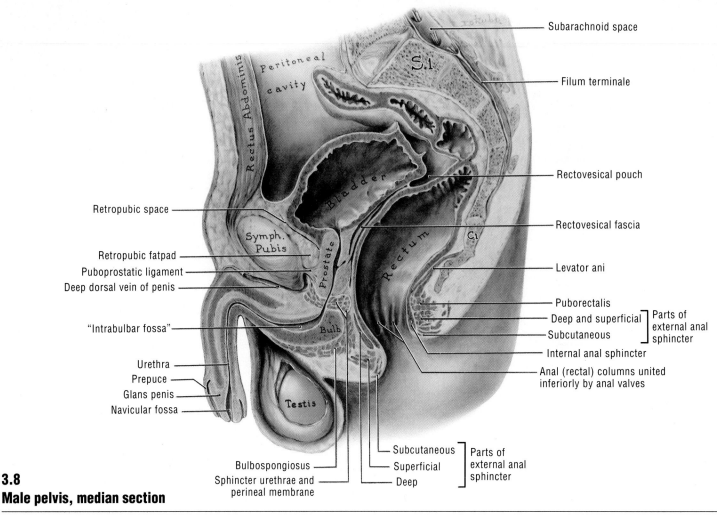

3.8
Male pelvis, median section

Observe:

1. The urinary bladder slightly distended and resting on the rectum; the prostatic urethra descending vertically through a somewhat elongated prostate and showing the prostatic utricle opening on to its posterior wall; the short membranous urethra passing through the deep perineal space; the spongy urethra with a low-lying dilation in the bulb and another in the glans penis; and the bulbospongiosus muscle that by contracting, empties the urethra;

2. The involuntary internal anal sphincter not descending as far as the voluntary external anal sphincter, and separated from it by an areolar layer;

3. The two layers of rectovesical fascia in the median plane between bladder and rectum; on each side it contains the deferent duct (vas deferens), seminal vesicle, and vesical vessels;

4. The peritoneum passing from the abdominal wall superior to the symphysis to the distended bladder, over the bladder to line the rectovesical pouch, and then to cover the anterior aspect of the rectum;

5. The tunica vaginalis (not labeled), opened in order to expose the testis, which here happens to be rotated so that the epididymis is anterior.

3.9
Diagram of the peritoneum covering the male pelvic organs, median section

The peritoneum passes:
1 from the anterior abdominal wall;
2 superior to the pubic bone;
3 on the superior surface of the urinary bladder;
4 2 cm inferiorly on the posterior surface of the urinary bladder;
5 on the superior ends of the seminal vesicles;
6 posteriorly to line the rectovesical pouch;
7 to cover the rectum;
8 posteriorly to become the sigmoid mesocolon.

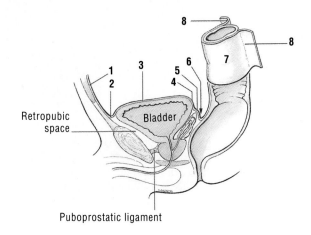

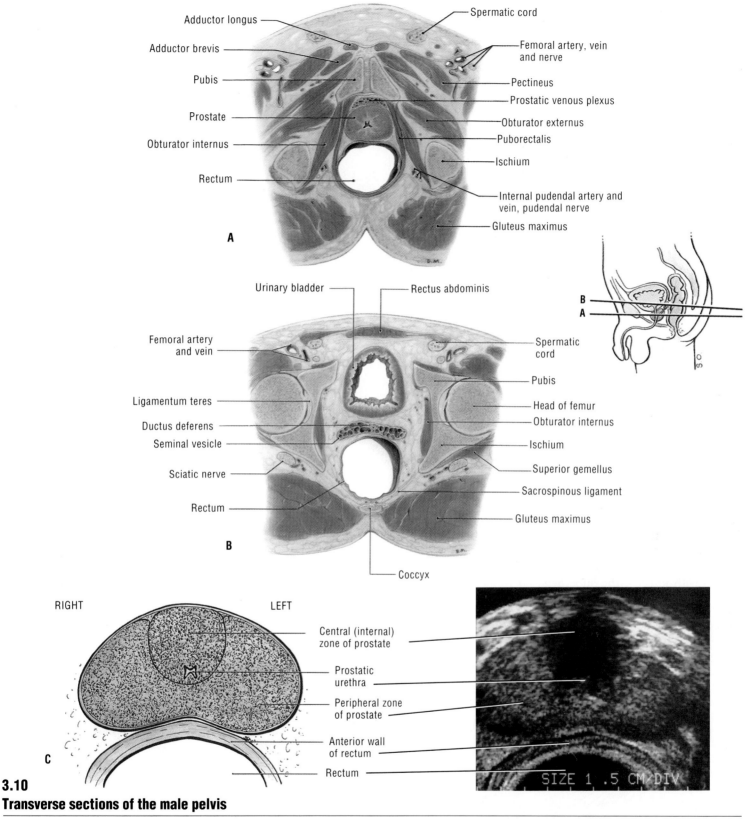

Adductor longus

Adductor brevis

Pubis

Prostate

Obturator internus

Rectum

Spermatic cord

Femoral artery, vein
and nerve

Pectineus

Prostatic venous plexus

Obturator externus

Puborectalis

Ischium

Internal pudendal artery and
vein, pudendal nerve

Gluteus maximus

A

Urinary bladder

Rectus abdominis

Femoral artery
and vein

Ligamentum teres

Ductus deferens

Seminal vesicle

Sciatic nerve

Rectum

Spermatic
cord

Pubis

Head of femur

Obturator internus

Ischium

Superior gemellus

Sacrospinous ligament

Gluteus maximus

B

Coccyx

RIGHT

LEFT

Central (internal)
zone of prostate

Prostatic
urethra

Peripheral zone
of prostate

Anterior wall
of rectum

Rectum

C

SIZE 1 .5 CM/DIV

3.10
Transverse sections of the male pelvis

A and **B**. Transverse sections of the male pelvis with orientation drawing on the right. **C**. Transverse (transrectal) ultrasound scan on the right and orientation drawing on the left. The probe was inserted into the rectum to scan the anteriorly located prostate. The ducts of the glands in the peripheral zone open into the prostatic sinuses, whereas the ducts of the glands in the central (internal) zone open into the prostatic sinuses and the seminal colliculus. The large peripheral zone is the usual site for carcinomas. (Courtesy of Dr. A.M. Arenson, Assistant Professor of Radiology, University of Toronto, Toronto, Ontario, Canada.)

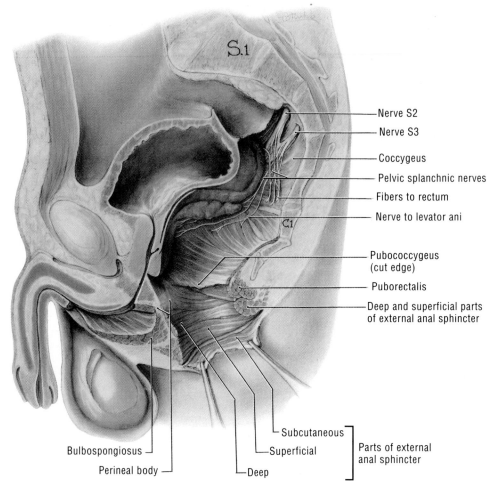

Nerve S2
Nerve S3
Coccygeus
Pelvic splanchnic nerves
Fibers to rectum
Nerve to levator ani

Pubococcygeus
(cut edge)
Puborectalis
Deep and superficial parts
of external anal sphincter

Bulbospongiosus
Perineal body

Subcutaneous
Superficial
Deep

Parts of external
anal sphincter

3.11
External anal sphincter and levator ani

This is Figure 3.8 from which the rectum, anal canal, and bulb of the penis are removed.

Observe:

1. The subcutaneous fibers of external anal sphincter held reflected with forceps; the superficial fibers mingling posteriorly with deep fibers; and deep fibers mingling posteriorly with puborectalis (inferior fibers of pubococcygeus), which forms a sling that occupies the angle between the rectum and the anal canal;

2. The pubococcygeus divided to allow the removal of the anal canal to which it is, in part, attached;

3. The ampulla of the deferent duct and seminal vesicle curving to fit the cyclindrical rectum.

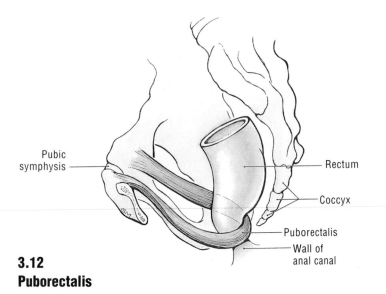

Pubic
symphysis
Rectum
Coccyx
Puborectalis
Wall of
anal canal

3.12
Puborectalis

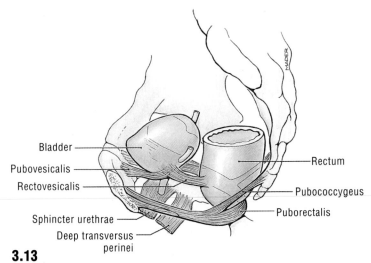

Bladder
Pubovesicalis
Rectovesicalis
Sphincter urethrae
Deep transversus
perinei
Rectum
Pubococcygeus
Puborectalis

3.13
Pubovesicalis and rectovesicalis

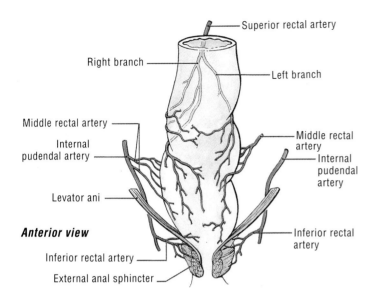

Anterior view

3.14
Arteries of the rectum and anal canal

The levator ani muscles are semidiagrammatic.

Observe:

1. The branches of the right and left divisions of the superior rectal artery obliquely encircling the rectum;

2. The middle rectal arteries (branches of the internal iliac arteries) are usually small; in this specimen the right artery is small, but the left one is large and partly replaces the left division of the superior rectal artery;

3. The inferior rectal arteries branching from the internal pudendal arteries;

4. Similarly, venous drainage is via superior, middle, and inferior rectal veins; there is a rich anastomosis between all three; since the superior rectal vein drains into the portal system while middle and inferior veins drain into the systemic, this is an important area of portal caval anastomosis.

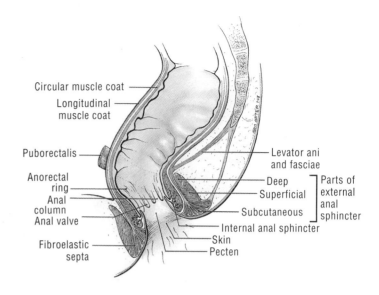

3.15
Anal sphincters and anal canal

In this median section, observe:

1. The internal anal sphincter is a thickening of the inner circular muscular coat of the canal;

2. The three parts of the external anal sphincter; its deep part is associated with the puborectalis muscle posteriorly;

3. Anal columns: vertical folds of mucosa containing twigs of superior rectal artery and vein; varicosity of these veins produces internal hemorrhoids;

4. Varicosity of the veins draining the end of the anal canal, inferior rectal veins, produces external hemorrhoids;

5. The pecten, or smooth zone of simple stratified epithelium, between the anal valves superiorly and the inferior border of the internal sphincter inferiorly; it is transitional between intestinal mucosa superiorly and skin having dermal papillae and appendages inferiorly.

3.16
Innervation of the rectum

In this schematic drawing, observe:
1. On the right: the voluntary external anal sphincter and skin around the anus innervated by the inferior rectal nerve, a branch of the pudendal nerve (S2, S3, and S4);

2. On the left: the autonomic innervation from the parasympathetic pelvic splanchnic nerves (S2, S3, and S4) and the sympathetic hypogastric nerves, from the superior hypogastric plexus, and the visceral (sacral) splanchnic nerves from the 2nd and 3rd sacral sympathetic ganglia; the sympathetic and parasympathetic fibers become intermingled in the inferior hypogastric plexus, located on the lateral walls of the rectum; the fibers are conveyed from the plexus to the wall of the rectum and the involuntary internal anal sphincter.

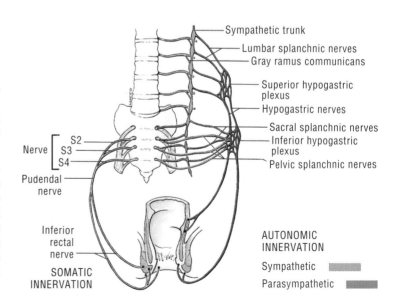

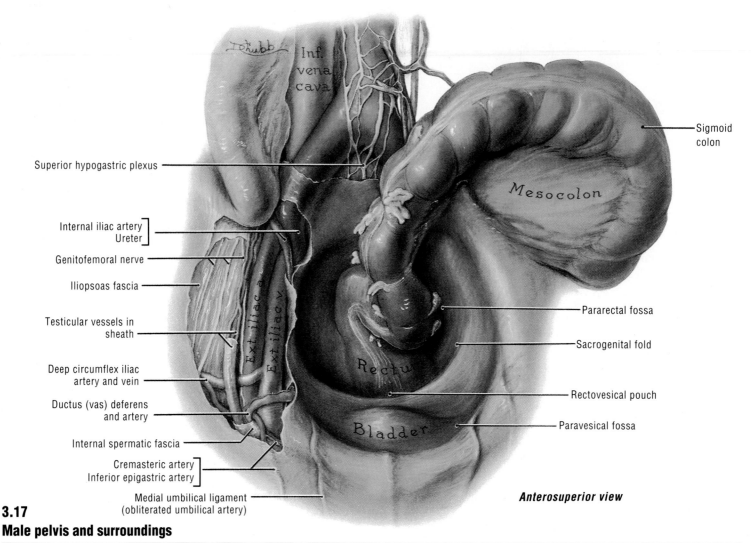

Superior hypogastric plexus

Internal iliac artery
Ureter

Genitofemoral nerve

Iliopsoas fascia

Testicular vessels in sheath

Deep circumflex iliac artery and vein

Ductus (vas) deferens and artery

Internal spermatic fascia

Cremasteric artery
Inferior epigastric artery

Medial umbilical ligament (obliterated umbilical artery)

Sigmoid colon

Mesocolon

Inf. vena cava

Rectum

Bladder

Pararectal fossa

Sacrogenital fold

Rectovesical pouch

Paravesical fossa

Anterosuperior view

3.17
Male pelvis and surroundings

Observe:

1. One limb of the inverted V-shaped root of the sigmoid mesocolon ascending near the external iliac vessels; the other descending to the sacrum;

2. The teniae coli forming two wide bands; one anterior to the rectum, the other posterior;

3. The superior hypogastric plexus lying in the fork of the aorta and anterior to the left common iliac vein;

4. The ureter adhering to the peritoneum, crossing the external iliac vessels, and descending anterior to the internal iliac artery; the ductus deferens and its artery also adhering to the peritoneum, crossing the external iliac vessels, and then hooking round the inferior epigastric artery to join the other constituents of the spermatic cord;

5. The genitofemoral nerve on the psoas fascia; its two lateral (femoral) branches become cutaneous; its medial (genital) branch supplies the cremaster muscle and becomes cutaneous.

3.18
Course of the ureter in the abdomen and pelvis

This diagram explains developmentally how the ureter comes to be crossed by testicular vessels in the abdomen and by the deferent duct in the pelvis.

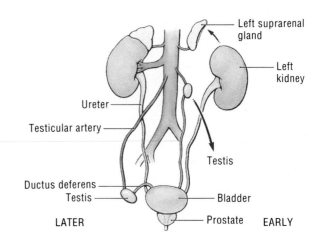

Left suprarenal gland

Left kidney

Ureter

Testicular artery

Testis

Ductus deferens
Testis

Bladder

Prostate

LATER

EARLY

Grant's Atlas of Anatomy

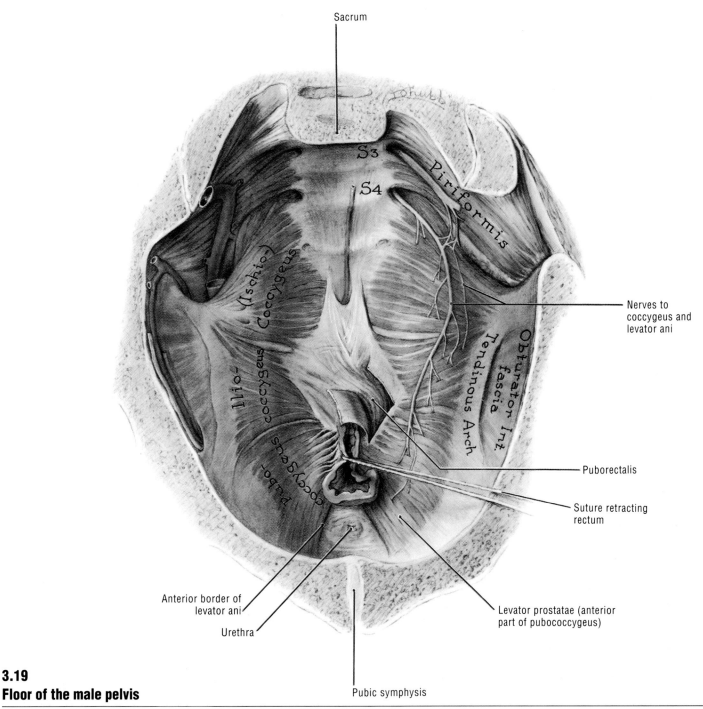

Sacrum

S3

S4

Piriformis

(Ischio) Coccygeus

Ilio-coccygeus

Pubo coccygeus

Coccygeus

Obturator Int. fascia Tendinous Arch

Nerves to coccygeus and levator ani

Puborectalis

Suture retracting rectum

Levator prostatae (anterior part of pubococcygeus)

Anterior border of levator ani

Urethra

Pubic symphysis

3.19
Floor of the male pelvis

The pelvic viscera are removed and the bony pelvis is sawn through transversely to demonstrate the levatores ani and coccygei muscles.

Observe:

1. The pubococcygeus muscle arising mainly from the pubic bone, the ischiococcygeus muscle from the ischial spine, and the iliococcygeus muscle from the tendinous arch in between; the pubococcygeus muscle is strong; the iliococcygeus muscle is weak; the ischiococcygeus muscle is largely transformed into the sacrospinous ligament; the pubo- and iliococcygei muscles together constitute the levator ani muscle;

2. The anterior free border of the pubococcygeus muscle, the posterior free border of the ischiococcygeus muscle; the clefts at the borders of the iliococcygeus muscle closed by areolar membranes;

3. The urethra passing between the anterior borders of the pubococcygei muscles; the rectum perforating the pubococcygei muscles, thus: (a) the anterior fibers of the muscles of opposite sides meet and unite in the central tendon of the perineum (perineal body) anterior to the rectum; (b) the posterior fibers unite posterior to the rectum in an aponeurosis that extends posteriorly to the anterior sacrococcygeal ligament; (c) the middle fibers blend with the outer wall of the anal canal and pass between internal and external anal sphincters;

4. Branches of S3 and S4 supplying the levator ani and coccygeus muscles; the pudendal nerve, via its perineal branch, also supplies the levator ani muscle.

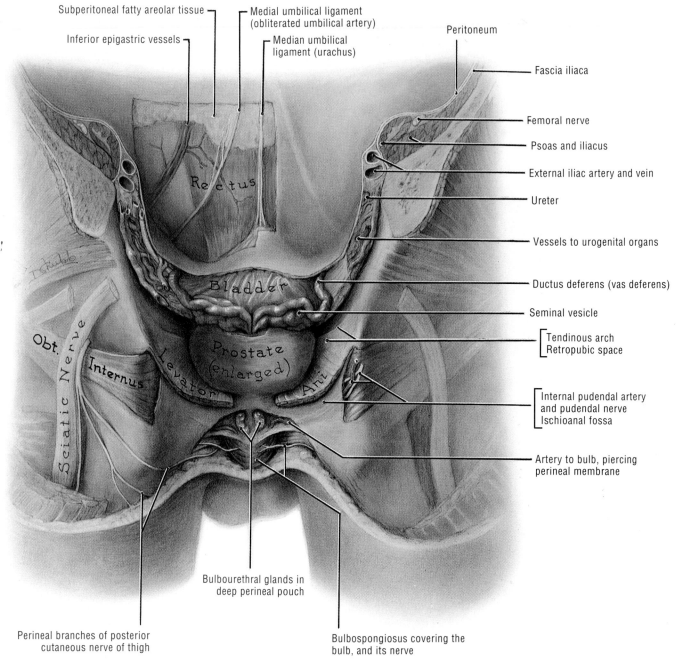

Subperitoneal fatty areolar tissue

Inferior epigastric vessels

Medial umbilical ligament
(obliterated umbilical artery)

Median umbilical
ligament (urachus)

Peritoneum

Fascia iliaca

Rectus

Femoral nerve

Psoas and iliacus

External iliac artery and vein

Ureter

Vessels to urogenital organs

Bladder

Ductus deferens (vas deferens)

Seminal vesicle

Tendinous arch
Retropubic space

Obt. Nerve

Sciatic Nerve

Internus

Levator

Prostate
(enlarged)

Ani

Internal pudendal artery
and pudendal nerve
Ischioanal fossa

Artery to bulb, piercing
perineal membrane

Bulbourethral glands in
deep perineal pouch

Bulbospongiosus covering the
bulb, and its nerve

Perineal branches of posterior
cutaneous nerve of thigh

3.20
Coronal section of the male pelvis

The section is through the pelvis just anterior to the rectum. The view is of the anterior portion from behind.

Observe:

1. The inferior epigastric artery and venae comitantes entering the rectus sheath, while the medial umbilical ligament (obliterated umbilical artery) and the median umbilical ligament (urachus), like the bladder, remain subperitoneal; the peritoneal folds having these three structures in their free edges are called: lateral, medial, and median umbilical folds.

2. The femoral nerve lying between psoas and iliacus muscles outside the psoas fascia, which is attached to the pelvic brim, while the external iliac artery and vein lie inside;

3. The ductus deferens and ureter, both subperitoneal; near the bladder, the ureter accompanying a leash of vesical vessels enclosed in rectovesical fascia;

4. The levator ani muscle and its fascial coverings separating the retropubic space from the ischioanal fossa;

5. The free, anterior borders of the levatores ani muscles;

6. The bulbourethral glands and the artery to the bulb lying superior to the perineal membrane (inferior fascia of the urogenital diaphragm), i.e., in the deep perineal space;

7. The obturator internus muscle making a right-angled turn as it escapes from its osseofascial pocket.

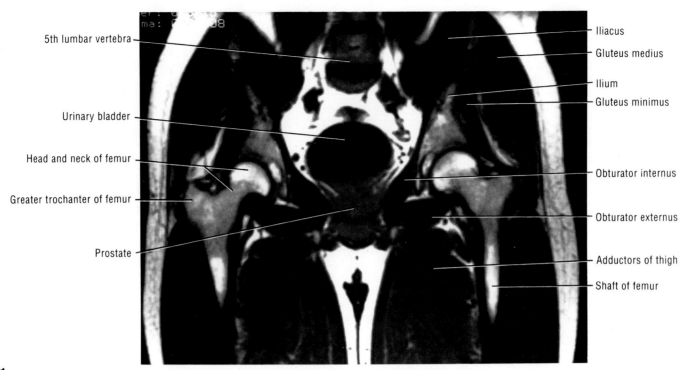

5th lumbar vertebra

Urinary bladder

Head and neck of femur

Greater trochanter of femur

Prostate

Iliacus

Gluteus medius

Ilium

Gluteus minimus

Obturator internus

Obturator externus

Adductors of thigh

Shaft of femur

3.21
Coronal MRI (magnetic resonance image) of the male pelvis

(Courtesy of Dr. W. Kucharczyk, Clinical Director of Tri-Hospital Resonance Centre, Toronto, Ontario, Canada.)

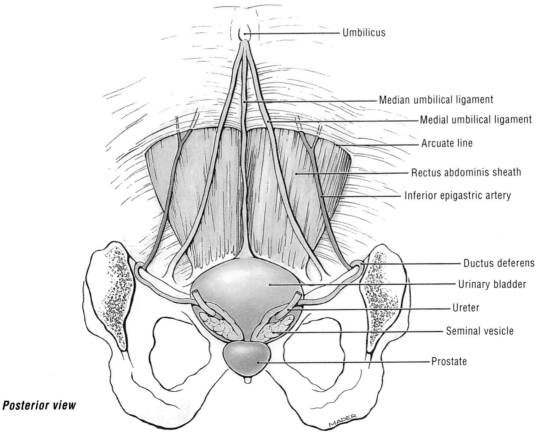

Umbilicus

Median umbilical ligament

Medial umbilical ligament

Arcuate line

Rectus abdominis sheath

Inferior epigastric artery

Ductus deferens

Urinary bladder

Ureter

Seminal vesicle

Prostate

Posterior view

3.22
Diagram of the anterior abdominal wall, bladder, and prostate

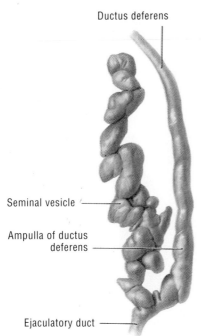

Ductus deferens

Seminal vesicle

Ampulla of ductus deferens

Ejaculatory duct

3.23
Seminal vesicle, unraveled

The vesicle is a tortuous tube with numerous outpouchings. The ampulla of the ductus deferens (vas deferens) has similar outpouchings.

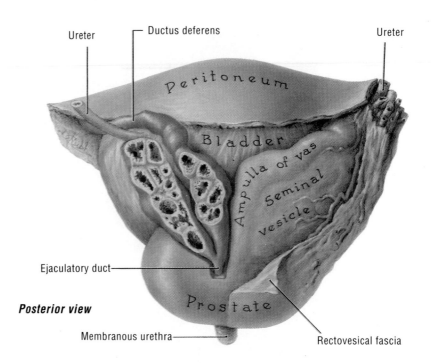

Ureter

Ductus deferens

Ureter

Peritoneum

Bladder

Ampulla of vas

Seminal vesicle

Ejaculatory duct

Posterior view

Prostate

Membranous urethra

Rectovesical fascia

3.24
Bladder, deferent ducts, seminal vesicles, and prostate

The left seminal vesicle and ampulla of the ductus deferens are dissected free and sliced open; part of the prostate is cut away to expose the ejaculatory duct.

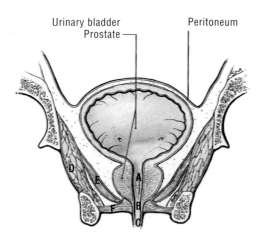

Urinary bladder
Prostate

Peritoneum

3.25
Coronal section of the male pelvis through the urinary bladder and prostate

Observe:
1. The parts of the urethra: prostatic *(A)*, membranous *(B)*, and spongy *(C)*;

2. The obturator internus *(D)* and levator ani *(E)* muscles and the urogenital diaphragm *(F)*.

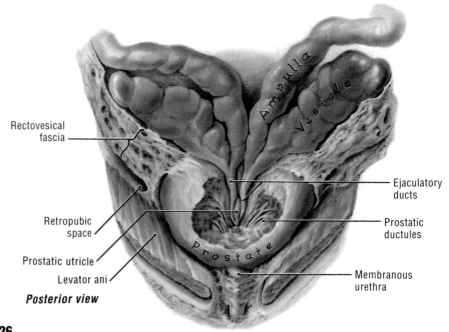

Rectovesical fascia

Ampulla

Vesicle

Ejaculatory ducts

Retropubic space

Prostatic ductules

Prostatic utricle

Levator ani

Prostate

Membranous urethra

Posterior view

3.26
Dissection of prostate

Observe:
1. The right and the left ejaculatory ducts, each formed where the duct of a seminal vesicle joins the ampullary end of a deferent duct;

2. The prostatic utricle, lying in between the ends of the two ejaculatory ducts, and all three are flattened from side to side; all three opened into the prostatic urethra;

3. The prostatic ductules, in all about 63 in number and mostly opening on to the prostatic sinus.

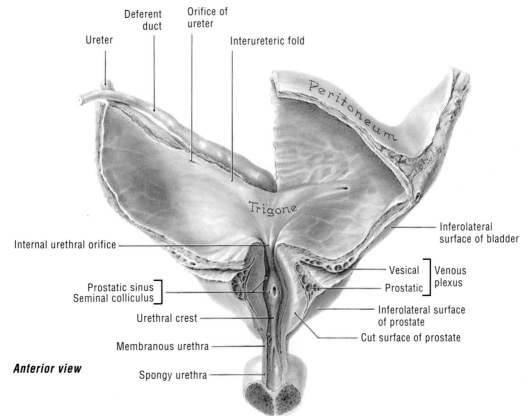

Ureter
Deferent duct
Orifice of ureter
Interureteric fold
Peritoneum
Trigone
Internal urethral orifice
Inferolateral surface of bladder
Prostatic sinus
Seminal colliculus
Vesical ⎤ Venous
Prostatic ⎦ plexus
Urethral crest
Inferolateral surface of prostate
Cut surface of prostate
Membranous urethra
Anterior view
Spongy urethra

3.27
Interior of the male urinary bladder and prostatic urethra

The anterior walls of the bladder, prostate, and urethra were cut away. The knife was then carried through the posterior wall of the bladder, at the right ureter and interureteric fold, which unites the two ureters along the superior limit of the smooth trigone.

Observe:
1. The right ureter not joining the bladder wall but traversing it obliquely as far as its slit-like orifice, which is situated 2-4 cm from the left orifice;

2. The mucous membrane, smooth over the trigone, but rugose elsewhere, especially when the bladder is empty;

3. The mouth of the prostatic utricle (not labeled) at the summit of the colliculus, on the urethral crest, and the orifice of an ejaculatory duct on each side of the utricle;

4. The urethral crest extending more superior than usual and bifurcating more inferior than usual;

5. The prostatic fascia enclosing a venous plexus.

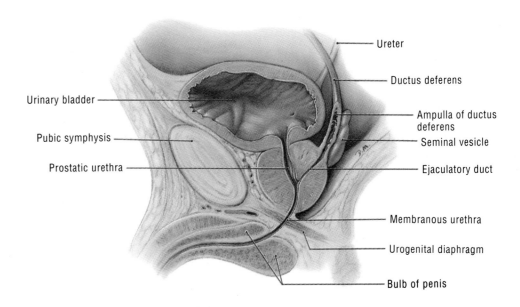

Ureter
Ductus deferens
Urinary bladder
Ampulla of ductus deferens
Pubic symphysis
Seminal vesicle
Prostatic urethra
Ejaculatory duct
Membranous urethra
Urogenital diaphragm
Bulb of penis

3.28
Sagittal section of bladder, prostate, and ductus deferens

Observe the ejaculatory duct (about 2 cm in length), formed by the union of the ductus deferens and the duct of the seminal vesicle, that passes anteriorly and inferiorly through the substance of the prostate to enter the prostatic urethra on the seminal colliculus.

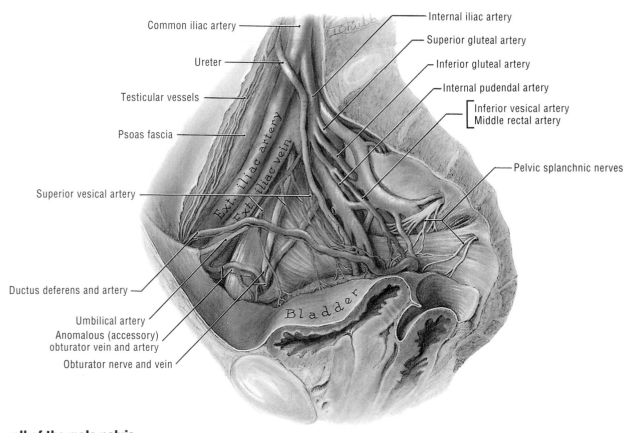

Common iliac artery

Ureter

Testicular vessels

Psoas fascia

Superior vesical artery

Ductus deferens and artery

Umbilical artery
Anomalous (accessory) obturator vein and artery

Obturator nerve and vein

Ext. iliac artery
Ext. iliac vein

Bladder

Internal iliac artery

Superior gluteal artery

Inferior gluteal artery

Internal pudendal artery

Inferior vesical artery
Middle rectal artery

Pelvic splanchnic nerves

3.29
Lateral wall of the male pelvis

Observe:

1. The ureter and ductus deferens running a strictly subperitoneal course across the external iliac vessels, umbilical artery, obturator nerve and vessels, and each receiving a branch from a vesical artery; the ureter crosses the exterior iliac artery at its origin (at common iliac bifurcation); the ductus crosses the external iliac artery at its termination (at the deep inguinal ring);

2. The umbilical artery, obliterated beyond the origin of the last superior vesical artery and creating a peritoneal fold;

3. An anomalous obturator artery here springing from the inferior epigastric artery; there are both a normal and an anomalous obturator vein;

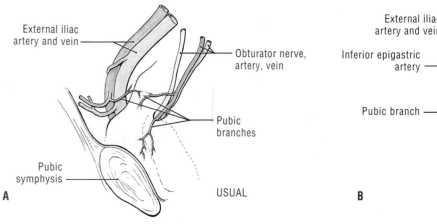

External iliac artery and vein

Obturator nerve, artery, vein

Pubic branches

Pubic symphysis

A   USUAL

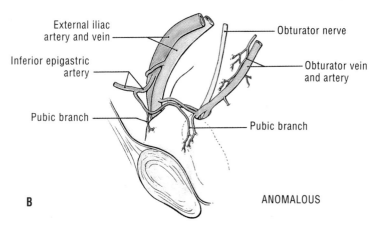

External iliac artery and vein

Inferior epigastric artery

Pubic branch

Obturator nerve

Obturator vein and artery

Pubic branch

B   ANOMALOUS

3.30
Usual and anomalous obturator arteries

A. The pubic branch of the obturator artery anastomoses posterior to the body of the pubis with the pubic branch of the inferior epigastric artery. **B.** The obturator artery arises from the inferior epigastric via the pubic anastomoses.

In a study of 283 limbs, the obturator artery arose from the internal iliac in 70%, from the inferior epigastric in 25.4%, and nearly equally from both in 4.6%.

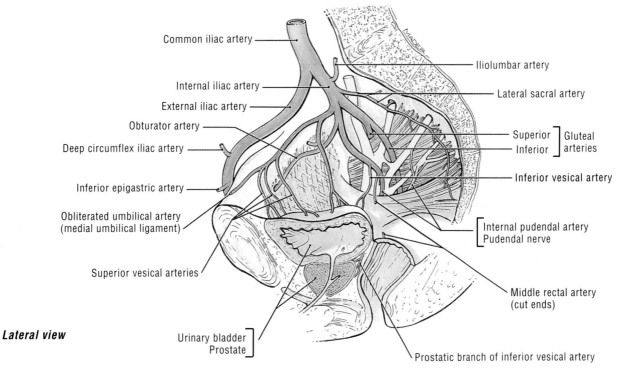

Common iliac artery

Internal iliac artery

External iliac artery

Obturator artery

Deep circumflex iliac artery

Inferior epigastric artery

Obliterated umbilical artery
(medial umbilical ligament)

Superior vesical arteries

Iliolumbar artery

Lateral sacral artery

Superior ⎤ Gluteal
Inferior ⎦ arteries

Inferior vesical artery

Internal pudendal artery
Pudendal nerve

Middle rectal artery
(cut ends)

Lateral view

Urinary bladder ⎤
Prostate ⎦

Prostatic branch of inferior vesical artery

3.31
Iliac arteries and their branches in the male

Observe:

1. The common iliac artery having two terminal branches, but no collateral branches;

2. The external iliac artery having two collateral branches, and ending as the femoral artery;

3. The internal iliac artery ending as an anterior and a posterior division; from these, branches arise variably; commonly, as here, the iliolumbar artery, lateral sacral artery, and superior gluteal artery spring from the posterior division; the others spring from the anterior division;

4. Of the 10 branches of the internal iliac artery, the obliterated umbilical, which in the fetus passed to the placenta, and three others are visceral; two supply the 5th lumbar and the sacral segments and are somatic segmental; three enter the gluteal region; and one passes to the anterior aspect of the thigh.

3.32
Iliac arteriogram

Injection has been made into the aorta in the lumbar region.

Observe:
1. The bifurcation of the aorta into right and left common iliac arteries (anterior to L4);

2. The bifurcation of the common iliacs into internal and external iliac arteries (opposite the sacroiliac joint, at the level of the lumbosacral disc). Consult Figure 3.31 for branches of the external and the internal iliac artery;

3. The *circled area* on the arteriogram indicates a site of narrowing (stenosis) of the right common iliac artery. (Courtesy of Dr. D. Sniderman, Associate Professor of Radiology, University of Toronto, Toronto, Ontario, Canada.)

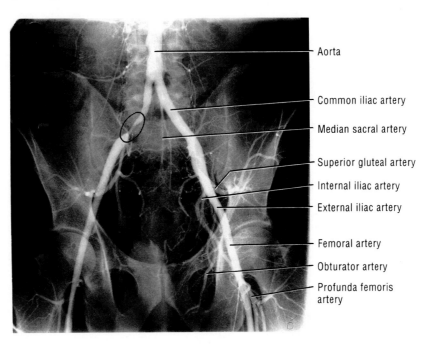

Aorta

Common iliac artery

Median sacral artery

Superior gluteal artery

Internal iliac artery

External iliac artery

Femoral artery

Obturator artery

Profunda femoris
artery

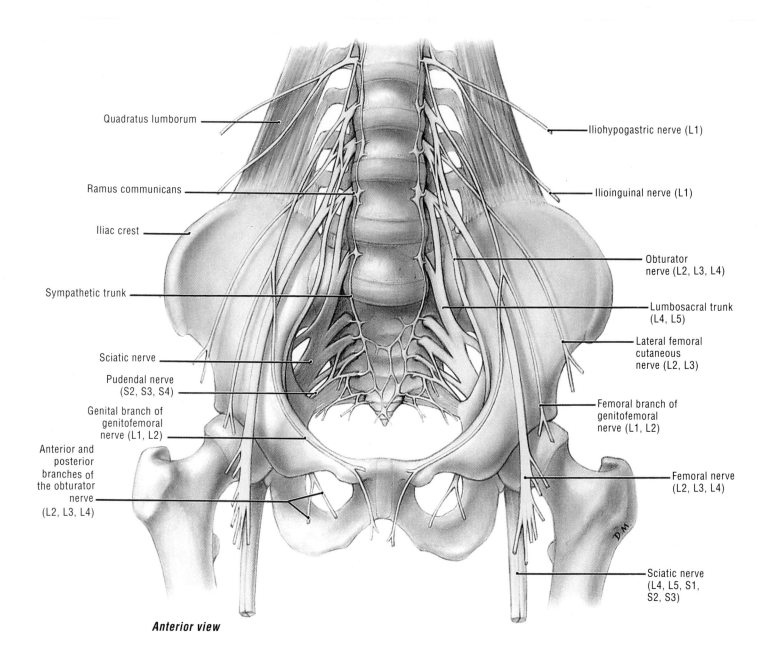

Quadratus lumborum

Ramus communicans

Iliac crest

Sympathetic trunk

Sciatic nerve

Pudendal nerve
(S2, S3, S4)

Genital branch of
genitofemoral
nerve (L1, L2)

Anterior and
posterior
branches of
the obturator
nerve
(L2, L3, L4)

Iliohypogastric nerve (L1)

Ilioinguinal nerve (L1)

Obturator
nerve (L2, L3, L4)

Lumbosacral trunk
(L4, L5)

Lateral femoral
cutaneous
nerve (L2, L3)

Femoral branch of
genitofemoral
nerve (L1, L2)

Femoral nerve
(L2, L3, L4)

Sciatic nerve
(L4, L5, S1,
S2, S3)

Anterior view

3.33
Overview of the lumbosacral plexus

Observe:

1. The lumbosacral trunk providing continuity between the lumbar and sacral plexuses;

2. The ventral primary rami of (T12), L1, L2, L3, and L4 forming the lumbar plexus and the ventral primary rami of L4, L5 and S1, S2, and S3 forming the sacral plexus;

3. The sciatic nerve, passing posteriorly through the greater sciatic foramen to the gluteal region;

4. The femoral nerve splitting into many branches in the femoral triangle just distal to the inguinal ligament; the obturator nerve passing through the obturator foramen with the obturator artery and vein to supply the medial aspect of the thigh;

5. The rami communicantes connecting the sympathetic trunk and ganglia with the ventral primary rami of the lumbosacral plexus.

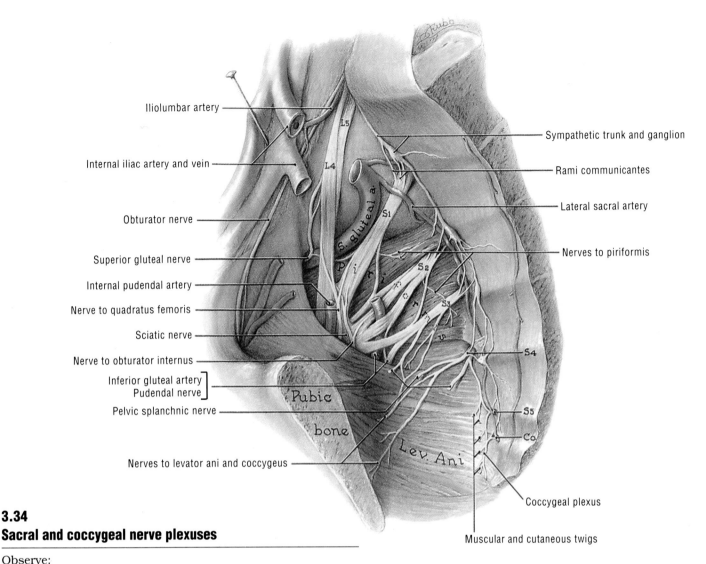

Iliolumbar artery

Internal iliac artery and vein

Obturator nerve

Superior gluteal nerve

Internal pudendal artery

Nerve to quadratus femoris

Sciatic nerve

Nerve to obturator internus

Inferior gluteal artery
Pudendal nerve

Pelvic splanchnic nerve

Nerves to levator ani and coccygeus

Sympathetic trunk and ganglion

Rami communicantes

Lateral sacral artery

Nerves to piriformis

Coccygeal plexus

Muscular and cutaneous twigs

3.34
Sacral and coccygeal nerve plexuses

Observe:

1. Either the sympathetic trunk or its ganglia sending gray rami communicantes to each sacral nerve and the coccygeal nerve;

2. The branch from L4 joining L5 to form the lumbosacral trunk;

3. The roots of S1 and S2 supplying the piriformis muscle; S3 and S4 supplying the coccygeus and levator ani muscles; S2, S3, and S4 each contributing a branch to the formation of the pelvic splanchnic nerves;

4. The sciatic nerve springing from segments L4, L5, S1, S2, and S3; the pudendal nerve from S2, S3, and S4; the coccygeal plexus from S4, S5, and coccygeal segments;

5. The iliolumbar artery accompanying nerve L5; the branches of the lateral sacral artery accompanying the sacral nerves; the superior gluteal artery passing posteriorly between L5 and S1, its position is not constant;

3.35
Sacral plexus

The sacral plexus is pierced by the superior and inferior gluteal arteries that turn posteriorly, whereas the pudendal artery continues anteroinferiorly toward the ischial spine.

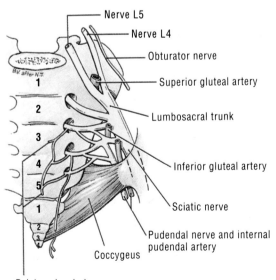

Nerve L5

Nerve L4

Obturator nerve

Superior gluteal artery

Lumbosacral trunk

Inferior gluteal artery

Sciatic nerve

Pudendal nerve and internal pudendal artery

Coccygeus

Pelvic splanchnic nerve

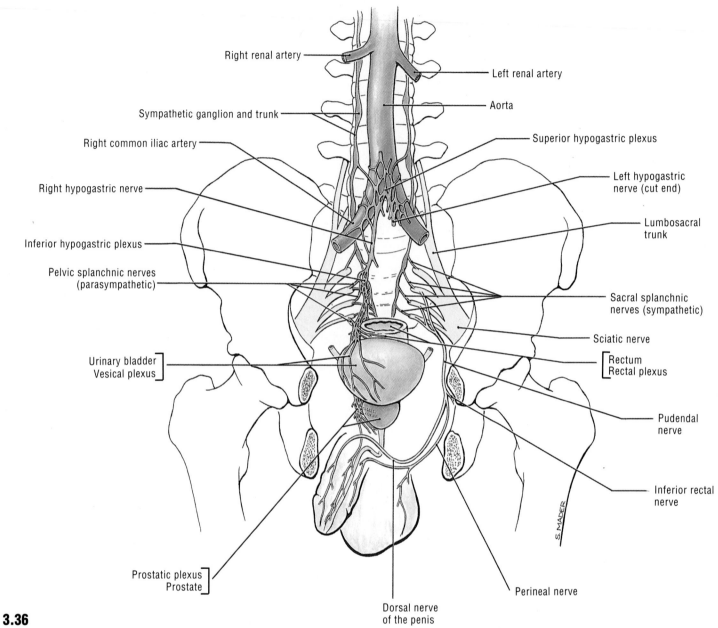

Right renal artery

Left renal artery

Aorta

Sympathetic ganglion and trunk

Superior hypogastric plexus

Right common iliac artery

Left hypogastric
nerve (cut end)

Right hypogastric nerve

Lumbosacral
trunk

Inferior hypogastric plexus

Pelvic splanchnic nerves
(parasympathetic)

Sacral splanchnic
nerves (sympathetic)

Sciatic nerve

Urinary bladder
Vesical plexus

Rectum
Rectal plexus

Pudendal
nerve

Inferior rectal
nerve

Prostatic plexus
Prostate

Perineal nerve

Dorsal nerve
of the penis

S. MADER

3.36
Innervation of the male pelvis

Observe:

1. The autonomic plexuses of the pelvis: the inferior hypogastric, the vesical, the middle rectal, and the prostatic; the pelvic plexuses consisting of both sympathetic and parasympathetic fibers; the right and left hypogastric nerves joining the superior hypogastric plexus to the inferior hypogastric plexus;

2. The right and left inferior hypogastric plexuses continuing as the vesical plexus supplying the urinary bladder, the seminal vesicles and deferent duct, as the middle rectal plexus supplying the rectum, and as the prostatic plexus supplying the prostate, seminal vesicles, corpus spongiosum, corpora cavernosum, and urethra;

3. The parasympathetic, pelvic splanchnic nerves arising

from the ventral primary rami of S2, S3, and S4 supplying motor fibers to the pelvic organs, and the sigmoid colon, splenic (left colic) flexure, and vasodilator fibers to the erectile tissue of the penis;

4. The sympathetic sacral splanchnic nerves arising from the sympathetic trunk and joining the inferior hypogastric plexuses; vasoconstrictor fibers innervating the male genital organs play an important role in ejaculation;

5. The pudendal nerve, a branch of the sacral plexus, arising from the ventral primary rami of S2, S3, and S4; this nerve is part of the voluntary somatic nervous system and can be seen innervating the perineal region.

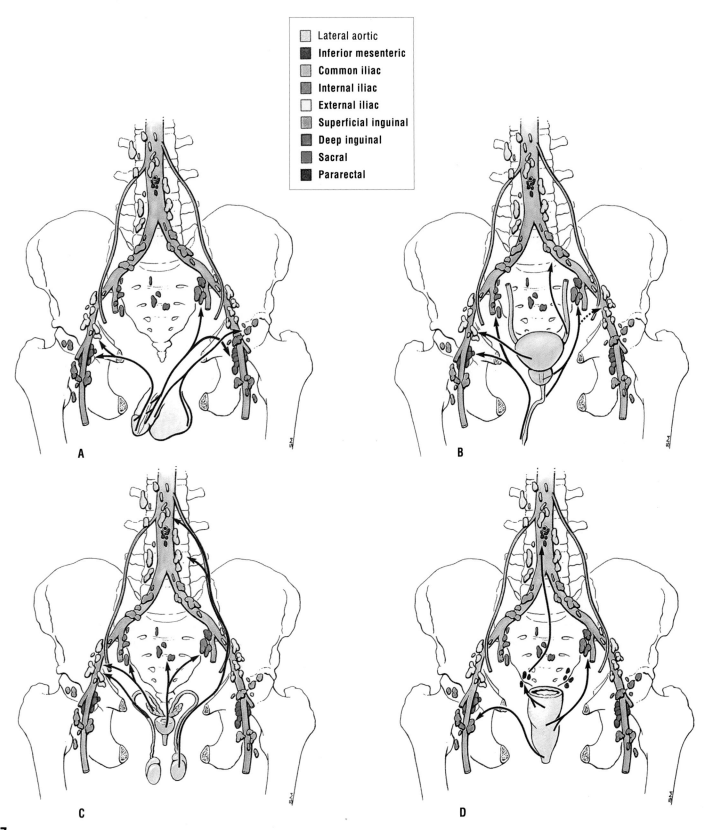

Lateral aortic
Inferior mesenteric
Common iliac
Internal iliac
External iliac
Superficial inguinal
Deep inguinal
Sacral
Pararectal

A

B

C

D

3.37
Lymphatic drainage of the male pelvis

A. Penis, scrotum and spongy urethra. **B**. Ureters, urinary bladder, prostate, and urethra. **C**. Testis, ductus deferens, prostate, and seminal vesicles. **D**. Rectum.

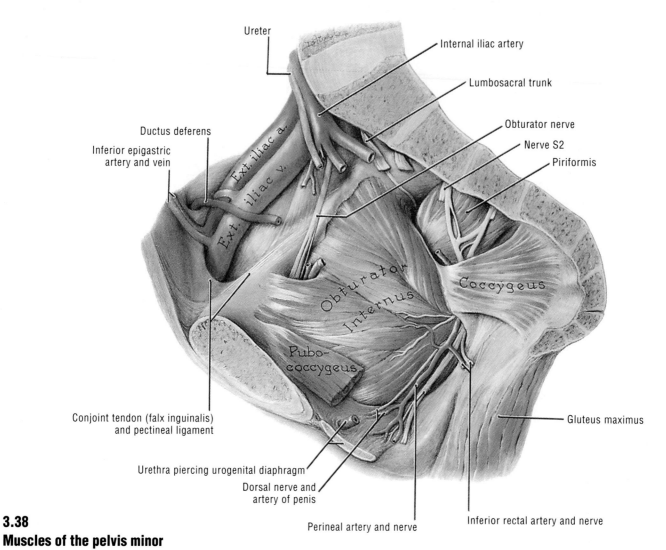

Ureter

Internal iliac artery

Lumbosacral trunk

Ductus deferens

Obturator nerve

Inferior epigastric
artery and vein

Nerve S2

Piriformis

Ext. iliac a.

Ext. iliac v.

Ext. iliac v.

Obturator
Internus

Coccygeus

Pubo-
coccygeus

Conjoint tendon (falx inguinalis)
and pectineal ligament

Gluteus maximus

Urethra piercing urogenital diaphragm

Dorsal nerve and
artery of penis

Perineal artery and nerve

Inferior rectal artery and nerve

3.38
Muscles of the pelvis minor

Observe:

1. The obturator internus muscle padding the side wall of the pelvis and escaping through the lesser sciatic foramen; its nerve is seen; the piriformis muscle padding the posterior wall and escaping through the greater sciatic foramen; the coccygeus muscle concealing the sacrospinous ligament; the pubococcygeus muscle, which is the chief and strongest part of levator ani muscle, springing from the body of the pubis;

2. The obturator nerve, artery, and vein escaping through the obturator foramen; the internal pudendal artery and the pudendal nerve making an exit through the greater sciatic foramen, and a re-entry through the lesser sciatic foramen, and then taking an anterior course (in the pudendal canal) within the obturator internus fascia to the urogenital diaphragm;

3. In the pelvis major, the deferent duct and the ureter descending across the external iliac artery and vein, the psoas fascia, and the pelvic brim to enter the pelvis minor (true pelvis).

3.39
Diagram of the pudendal nerve

Observe:
1. The five regions in which it runs:
Pelvis
Gluteal region
Pudendal canal
Urogenital diaphragm
Dorsum of penis

2. The three divisions into which it divides: inferior rectal nerve, perineal nerve, and dorsal nerve of penis.

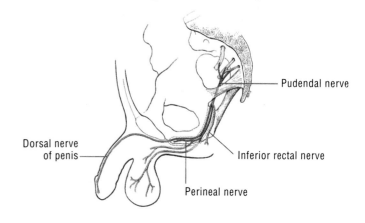

Pudendal nerve

Dorsal nerve
of penis

Inferior rectal nerve

Perineal nerve

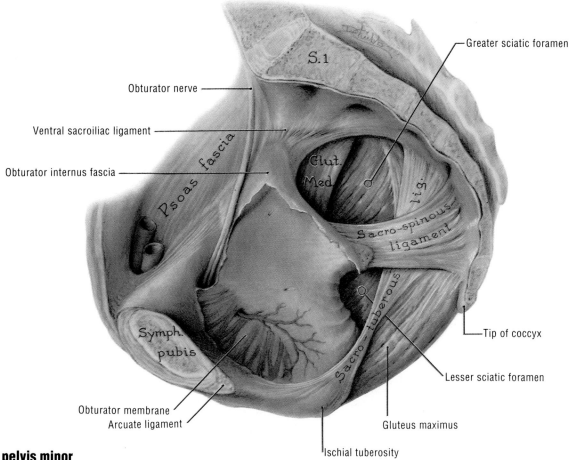

Greater sciatic foramen

Obturator nerve

Ventral sacroiliac ligament

Obturator internus fascia

S.1

Glut. Med.

Psoas fascia

Sacro-spinous-ligament

lig.

Tip of coccyx

Symph. pubis

Sacro-tuberous

Lesser sciatic foramen

Obturator membrane
Arcuate ligament

Gluteus maximus

Ischial tuberosity

3.40
Walls of the pelvis minor

Observe:

1. Anteriorly, the pubis; posteriorly, the sacrum and coccyx; posterolaterally, the coccyx and inferior part of the sacrum fastened to the ischial tuberosity by the sacrotuberous ligament and to the ischial spine by the sacrospinous ligament; the superior part of the sacrum joined to the ilium by the ventral sacroiliac ligament;

2. Anterosuperior to the sacrotuberous ligament, the greater and lesser sciatic foramina, the greater sciatic foramen being superior, and the lesser sciatic foramen inferior to the sacrospinous ligament;

3. Anterolaterally, the fascia covering the obturator internus muscle snipped away and the obturator internus muscle removed from its osseofascial pocket, thereby exposing the ischium and obturator membrane; the mouth of this pocket is the lesser sciatic foramen; through it the obturator internus muscle escapes from the pelvis, and the grooves made by its tendon are conspicuous;

4. Obturator internus fascia attached along the line of the obturator nerve superiorly; to the sacrotuberous ligament inferiorly; and to the posterior border of the body of the ischium posteriorly.

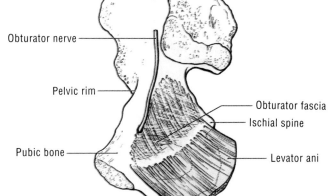

Obturator nerve

Pelvic rim

Pubic bone

Obturator fascia
Ischial spine

Levator ani

3.41
Origin of levator ani

The origin is from the body of the pubis, the ischial spine, and the tendinous arch in between.

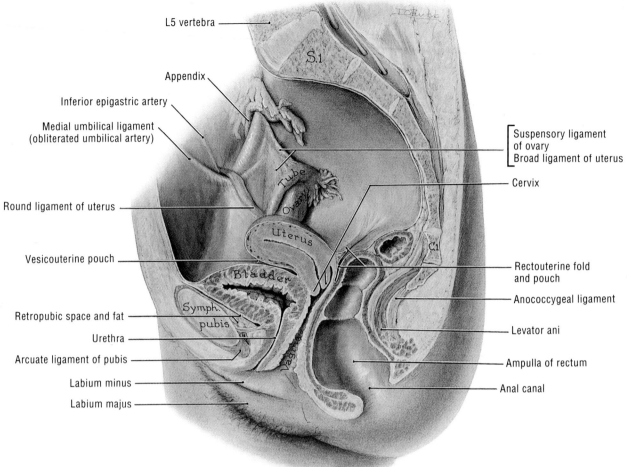

L5 vertebra

Appendix

Inferior epigastric artery

Medial umbilical ligament
(obliterated umbilical artery)

Round ligament of uterus

Vesicouterine pouch

Retropubic space and fat

Urethra

Arcuate ligament of pubis

Labium minus

Labium majus

Suspensory ligament
of ovary
Broad ligament of uterus

Cervix

Rectouterine fold
and pouch

Anococcygeal ligament

Levator ani

Ampulla of rectum

Anal canal

3.42
Female pelvis, median section

The uterus was sectioned in its own median plane and depicted as though this coincided with the median plane of the body, which is seldom the case.

Observe:
1. The uterine tube and the ovary, on the lateral wall of the pelvis, i.e., in the angle between ureter and the umbilical artery, and medial to the obturator nerve and vessels;

2. The uterus, bent on itself at the junction of body and cervix; the cervix, opening on the anterior wall of the vagina, and having a short, round, anterior lip and a long, thinner, posterior lip;

3. The ostium (external os) of the uterus, at the level of the superior aspect of the symphysis pubis;

4. The anterior fornix of the vagina, 1 cm or more from the vesicouterine pouch; the posterior fornix covered with 1 cm or more of the rectouterine pouch, which is the most inferior part of the peritoneal cavity, when the subject is erect;

5. The urethra (3 cm long), the vagina, and the rectum parallel to one another and to the pelvic brim; the uterus, nearly at right angles to them, when the bladder is empty.

3.43
Diagram of peritoneum covering the female pelvic organs

The peritoneum passes:
1 from the anterior abdominal wall;
2 superior to the pubic bone;
3 on the superior surface of the urinary bladder;
4 from the bladder to the uterus (vesicouterine pouch);
5 on the fundus and body of the uterus, the posterior fornix, and the wall of the vagina;
6 between the rectum and uterus (rectouterine pouch);
7 on the anterior and lateral sides of the rectum;
8 posteriorly to become the sigmoid mesocolon.

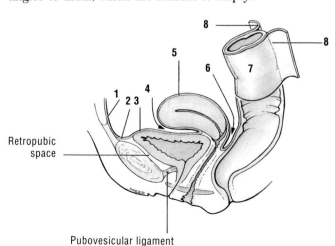

Retropubic space

Pubovesicular ligament

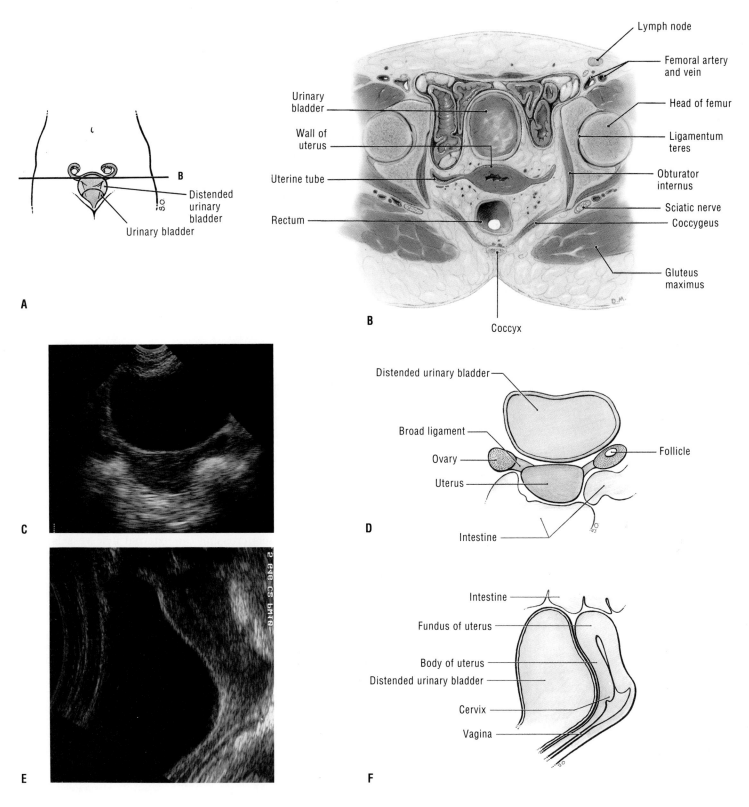

A. Level of section shown in **B**. **B**. Distended urinary bladder. Urinary bladder.

Labels in figure:
- Lymph node
- Femoral artery and vee
- Head of femur
- Ligamentum teres
- Obturator internus
- Sciatic nerve
- Coccygeus
- Gluteus maximus
- Coccyx
- Urinary bladder
- Wall of uterus
- Uterine tube
- Rectum
- Distended urinary bladder
- Broad ligament
- Ovary
- Uterus
- Follicle
- Intestine
- Fundus of uterus
- Body of uterus
- Distended urinary bladder
- Cervix
- Vagina

3.44
Female pelvis

A. Level of section shown in **B. B.** Transverse section. **C.** Transverse ultrasound scan. **D.** Diagram of transverse ultrasound scan shown in **C. E.** Sagittal ultrasound scan. The scan has been put in the same orientation as Figure 3.42. Note the distended bladder in the scan. **F.** Diagram of sagittal ultrasound scan shown in **E.** (Courtesy of Dr. A.M. Arenson, Assistant Professor of Radiology, University of Toronto, Toronto, Ontario, Canada.)

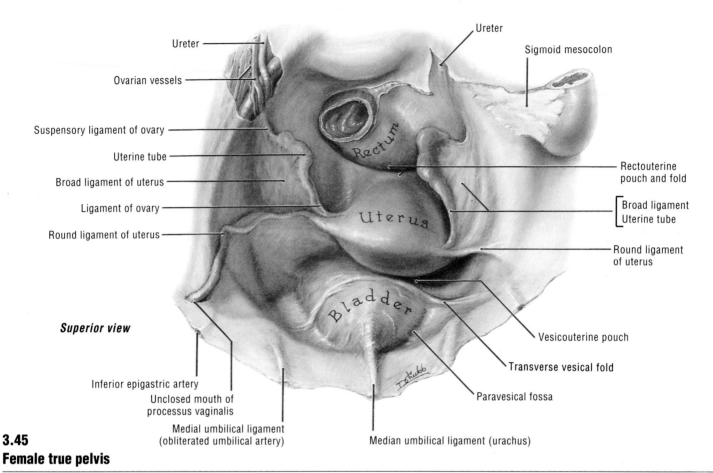

Ureter

Ureter

Sigmoid mesocolon

Ovarian vessels

Suspensory ligament of ovary

Uterine tube

Broad ligament of uterus

Ligament of ovary

Round ligament of uterus

Rectum

Uterus

Rectouterine pouch and fold

Broad ligament
Uterine tube

Round ligament of uterus

Bladder

Superior view

Vesicouterine pouch

Transverse vesical fold

Inferior epigastric artery

Unclosed mouth of processus vaginalis

Paravesical fossa

Medial umbilical ligament (obliterated umbilical artery)

Median umbilical ligament (urachus)

3.45
Female true pelvis

Observe:

1. The pear-shaped uterus asymmetrically placed, as usual; here leaning to the left;

2. The right round ligament of the uterus; here longer than the left and having an acquired "mesentery"; the round ligament of the female takes the same subperitoneal course as the deferent duct of the male;

3. The free edge of the medial four-fifths of the broad ligament occupied by the uterine tube (fallopian tube); the lateral one-fifth, occupied by the ovarian vessels, is the suspensory ligament of the ovary;

4. The ovarian vessels crossing the external iliac vessels very close to the ureter; the left ureter crossing at the apex of the inverted V-shaped root of the sigmoid mesocolon.

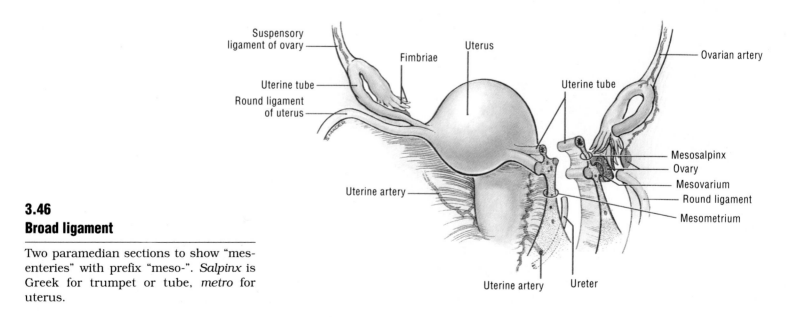

Suspensory ligament of ovary

Fimbriae

Uterus

Ovarian artery

Uterine tube

Round ligament of uterus

Uterine tube

Mesosalpinx

Ovary

Mesovarium

Round ligament

Uterine artery

Mesometrium

Uterine artery

Ureter

3.46
Broad ligament

Two paramedian sections to show "mesenteries" with prefix "meso-". *Salpinx* is Greek for trumpet or tube, *metro* for uterus.

Grant's Atlas of Anatomy

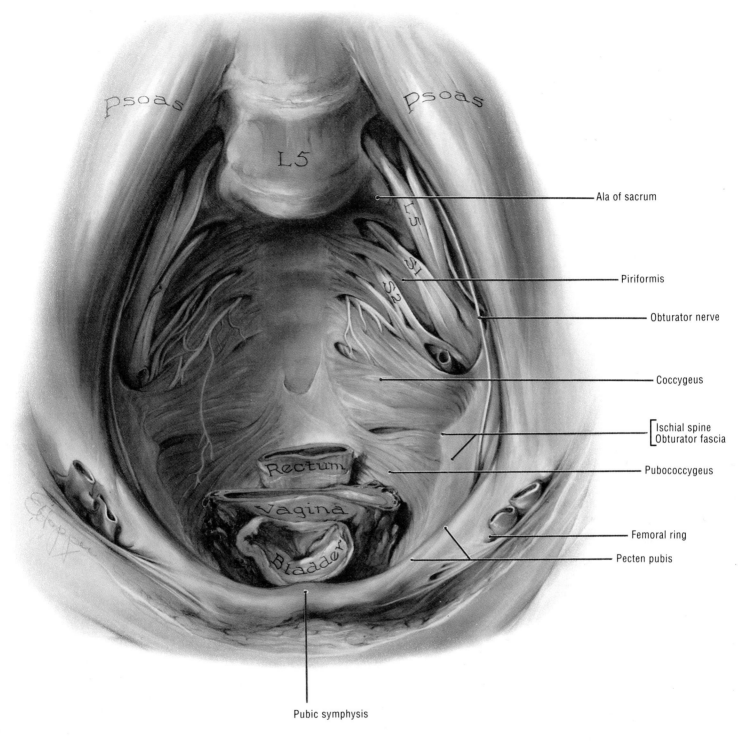

Psoas — Psoas

L5

L5
S1
S2

Ala of sacrum

Piriformis

Obturator nerve

Coccygeus

Ischial spine
Obturator fascia

Rectum

Vagina

Bladder

Pubococcygeus

Femoral ring

Pecten pubis

Pubic symphysis

3.47
Floor of the female pelvis

Observe:

1. The muscles of the pelvic floor;

2. The relative positions of the bladder, vagina, and rectum;

3. The obturator nerve, derived from lumbar nerves 2, 3, and 4, running along the lateral wall of the pelvis to enter the thigh through the obturator foramen;

4. The femoral ring, the doorway into the femoral canal, the site of femoral hernia.

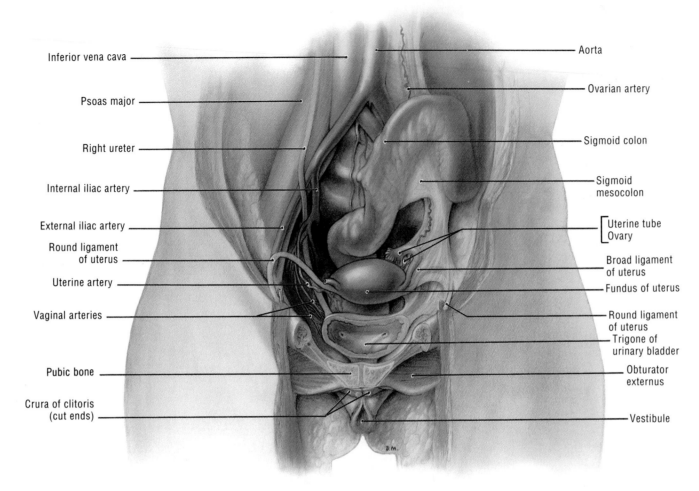

Inferior vena cava

Psoas major

Right ureter

Internal iliac artery

External iliac artery

Round ligament of uterus

Uterine artery

Vaginal arteries

Pubic bone

Crura of clitoris (cut ends)

Aorta

Ovarian artery

Sigmoid colon

Sigmoid mesocolon

Uterine tube
Ovary

Broad ligament of uterus

Fundus of uterus

Round ligament of uterus

Trigone of urinary bladder

Obturator externus

Vestibule

Anterosuperior view

3.48
Female genital organs

Part of the pubic bones, the anterior aspect of the bladder, and on the right side the uterine tube, ovary, broad ligament, and peritoneum covering the lateral wall of the pelvis have been removed. On the right, note the cut end of the uterine tube and the intact round ligament.

Observe:

1. The uterus asymmetrically placed, here leaning slightly to the left;

2. The uterine artery, lying with its veins in the base of the broad ligament and running superiorly along the lateral margin of the uterus;

3. The vaginal artery, a branch of the uterine artery, supplying the cervix and the anterior surface of the vagina; the vaginal artery arising from the internal iliac artery and supplying the posterior surface of the vagina.

4. The root of the sigmoid mesocolon situated anterior to the left ureter, and acting as a guide to it;

5. The left ureter, crossing the external iliac artery at the bifurcation of the common iliac artery and descending anterior to the internal iliac artery; its subperitoneal course from where it enters the pelvis to where it passes deep to the broad ligament; the close proximity of the left ureter to the cervix of the uterus and lateral fornix of the vagina, where it is crossed by the uterine artery.

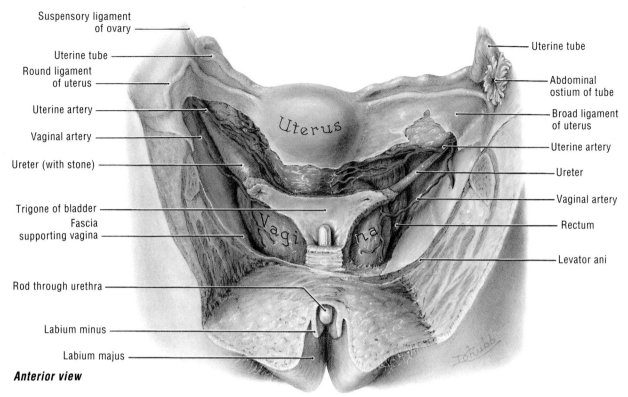

Suspensory ligament of ovary

Uterine tube

Round ligament of uterus

Uterine artery

Vaginal artery

Ureter (with stone)

Trigone of bladder

Fascia supporting vagina

Rod through urethra

Labium minus

Labium majus

Uterine tube

Abdominal ostium of tube

Broad ligament of uterus

Uterine artery

Ureter

Vaginal artery

Rectum

Levator ani

Uterus

Vagina

Anterior view

3.49
Uterus in situ

The pubic bones and the bladder, trigone excepted, are removed.

Observe:

1. Ureters, trigone of bladder, and urethra in relation to the asymmetrically placed uterus and vagina;

2. Ostium of the left uterine tube here happens to face anteriorly.

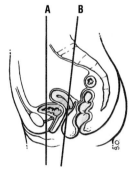

3.50
Orientation drawing for Figure 3.51A and B

3.51
Coronal MRIs (magnetic resonance images) of the female pelvis

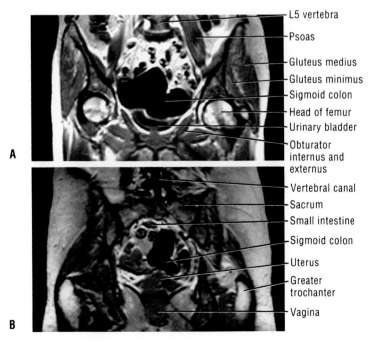

L5 vertebra

Psoas

Gluteus medius

Gluteus minimus

Sigmoid colon

Head of femur

Urinary bladder

Obturator internus and externus

Vertebral canal

Sacrum

Small intestine

Sigmoid colon

Uterus

Greater trochanter

Vagina

A

B

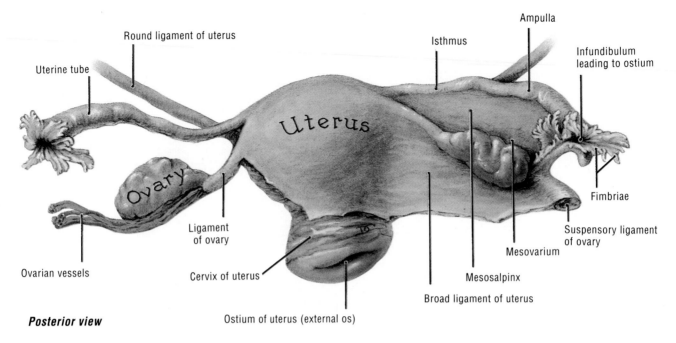

Posterior view

3.52
Uterus and its adenexa

On the left side:
The broad ligament of the uterus is removed, thereby setting free: the uterine tube, the round ligament of uterus, and the ligament of ovary; these three are attached, close together, to the lateral wall of the uterus, at the junction of its fundus and body.

On the right side:
The "mesentery" of the uterus and tube is called the broad

ligament; the ovary is attached (a) to the broad ligament by a "mesentery" of its own, called the mesovarium; (b) to the uterus by the ligament of the ovary; and (c) near the pelvic brim, by the suspensory ligament of the ovary, which transmits the ovarian vessels; the part of the broad ligament superior to the level of the mesovarium is called the mesosalpinx.

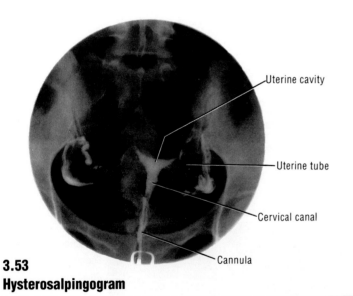

3.53
Hysterosalpingogram

Radiopaque contrast medium has been injected via a cannula into the uterus through the external os. The triangular uterine cavity is clearly outlined. Contrast medium has traveled through the uterine tubes to the infundibulum and leaked into the peritoneal cavity on both sides. (Courtesy of Dr. E.L. Lansdown, Professor of Radiology, University of Toronto, Toronto, Ontario, Canada.)

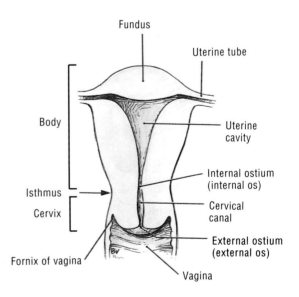

3.54
Parts of the uterus

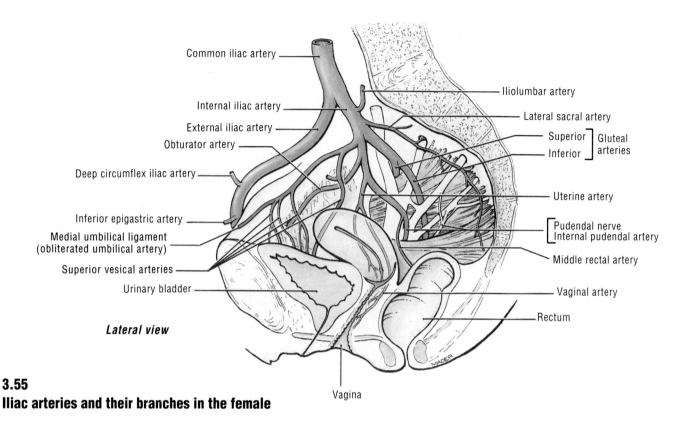

Common iliac artery

Internal iliac artery

External iliac artery

Obturator artery

Deep circumflex iliac artery

Inferior epigastric artery

Medial umbilical ligament
(obliterated umbilical artery)

Superior vesical arteries

Urinary bladder

Lateral view

Iliolumbar artery

Lateral sacral artery

Superior ⎤ Gluteal
Inferior ⎦ arteries

Uterine artery

Pudendal nerve
Internal pudendal artery

Middle rectal artery

Vaginal artery

Rectum

Vagina

3.55
Iliac arteries and their branches in the female

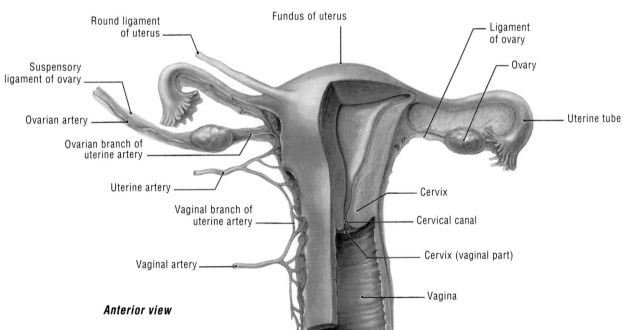

Round ligament
of uterus

Fundus of uterus

Ligament
of ovary

Ovary

Suspensory
ligament of ovary

Ovarian artery

Ovarian branch of
uterine artery

Uterine artery

Vaginal branch of
uterine artery

Vaginal artery

Uterine tube

Cervix

Cervical canal

Cervix (vaginal part)

Vagina

Anterior view

3.56
Blood supply of the uterus, vagina, and the ovaries

Observe:

1. On the left side, part of the uterine and vaginal walls have been cut away, to expose the cervix, the slit-like uterine cavity, and the thick muscular wall of the uterus, the myometrium;

2. On the right side, the ovarian artery (from the aorta) and the uterine artery (from the internal iliac) supplying the ovary, uterine tube, and the uterus, and anastomosing in the broad ligament along the lateral aspect of the uterus; the uterine artery sending a uterine branch to supply the body and fundus of the uterus and a vaginal branch to supply the cervix and vagina; the vaginal artery anastomosing with the vaginal branch of the uterine artery.

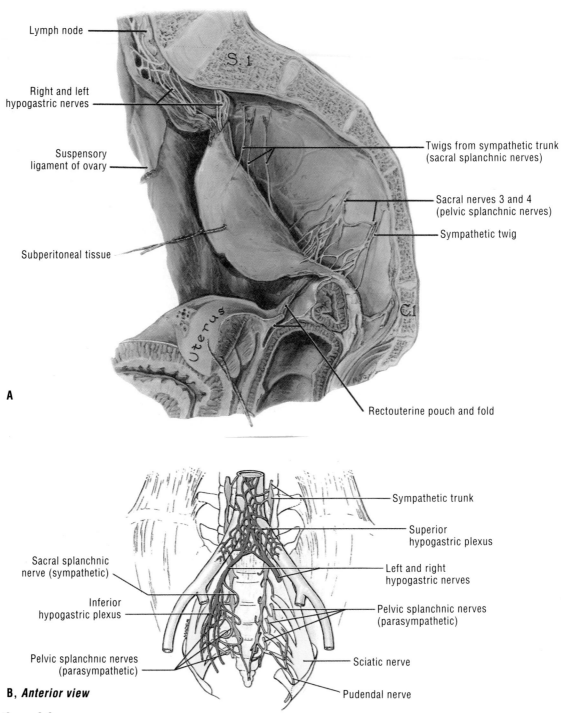

Lymph node

Right and left
hypogastric nerves

Suspensory
ligament of ovary

Subperitoneal tissue

S.1

Twigs from sympathetic trunk
(sacral splanchnic nerves)

Sacral nerves 3 and 4
(pelvic splanchnic nerves)

Sympathetic twig

C.1

Uterus

Rectouterine pouch and fold

A

Sacral splanchnic
nerve (sympathetic)

Inferior
hypogastric plexus

Pelvic splanchnic nerves
(parasympathetic)

Sympathetic trunk

Superior
hypogastric plexus

Left and right
hypogastric nerves

Pelvic splanchnic nerves
(parasympathetic)

Sciatic nerve

Pudendal nerve

B, *Anterior view*

3.57
Autonomic nerves of the pelvis

A. Median section, rectum and subperitoneal tissue, reflected anteriorly. Observe:

1. The rectum and subperitoneal fatty areolar tissue pulled anteriorly, thus rendering taut the pelvic splanchnic nerves from S2, S3 and S4, sympathetic fibers, and the right hypogastric nerve;

2. The parasympathetic, pelvic splanchnic nerves arising from the ventral primary rami of S2, S3, and S4 supplying motor fibers to the pelvic organs, and the sigmoid colon, and vasodilator fibers to the erectile tissue of the clitoris and bulb of the vestibule;

3. The sympathetic sacral splanchnic nerves arising from the sympathetic trunk and joining the inferior hypogastric plexuses.

B. Superior and inferior hypogastric plexuses. Observe:

1. The right and left hypogastric nerves joining the superior hypogastric plexus to the inferior hypogastric plexus; the pelvic plexuses, including the large inferior hypogastric plexus, consisting of both sympathetic and parasympathetic fibers;

2. The pudendal nerve, a branch of the sacral plexus, arising from the ventral primary rami of S2, S3, and S4; this nerve is part of the voluntary somatic nervous system and innervates the perineal region.

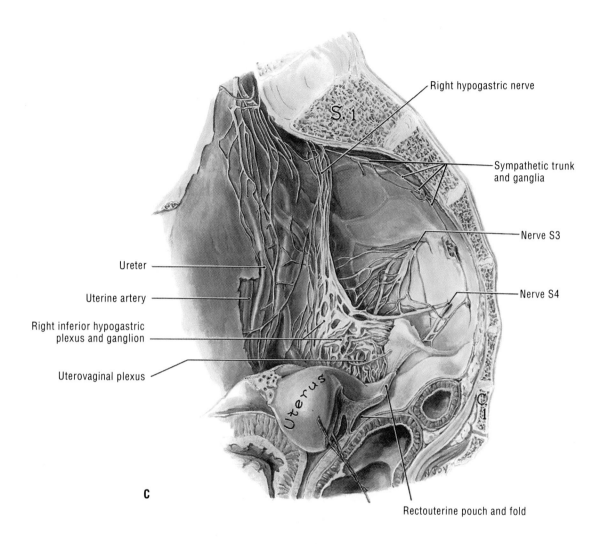

Right hypogastric nerve

S. 1

Sympathetic trunk
and ganglia

Nerve S3

Ureter

Uterine artery

Nerve S4

Right inferior hypogastric
plexus and ganglion

Uterovaginal plexus

Uterus

C

C. 1

Rectouterine pouch and fold

3.57

Autonomic nerves of the pelvis *(continued)*

C. Median section, subperitoneal tissue removed. This is a latter stage in dissection of Figure 3.57**A**. Observe:

1. The right and left inferior hypogastric plexuses continuing as: the vesical plexus supplying the urinary bladder, the middle rectal plexus supplying the rectum, the uterovaginal plexus supplying the uterus, the uterine tubes, the vagina, the urethra, the greater vestibular glands, and the erectile tissue of the clitoris and the bulb of the vestibule;

2. The ovaries and distal part of the uterine tubes are supplied by the ovarian plexuses which accompany the ovarian arteries.

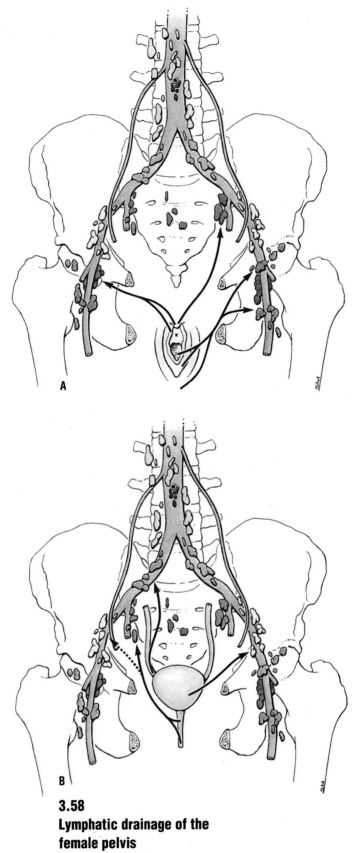

3.58
Lymphatic drainage of the female pelvis

A. External genitalia. B. Ureters, urinary bladder, and urethra.

	Lateral aortic
	Inferior mesenteric
	Common iliac
	Internal iliac
	External iliac
	Superficial inguinal
	Deep inguinal
	Sacral
	Pararectal

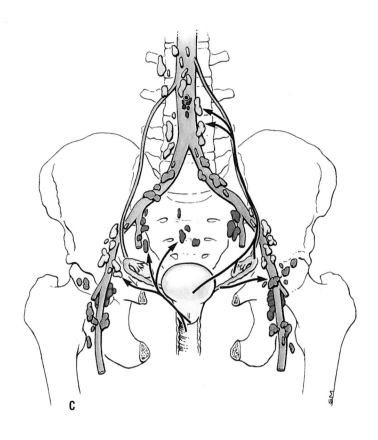

C

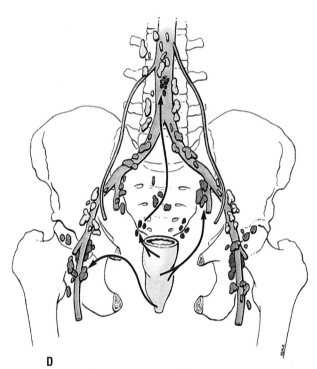

D

3.58
Lymphatic drainage of the
female pelvis *(continued)*

C. Uterus, vagina, uterine tubes, and ovaries. **D.** Rectum.

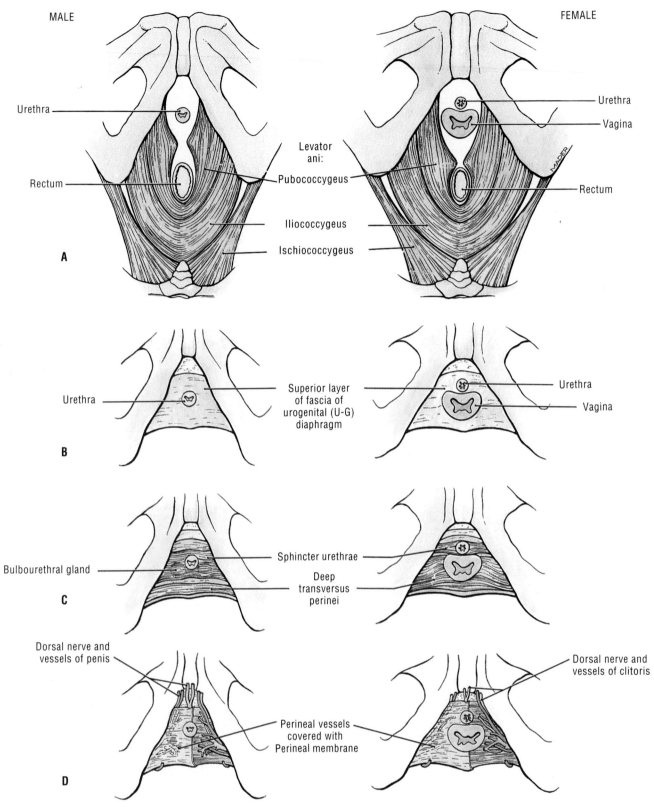

MALE

FEMALE

Urethra

Rectum

A

Levator
ani:

Pubococcygeus

Iliococcygeus

Ischiococcygeus

Urethra

Vagina

Rectum

Urethra

B

Superior layer
of fascia of
urogenital (U-G)
diaphragm

Urethra

Vagina

Bulbourethral gland

C

Sphincter urethrae

Deep
transversus
perinei

Dorsal nerve and
vessels of penis

D

Perineal vessels
covered with
Perineal membrane

Dorsal nerve and
vessels of clitoris

3.59
Layers of the perineum in the male and female

These schematic diagrams show layers of the perineum built up from deep to superficial. In **A**, the pelvic diaphragm, the angle between the two ischiopubic rami is almost filled by the levator ani (three coccygeus) muscles. The urethra (and vagina in the female) peer through anteriorly, the rectum posteriorly. A superior layer of fascia of the urogenital (U-G) diaphragm, **B**, and an inferior layer of fascia, the perineal membrane, **D**, enclose a deep perineal space or pouch, **C**, containing two muscles and, in the male, the bulbourethral glands. The sandwich formed by the two layers of fascia and the contents of the deep pouch comprise the urogenital diaphragm.

Grant's Atlas of Anatomy

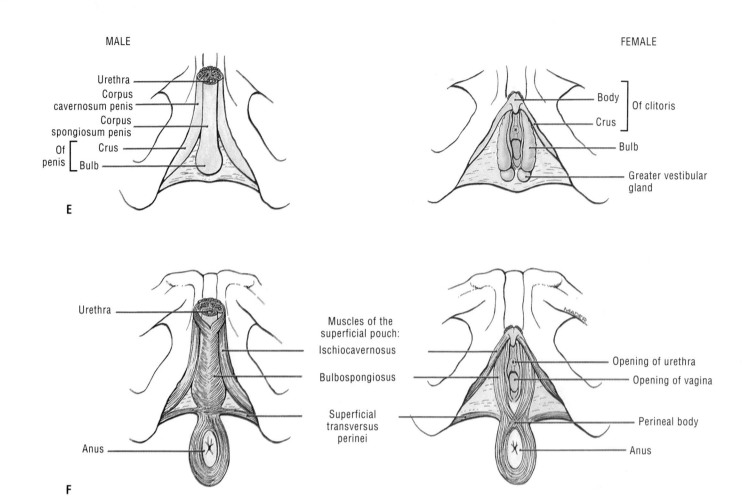

MALE

Urethra
Corpus
cavernosum penis
Corpus
spongiosum penis
Of penis { Crus
Bulb

E

FEMALE

Body } Of clitoris
Crus
Bulb
Greater vestibular gland

Urethra

Anus

F

Muscles of the superficial pouch:
Ischiocavernosus
Bulbospongiosus
Superficial transversus perinei

Opening of urethra
Opening of vagina
Perineal body
Anus

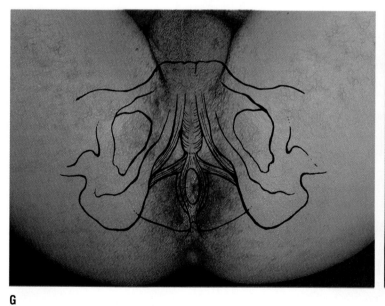

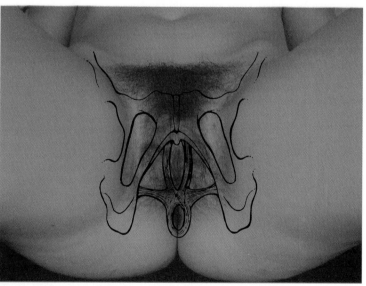

G

3.59
Layers of the perineum in the male and female *(continued)*

Superficial and deep layers of perineal fascia attach to the ischiopubic ramus and to the posterior margin of the urogenital diaphragm and so enclose the superficial perineal space or pouch that contains the structures shown in **E** and the muscles shown in **F**. In the female, greater vestibular glands lie posterior to the bulb of the vestibule. **G** shows an overview of the U-G diaphragm and related structures.

3.60
Pelvic diaphragm and ischioanal fossa, schematic diagrams

Observe:

1. The funnel-shaped levator ani muscles forming the internal (pelvic) aspect of the pelvic diaphragm (**A**); the brim of the funnel attaching to the pubis anteriorly, the obturator internus fascia, and the coccyx posteriorly; the tubular end of the funnel representing the anal canal; anteriorly, the margins of the deficiency in the levator ani muscles blending with the wall of the prostate in the male or vagina and urethra in the female;

2. The pelvic diaphragm consisting of the levator ani muscles and the inferior and superior layers of fascia covering the muscles (**A**);

3. The levator ani muscle consisting of: (a) the levator prostatae muscle or the pubovaginalis muscle around the anteriorly located deficiency, (b) the puborectalis muscle, (c) the pubococcygeus muscle, and (d) the iliococcygeus muscle (**C**);

4. The ischioanal (ischiorectal) fossae (**B**) are fat-filled spaces around the wall of the anal canal; the anterior recess of the ischioanal fossa lying superior to the urogenital diaphragm; the posterior recess of the fossa bounded superolaterally by the gluteus maximus muscle; the inferior rectal nerve, artery, and vein crossing the fossa to supply the anal region; the inferior rectal nerve innervating the voluntary external anal sphincter.

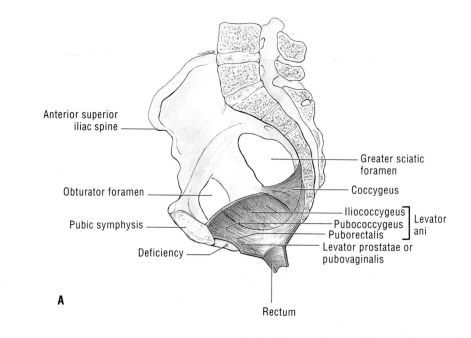

A

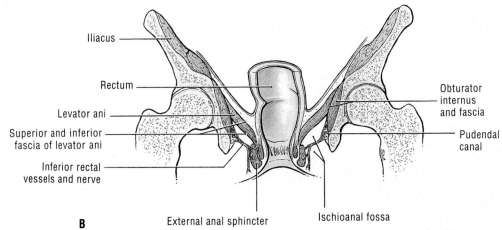

B

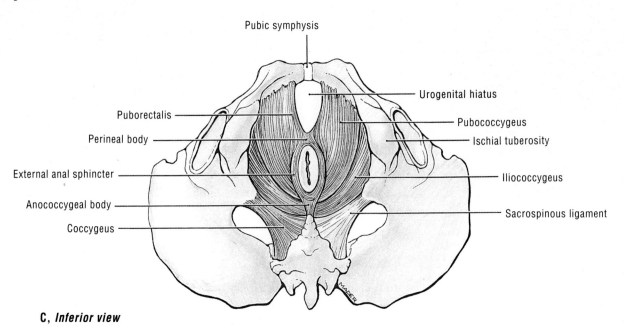

C, *Inferior view*

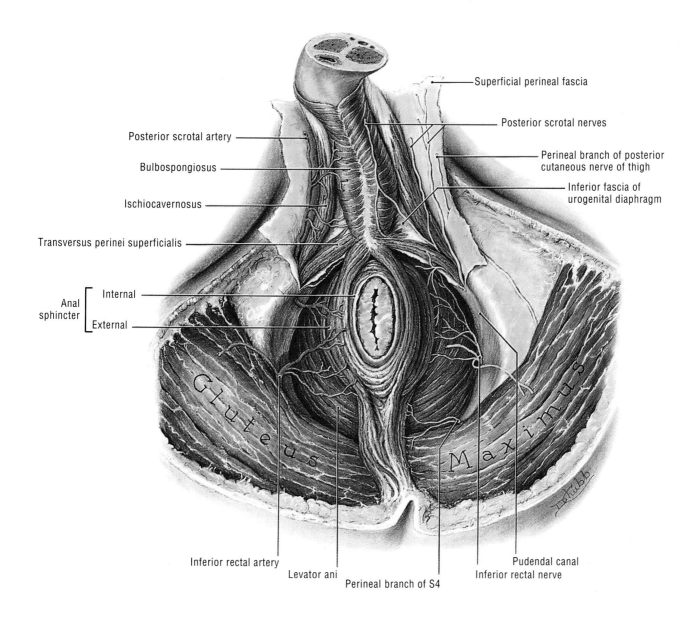

Posterior scrotal artery

Bulbospongiosus

Ischiocavernosus

Transversus perinei superficialis

Anal sphincter — Internal

Anal sphincter — External

Superficial perineal fascia

Posterior scrotal nerves

Perineal branch of posterior cutaneous nerve of thigh

Inferior fascia of urogenital diaphragm

Inferior rectal artery

Levator ani

Perineal branch of S4

Pudendal canal
Inferior rectal nerve

3.61
Male perineum

Observe in the anal region:

1. The anal orifice at the center of the anal triangle, surrounded by external anal sphincter, and an ischioanal (ischiorectal) fossa on each side;

2. The superficial fibers of external anal sphincter anchoring the anus anteriorly to the perineal body, or central tendon of the perineum, and posteriorly to the coccyx, here to the skin;

3. The ischioanal fossa, filled with fat, bounded medially by the levator ani muscle; laterally by obturator internus fascia; posteriorly by the gluteus maximus muscle lying superficial to the sacrotuberous ligament; anteriorly by the perineal membrane;

4. The inferior rectal nerve leaving the pudendal canal and, with the perineal branch of S4, supplying the external anal sphincter; its cutaneous twigs to the anus are removed; the branch hooking

around the gluteus maximus muscle is replacing the perforating cutaneous nerve.

Observe in the urogenital region:

5. The superficial perineal (Colles') fascia incised in the midline, freed from its attachment to the base of the perineal membrane, and reflected;

6. The cutaneous nerves and artery in the superficial perineal space (pouch);

7. The three paired superficial perineal muscles: the bulbospongiosus, the ischiocavernosus, and the superficial transversus perinei;

8. The exposed triangular portion of the perineal membrane or inferior fascia of the urogenital diaphragm.

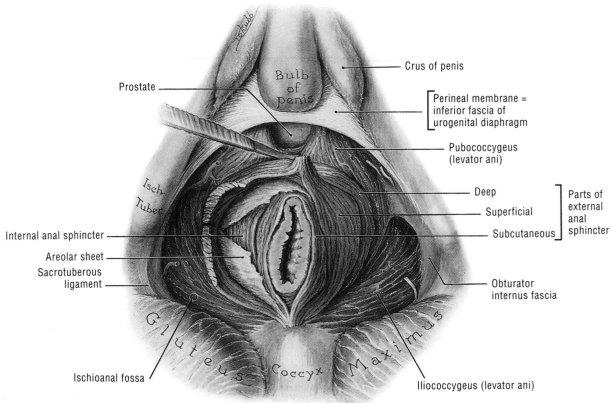

3.62

Dissection of the external anal sphincter

Observe:

1. The three parts of this voluntary sphincter: (a) subcutaneous, encircling the anal orifice; (b) superficial, anchoring the anus in the median plane, to the perineal body anteriorly and to the coccyx posteriorly, and (c) deep, forming a wide encircling band;

2. On the left of the figure: the superficial and deep parts of the sphincter are reflected, and the underlying sheet, consisting of

areolar tissue, levator ani fibers, and outer longitudinal muscular coat of the gut, is cut, in order to reveal the inner circular muscular coat of the gut, which is thickened to form the involuntary internal anal sphincter;

3. The anterior free borders of levator ani muscles meeting anterior to the anal canal, and pushed posteriorly in order to expose the prostate;

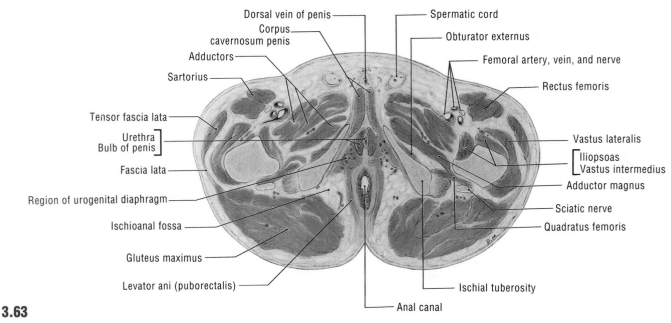

3.63

Transverse section of the male pelvis and perineum

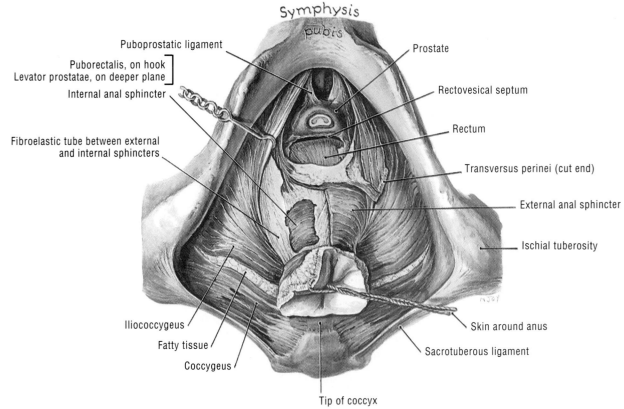

Symphysis pubis

Puboprostatic ligament

Puborectalis, on hook
Levator prostatae, on deeper plane

Internal anal sphincter

Fibroelastic tube between external
and internal sphincters

Iliococcygeus

Fatty tissue

Coccygeus

Tip of coccyx

Prostate

Rectovesical septum

Rectum

Transversus perinei (cut end)

External anal sphincter

Ischial tuberosity

Skin around anus

Sacrotuberous ligament

3.64

Levator ani and coccygei muscles, the exposure of the prostate

The urogenital diaphragm and its fasciae have been removed.

Observe:

1. The anal canal guarded by two sphincters: the internal anal sphincter, a continuation of the circular muscle coat of the gut; it is smooth muscle; the external anal sphincter, extending inferior to the internal sphincter and having three parts; it is skeletal muscle;

2. The longitudinal muscle coat of the rectum and its fascia blending with the levator ani muscle and its fasciae to form a fibroelastic tube that descends between the two sphincters; from this tube, septa pass through the internal sphincter to the submucous coat, through the external sphincter to the skin, and, as the anal intermuscular septum, inferior to the internal sphincter.

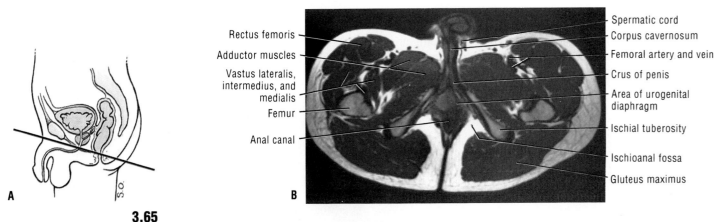

Rectus femoris

Adductor muscles

Vastus lateralis, intermedius, and medialis

Femur

Anal canal

Spermatic cord

Corpus cavernosum

Femoral artery and vein

Crus of penis

Area of urogenital diaphragm

Ischial tuberosity

Ischioanal fossa

Gluteus maximus

A

B

3.65

Transverse MRI (magnetic resonance image) of the male pelvis and perineum

A. Orientation drawing for Figures 3.63 and 3.65**B**. **B**. Compare this MRI to Figure 3.63. (Courtesy of Dr. W. Kucharczyk, Clinical Director of Tri-Hospital Resonance Centre, Toronto, Ontario, Canada.)

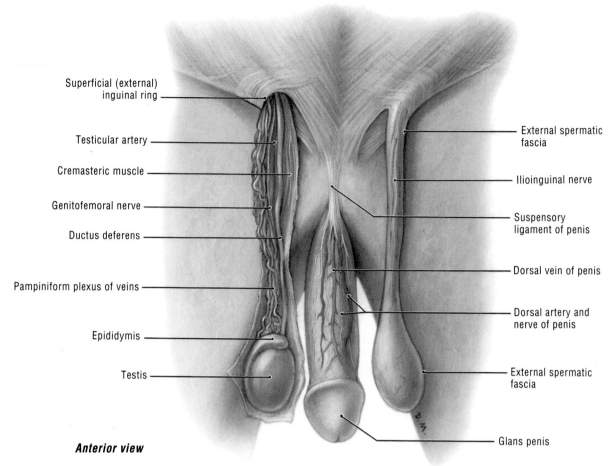

Superficial (external)
inguinal ring

Testicular artery

Cremasteric muscle

Genitofemoral nerve

Ductus deferens

Pampiniform plexus of veins

Epididymis

Testis

External spermatic
fascia

Ilioinguinal nerve

Suspensory
ligament of penis

Dorsal vein of penis

Dorsal artery and
nerve of penis

External spermatic
fascia

Glans penis

Anterior view

3.66

Vessels and nerves of the penis and contents of the spermatic cord

Observe:

1. The superficial fascia covering the penis is removed to expose the midline deep dorsal vein, and the bilateral dorsal arteries and nerves of the penis; the triangular suspensory ligament of the penis attaching to the region of the pubic symphysis and blending with the deep fascia of the penis;

2. On the left, the spermatic cord passing through the external inguinal ring and picking up a covering of external spermatic fascia from the margins of the external inguinal ring; the ilioinguinal nerve, supplying the skin at the base of the penis and the anterior aspect of the scrotum, and the cremasteric vessels, supplying the coverings of the cord and cremaster muscle, lying superficially on the spermatic cord;

3. On the right, the coverings of the spermatic cord and testis have been reflected and the contents of the cord separated; the spermatic cord containing: the ductus deferens (with its vessels), the testicular artery dissected away from the surrounding pampiniform plexus of veins, the genital branch of the genitofemoral nerve and fibers of the cremaster muscle; lymphatic vessels and autonomic nerve fibers, not shown here, are also present.

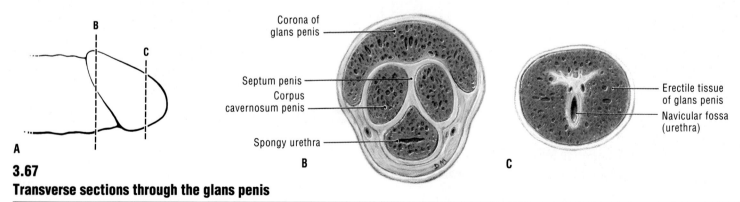

Corona of
glans penis

Septum penis
Corpus
cavernosum penis

Spongy urethra

Erectile tissue
of glans penis
Navicular fossa
(urethra)

A   B   C

3.67

Transverse sections through the glans penis

A shows the levels of sections illustrated in **B** and **C**. One section is taken through the glans penis more proximally (**B**) and the other more distally (**C**), as indicated by the orientation drawing (**A**).

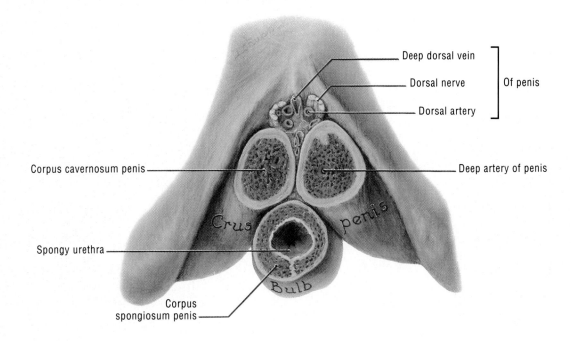

3.68
Transverse section through the root of the penis

Observe that the urethra is dilated within the bulb of the penis.

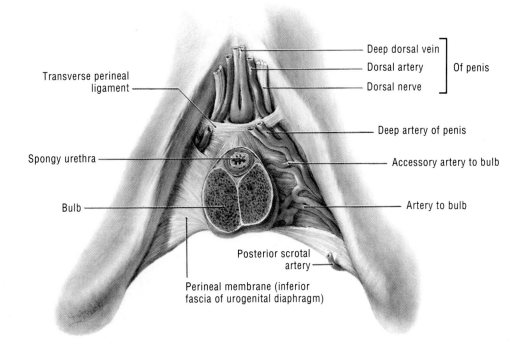

3.69
Deep perineal region

The crura are removed and the bulb is cut shorter than in Figure 3.68 and viewed more inferiorly.

On the right, the perineal membrane is, in part, removed and the deep perineal space is thereby opened.

Observe:
1. The fibers of the perineal membrane converging on the bulb and mooring it to the pubic arch;

2. The urethra, still membranous and bound to the dorsum of the bulb;

3. The septum in the bulb indicating its bilateral origin;

4. The artery to the bulb (here double); the artery to the crus, called the deep artery; and the dorsal artery that ends in the glans penis; the deep dorsal vein, originally double, which ends in the prostatic plexus.

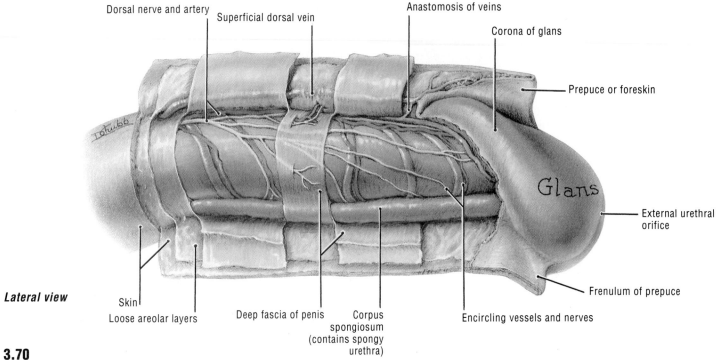

Lateral view

3.70
Penis

The three tubular envelopes of the penis are reflected; so also is the prepuce.

Observe:

1. The skin carried forward as the prepuce;

2. The loose, laminated, subcutaneous, areolar tissue, called the superficial fascia of the penis, carried forward into the prepuce, and containing the superficial dorsal vein; this vein begins in the prepuce, anastomoses with the deep dorsal vein from the glans, and ends in the superficial inguinal veins;

3. The deep fascia penis; it ends at the glans penis;

4. Large encircling tributaries of the deep dorsal vein; thread-like companion arteries; numerous oblique nerves;

5. The vessels and nerves at the neck plunging into the glans penis.

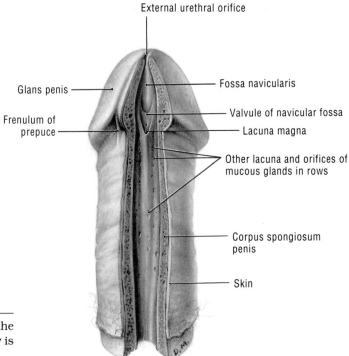

3.71
Interior of the spongy urethra

A longitudinal incision was made on the urethral surface of the penis and carried through the floor of the urethra, so the view is of the dorsal surface of the interior of the urethra.

3.72
Male genital and urinary tracts

Observe:

1. The ureters opening into the urinary bladder at the superior angles of the trigone; the urethra leaving the bladder at the inferior angle of the trigone;

2. Within the prostate gland, the ejaculatory ducts from the seminal vesicles entering the urethra;

3. The efferent ductules at the superior pole of the testis emptying into the head of the epididymis;

4. The ductus deferens ascending from the scrotum, entering the inguinal canal through the superficial ring, and exiting through the deep ring, hooking around the lateral side of the inferior epigastric artery.

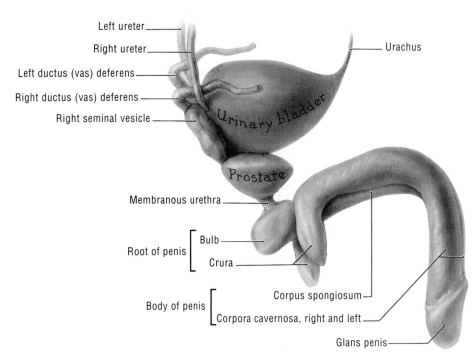

3.73
Diagram of male urogenital system, median section

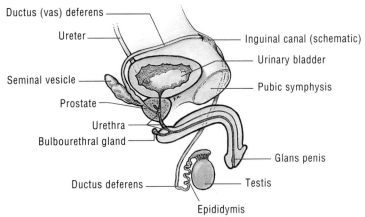

3.74
Dissection of the penis

The corpus spongiosum is separated from the corpora cavernosa penis. The natural flexures are preserved.

Observe:

1. The corpora cavernosa penis bent where that organ is slung by the suspensory ligament of the penis to the pubic symphysis, and grooved by encircling vessels;

2. The corpus spongiosum penis massed (a) posteriorly to form the bulb of the penis, and (b) anteriorly to form the glans that fits like a cap on the blunt ends of the corpora cavernosa penis.

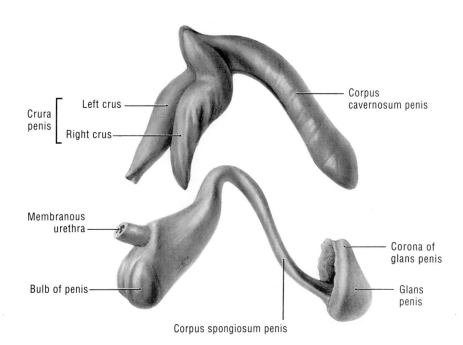

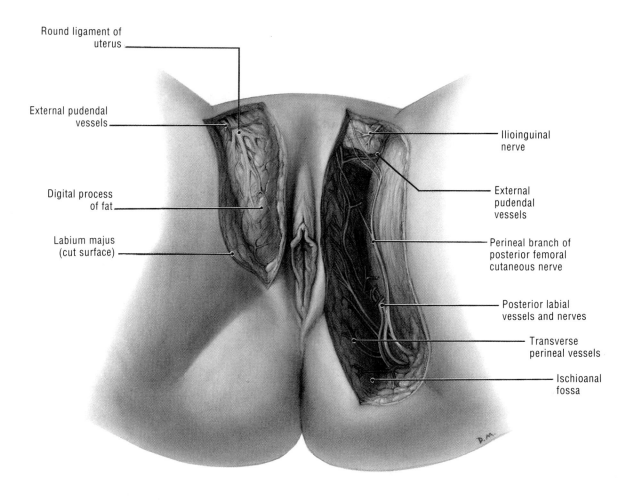

Round ligament of
uterus

External pudendal
vessels

Digital process
of fat

Labium majus
(cut surface)

Ilioinguinal
nerve

External
pudendal
vessels

Perineal branch of
posterior femoral
cutaneous nerve

Posterior labial
vessels and nerves

Transverse
perineal vessels

Ischioanal
fossa

3.75
Female perineum–I

Observe on the right:

1. A long digital, or finger-like, process of fat lying deep to the subcutaneous fatty tissue and descending far into the labium majus;

2. The round ligament of the uterus ending as a branching band of fascia that spreads out superficial to the digital process; and the external pudendal vessels crossing the process;

3. The vestibule of the vagina is the region between the labia minora and external to the hymen.

Observe, on the left:

1. The digital process of fat is largely removed;

2. The posterior labial vessels and nerves (S2, S3), joined by the perineal branch of the posterior femoral cutaneous nerve (S1, S2, S3) running anteriorly almost to the mons pubis; the vessels there anastomosing with the external pudendal vessels, and the nerves meeting the ilioinguinal nerve (L1).

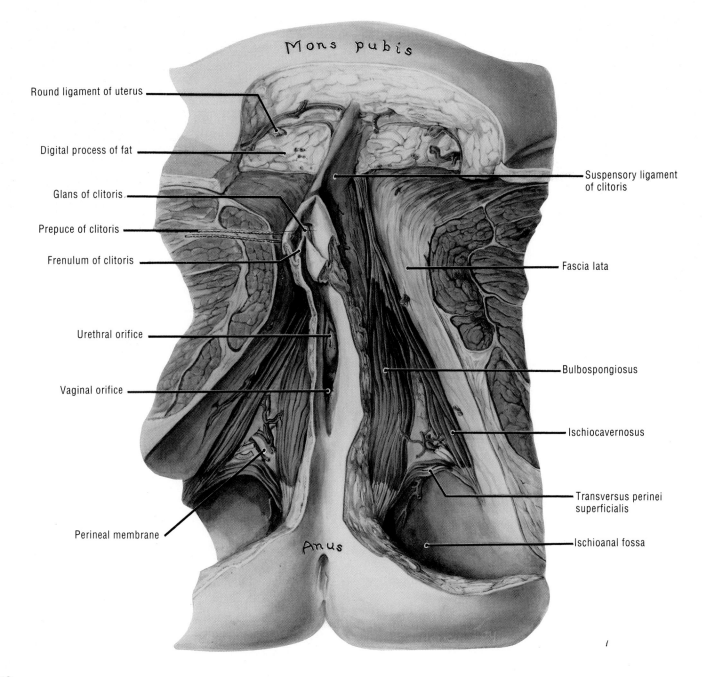

Mons pubis

Round ligament of uterus

Digital process of fat

Glans of clitoris

Prepuce of clitoris

Frenulum of clitoris

Urethral orifice

Vaginal orifice

Perineal membrane

Anus

Suspensory ligament
of clitoris

Fascia lata

Bulbospongiosus

Ischiocavernosus

Transversus perinei
superficialis

Ischioanal fossa

3.76
Female perineum–II

Observe:

1. The thickness of the superficial fatty tissue at the mons pubis and the encapsulated digital process of fat deep to this; the suspensory ligament of the clitoris descending from the linea alba and symphysis pubis;

2. The prepuce of the clitoris, thrown like a hood over the clitoris, and the anterior ends of the labia minora uniting to form the frenulum of the clitoris;

3. The three muscles on each side: bulbospongiosus, ischiocavernosus, and transversus perinei superficialis, which when slightly separated reveal the perineal membrane; the bulbospongiosus muscle overlies the bulb of the vestibule; in the male, the muscles of the two sides are united by a median raphe (Fig. 3.61); in the female, the orifice of the vagina separates the two;

4. The pinpoint orifices of the right and the left paraurethral duct below the urethral orifice;

5. The anterior recess of the ischioanal fossa lying deep to the urogenital diaphragm.

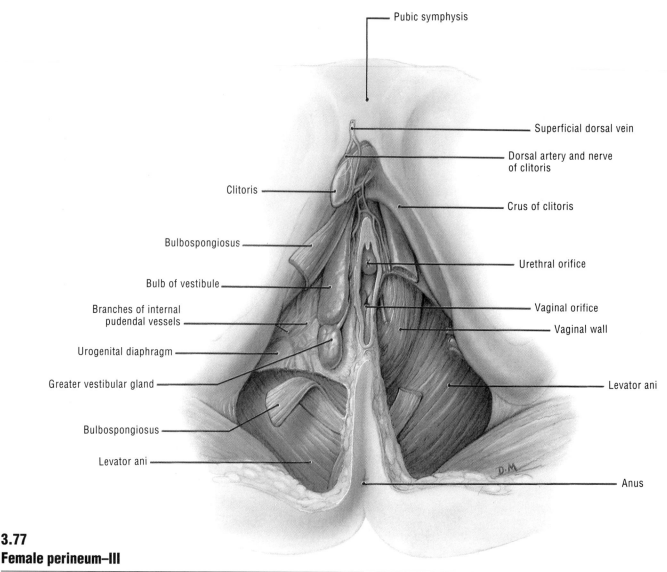

Pubic symphysis

Superficial dorsal vein

Dorsal artery and nerve of clitoris

Clitoris

Crus of clitoris

Bulbospongiosus

Urethral orifice

Bulb of vestibule

Branches of internal pudendal vessels

Vaginal orifice

Vaginal wall

Urogenital diaphragm

Greater vestibular gland

Levator ani

Bulbospongiosus

Levator ani

Anus

3.77
Female perineum–III

Observe:

1. The bulbospongiosus muscle is divided and reflected on the right side, and largely excised on the left side;

2. The glans clitoris, pulled over to the right side, and the dorsal vessels and nerve of the clitoris running to it;

3. The bulb of the vestibule, one on each side of the vestibule of the vagina and therein differing from the bulb of the penis, which is unpaired; the bulb on the left has been partially removed;

4. Veins connecting the bulbs of the vestibule to the glans of the clitoris;

5. On the right, the greater vestibular gland situated at the posterior end of the bulb and like it covered with bulbospongiosus muscle, and having a long duct (about 1.9 mm) that opens into the vestibule;

6. On the left side, the perineal membrane is cut away, thereby revealing the vessels of the bulb and the dorsal nerve and vessels of the clitoris within the deep perineal space.

3.78
Clitoris

The body of the clitoris comprises two corpora cavernosa that are bent, suspended by a suspensory ligament, and capped by a glans. The crura are covered by the paired ischiocavernosus muscles. The bulbs of the vestibule and the commissure of the bulbs are represented in the male by the bulb and body of the corpus spongiosum. These, however, are not regarded as part of the clitoris and are not traversed by the urethra.

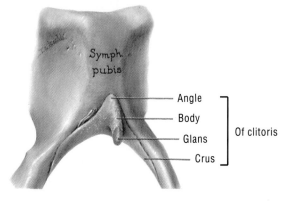

Symph. pubis

Angle
Body
Glans
Crus

} Of clitoris

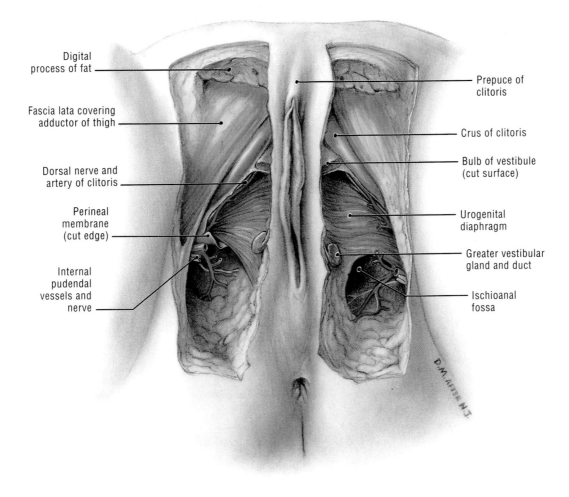

Digital process of fat

Fascia lata covering adductor of thigh

Dorsal nerve and artery of clitoris

Perineal membrane (cut edge)

Internal pudendal vessels and nerve

Prepuce of clitoris

Crus of clitoris

Bulb of vestibule (cut surface)

Urogenital diaphragm

Greater vestibular gland and duct

Ischioanal fossa

3.79
Female perineum–IV

Observe:

1. The bulbs of the vestibule are removed, except at their pubic ends; the greater vestibular glands and ducts remain; the perineal membrane is removed except for a marginal fringe;

2. The urogenital diaphragm, shown on both sides as a thin sheet of striated muscle;

3. Between the perineal membrane and the muscle of the uro-genital diaphragm, the dorsal nerve and artery to the clitoris running anteriorly and giving twigs to the bulb and crus;

4. The tough fatty areolar tissue that lies between the vagina and anus called the perineal body; in it lie veins that connect the veins of the bulb to the inferior rectal veins.

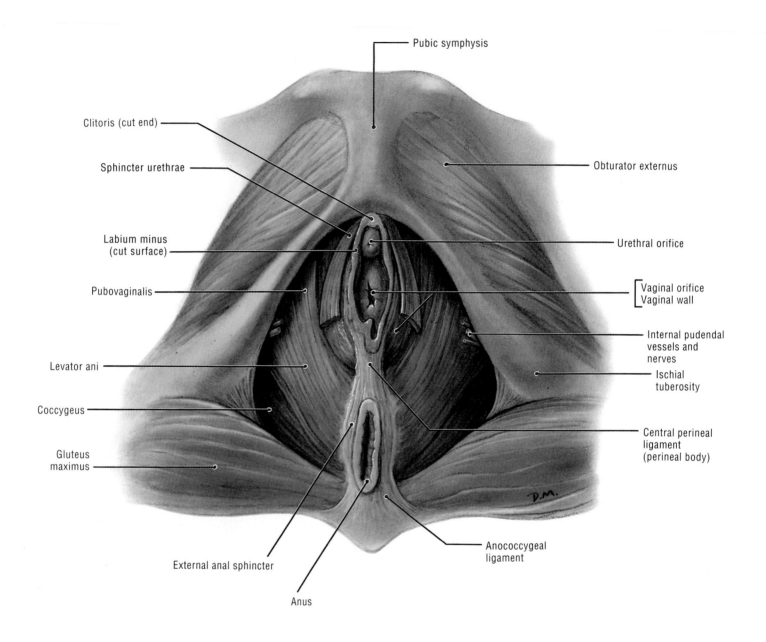

Pubic symphysis

Clitoris (cut end)

Sphincter urethrae

Labium minus
(cut surface)

Pubovaginalis

Levator ani

Coccygeus

Gluteus
maximus

External anal sphincter

Anus

Obturator externus

Urethral orifice

Vaginal orifice
Vaginal wall

Internal pudendal
vessels and
nerves

Ischial
tuberosity

Central perineal
ligament
(perineal body)

Anococcygeal
ligament

3.80
Female perineum–V

Observe:

1. The urogenital diaphragm and its fasciae have been removed from the sloping interior surface of the levator ani muscle and detached from the sloping outer wall of vagina with which it fuses;

2. The anterior parts of the levator ani (pubovaginales) muscle meeting posterior to the vaginal orifice;

3. The laminated nature of this part of the wall of the vagina; it is laminated because several layers of fascia fuse with it and lose their identity in it, namely, the superficial perineal fascia, the

urogenital diaphragm and its fasciae, and the fasciae of the levator ani muscles;

4. The sphincter urethrae, of striated muscle, resting on the urethra and straddling the vagina;

5. The labia minora, cut short, bounding the vestibule of the vagina, and the hymen, separating the vestibule from the cavity of the vagina.

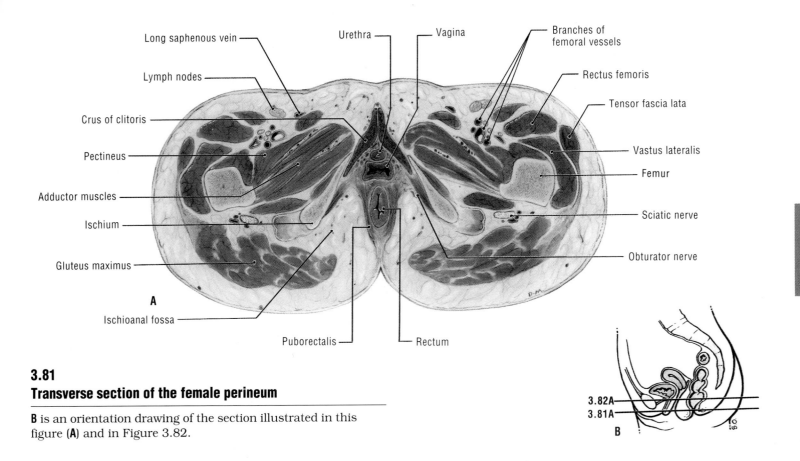

Long saphenous vein
Lymph nodes
Crus of clitoris
Pectineus
Adductor muscles
Ischium
Gluteus maximus

Urethra
Vagina
Branches of femoral vessels
Rectus femoris
Tensor fascia lata
Vastus lateralis
Femur
Sciatic nerve
Obturator nerve

A

Ischioanal fossa
Puborectalis
Rectum

3.81
Transverse section of the female perineum

B is an orientation drawing of the section illustrated in this figure (**A**) and in Figure 3.82.

3.82A
3.81A
B

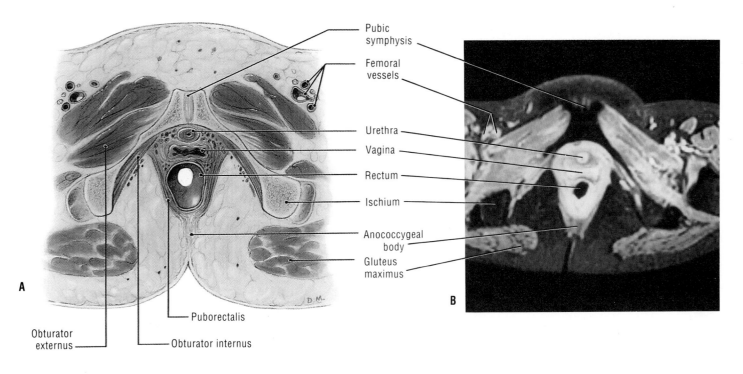

Pubic symphysis
Femoral vessels
Urethra
Vagina
Rectum
Ischium
Anococcygeal body
Gluteus maximus

A

Obturator externus
Puborectalis
Obturator internus

B

3.82
Transverse section of the female pelvis

Compare Figure 3.81A to this figure (**A**). **B**. Transverse MRI (magnetic resonance image) of the female pelvis. (Courtesy of Dr. W. Kucharczyk, Clinical Director of Tri-Hospital Resonance Centre, Toronto, Ontario, Canada.)

3.83
Radiograph of fetus

Observe:
In this view of a fetus in utero, that the head is framed by the pelvic brim, the incompletely ossified vertebral column arches to the mother's left side; at the top of the radiograph, the flexed lower limb is visible. (Courtesy of Dr. E.L. Lansdown, Professor of Radiology, University of Toronto, Toronto, Ontario, Canada.)

3.84
Radiograph of twins

(Courtesy of Dr. J. Heslin, Assistant Professor of Anatomy, University of Toronto, Toronto, Ontario, Canada.)

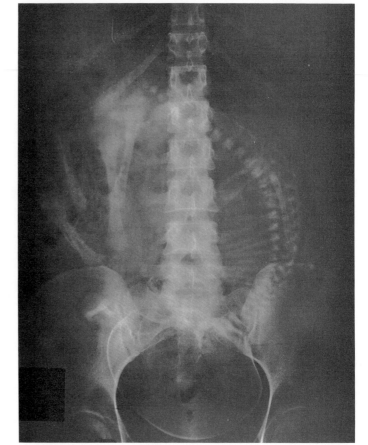

Anteroposterior view

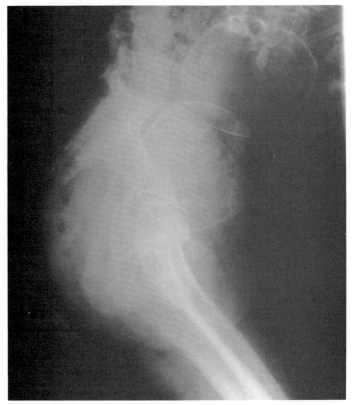

Lateral view

4   The Back

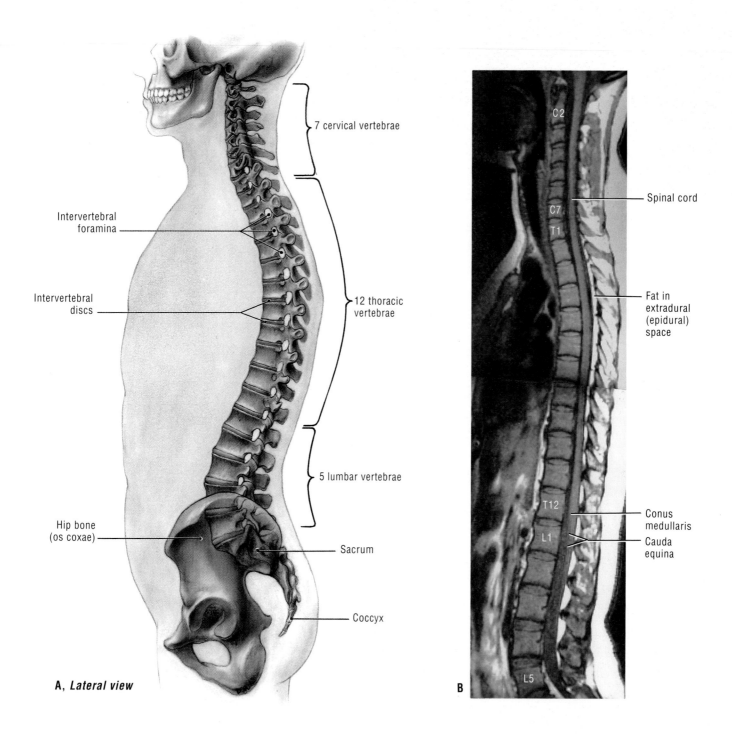

A, Lateral view

7 cervical vertebrae

Intervertebral foramina

Intervertebral discs

12 thoracic vertebrae

5 lumbar vertebrae

Hip bone (os coxae)

Sacrum

Coccyx

B

C2

Spinal cord

C7

T1

Fat in extradural (epidural) space

T12

Conus medullaris

L1

Cauda equina

L5

4.1
Vertebral column

Compare **A** and **B**.

A. Note the intervertebral foramina where the spinal nerves exit the vertebral (spinal) canal.

B. Sagittal MRI (magnetic resonance image). (Courtesy of Dr. W. Kucharczyk, Clinical Director of Tri-Hospital Resonance Centre, Toronto, Ontario, Canada.)

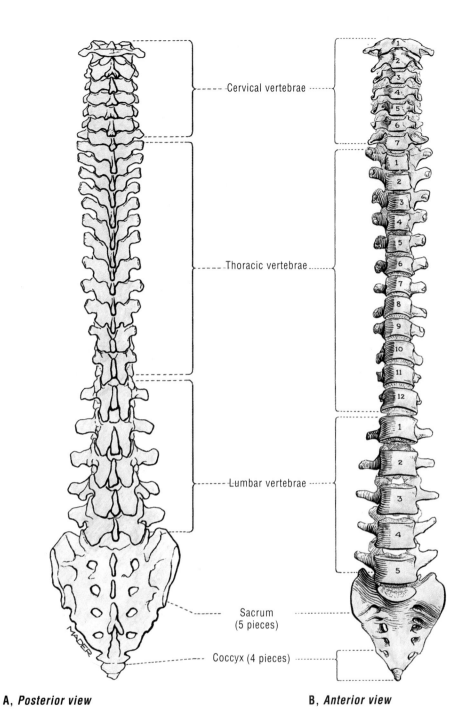

Cervical vertebrae

Thoracic vertebrae

Lumbar vertebrae

Sacrum
(5 pieces)

Coccyx (4 pieces)

A, Posterior view

B, Anterior view

4.2
Vertebral column

Observe:

1. The vertebral column comprises 24 separate (presacral) vertebrae and two composite vertebrae, the sacrum, and the coccyx; of the 24 separate vertebrae, 12 support ribs and, therefore, are thoracic; of the other 12, seven are in the neck (cervical) and five are in the lumbar region (lumbar);

2. Vertebrae forming the posterior walls of the bony cavities (the thoracic vertebrae posterior to the thoracic cavity, and the sacrum and coccyx posterior to the pelvic cavity) are concave anteriorly, but elsewhere (in the cervical and lumbar regions), by way of compensation, they are convex anteriorly;

3. The transverse processes of the atlas spread widely; those of C7 spread almost as far; those of C2 to C6 much less; the spread diminishes progressively from T1 to T12; in the lumbar region, it is greatest at L3.

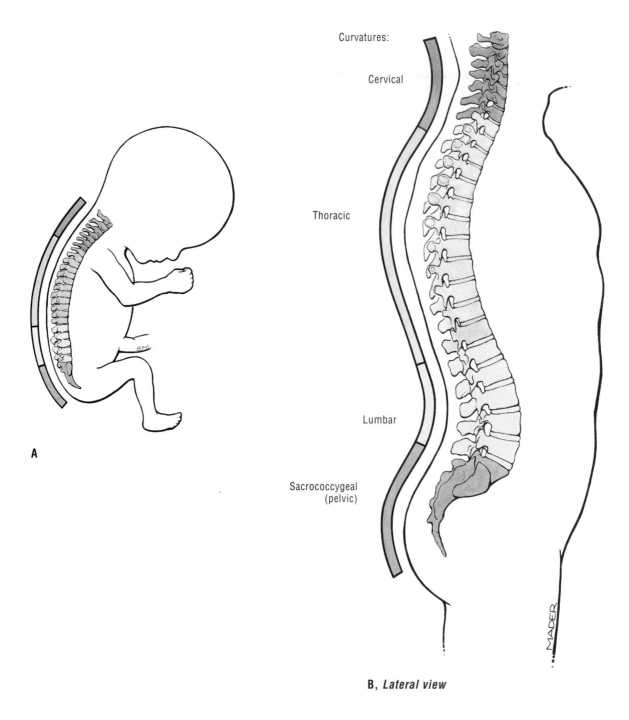

A

Curvatures:

Cervical

Thoracic

Lumbar

Sacrococcygeal
(pelvic)

B, *Lateral view*

4.3
Curvatures of the vertebral column

A. Fetus. **B.** Adult.

Observe:

1. The four curvatures of the adult vertebral column (**B**) include: (a) the cervical curve, which is convex anteriorly and lies between vertebrae C1 and T2, (b) the thoracic curve, which is concave anteriorly, between vertebrae T2 to T12, (c) the lumbar curve, convex anteriorly and lying between T12 and the lumbosacral joint, (d) the sacrococcygeal (pelvic) curve, concave anteriorly and spanning between the lumbosacral joint and the tip of the coccyx;

2. The C-shaped curvature of the spine during fetal life (**A**), the curvature is concave anteriorly;

3. The thoracic and sacrococcygeal curves are primary curves; the cervical curve appears before birth but develops extensively when the child begins to hold the head up; the lumbar curve develops when the child begins to walk; the cervical and lumbar curves are known as secondary curves since they develop after birth.

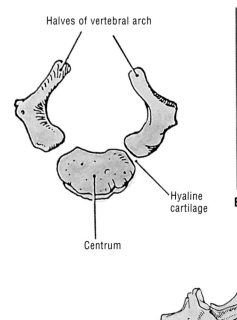

Halves of vertebral arch

Hyaline cartilage

Centrum

A

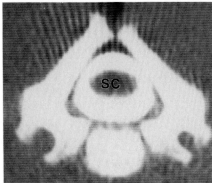

B, *Transverse scan*

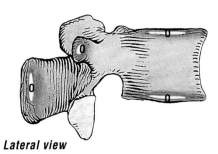

Lateral view

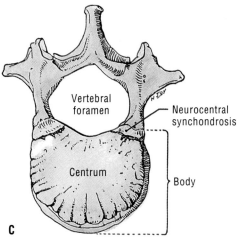

Vertebral foramen

Neurocentral synchondrosis

Centrum

Body

C

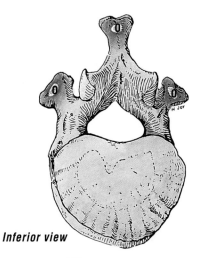

Inferior view

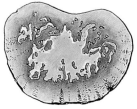

EPIPHYSEAL PLATE REMOVED FROM THE VERTEBRA ABOVE

D

4.4
Development of vertebrae

A. At birth, a vertebra consists of three bony parts, united by hyaline cartilage;

B. The computed tomographic (CT) scan shows the three bony parts of a vertebra at birth; also note the contrast material around the spinal cord *(SC)* filling the dural sac;

C. From age 2, the halves of each vertebral (neural) arch begin to fuse to each other, from the lumbar to the cervical region; from about age 7, the arches fuse to the centrum in sequence from cervical to lumbar regions;

D. During puberty, secondary centers of ossification *(O)* appear for the tips of spinous and transverse processes; epiphyseal plates for the body consist of a plate of hyaline cartilage and circumferential bony ring.

4.5
Three-dimensional computer-generated image of a vertebra

In this image of the vertebra of an 18-year-old person, the secondary centers of ossification have fused. (Scans courtesy of Dr. D. Armstrong, Associate Professor of Radiology, University of Toronto, Toronto, Ontario, Canada.)

Superior articular process of vertebra below

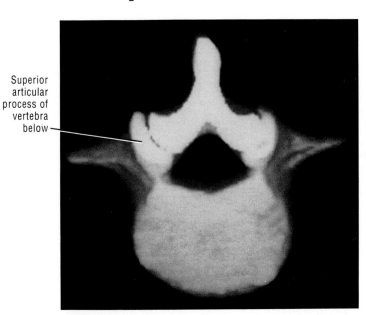

Inferior view

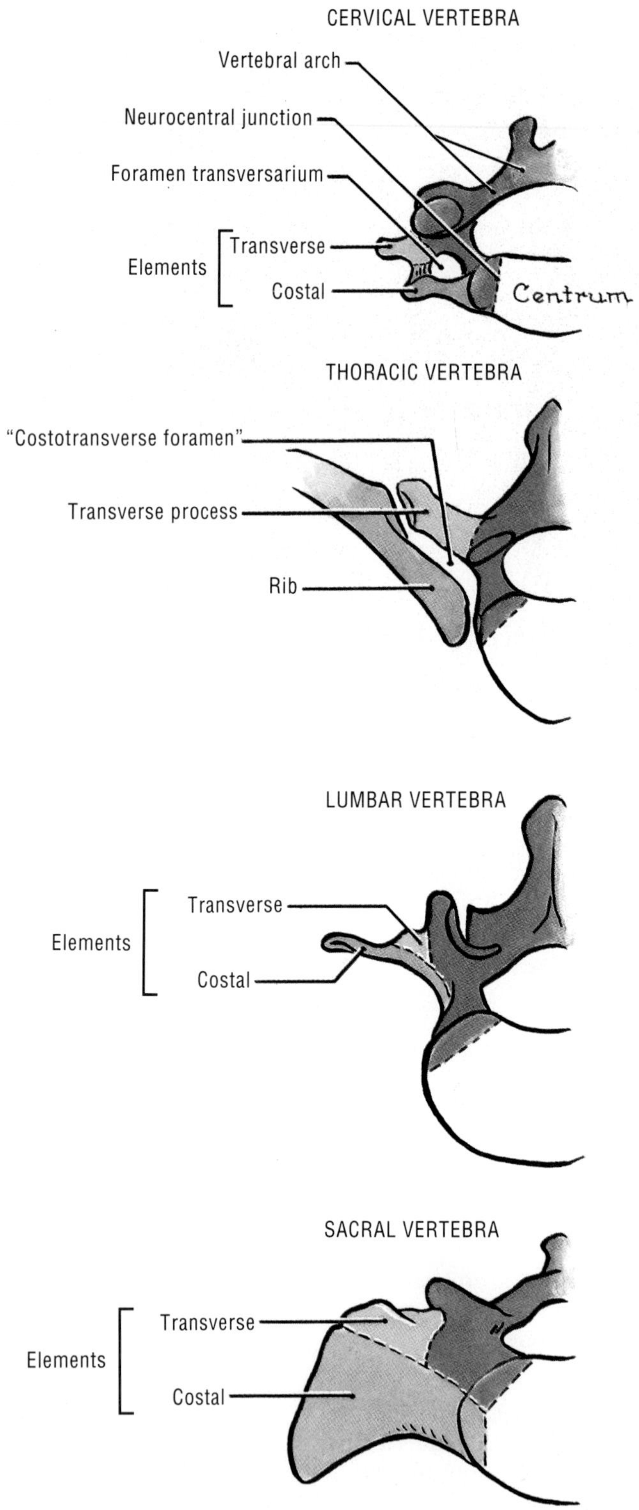

CERVICAL VERTEBRA

Vertebral arch

Neurocentral junction

Foramen transversarium

Elements [Transverse

Costal

Centrum

THORACIC VERTEBRA

"Costotransverse foramen"

Transverse process

Rib

LUMBAR VERTEBRA

Elements [Transverse

Costal

SACRAL VERTEBRA

Elements [Transverse

Costal

4.6
Diagram of the homologous parts of the vertebrae

Observe:

1. The centrum (uncolored), the vertebral (neural) arch (dark pink) and its process (pink), and the rib or costal element (yellow);

2. A rib or costa is a free element in the thoracic region; in the cervical region, it is represented by the anterior part of a transverse process; in the lumbar region, by the anterior part of a transverse process; and in the sacrum, by the anterior part of the lateral mass;

3. The heads of the ribs (thoracic region) articulate with the sides of the bodies of the vertebrae posterior to the neurocentral junctions, i.e., not with the centra, but with the neural arches.

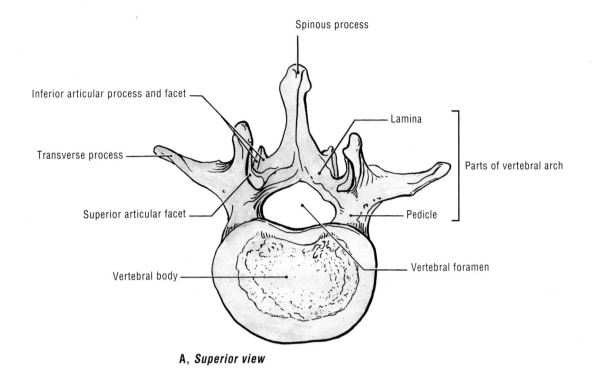

Spinous process

Inferior articular process and facet

Lamina

Transverse process

Parts of vertebral arch

Superior articular facet

Pedicle

Vertebral foramen

Vertebral body

A, *Superior view*

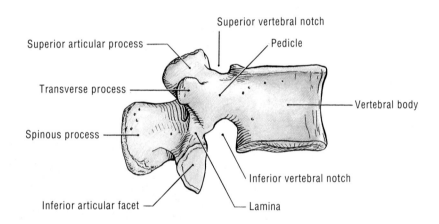

Superior vertebral notch

Superior articular process

Pedicle

Transverse process

Vertebral body

Spinous process

Inferior vertebral notch

Inferior articular facet

Lamina

B, *Lateral view*

4.7
Typical vertebra

A typical vertebra (2nd lumbar vertebra) comprises the following parts:

1. A columnar body, situated anteriorly; its function is to support weight; like other long bones, it is narrow about its middle and expanded at both ends; these ends are articular and during growth have epiphyses;

2. A vertebral arch, posterior to the body; with the body this arch encloses the vertebral foramen; collectively, the vertebral foramina constitute the vertebral canal wherein lodges the spinal cord; the function of a vertebral arch is to afford protection to the cord; the vertebral arch consists of two stout, rounded pedicles, one on each side, that spring from the body and that are united posteriorly by two flat plates or laminae;

3. Three processes, two transverse and one spinous; these project from the vertebral arch like spokes from a capstan; they afford attachment to muscles and are the levers that help move the vertebrae;

4. Four articular processes: two superior and two inferior; each articular process has an articular facet; the articular processes project superiorly and inferiorly, respectively, from the vertebral arch and come into apposition with the articular facet of the corresponding processes of the vertebrae above and below; their function is to restrict movements to certain directions, or at least to decree in what directions movements may be permitted; also, they prevent the vertebrae from slipping anteriorly.

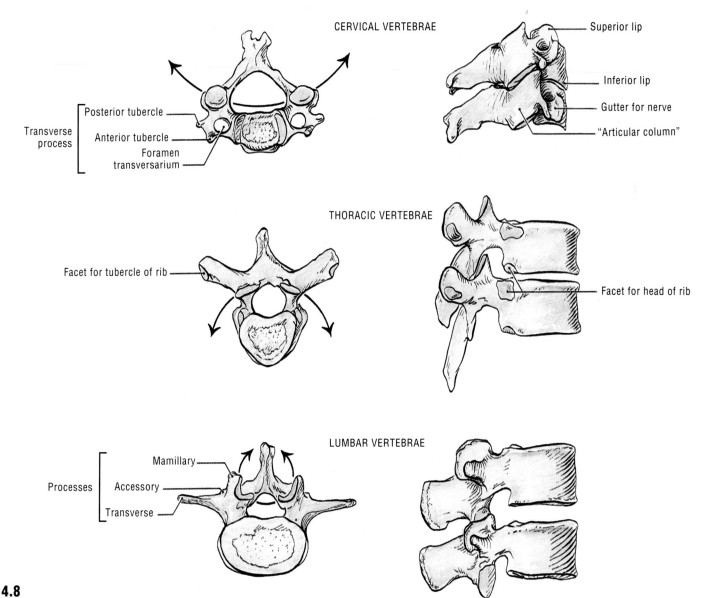

CERVICAL VERTEBRAE

Transverse process
- Posterior tubercle
- Anterior tubercle
- Foramen transversarium

- Superior lip
- Inferior lip
- Gutter for nerve
- "Articular column"

THORACIC VERTEBRAE

Facet for tubercle of rib

Facet for head of rib

LUMBAR VERTEBRAE

Processes
- Mamillary
- Accessory
- Transverse

4.8
Distinguishing features and movements

Observe:

1. The most distinctive feature of the cervical vertebrae is the presence of foramina transversaria; all thoracic vertebrae have facets for articulation with the heads of ribs; the absence of these two features is distinctive of the large lumbar vertebrae;

2. The bodies of cervical and lumbar vertebrae are greater in the transverse diameter than in the anteroposterior, and the vertebral foramina are triangular; in thoracic vertebrae, the two diameters are about equal and the foramen is circular; further, the superior surface of the body of a cervical vertebra ends at each side in an upturned superior lip, hence it is concave from side to side, and the inferior surface ends anteriorly in a downturned inferior lip; the superior and inferior surfaces of thoracic and lumbar bodies are flat;

3. A transverse process in the cervical region points laterally, inferiorly, and anteriorly, and ends in two tubercles with a gutter between them; in the thoracic region, it points laterally, posteriorly, and superiorly, has a facet for the tubercle of a rib, and is stout;

in the lumbar region, it points laterally, and is long and slender;

4. Spinous processes are bifid if cervical, spine-like if thoracic, and oblong if lumbar;

5. Articular processes in the cervical region collectively form a cylinder that is, in part, weight-bearing; it is cut obliquely into segments; in the thoracic and lumbar regions, the superior articular facets lie posterior to the pedicles, and the inferior facets are anterior to the laminae; superior articular facets in the cervical region face mainly superiorly; in the thoracic region, mainly posteriorly; in the lumbar region, mainly medially; the change in direction is gradual from cervical to thoracic, but from thoracic to lumbar it is abrupt;

6. Movements: in all three regions, the articular processes permit flexion and extension and side to side movement; cervical vertebrae allow one to look sideways up; thoracic vertebrae allow medial and lateral rotation, but lumbar vertebrae do not.

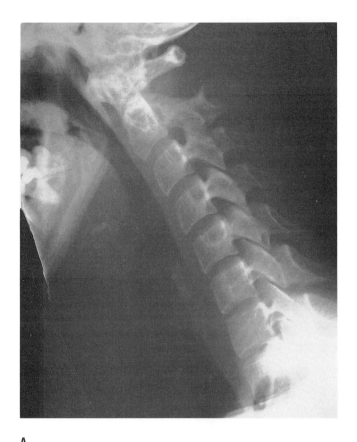

A

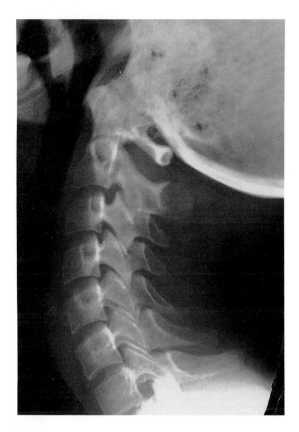

B

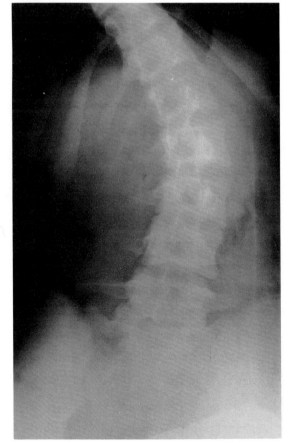

C

4.9
Movements of the vertebral column

A. Lateral radiograph of the flexed cervical spine. **B.** Lateral radiograph of the extended cervical spine. **C.** Anteroposterior radiograph of the lumbar spine during lateral bending. (Courtesy of Dr. E. Becker, Associate Professor of Radiology, and Dr. P. Bobechko, Assistant Professor of Radiology, University of Toronto, Toronto, Ontario, Canada.)

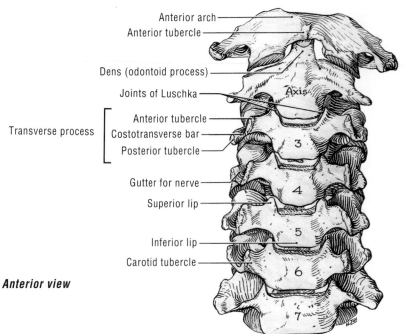

Anterior arch
Anterior tubercle

Dens (odontoid process)

Joints of Luschka

Transverse process [
Anterior tubercle
Costotransverse bar
Posterior tubercle

Gutter for nerve

Superior lip

Inferior lip

Carotid tubercle

Axis

3

4

5

6

7

Anterior view

4.10
Articulated cervical vertebrae

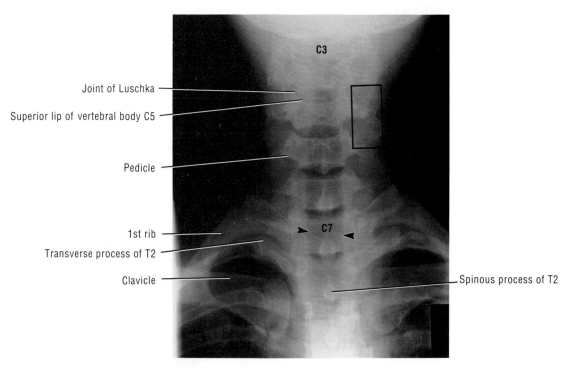

Joint of Luschka

Superior lip of vertebral body C5

Pedicle

1st rib

Transverse process of T2

Clavicle

C3

C7

Spinous process of T2

4.11
Anteroposterior radiograph of the cervical spine

Observe:

1. The bifid spinous processes of cervical vertebrae;

2. The margins of the (black) column of air in the trachea *(arrowheads)*;

3. The laterally located column of articular processes and the overlapping transverse processes indicated by the boxed area.

4. The superior surface of vertebral bodies C3 to C7 have lateral upturned lips which articulate with the vertebra above (joints of Luschka). (Courtesy of Dr. J. Heslin, Assistant Professor of Anatomy, University of Toronto, Toronto, Ontario, Canada.)

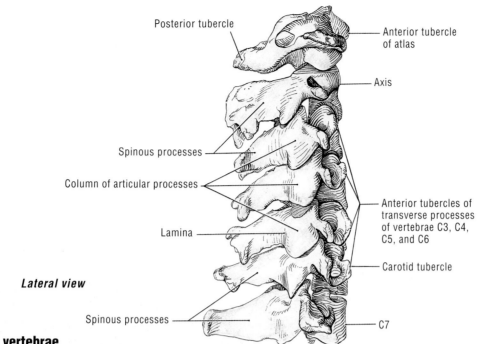

Posterior tubercle

Anterior tubercle
of atlas

Axis

Spinous processes

Column of articular processes

Anterior tubercles of
transverse processes
of vertebrae C3, C4,
C5, and C6

Lamina

Carotid tubercle

Lateral view

4.12
Articulated cervical vertebrae

Spinous processes

C7

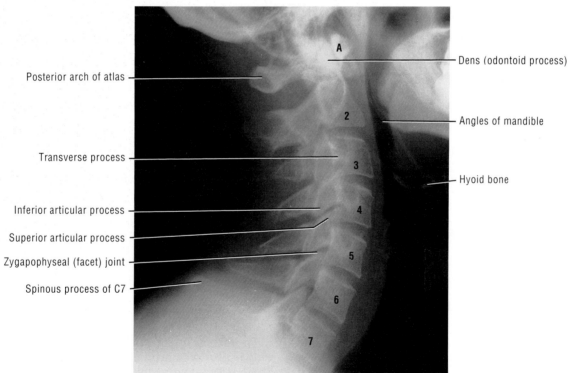

Posterior arch of atlas

Dens (odontoid process)

Angles of mandible

Transverse process

Hyoid bone

Inferior articular process

Superior articular process

Zygapophyseal (facet) joint

Spinous process of C7

4.13
Lateral radiograph of the cervical spine

Observe:

1. The bodies of 2nd to 7th cervical vertebrae have been numbered;

2. The anterior arch of the atlas (*A*) is in a plane anterior to a curved line joining the anterior borders of the bodies of the vertebrae;

3. The spinous process of C7, the vertebra prominens. (Courtesy of Dr. J. Heslin, Assistant Professor of Anatomy, University of Toronto, Toronto, Ontario, Canada.)

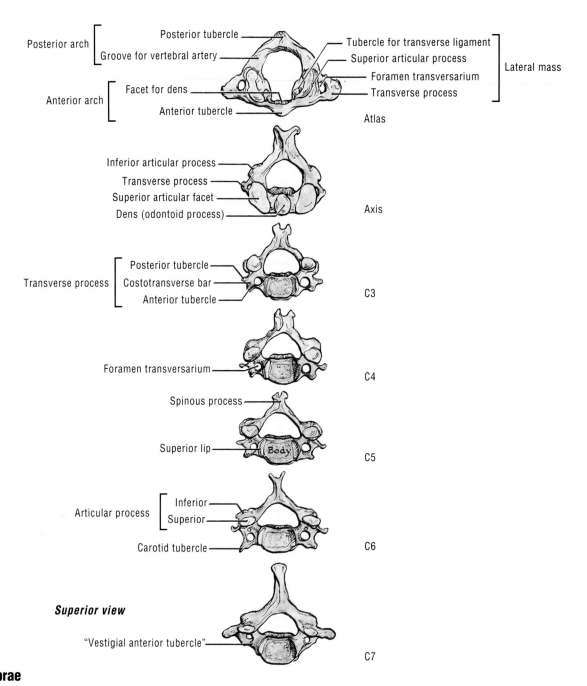

Posterior arch {
Posterior tubercle
Groove for vertebral artery

Tubercle for transverse ligament
Superior articular process
Foramen transversarium
Transverse process
} Lateral mass

Anterior arch {
Facet for dens
Anterior tubercle

Atlas

Inferior articular process
Transverse process
Superior articular facet
Dens (odontoid process)

Axis

Transverse process {
Posterior tubercle
Costotransverse bar
Anterior tubercle

C3

Foramen transversarium

C4

Spinous process

Superior lip — Body

C5

Articular process {
Inferior
Superior

Carotid tubercle

C6

Superior view

"Vestigial anterior tubercle"

C7

4.14
Cervical vertebrae

Observe:

1. The 3rd, 4th, 5th, and 6th cervical vertebrae are "typical"; the 1st, 2nd, and 7th are "atypical";

2. The body, transversely elongated, is of equal depth anteriorly and posteriorly; its superior surface with lateral lips, resembling a seat with upturned side arms, bears facets that articulate with the vertebra above; arthritic expansion of these joints encroach on the vertebral canal (spinal cord) and the foramen transversarium (vertebral artery) (see Hall MC. *Luschka's joint.* Springfield, IL: Charles C Thomas, 1965);

3. The body of the atlas is missing: it is joined to the axis as the dens; the anterior arch on the atlas lies anterior to the dens and articulates with it;

4. The vertebral foramen is large and triangular;

5. The superior and inferior vertebral notches, nearly equal in depth;

6. The spinous process, short and bifid, except that of the atlas, which is reduced to a tubercle, and that of C7 (vertebra prominens), which is long and nonbifid; that of the axis is massive;

7. The transverse processes, short, perforated, and ending laterally in anterior and posterior tubercles with a gutter between them; those of the atlas and of C7 are long and have but one (posterior) tubercle; so has the axis, but it is short;

8. The superior facets of the axis and the inferior and superior facets of the atlas are in series with the facets at the lateral aspects of the superior and inferior surfaces of the bodies.

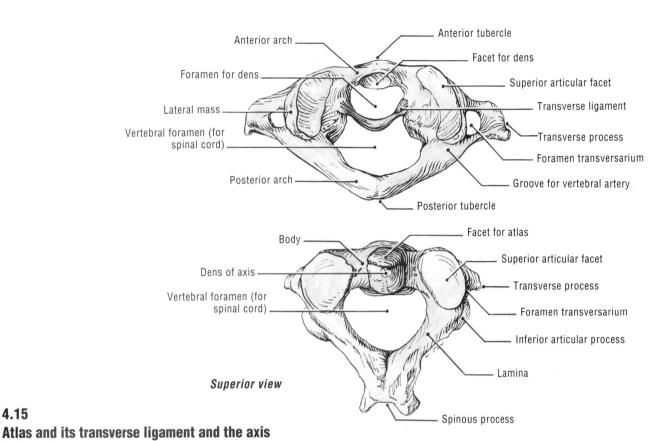

Superior view

4.15
Atlas and its transverse ligament and the axis

Observe:

1. The large vertebral foramen of the atlas that is divided into two foramina by the transverse ligament of the atlas; in the larger, posterior foramen, the spinal cord lies loosely; in the smaller, anterior foramen, the dens of the axis fits tightly;

2. The dens articulates anteriorly with the anterior arch of the atlas and posteriorly with the transverse ligament that, like the anular ligament of the radius, forms an arc of a circle.

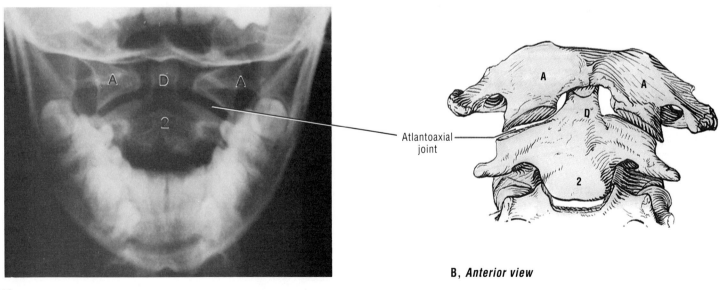

A

B, Anterior view

4.16
The atlantoaxial joint

A. Anteroposterior radiograph.

Observe:

1. The radiograph was taken through the open mouth;

2. The body of the axis *(2)* with the dens (odontoid process) *(D)* projecting superiorly between the lateral masses of the atlas *(A).*

B. Articulated atlas and axis.

4.17
Thoracic vertebrae

Observe:

1. The middle four are typically thoracic; the superior four have some cervical features; and the inferior four some lumbar features;

2. The body, deeper posteriorly than anteriorly, with flat superior and inferior surfaces; the surface area (weight-bearing surface) increasing from T1 to T12; the triangular shape of the middle four, which have almost equal transverse and anteroposterior diameters; the transverse diameter increases toward the cervical and lumbar ends of the series;

3. The rib facet at the superior posterolateral angle of the body encroaching on the inferior posterolateral angle of the body above, except for the facets of T10, T11, and T12, which are on the pedicles;

4. The superior vertebral notch present on T1 only;

5. The vertebral foramen circular and becoming triangular toward the cervical and lumbar ends;

6. The spinous processes of the middle four, which are long, overlapping, and nearly vertical; those of the 1st, 2nd, and 11th, 12th are nearly horizontal, and those of 3rd, 4th and 9th, 10th are oblique;

7. The length of the transverse processes diminishes progressively from T1 to T12; T1 to T10 have rib facets on their transverse processes; these are concave and placed anteriorly on T1 to T7, flat and superiorly placed on T8 to T10;

8. The cervical features of T1 include the superior vertebral notches and the upturned lateral lips on the body;

9. The lumbar features of T12 include the lateral direction of the inferior articular processes and possession of mamillary, accessory, and lateral tubercles.

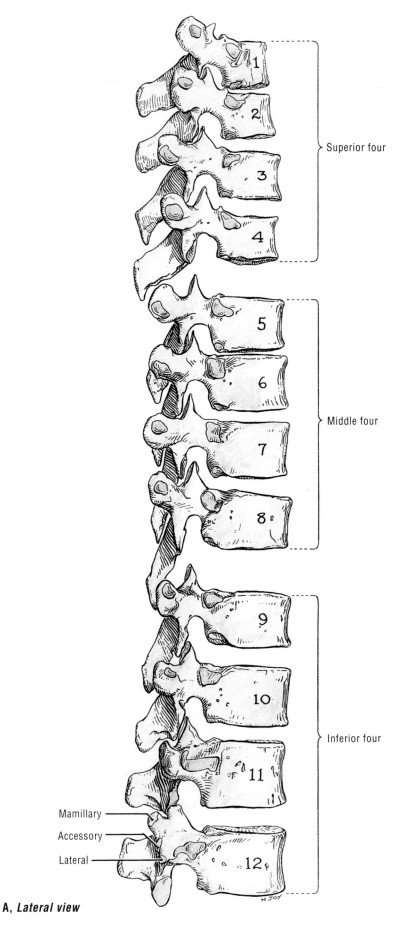

Superior four

Middle four

Inferior four

Mamillary

Accessory

Lateral

A, Lateral view

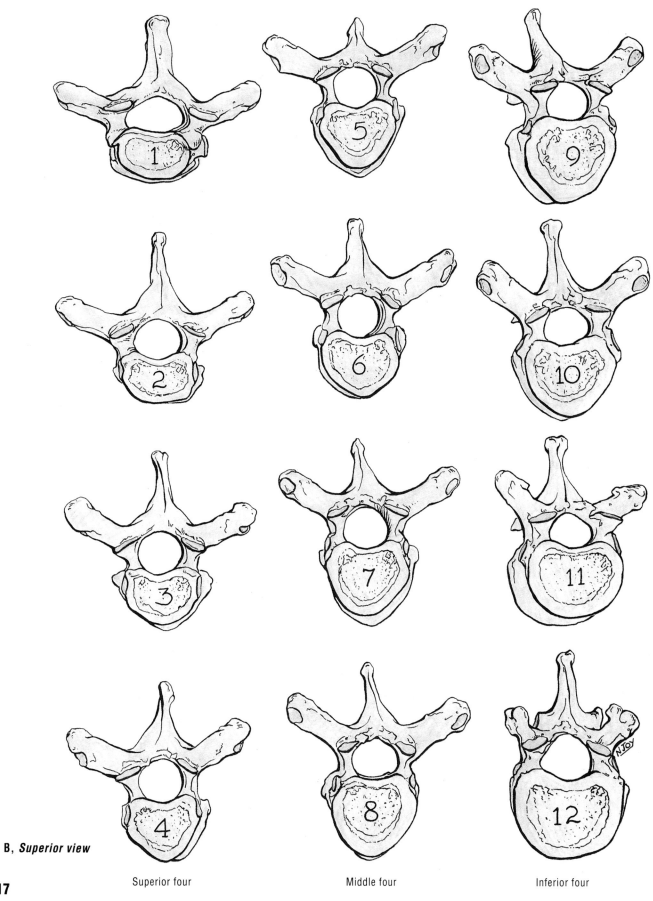

B, *Superior view*

4.17
Thoracic vertebrae *(continued)*

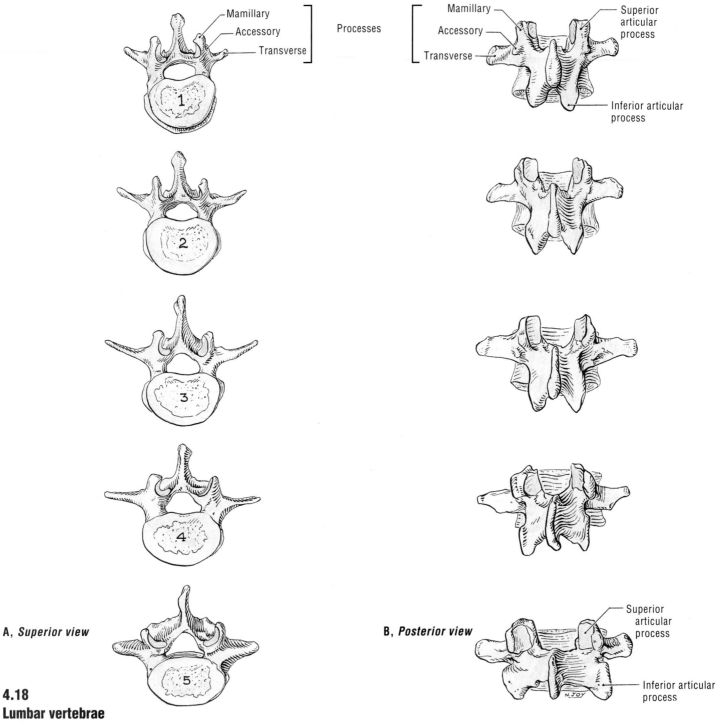

Processes
Mamillary
Accessory
Transverse

Mamillary — Superior articular process
Accessory
Transverse — Inferior articular process

Superior articular process
Inferior articular process

A, *Superior view*

B, *Posterior view*

4.18
Lumbar vertebrae

Observe:

1. The kidney-shaped bodies, greater in transverse than in anteroposterior diameter; bodies of L1 and L2 are deeper posteriorly; L4 and L5 are deeper anteriorly; L3 is transitional;

2. The vertebral foramina, small and triangular, and having pinched lateral angles in L5;

3. The slight superior vertebral notches;

4. The large, oblong, and horizontal spinous processes;

5. The long, slender, horizontal transverse processes; that of L3 projects farthest; that of L5 spreads anteriorly onto the body, is conical, and its apex has a superior tilt; the mamillary process (for the origin of the multifidus muscle) on the superior articular process; the accessory process (for insertion of the longissimus muscle) on the transverse process;

6. The superior articular processes, facing each other and grasping the inferior processes of the vertebra above; the inferior articular processes, close together in L1, but far apart in L5 and facing more anteriorly.

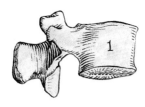

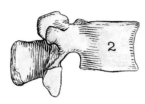

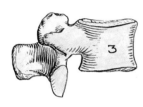

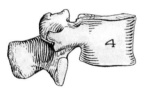

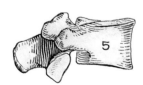

Lateral view

4.19
Lumbar vertebrae

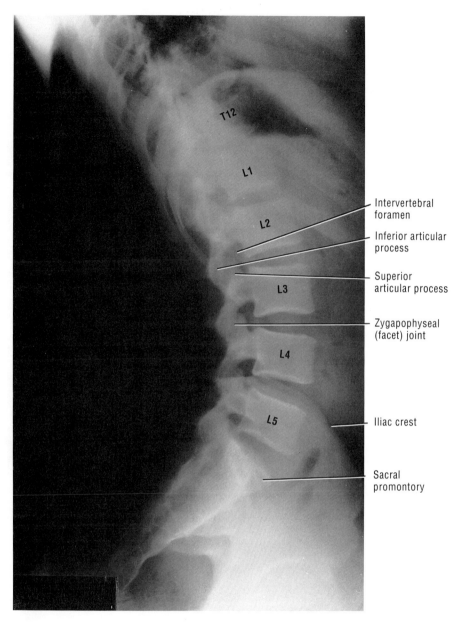

Intervertebral foramen

Inferior articular process

Superior articular process

Zygapophyseal (facet) joint

Iliac crest

Sacral promontory

Lateral view

4.20
Radiograph of lumbosacral spine

Observe:

1. The spaces for intervertebral discs;

2. The angulation at the lumbosacral junction producing the sacral promontory;

3. The facet joint between the superior articular process of L4 and the inferior articular process of L3;

4. The anterior margin of the vertebral canal; an intervertebral foramen bounded superiorly and inferiorly by the pedicles, anteriorly by the vertebral bodies and the intervertebral disc, and posteriorly by the articular process. (Courtesy of Dr. J. Heslin, Assistant Professor of Anatomy, University of Toronto, Toronto, Ontario, Canada.)

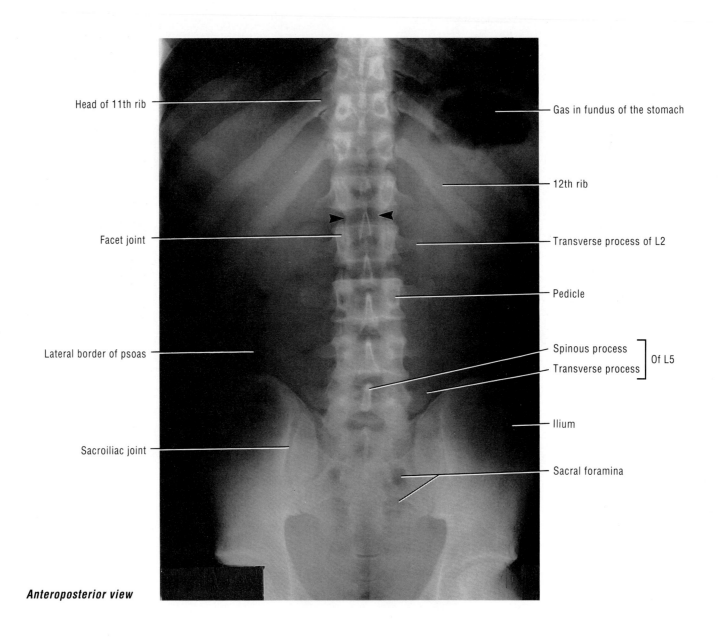

Head of 11th rib

Gas in fundus of the stomach

12th rib

Facet joint

Transverse process of L2

Pedicle

Lateral border of psoas

Spinous process ⎤
Transverse process ⎦ Of L5

Ilium

Sacroiliac joint

Sacral foramina

Anteroposterior view

4.21
Radiograph of inferior thoracic and lumbosacral spine

Observe:

1. The articulation of the 12th rib with the 12th thoracic vertebra;

2. The bodies and processes of the five lumbar vertebrae; the spinous process and transverse process of L5 are labeled;

3. The sinuous sacroiliac joint;

4. The lateral margin of right and left psoas major muscles;

5. The vertebral canal indicated by *arrowheads*.

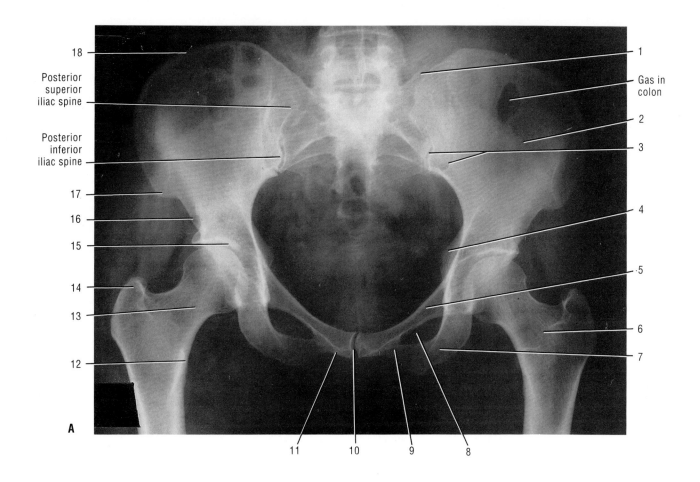

18

Posterior
superior
iliac spine

Posterior
inferior
iliac spine

17

16

15

14

13

12

A

1

Gas in
colon

2

3

4

5

6

7

11   10   9   8

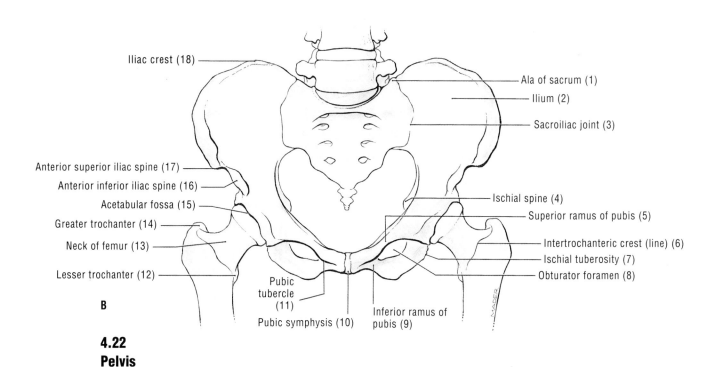

Iliac crest (18)

Ala of sacrum (1)

Ilium (2)

Sacroiliac joint (3)

Anterior superior iliac spine (17)

Anterior inferior iliac spine (16)

Acetabular fossa (15)

Greater trochanter (14)

Neck of femur (13)

Lesser trochanter (12)

Ischial spine (4)

Superior ramus of pubis (5)

Intertrochanteric crest (line) (6)

Ischial tuberosity (7)

Obturator foramen (8)

Pubic
tubercle
(11)

Pubic symphysis (10)

Inferior ramus of
pubis (9)

B

4.22
Pelvis

Compare the radiograph of the pelvis (**A**) to the diagram of the bony pelvis with articulated femora (**B**). (Courtesy of Dr. E.L. Lansdown, Professor of Radiology, University of Toronto, Toronto, Ontario, Canada.)

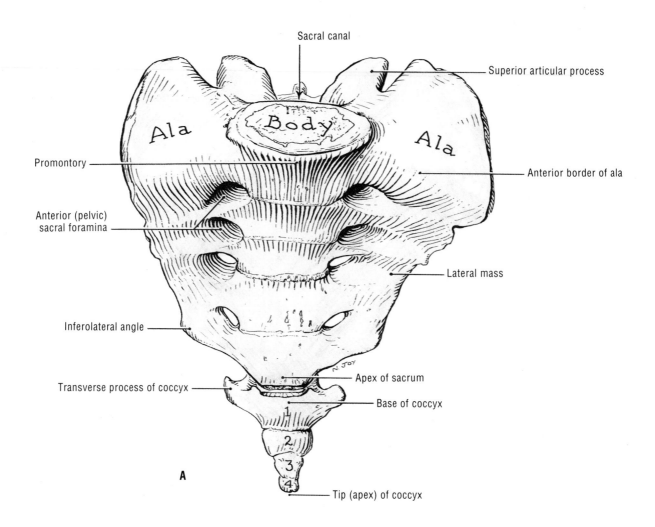

Sacral canal

Superior articular process

Body

Ala

Ala

Promontory

Anterior border of ala

Anterior (pelvic) sacral foramina

Lateral mass

Inferolateral angle

Apex of sacrum

Transverse process of coccyx

Base of coccyx

Tip (apex) of coccyx

A

4.23
Sacrum and coccyx

Observe in **A** (pelvic surface and base):

1. The five sacral bodies, demarcated by four transverse lines that end laterally in four pairs of anterior sacral foramina;

2. The foramina of the two sides, approximately equidistant throughout; their margins are rounded laterally but sharp elsewhere, indicating the courses of the emerging nerves;

3. The coccyx has four pieces; the first piece bears a pair of transverse processes and a pair of cornua; the other three pieces are nodular.

Observe in **B** (lateral view):

1. Anterosuperiorly, the auricular, ear-shaped surface that articulates with the ilium of the hip bone (os coxae);

2. Posterosuperiorly, the sacral tuberosity for the attachment of the dorsal sacroiliac and interosseous sacroiliac ligaments;

3. Inferiorly, the apex of the sacrum articulating with the coccyx, which is concave anteriorly.

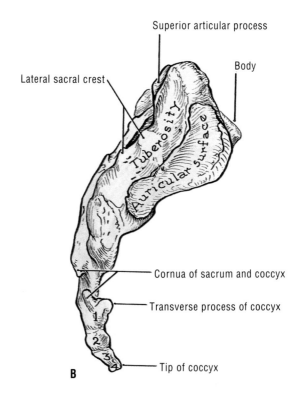

Superior articular process

Body

Lateral sacral crest

Cornua of sacrum and coccyx

Transverse process of coccyx

Tip of coccyx

B

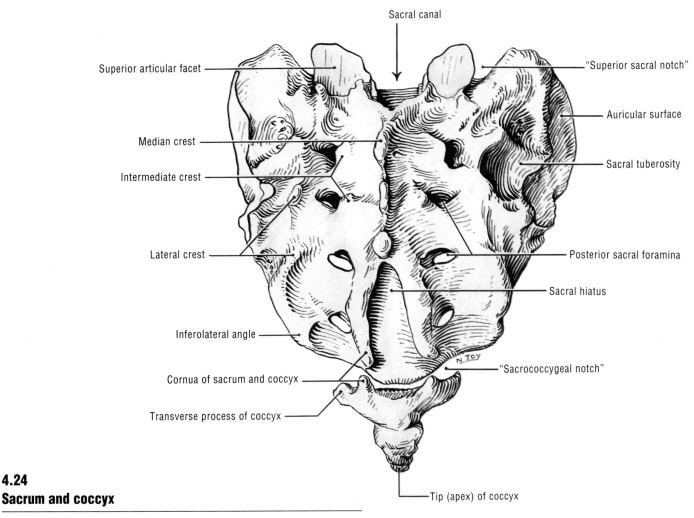

Sacral canal

Superior articular facet

"Superior sacral notch"

Auricular surface

Median crest

Sacral tuberosity

Intermediate crest

Lateral crest

Posterior sacral foramina

Sacral hiatus

Inferolateral angle

"Sacrococcygeal notch"

Cornua of sacrum and coccyx

Transverse process of coccyx

Tip (apex) of coccyx

4.24
Sacrum and coccyx

Observe (posterior surface):
1. The absence of the 4th and 5th sacral spines and laminae;

2. The superior articular processes, the intermediate crest, and the sacral and coccygeal cornua are serially homologous; so, likewise, are the "superior sacral notch," the four dorsal sacral foramina, and the "sacrococcygeal notch";

3. A straight probe can be passed through a lower posterior sacral foramen, across the sacral canal, and through an anterior sacral foramen.

4.25
Sacrum in youth

The costal elements begin to fuse with each other about puberty. The bodies begin to fuse with each other from inferior to superior about the 17th to 18th year, fusion being complete by the 24th year, and between the 2nd and 1st bodies until the 33rd year (see McKern TW, Stewart TD. *Skeletal Age Changes in Young American Males.* Natick, MA: Quartermaster Research & Development Center, 1957).

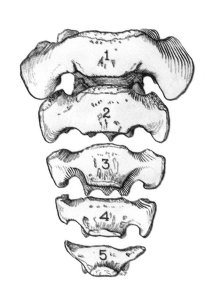

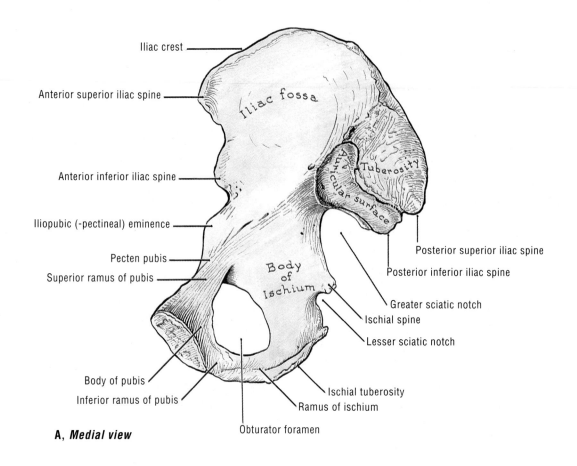

Iliac crest

Anterior superior iliac spine

Iliac fossa

Auricular surface

Tuberosity

Anterior inferior iliac spine

Iliopubic (-pectineal) eminence

Pecten pubis

Superior ramus of pubis

Body of Ischium

Posterior superior iliac spine

Posterior inferior iliac spine

Greater sciatic notch

Ischial spine

Lesser sciatic notch

Body of pubis

Inferior ramus of pubis

Ischial tuberosity

Ramus of ischium

Obturator foramen

A, *Medial view*

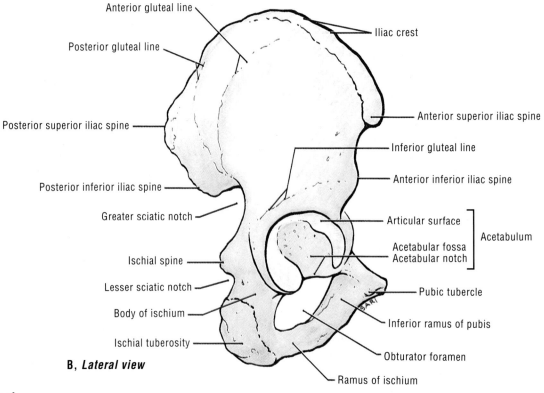

Anterior gluteal line

Posterior gluteal line

Iliac crest

Posterior superior iliac spine

Anterior superior iliac spine

Inferior gluteal line

Anterior inferior iliac spine

Posterior inferior iliac spine

Greater sciatic notch

Articular surface

Acetabulum

Acetabular fossa

Acetabular notch

Ischial spine

Lesser sciatic notch

Pubic tubercle

Body of ischium

Inferior ramus of pubis

Ischial tuberosity

Obturator foramen

B, *Lateral view*

Ramus of ischium

4.26
Hip bone (os coxae)

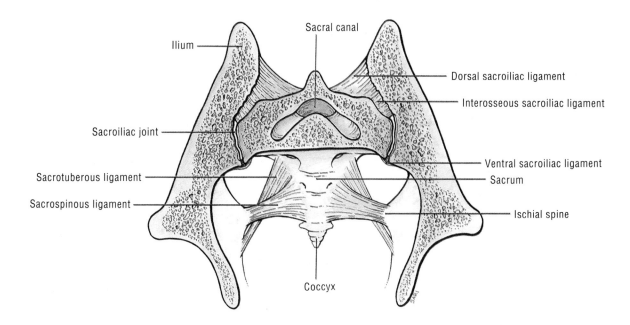

4.27
Coronal section of the pelvis to illustrate the transversely oriented sacroiliac joints

Note that the strong interosseous sacroiliac ligament lies anterior to the dorsal sacroiliac ligament and consists of short fibers connecting the tuberosity of the sacrum to the ilium.

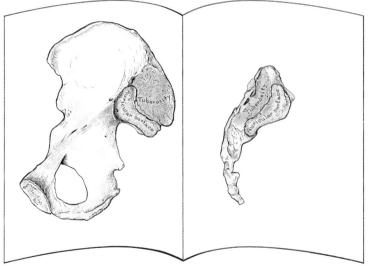

A, *Medial view*   **B,** *Lateral view*

4.28
Articular surfaces of the sacroiliac joint

Observe:

1. The auricular surface (articular area) of the sacrum and hip bone (os coxae) (**A**);

2. The roughened areas superior and posterior to the auricular areas (orange) for the attachment of the interosseous sacroiliac ligament.

A, *Oblique view*

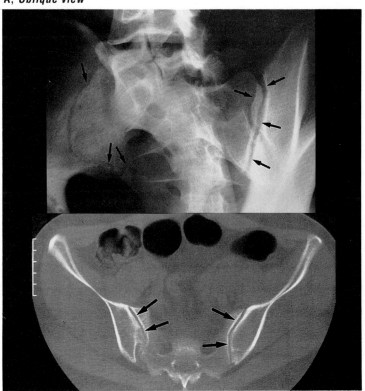

B, *Transverse scan*

4.29
Radiograph and CT (computed tomographic) scan of the sacroiliac joint

The sacroiliac joint is indicated by *arrows*. (Radiograph courtesy of Dr. J. Heslin, and CT scan courtesy of Dr. E. Becker, University of Toronto, Toronto, Ontario, Canada.)

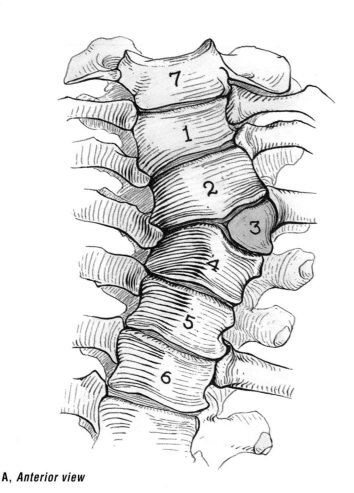

A, *Anterior view*

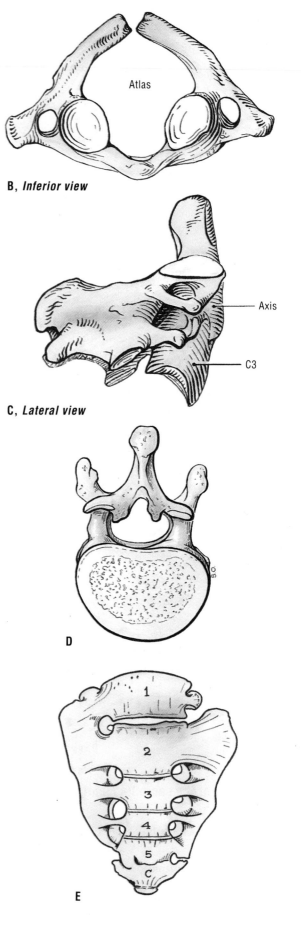

B, *Inferior view*

C, *Lateral view*

D

E

4.30
Anomalies of the vertebrae

A. Hemivertebra. The entire right half of the 3rd thoracic vertebra and the corresponding rib are absent. The left lamina and the spine are fused with those of T4, and the left intervetebral foramen is reduced in size. Observe the associated scoliosis (lateral curvature of the spine). **B.** Unfused posterior arch of the atlas. Of the three vertebral components at birth, the centrum has fused to the right and left halves of the vertebral arch, but the arch has not fused in the midline posteriorly. **C.** Synostosis of vertebrae C2 (axis) and C3. Congenital synostosis of two vertebrae is relatively common, especially these two. **D.** Ossifying ligamenta flava. Sharp, bony spurs commonly grow from the laminae inferiorly into the ligamenta flava, thereby reducing the lengths of these elastic bands. Hence, when the vertebral column is flexed, they are likely to be torn. Restricted to the thoracic and lumbar regions, most common and largest on T11, they diminish in size and frequency cranially to T1 and caudally to L5. **E.** Transitional lumbosacral vertebra. In this instance, the 1st sacral vertebra is partly free (lumbarized). Not uncommonly, the 5th lumbar vertebra is partly fused to the sacrum (sacralized).

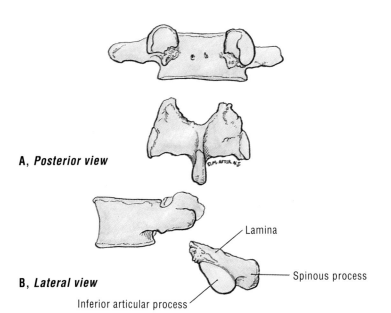

A, *Posterior view*

B, *Lateral view*

Lamina

Spinous process

Inferior articular process

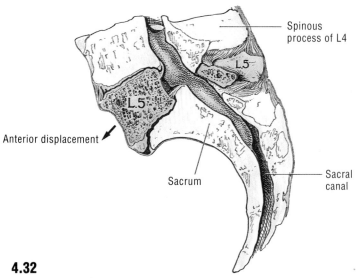

Spinous process of L4

L5

Anterior displacement

L5

Sacrum

Sacral canal

4.31
Spondylolysis of L5

In this case, the 5th lumbar vertebra has an oblique defect, spondylolysis, through the pars interarticularis. The defect may be traumatic or embryologic in origin. The two elements are usually held together by fibrous tissue and separation of these elements is called spondylolisthesis.

4.32
Spondylolisthesis

The anterior element of L5 has slipped anteriorly, but the posterior elements have remained normally aligned.

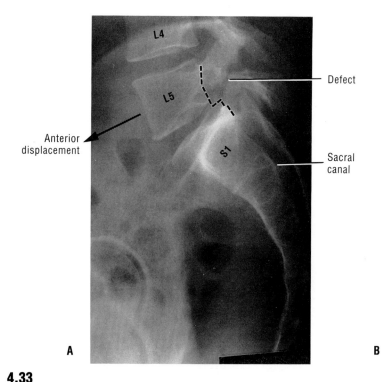

L4

L5

Defect

Anterior displacement

S1

Sacral canal

A

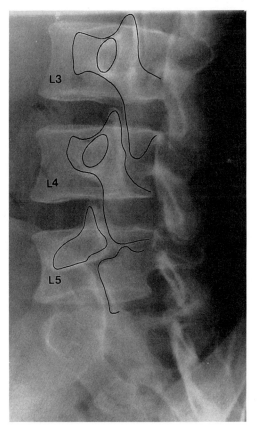

L3

L4

L5

B

4.33
Radiographic study of spondylolisthesis

A. Lateral radiograph. The *dotted line* following the posterior vertebral margins of L5 and the sacrum shows the anterior displacement of L5. **B.** Oblique radiograph. Note the superimposed outline of a dog, the head consisting of the transverse process, the eye of the pedicle and the ear of the superior articular process. The lucent cleft across the "neck" of the dog is called spondylolysis. (Courtesy of Dr. E. Becker, Associate Professor of Radiology, University of Toronto, Toronto, Ontario, Canada.)

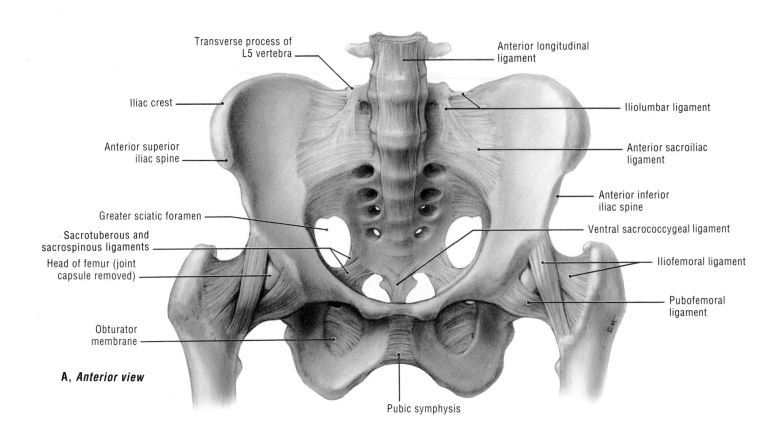

Transverse process of L5 vertebra

Iliac crest

Anterior superior iliac spine

Greater sciatic foramen

Sacrotuberous and sacrospinous ligaments

Head of femur (joint capsule removed)

Obturator membrane

Anterior longitudinal ligament

Iliolumbar ligament

Anterior sacroiliac ligament

Anterior inferior iliac spine

Ventral sacrococcygeal ligament

Iliofemoral ligament

Pubofemoral ligament

Pubic symphysis

A, *Anterior view*

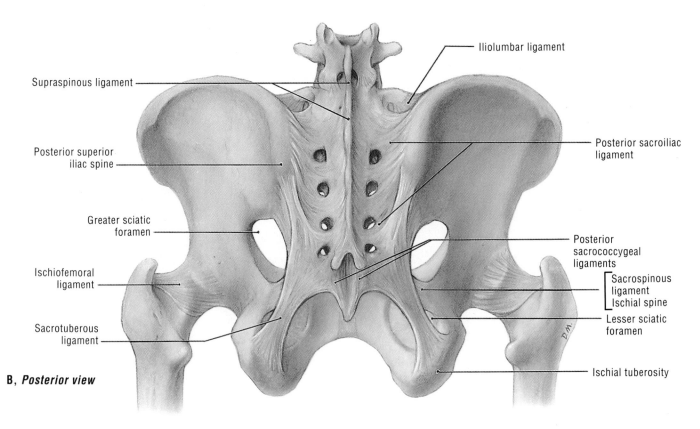

Supraspinous ligament

Posterior superior iliac spine

Greater sciatic foramen

Ischiofemoral ligament

Sacrotuberous ligament

Iliolumbar ligament

Posterior sacroiliac ligament

Posterior sacrococcygeal ligaments

Sacrospinous ligament
Ischial spine

Lesser sciatic foramen

Ischial tuberosity

B, *Posterior view*

4.34
Lumbar and pelvic ligaments

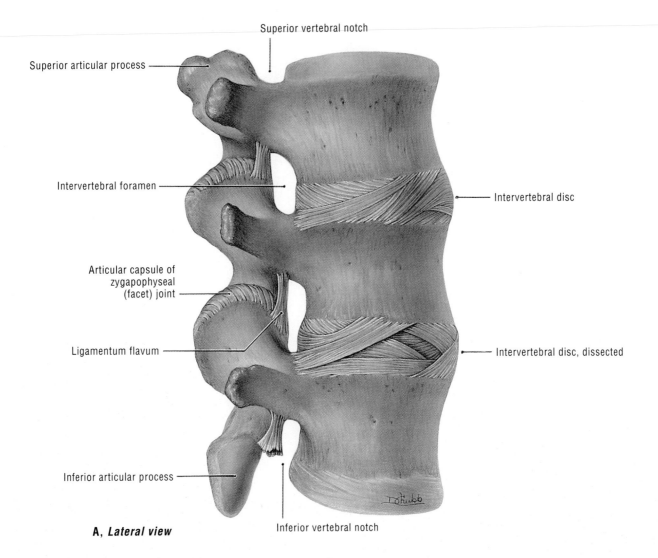

Superior vertebral notch

Superior articular process

Intervertebral foramen

Articular capsule of
zygapophyseal
(facet) joint

Ligamentum flavum

Inferior articular process

Intervertebral disc

Intervertebral disc, dissected

Inferior vertebral notch

A, *Lateral view*

4.35
Intervertebral disc

A. Sections have been removed from the superficial layers of the inferior disc in order to show the directions of the fibers.

Observe:

1. The anulus fibrosus arranged in layers of parallel fibers that criss-cross those of the next layer;

2. An intervertebral foramen, resulting from the apposition of a superior and an inferior vertebral notch, bounded superiorly and inferiorly by pedicles, anteriorly by an intervertebral disc and parts of the two bodies united by that disc, and posteriorly by a capsular ligament and parts of the two articular processes united by that capsular ligament; further, the anterior part of the capsule is strengthened by the lateral border of the ligamentum flavum;

3. The vulnerability of a spinal nerve to the pressure of an extruded nucleus pulposus through a torn anulus fibrosus; the most common site of a disc lesion is between L5 and S1.

B. Diagram. Note that the center of the disc is filled with fibrogelatinous pulp, the nucleus pulposus, which acts as a shock absorber. As a result of aging, the nucleus pulposus becomes increasingly fibrocartilaginous and contains less water.

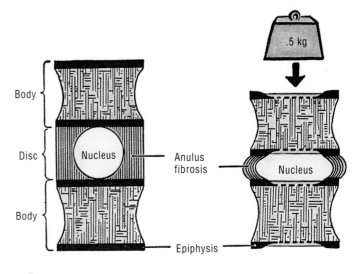

Body

Disc

Body

.5 kg

Nucleus

Anulus
fibrosis

Nucleus

Epiphysis

B

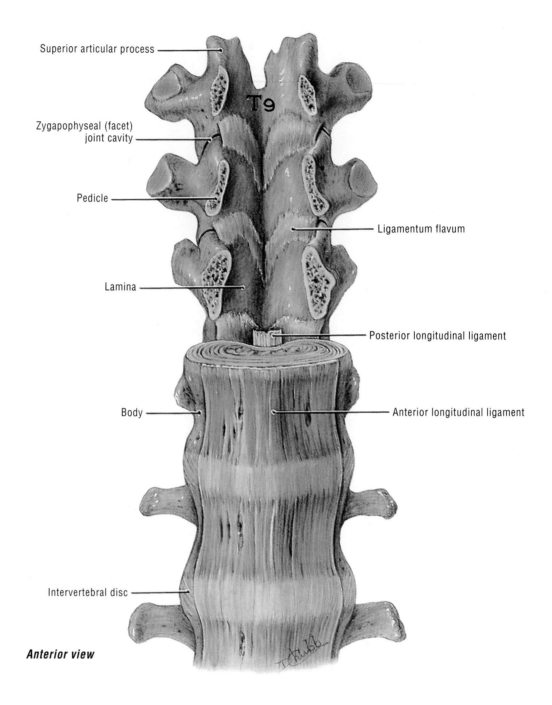

Superior articular process

Zygapophyseal (facet)
joint cavity

Pedicle

Lamina

Body

Intervertebral disc

Anterior view

T9

Ligamentum flavum

Posterior longitudinal ligament

Anterior longitudinal ligament

4.36
Anterior longitudinal ligament and the ligamenta flava

The pedicles of the 9th, 10th, and 11th thoracic vertebrae have been sawn through and their bodies viewed in Figure 4.37.

Observe:

1. The anterior and posterior longitudinal ligaments are ligaments of the bodies; the ligamenta flava are ligaments of the vertebral arches;

2. The anterior longitudinal ligaments are broad, strong, fibrous bands; they are attached to the intervertebral discs and the vertebral bodies anteriorly; they have foramina for arteries and veins passing to and from the vertebral bodies;

3. The ligamenta flava, composed of yellow or elastic fibers, extend between adjacent laminae; those of opposite sides meet and blend in the median plane; they extend laterally to the articular processes where they blend with the anterior fibers of the capsule of the joint; being elastic, they tend, at all times, to restore the vertebral column to the extended or erect position; cranially, they are in series with the posterior atlantoaxial and posterior atlanto-occipital membranes.

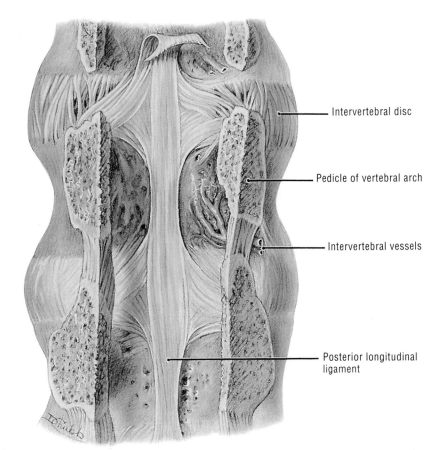

Intervertebral disc

Pedicle of vertebral arch

Intervertebral vessels

Posterior longitudinal ligament

Posterior view

4.37
Posterior longitudinal ligament

The vertebral arches have been sawn through and are shown in the superior part of Figure 4.36.

Observe:

1. This taut but somewhat flimsy band passing from disc to disc, spanning the posterior surfaces of the bodies of the vertebrae, and rendering smooth the anterior wall of the vertebral canal;

2. The diamond shape taken by the ligament posterior to each disc, where it both gives and receives fibers;

4.38
Transverse section of an intervertebral disc and ligaments

The nucleus pulposus has been scooped out and the cartilaginous epiphyseal plate exposed.

Observe:

1. The rings of the anulus fibrosus, least numerous posteriorly;

2. The continuity of the following ligaments: capsular, flavum, interspinous, and supraspinous;

3. The synovial fold, containing a pad of fat, such as is present in all synovial joints;

4. The longitudinal vertebral venous sinuses that extend extradurally throughout the length of the vertebral canal (Fig. 4.40).

5. The cauda equina of the spinal cord (not labeled) lying free within the subarachnoid space.

3. Between the ligament and a vertebral body, a plexus of veins that receives the basivertebral vein from the body, communicates with the longitudinal vertebral venous sinus on each side, and drains by way of the intervertebral veins; the ligament extends to the sacrum inferiorly; it becomes the strong tectorial membrane cranially.

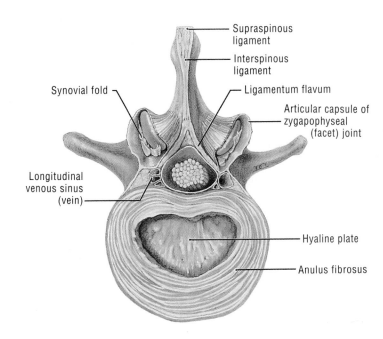

Supraspinous ligament

Interspinous ligament

Synovial fold

Ligamentum flavum

Articular capsule of zygapophyseal (facet) joint

Longitudinal venous sinus (vein)

Hyaline plate

Anulus fibrosus

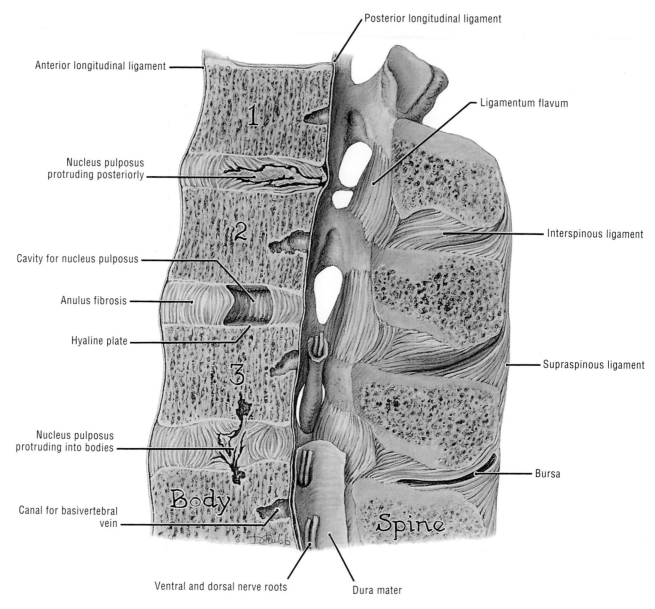

Anterior longitudinal ligament

Nucleus pulposus protruding posteriorly

Cavity for nucleus pulposus

Anulus fibrosis

Hyaline plate

Nucleus pulposus protruding into bodies

Canal for basivertebral vein

Ventral and dorsal nerve roots

Posterior longitudinal ligament

Ligamentum flavum

Interspinous ligament

Supraspinous ligament

Bursa

Dura mater

Body

Spine

4.39
Median section of the vertebral column and ligaments

Observe:

1. The nucleus pulposus of the normal disc between the 2nd and 3rd vertebrae has been scooped out from the enclosing anulus fibrosus;

2. The ligamentum flavum, extending from the superior border and adjacent part of the posterior aspect of one lamina to the inferior border and adjacent part of the anterior aspect of the lamina above, and extending laterally to the intervertebral foramen;

3. The interspinous ligament, uniting obliquely the superior and inferior borders of two adjacent spines; elastic fibers are sparse;

4. The supraspinous ligament extending as far inferiorly as L4 or L5; many of the fibers shown above are not ligamentous, but the

fibrous attachments of thoracolumbar fascia and the deep back muscles;

5. The adventitious bursa between the 3rd and 4th lumbar spines, acquired presumably as the result of habitual hyperextension that brings the lumbar spines into contact;

6. Two degenerative changes: (a) The pulp of the disc between the 1st and 2nd vertebrae has herniated posteriorly through the anulus; the vulnerability of a spinal nerve to the pressure of an extruded nucleus pulposus through a torn anulus fibrosus, and (b) the pulp of the disc between the 3rd and 4th vertebrae has herniated through the cartilaginous epiphyseal plates into the bodies of the vertebrae superiorly and inferiorly.

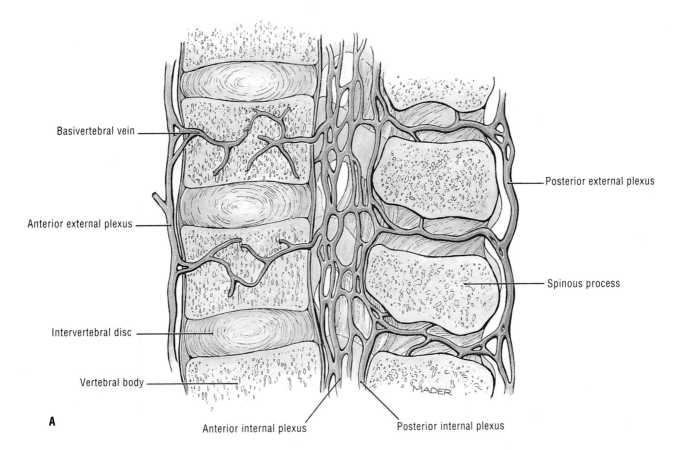

Basivertebral vein

Anterior external plexus

Intervertebral disc

Vertebral body

A

Anterior internal plexus

Posterior external plexus

Spinous process

Posterior internal plexus

4.40
Vertebral venous plexuses

A. Median section. **B.** Superior view. Note the vertebral body is sectioned transversely. There is an internal and an external plexus, communicating with each other and with both segmental systemic veins and the portal system. Infection and tumors may spread from systemic and portal areas (e.g., prostate, breast) to the vertebral venous system and lodge in vertebrae, spinal cord, brain, or skull.

The internal plexus: The vertebral canal contains a plexus of thin-walled, valveless veins that surround like a basketwork the dura mater of the spinal cord and the posterior longitudinal ligament; anterior and posterior longitudinal channels (venous sinuses) can be discerned in this plexus; cranially, this plexus communicates through the foramen magnum with the occipital and basilar sinuses; at each spinal segment, the plexus receives veins from the spinal cord and a basivertebral vein from the body of a vertebra; the plexus, in turn, is drained by intervertebral veins that pass through the intervertebral and sacral foramina to the vertebral, intercostal, lumbar, and lateral sacral veins.

The external plexus: Through the body of each vertebra come veins that form a meager anterior vertebral plexus, and through the ligamenta flava pass veins that form a well-marked posterior vertebral plexus; in the cervical region, these plexuses communicate freely with the occipital and profunda cervicis veins, which receive from the sigmoid sinus the mastoid and condyloid emissary veins; in the thoracic, lumbar, and pelvic regions the azygos (or hemiazygos), the ascending lumbar, and the lateral sacral veins, respectively, further link segment to segment.

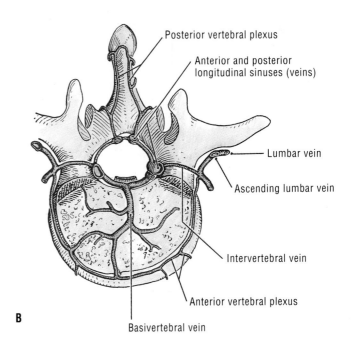

Posterior vertebral plexus

Anterior and posterior longitudinal sinuses (veins)

Lumbar vein

Ascending lumbar vein

Intervertebral vein

Anterior vertebral plexus

Basivertebral vein

B

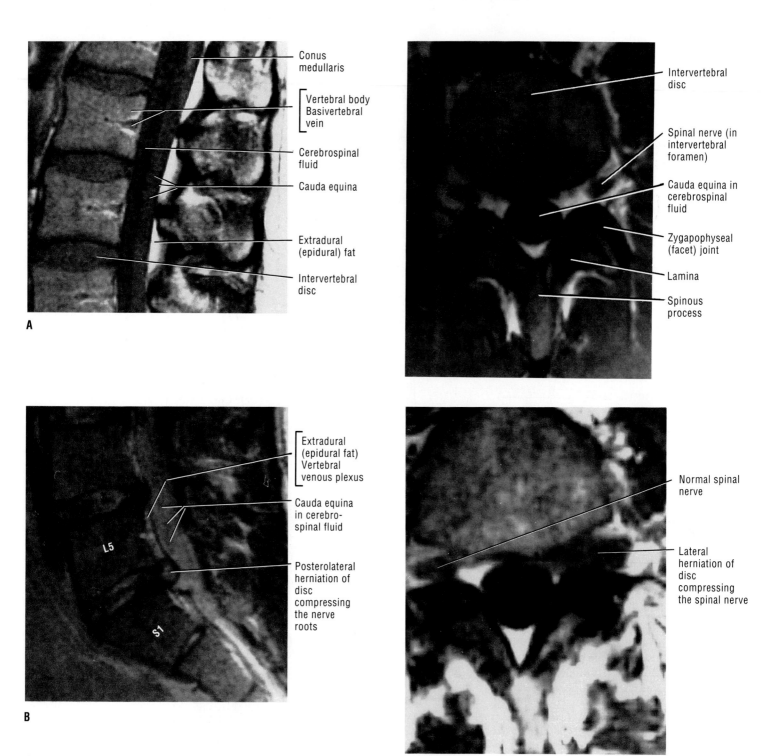

Conus medullaris

Vertebral body
Basivertebral vein

Cerebrospinal fluid

Cauda equina

Extradural (epidural) fat

Intervertebral disc

A

Intervertebral disc

Spinal nerve (in intervertebral foramen)

Cauda equina in cerebrospinal fluid

Zygapophyseal (facet) joint

Lamina

Spinous process

Extradural (epidural fat)
Vertebral venous plexus

Cauda equina in cerebro-spinal fluid

Posterolateral herniation of disc compressing the nerve roots

B

Normal spinal nerve

Lateral herniation of disc compressing the spinal nerve

4.41

MRIs (magnetic resonance images) of the vertebral column and the intervertebral discs

A. Normal intervertebral disc: sagittal scan (*left*) and transverse scan (*right*). **B.** Herniated (ruptured) intervertebral disc: sagittal scan (*left*) and transverse scan (*right*). Protrusion or rupture (herniation) of the nucleus pulposis through the anulus fibrosis occurs most frequently at the lumbar (lumbosacral) levels and is usually posterolateral in direction. The disc may also rupture through the lateral (weaker) part of the posterior longitudinal ligament. Herniation of the disc usually causes impingement of the nerve roots and/or spinal nerve and, therefore, results in sensory loss, numbness, and muscle weakness in the dermatomal and myotomal distribution of the affected nerve roots and/or spinal nerve. (Courtesy of Dr. W. Kucharczyk, Clinical Director of Tri-Hospital Resonance Centre, Toronto, Ontario, Canada.)

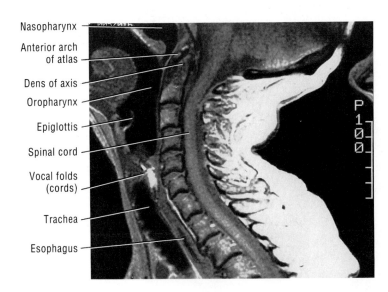

Nasopharynx
Anterior arch of atlas
Dens of axis
Oropharynx
Epiglottis
Spinal cord
Vocal folds (cords)
Trachea
Esophagus

4.42
Sagittal MRI (magnetic resonance image) of the cervical spine

(Courtesy of Dr. W. Kucharczyk, Clinical Director of Tri-Hospital Resonance Centre, Toronto, Ontario, Canada.)

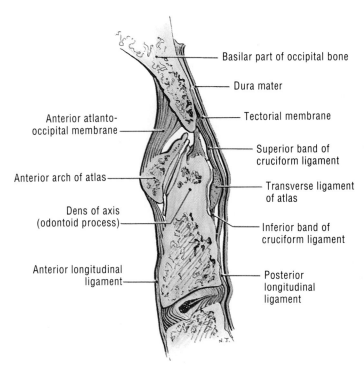

Basilar part of occipital bone
Dura mater
Tectorial membrane
Anterior atlanto-occipital membrane
Superior band of cruciform ligament
Anterior arch of atlas
Transverse ligament of atlas
Dens of axis (odontoid process)
Inferior band of cruciform ligament
Anterior longitudinal ligament
Posterior longitudinal ligament

4.43
Median section through the dens (odontoid process)

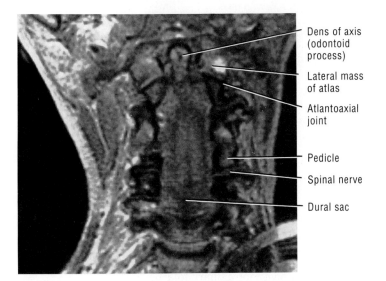

Dens of axis (odontoid process)
Lateral mass of atlas
Atlantoaxial joint
Pedicle
Spinal nerve
Dural sac

4.44
Coronal MRI (magnetic resonance image) of the cervical spine

(Courtesy of Dr. W. Kucharczyk, Clinical Director of Tri-Hospital Resonance Centre, Toronto, Ontario, Canada.)

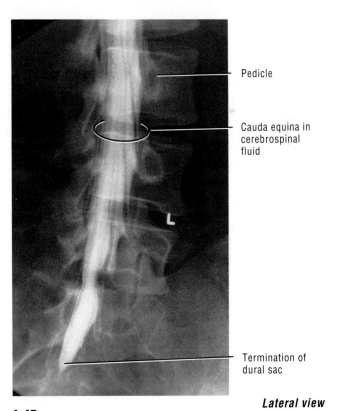

Pedicle
Cauda equina in cerebrospinal fluid
Termination of dural sac

Lateral view

4.45
Myelogram

(Courtesy of Dr. M. Keller, Assistant Professor of Radiology, University of Toronto, Toronto, Ontario, Canada.)

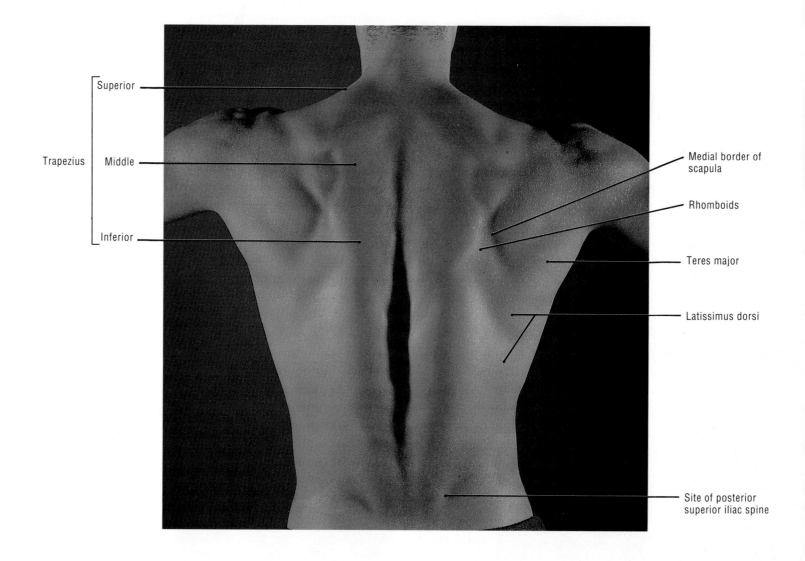

Superior ⌐
Trapezius ⎱ Middle
Inferior ⌐

Medial border of scapula

Rhomboids

Teres major

Latissimus dorsi

Site of posterior superior iliac spine

4.46
Surface anatomy of the back

Observe:

1. The upper limbs are elevated, therefore the scapulae have moved laterally on the thoracic wall, enabling the visualization of the rhomboid muscles;

2. The superior, middle, and inferior parts of the trapezius muscle;

3. The latissimus dorsi and teres major muscles forming the posterior axillary fold;

4. The deep midline furrow separating the lateral bulges of the erector spinae group of muscles;

5. The dimples (depressions) indicating the site of the posterior superior iliac spines, which usually lie at the level of the sacroiliac joint.

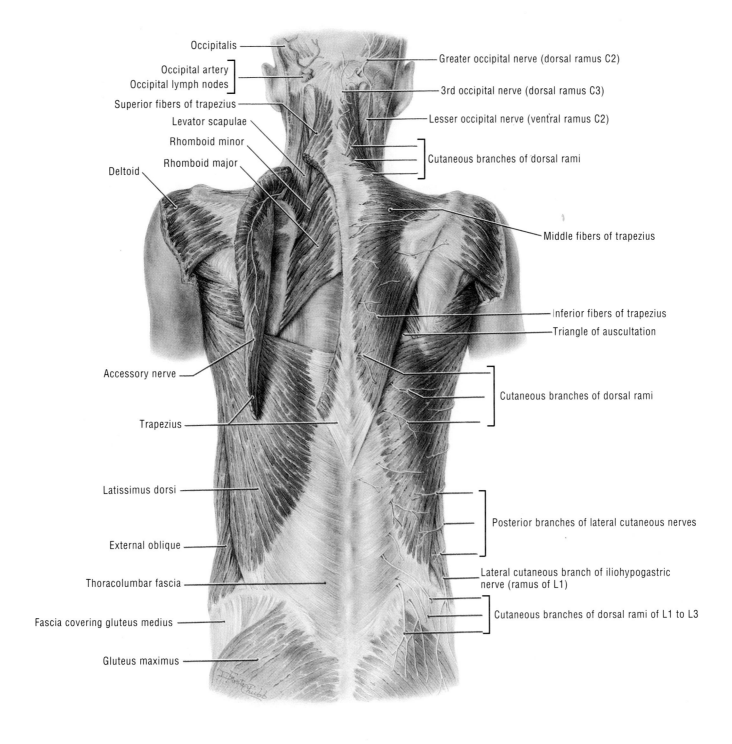

Occipitalis

Occipital artery
Occipital lymph nodes

Superior fibers of trapezius

Levator scapulae

Rhomboid minor

Rhomboid major

Deltoid

Accessory nerve

Trapezius

Latissimus dorsi

External oblique

Thoracolumbar fascia

Fascia covering gluteus medius

Gluteus maximus

Greater occipital nerve (dorsal ramus C2)

3rd occipital nerve (dorsal ramus C3)

Lesser occipital nerve (ventral ramus C2)

Cutaneous branches of dorsal rami

Middle fibers of trapezius

Inferior fibers of trapezius

Triangle of auscultation

Cutaneous branches of dorsal rami

Posterior branches of lateral cutaneous nerves

Lateral cutaneous branch of iliohypogastric
nerve (ramus of L1)

Cutaneous branches of dorsal rami of L1 to L3

4.47
Superficial muscles of the back

On the left side, the trapezius muscle is reflected.

Observe two layers:
1. The trapezius and latissimus dorsi muscles;

2. The levator scapulae and rhomboids minor and major; these muscles help attach the upper limb to the trunk.

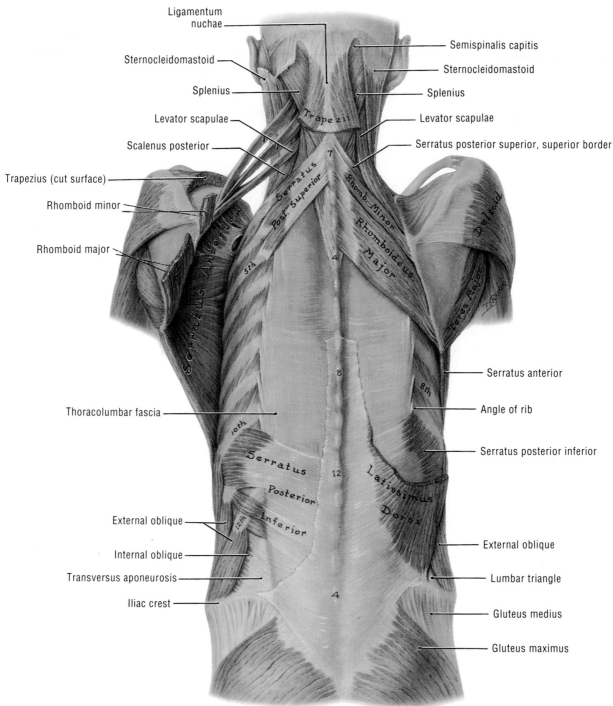

Ligamentum nuchae

Sternocleidomastoid

Splenius

Levator scapulae

Scalenus posterior

Trapezius (cut surface)

Rhomboid minor

Rhomboid major

Thoracolumbar fascia

External oblique

Internal oblique

Transversus aponeurosis

Iliac crest

Semispinalis capitis

Sternocleidomastoid

Splenius

Levator scapulae

Serratus posterior superior, superior border

Serratus anterior

Angle of rib

Serratus posterior inferior

External oblique

Lumbar triangle

Gluteus medius

Gluteus maximus

4.48
Intermediate muscles of the back

The trapezius and latissimus dorsi muscles are largely cut away on both sides.

Observe:

1. On the right side: the levator scapulae and rhomboid muscles; the serratus posterior superior, extending superior to rhomboid minor muscles;

2. On the left side: the rhomboid muscles have been severed allowing the vertebral border of the scapula to be raised from the thoracic wall; the digitations of levator scapulae muscles;

3. Serratus posterior superior and inferior are the intermediate layer of muscles, passing from spines of the vertebrae to the ribs; the two muscles slope in opposite directions and are muscles of inspiration;

4. The thoracolumbar fascia, extending laterally to the angles of the ribs, becoming thin superiorly, passing deep to serratus posterior superior muscle, and reinforced inferiorly by latissimus dorsi and serratus posterior inferior muscles.

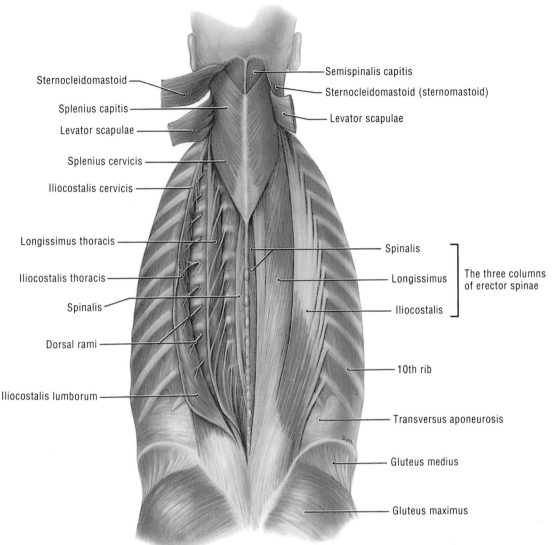

Sternocleidomastoid

Splenius capitis

Levator scapulae

Splenius cervicis

Iliocostalis cervicis

Longissimus thoracis

Iliocostalis thoracis

Spinalis

Dorsal rami

Iliocostalis lumborum

Semispinalis capitis

Sternocleidomastoid (sternomastoid)

Levator scapulae

Spinalis

Longissimus — The three columns of erector spinae

Iliocostalis

10th rib

Transversus aponeurosis

Gluteus medius

Gluteus maximus

4.49
Deep muscles of the back: splenius and erector spinae

Observe:

1. The splenius capitis muscle attaching to the mastoid process deep to the sternocleidomastoid muscle; the splenius cervicis muscle to the 1st, 2nd, (and 3rd) cervical transverse processes deep to the levator scapulae muscle;

2. On the right side: the erector spinae muscles in situ, lying between the spinous processes medially and the angles of the ribs laterally and splitting into three longitudinal columns: iliocostalis laterally, longissimus in the middle, and spinalis medially;

3. On the left side, the spinalis muscle, the thinnest and most medial of the erector spinae muscles, running from inferior to more superior spinous processes, inconstantly extending as high as the cervical region; the longissimus muscle, the intermediate column, pulled laterally to show the insertion into transverse processes and ribs; not shown here are its extensions to neck and head, longissimus cervicis and capitis; the iliocostalis muscle, the most lateral, consisting of three parts: iliocostalis lumborum, iliocostalis thoracis, and the iliocostalis cervicis, inserting on the posterior tubercles of inferior cervical vertebrae.

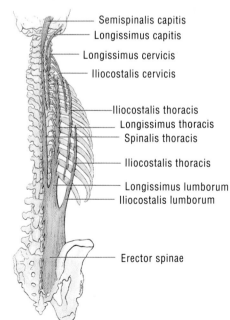

Semispinalis capitis
Longissimus capitis

Longissimus cervicis
Iliocostalis cervicis

Iliocostalis thoracis
Longissimus thoracis
Spinalis thoracis

Iliocostalis thoracis

Longissimus lumborum
Iliocostalis lumborum

Erector spinae

4.50
Erector spinae and semispinalis

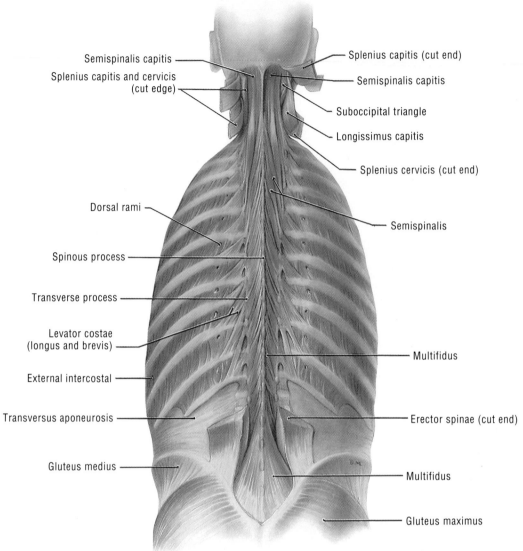

Semispinalis capitis

Splenius capitis and cervicis (cut edge)

Dorsal rami

Spinous process

Transverse process

Levator costae (longus and brevis)

External intercostal

Transversus aponeurosis

Gluteus medius

Splenius capitis (cut end)

Semispinalis capitis

Suboccipital triangle

Longissimus capitis

Splenius cervicis (cut end)

Semispinalis

Multifidus

Erector spinae (cut end)

Multifidus

Gluteus maximus

4.51
Deep muscles of the back: semispinalis and multifidus

The semispinalis, multifidus, and rotatores muscles constitute the transversospinalis group of deep muscles. In general, their bundles pass obliquely in a superomedial direction, from transverse processes to spinous processes, in successively deeper layers. The bundles of semispinalis span about five interspaces, those of multifidus about three, and those of rotatores, one or two (Fig. 4.52).

Observe:

1. The semispinalis (thoracis, cervicis, and capitis) muscles extending from the lower thoracic region to the skull; the semispinalis capitis, a powerful extensor muscle, originates from the lower cervical and upper thoracic vertebrae and inserts into the occipital bone between the superior and inferior nuchal lines;

2. The multifidus muscle, extending from the sacrum to the spine of the axis, arising in the lumbosacral region from the aponeurosis of erector spinae, from the sacrum, and from mamillary processes of the lumbar vertebrae and inserting into spinous processes about three segments higher up.

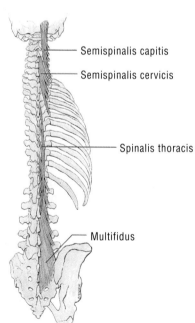

Semispinalis capitis

Semispinalis cervicis

Spinalis thoracis

Multifidus

4.52
Semispinalis, multifidus, and spinalis

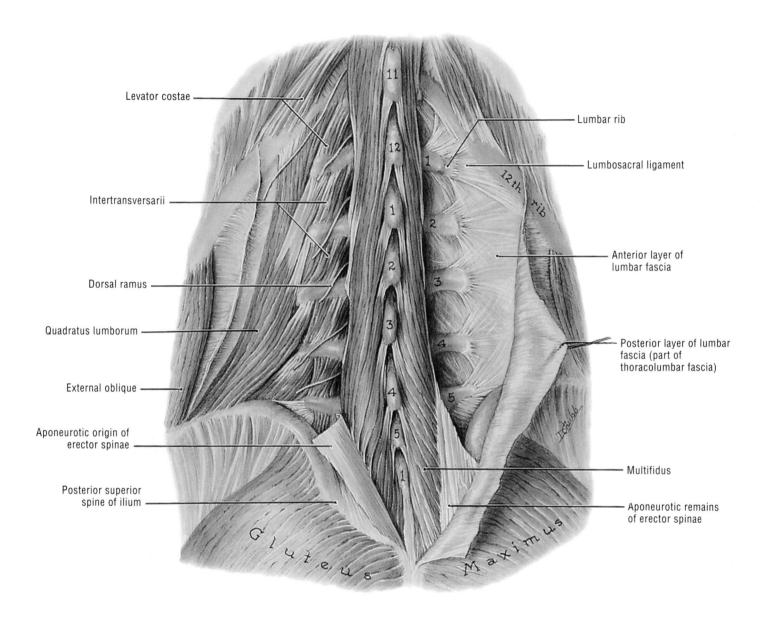

Levator costae

Intertransversarii

Dorsal ramus

Quadratus lumborum

External oblique

Aponeurotic origin of erector spinae

Posterior superior spine of ilium

Lumbar rib

Lumbosacral ligament

Anterior layer of lumbar fascia

Posterior layer of lumbar fascia (part of thoracolumbar fascia)

Multifidus

Aponeurotic remains of erector spinae

Gluteus Maximus

4.53

The back: multifidus, quadratus lumborum, lumbar fascia

Observe:

1. The multifidus muscle originating from the aponeurosis of erector spinae, from the sacrum, and from mamillary processes of the lumbar vertebrae and passing superomedially to spinous processes;

2. On the right side, after removal of erector spinae, the anterior layer of thoracolumbar fascia attached in a fan-shaped manner to

the tips of transverse processes; also, a short lumbar rib;

3. On the left side, after removal of the anterior layer of thoracolumbar fascia, the lateral border of the quadratus lumborum muscle is oblique, and the medial border is in continuity with the intertransversarii.

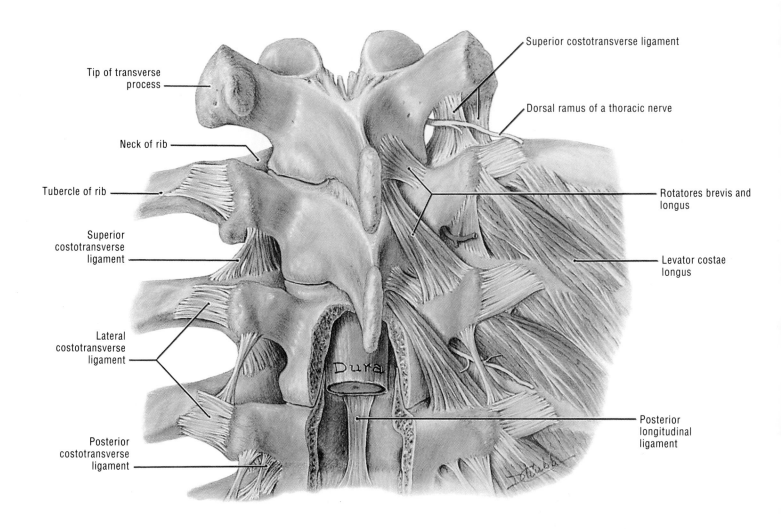

Tip of transverse process

Neck of rib

Tubercle of rib

Superior costotransverse ligament

Lateral costotransverse ligament

Posterior costotransverse ligament

Dura

Superior costotransverse ligament

Dorsal ramus of a thoracic nerve

Rotatores brevis and longus

Levator costae longus

Posterior longitudinal ligament

4.54
Rotatores and the costotransverse ligaments

Observe:

1. Of the three layers of transversospinalis or oblique muscles of the back (semispinalis, multifidus, rotatores), the rotatores are the deepest and shortest; they pass from the root of one transverse process superomedially to the junction of the transverse process and lamina of the vertebra above; some (rotatores longi) span two vertebrae;

2. Similarly, the levatores costarum pass from the tip of one transverse process inferiorly to the rib below; some (levatores longi) span across two ribs;

3. Of the three sets of costotransverse ligaments, superior, lat-

eral, and medial: (a) The superior ligament splits laterally into two sheets between which lie the levator costae and external intercostal; the dorsal ramus of a thoracic nerve passes posterior to this ligament and the ventral ramus (intercostal nerve) passes anterior; (b) The lateral ligament is strong and, if there were no joint cavity between transverse process and rib, it would be continuous with the medial ligament; (c) The medial ligament passes between the anterior aspect of a transverse process and the posterior aspect of the neck of its own rib; it is called the costotransverse ligament; a few fibers lying posteromedial to the superior ligament, constitute a posterior costotransverse ligament.

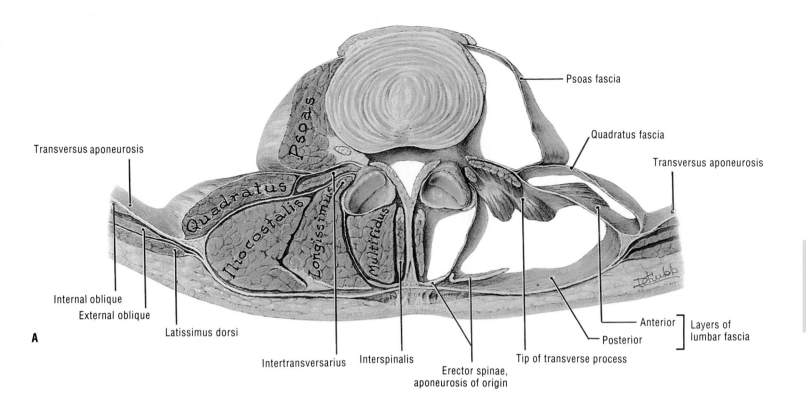

Transversus aponeurosis

Psoas

Quadratus

Iliocostalis

Longissimus

Multifidus

Psoas fascia

Quadratus fascia

Transversus aponeurosis

Internal oblique

External oblique

Latissimus dorsi

Intertransversarius

Interspinalis

Erector spinae,
aponeurosis of origin

Tip of transverse process

Anterior
Posterior

Layers of
lumbar fascia

A

4.55
Transverse section of the muscles of the back

A. On the left side, the muscles are seen within their sheaths or compartments. On the right side, the empty sheaths are shown.

Observe:

1. The posterior aponeurosis of transversus abdominis muscle, splitting into two strong sheets the anterior and the posterior layers of the thoracolumbar fascia, which enclose the deep muscles of the back;

2. The posterior layer of the thoracolumbar fascia, reinforced by the latissimus dorsi muscle and, at a higher level, by the serratus posterior inferior muscle;

3. The weaker areolar layer covering the quadratus lumborum muscle and that covering the psoas muscle;

4. The ends of intertransversarius, longissimus, and quadratus lumborum muscles, attached to a transverse process.

B. This transverse section shows erector spinae muscles in three columns and the transversospinalis muscle in three layers.

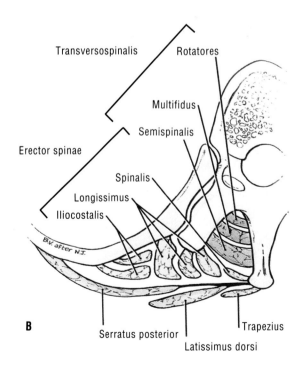

Transversospinalis

Rotatores

Multifidus

Semispinalis

Erector spinae

Spinalis

Longissimus

Iliocostalis

B

Serratus posterior

Latissimus dorsi

Trapezius

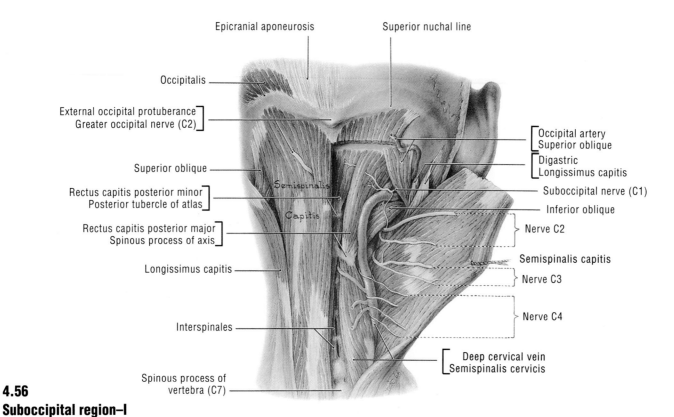

Epicranial aponeurosis

Superior nuchal line

Occipitalis

External occipital protuberance
Greater occipital nerve (C2)

Superior oblique

Rectus capitis posterior minor
Posterior tubercle of atlas

Rectus capitis posterior major
Spinous process of axis

Longissimus capitis

Interspinales

Spinous process of
vertebra (C7)

Semispinalis

Capitis

Occipital artery
Superior oblique
Digastric
Longissimus capitis

Suboccipital nerve (C1)

Inferior oblique

Nerve C2

Semispinalis capitis

Nerve C3

Nerve C4

Deep cervical vein
Semispinalis cervicis

4.56
Suboccipital region–I

The trapezius, sternocleidomastoid, and splenius muscles are removed.

Observe:

1. Semispinalis capitis, the great extensor muscle of the head and neck, forming the posterior wall of the suboccipital region, pierced by the greater occipital nerve (C2, dorsal ramus), and having free medial and lateral borders at this high level; the right semispinalis muscle is divided and turned laterally;

2. The greater occipital nerve, when followed caudally, leads to the inferior border of inferior oblique muscle around which it turns; following the inferior border of inferior oblique muscle

medially from the nerve leads to the spinous process of the axis, and, followed laterally, leads to the transverse process of the atlas;

3. Five muscles (all paired) attached to the spinous process of the axis: inferior oblique, rectus capitis posterior major, semispinalis cervicis, which largely conceals multifidus, and interspinalis;

4. Occipital veins emerging through the suboccipital triangle to join the deep cervical vein and, with it, the suboccipital nerve (C1, dorsal ramus);

5. The suboccipital triangle bounded by three muscles: inferior oblique, superior oblique, and rectus major.

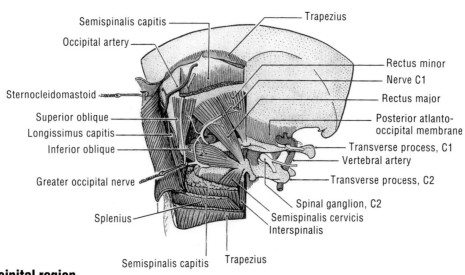

Semispinalis capitis

Occipital artery

Sternocleidomastoid

Superior oblique
Longissimus capitis
Inferior oblique

Greater occipital nerve

Splenius

Semispinalis capitis

Trapezius

Rectus minor
Nerve C1
Rectus major
Posterior atlanto-occipital membrane
Transverse process, C1
Vertebral artery
Transverse process, C2
Spinal ganglion, C2
Semispinalis cervicis
Interspinalis

Trapezius

4.57
Diagram of the suboccipital region

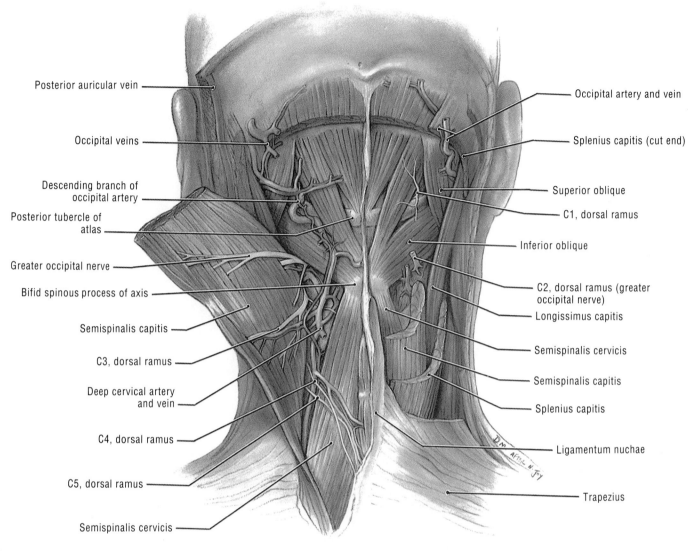

Posterior auricular vein

Occipital veins

Descending branch of occipital artery

Posterior tubercle of atlas

Greater occipital nerve

Bifid spinous process of axis

Semispinalis capitis

C3, dorsal ramus

Deep cervical artery and vein

C4, dorsal ramus

C5, dorsal ramus

Semispinalis cervicis

Occipital artery and vein

Splenius capitis (cut end)

Superior oblique

C1, dorsal ramus

Inferior oblique

C2, dorsal ramus (greater occipital nerve)

Longissimus capitis

Semispinalis cervicis

Semispinalis capitis

Splenius capitis

Ligamentum nuchae

Trapezius

4.58
Suboccipital region–II

Observe:

1. The suboccipital region contains four pairs of structures: two straight muscles: rectus major and minor; two oblique muscles: superior oblique and inferior oblique; two nerves (dorsal primary rami): C1 suboccipital (motor) and C2 greater occipital (sensory); two arteries: occipital and vertebral;

2. The ligamentum nuchae, which represents the cervical part of the supraspinous ligament, is a median, thin, fibrous partition attached to the spinous processes of the cervical vertebrae and the external occipital crest; its posterior border gives origin to the trapezius muscle and extends superiorly to the inion or external occipital protuberance;

3. The rectus capitis posterior minor muscle arising from the posterior tubercle of the atlas and, therefore, lying on a deeper plane than the posterior major muscle, which arises from a spinous process;

4. The suboccipital nerve (C1, dorsal ramus) supplying the three muscles bounding the suboccipital triangle, also the rectus capitis minor muscle, and communicating with the greater occipital nerve;

5. The descending branch of the occipital artery anastomosing with the deep cervical artery, a branch of the subclavian;

6. The posterior vertebral venous plexus; this plexus is largely embedded in fascia, is usually empty, and therefore, inconspicuous, and hence is removed unnoticed with the fascia unless specially injected, as here, or engorged with blood;

7. The longissimus capitis muscle being the only section of erector spinae to reach the skull;

8. The posterior arch of the atlas forming the floor of the suboccipital triangle.

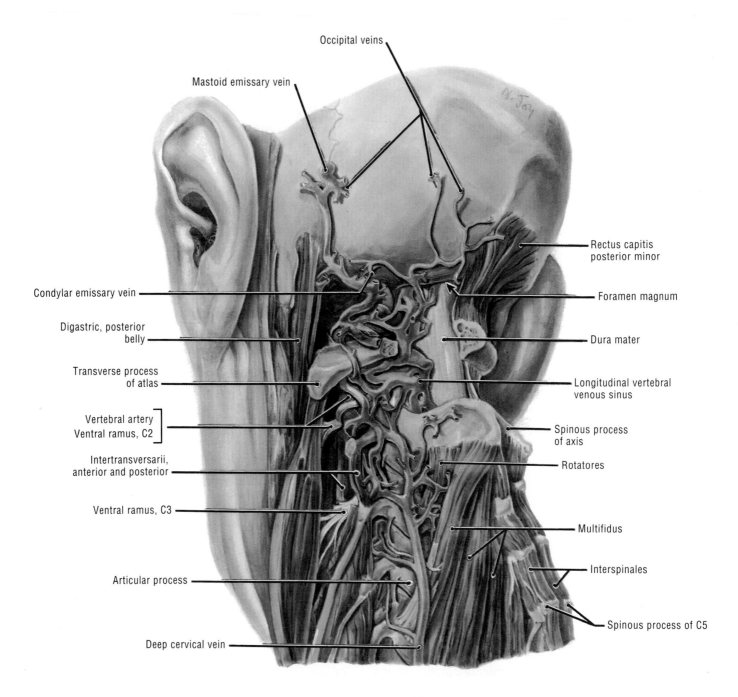

Occipital veins

Mastoid emissary vein

Rectus capitis
posterior minor

Condylar emissary vein

Foramen magnum

Digastric, posterior
belly

Dura mater

Transverse process
of atlas

Longitudinal vertebral
venous sinus

Vertebral artery
Ventral ramus, C2

Spinous process
of axis

Intertransversarii,
anterior and posterior

Rotatores

Ventral ramus, C3

Multifidus

Interspinales

Articular process

Spinous process of C5

Deep cervical vein

4.59
Suboccipital region—III

In this posterolateral view, the posterior arch of the atlas, the atlanto-occipital, and atlantoaxial membranes have been removed.

Observe:
1. The vertebral venous system of veins and its numerous intercommunications and connections, e.g., through the foramen magnum and the mastoid foramen and condylar canal with the intracranial venous sinuses; between the laminae and through the intervertebral foramina with the longitudinal vertebral venous sinuses; communicating with the veins of the scalp, with the veins around the vertebral artery and, via the deep cervical vein, with the brachiocephalic vein inferiorly;

2. The interspinales and the multifidi muscles extending to, but not superior to, the spinous process of the axis.

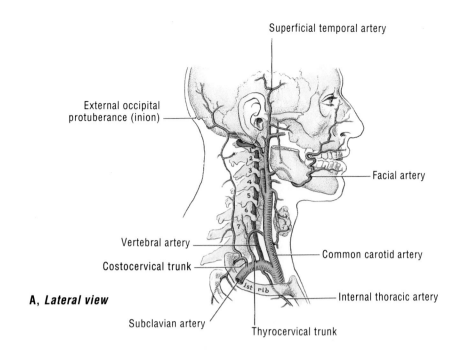

Superficial temporal artery

External occipital
protuberance (inion)

Facial artery

Vertebral artery

Common carotid artery

Costocervical trunk

1st rib

Internal thoracic artery

Subclavian artery

Thyrocervical trunk

A, *Lateral view*

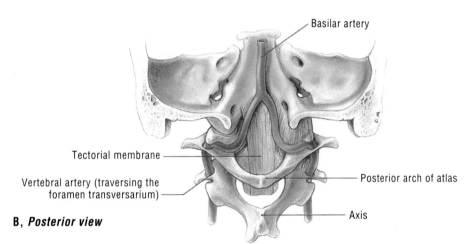

Basilar artery

Tectorial membrane

Posterior arch of atlas

Vertebral artery (traversing the
foramen transversarium)

Axis

B, *Posterior view*

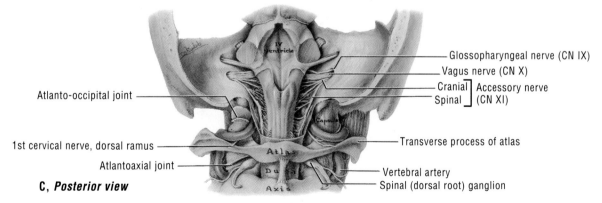

IV
Ventricle

Glossopharyngeal nerve (CN IX)

Vagus nerve (CN X)

Cranial ⎤ Accessory nerve
Spinal ⎦ (CN XI)

Atlanto-occipital joint

Capsule

1st cervical nerve, dorsal ramus

Transverse process of atlas

Atlas

Atlantoaxial joint

Dura

Vertebral artery

C, *Posterior view*

Axis

Spinal (dorsal root) ganglion

4.60

Course of the vertebral artery in the cervical region

Observe:

A. The vertebral artery arising from the subclavian artery and passing through the foramina transversaria of the upper six cervical vertebrae;

B. The vertebral arteries entering the skull through the foramen

magnum and joining to form the basilar artery;

C. The relationship of the spinal cord, brainstem, and cranial nerves to the vertebral arteries; the vertebral arteries raised from their grooves on the atlas.

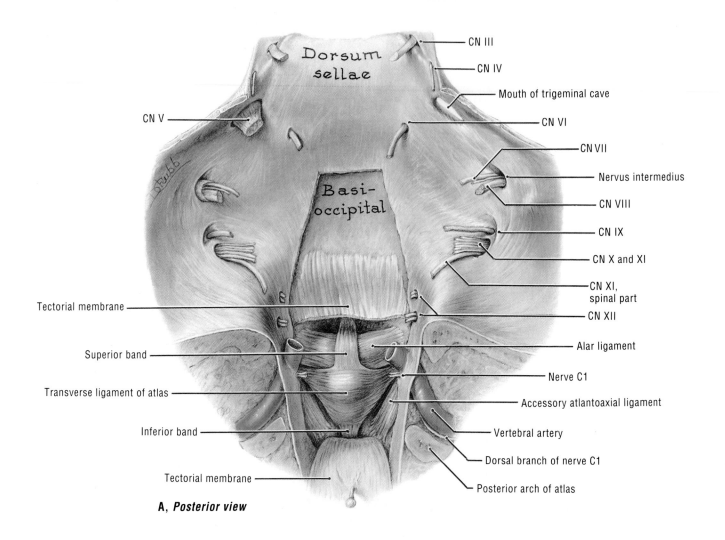

A, Posterior view

Labels on figure A:
- Dorsum sellae
- CN III
- CN IV
- Mouth of trigeminal cave
- CN V
- CN VI
- Basi-occipital
- CN VII
- Nervus intermedius
- CN VIII
- CN IX
- CN X and XI
- CN XI, spinal part
- Tectorial membrane
- CN XII
- Superior band
- Alar ligament
- Transverse ligament of atlas
- Nerve C1
- Accessory atlantoaxial ligament
- Inferior band
- Vertebral artery
- Dorsal branch of nerve C1
- Tectorial membrane
- Posterior arch of atlas

4.61
Craniovertebral joints

Observe:

1. The bow-shaped transverse ligament of the atlas, which, by the addition of a superior and an inferior longitudinal band, becomes a cruciform ligament stretching from the axis to the occipital bone;

2. The alar ligament passing from the sides of the apex of the dens postero-laterally, superior to the transverse ligament, to the medial sides of the occipital condyles;

3. The sites where the last 10 pairs of cranial nerves and the first pair of cervical nerves pass through the dura, noting: (a) they are in numerical sequence, craniocaudally, and (b) nerves III, IV, and VI, which supply the muscles of the eye, and XII, which supplies the muscles of the tongue, are nearly in vertical line with each other and with the ventral or motor root of C1 (**A**).

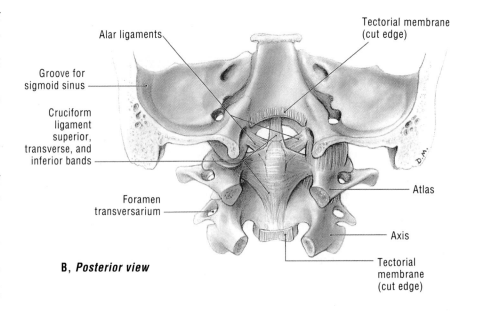

Labels on figure B:
- Alar ligaments
- Tectorial membrane (cut edge)
- Groove for sigmoid sinus
- Cruciform ligament superior, transverse, and inferior bands
- Atlas
- Foramen transversarium
- Axis
- Tectorial membrane (cut edge)

B, Posterior view

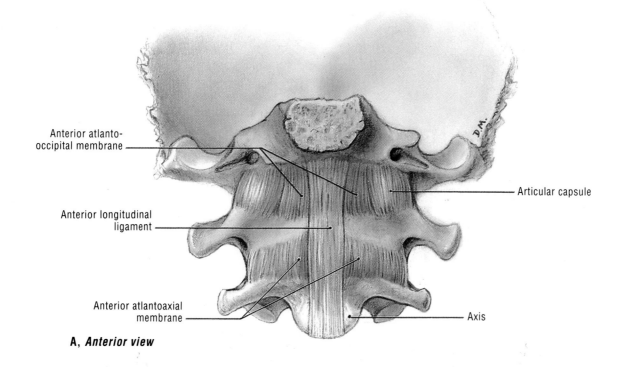

Anterior atlanto-occipital membrane

Anterior longitudinal ligament

Anterior atlantoaxial membrane

Articular capsule

Axis

A, Anterior view

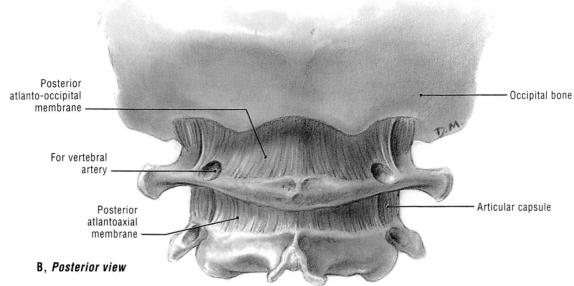

Posterior atlanto-occipital membrane

For vertebral artery

Posterior atlantoaxial membrane

Occipital bone

Articular capsule

B, Posterior view

4.62

Ligaments of the atlanto-occipital and atlantoaxial joints

Observe:

1. The anterior longitudinal ligament blending in the midline with the anterior atlanto-occipital and anterior atlantoaxial membranes and laterally with the facet joints (**A**);

2. The posterior atlanto-occipital membrane lying between the foramen magnum and the superior surface of the posterior arch of the atlas; the posterior atlantoaxial membrane lying between the inferior surface of the posterior arch of the atlas and the laminae of the axis; it is continuous with the ligamentum flava (**B**);

3. The large vertebral foramen of the atlas that is divided into two foramina by the transverse ligament of the atlas; in the larger, posterior foramen, the spinal cord lies loosely; in the smaller, anterior foramen, the dens of the axis fits tightly (**C**).

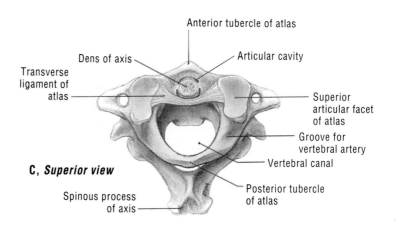

Anterior tubercle of atlas

Dens of axis

Transverse ligament of atlas

Articular cavity

Superior articular facet of atlas

Groove for vertebral artery

Vertebral canal

Posterior tubercle of atlas

C, Superior view

Spinous process of axis

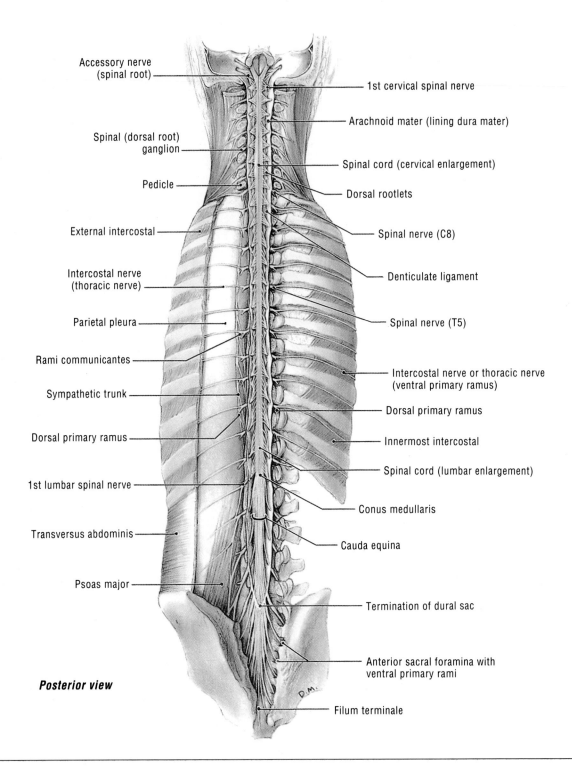

Accessory nerve (spinal root)

1st cervical spinal nerve

Arachnoid mater (lining dura mater)

Spinal (dorsal root) ganglion

Spinal cord (cervical enlargement)

Pedicle

Dorsal rootlets

External intercostal

Spinal nerve (C8)

Intercostal nerve (thoracic nerve)

Denticulate ligament

Parietal pleura

Spinal nerve (T5)

Rami communicantes

Intercostal nerve or thoracic nerve (ventral primary ramus)

Sympathetic trunk

Dorsal primary ramus

Dorsal primary ramus

Innermost intercostal

1st lumbar spinal nerve

Spinal cord (lumbar enlargement)

Conus medullaris

Transversus abdominis

Cauda equina

Psoas major

Termination of dural sac

Anterior sacral foramina with ventral primary rami

Posterior view

Filum terminale

4.63
Spinal cord in situ

Observe:

1. The vertebral (neural) arches of the vertebrae and the posterior aspect of the sacrum have been removed to expose the vertebral canal; also, the dural sac has been cut open posteriorly to reveal the spinal cord and nerve roots; the termination of the spinal cord between the 1st and 2nd lumbar vertebrae and the dural sac at the 2nd sacral segment;

2. On the left: (a) the ribs articulating with the transverse processes of the thoracic vertebrae, (b) the intercostal nerves (ventral primary rami) passing posterior to the innermost inter-

costal muscles, and (c) the dorsal primary rami innervating the deep back muscles;

3. On the right: (a) the formation of the brachial and lumbosacral plexuses by the ventral primary rami of the spinal nerves, (b) the ribs and intercostal muscles have been removed posteriorly to expose the parietal pleura and the sympathetic trunk, and (c) the spinal (dorsal root) ganglia located at the intervertebral foramina, bounded superiorly and inferiorly by the pedicles.

4.64
Spinal cord within its membranes

Observe:

1. The denticulate ligament, running like a band along each side of the spinal cord and, by means of strong, tooth-like processes, anchoring the cord to the dura between successive nerve roots;

2. The ventral nerve roots, lying anterior to the denticulate ligament and the dorsal nerve roots posterior to the ligament;

3. The ventral and the dorsal root of each nerve, leaving the dura by a separate opening;

4. The fila of the various dorsal roots, having a linear attachment to the cord;

5. One filum of the inferior left dorsal root, deserting its own root and joining the root superior to it.

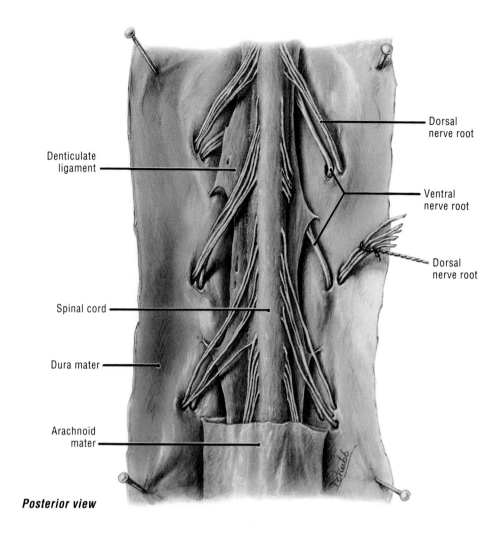

Denticulate ligament

Spinal cord

Dura mater

Arachnoid mater

Dorsal nerve root

Ventral nerve root

Dorsal nerve root

Posterior view

4.65
Formation of spinal nerves

Observe:

1. The dural sac consisting of the dura mater and the arachnoid mater; the pia mater covering the spinal cord and projecting laterally as the denticulate ligaments separating the rows of dorsal and ventral rootlets;

2. Cerebrospinal fluid circulates between pia and arachnoid, in the subarachnoid space;

3. On each side, two rows of rootlets attach to the cord; the dorsal filaments carry sensory information to the central nervous system; the ventral filaments convey motor information from the central nervous system to the periphery;

4. A number of rootlets combine to form at each segment dorsal and ventral roots;

5. The swollen area on the dorsal root, the spinal (dorsal root) ganglion, contains cell bodies of sensory neurons;

6. Dorsal and ventral roots unite to form a spinal nerve;

7. Dura (and arachnoid) continues as a sheath around nerves leaving the spinal cord.

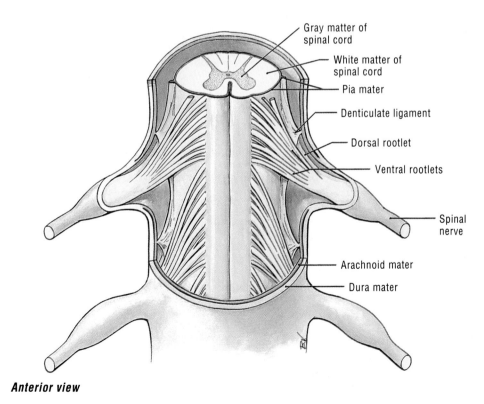

Gray matter of spinal cord

White matter of spinal cord

Pia mater

Denticulate ligament

Dorsal rootlet

Ventral rootlets

Spinal nerve

Arachnoid mater

Dura mater

Anterior view

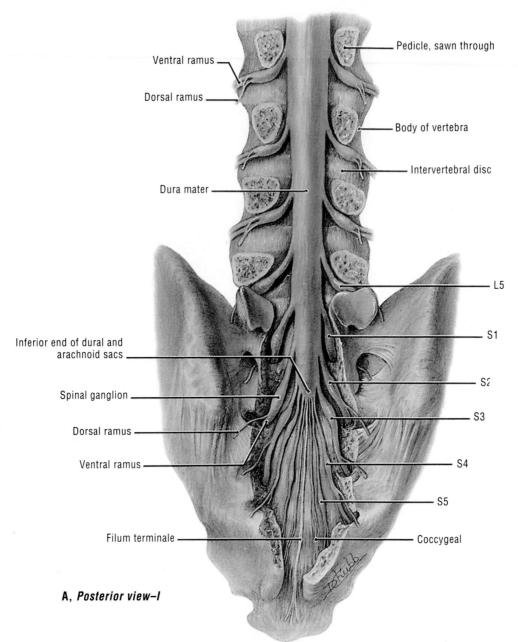

Ventral ramus

Dorsal ramus

Dura mater

Inferior end of dural and
arachnoid sacs

Spinal ganglion

Dorsal ramus

Ventral ramus

Filum terminale

Pedicle, sawn through

Body of vertebra

Intervertebral disc

L5

S1

S2

S3

S4

S5

Coccygeal

A, *Posterior view–I*

4.66
Inferior end of the dural sac

A. The posterior parts of the lumbar and sacral vertebrae are sawn and nibbled away. Observe:

1. The inferior limit of the dural (and the contained arachnoid) sac, at the level of the posterior superior iliac spine (body of 2nd sacral vertebra), and the continuation of the dura as the filum of spinal dura mater;

2. The lumbar spinal ganglia in the intervertebral foramina; the sacral spinal ganglia, somewhat asymmetrical, within the sacral canal;

3. The dorsal nerve rami, smaller than ventral rami, and having both efferent and afferent components.

Observe in **B**:

1. The inferior margin of the denticulate ligament, variable in level and asymmetrical;

2. A radicular branch of a spinal vein accompanying the dorsal root of nerve L1; there are only four or five radicular veins and arteries on each side of the cord to accompany the 31 pairs of spinal nerves;

3. The conus medullaris, or conical lower end of the spinal medulla, continued as a glistening thread, the filum terminale, which descends with the posterior and anterior nerve roots; these constitute the cauda equina;

4. The subarachnoid space enclosed by arachnoid mater; the subdural space, which is the potential space between the dural and arachnoid maters.

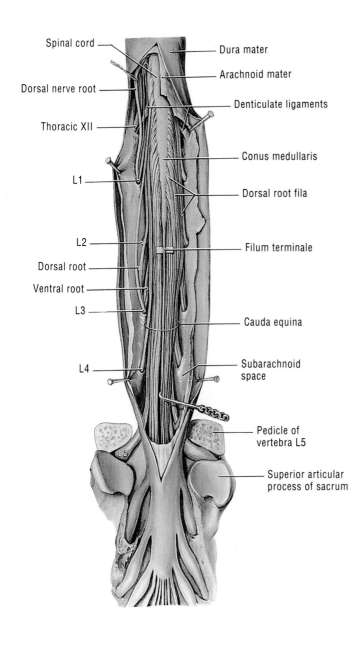

Spinal cord — Dura mater

Dorsal nerve root — Arachnoid mater

— Denticulate ligaments

Thoracic XII —

Conus medullaris

L1 —

Dorsal root fila

L2 — Filum terminale

Dorsal root —

Ventral root —

L3 — Cauda equina

Subarachnoid
space

L4 —

Pedicle of
vertebra L5

Superior articular
process of sacrum

B, *Posterior view–II*

4.66
Inferior end of the dural sac *(continued)*

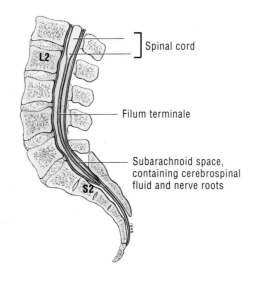

Spinal cord

Filum terminale

Subarachnoid space,
containing cerebrospinal
fluid and nerve roots

4.67
Spinal cord in situ

Observe:

1. The spinal cord, in the adult, usually ends at the level of the disc between the 1st and 2nd lumbar vertebrae;

2. The subarachnoid space usually ends at the level of the disc between the 1st and 2nd sacral vertebrae, but it may be more inferior;

3. Variations: 95% of cords end within the limits of the bodies of verterbrae L1 and L2, whereas 3% end posterior to the inferior half of vertebra T12, and 2% posterior to vertebra L3 (see Jit I, Charnakia VM. *The vertebral level of the termination of the spinal cord.* J Anat Soc India 1959; 8:93).

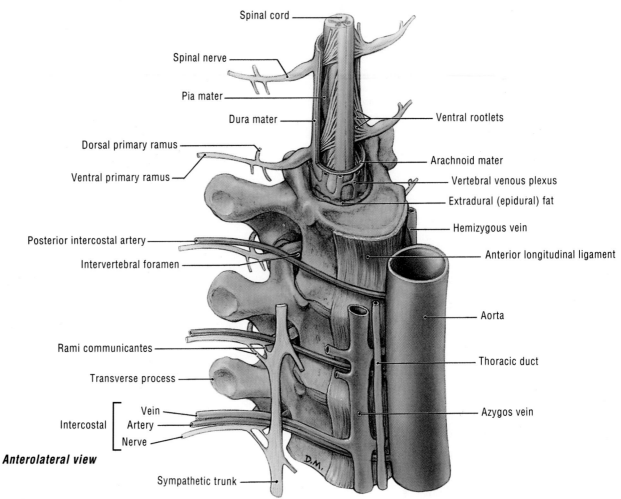

Spinal cord
Spinal nerve
Pia mater
Dura mater
Dorsal primary ramus
Ventral primary ramus
Posterior intercostal artery
Intervertebral foramen
Rami communicantes
Transverse process
Intercostal { Vein / Artery / Nerve }
Anterolateral view
Sympathetic trunk

Ventral rootlets
Arachnoid mater
Vertebral venous plexus
Extradural (epidural) fat
Hemizygous vein
Anterior longitudinal ligament
Aorta
Thoracic duct
Azygos vein

4.68
Spinal cord and prevertebral structures

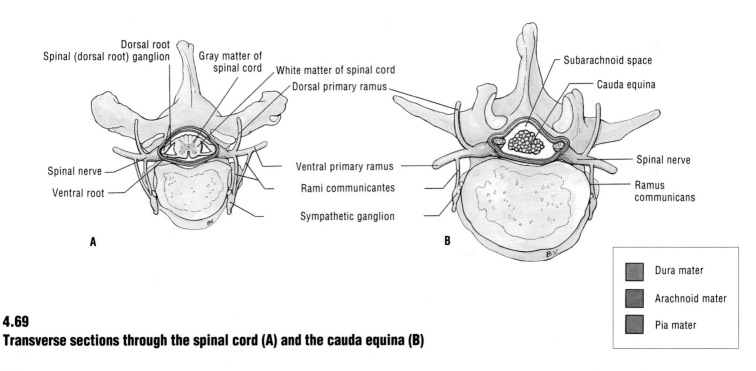

Dorsal root
Spinal (dorsal root) ganglion
Gray matter of spinal cord
White matter of spinal cord
Dorsal primary ramus
Spinal nerve
Ventral root
Ventral primary ramus
Rami communicantes
Sympathetic ganglion

Subarachnoid space
Cauda equina
Spinal nerve
Ramus communicans

A

B

Dura mater
Arachnoid mater
Pia mater

4.69
Transverse sections through the spinal cord (A) and the cauda equina (B)

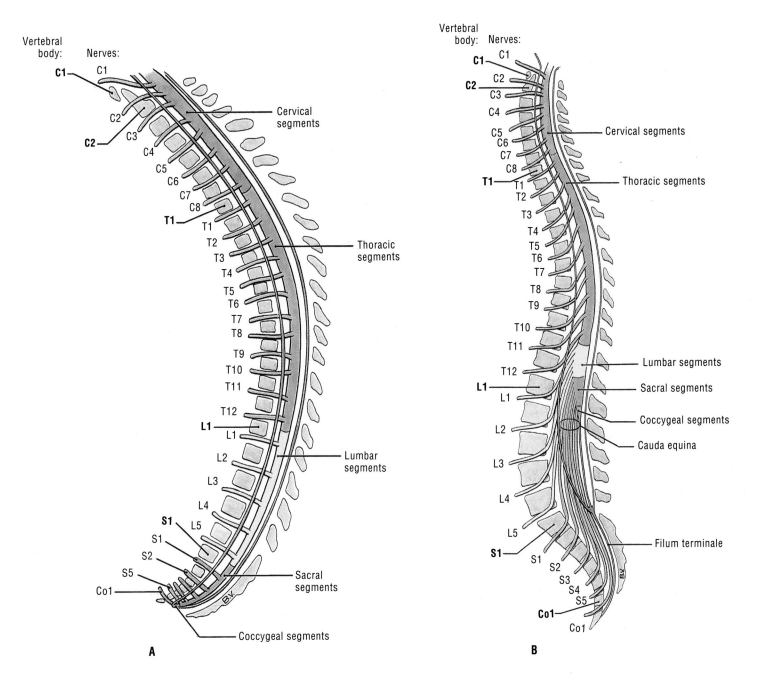

Vertebral body: Nerves:

C1 — C1
C2 — C2
C3
C4
C5
C6
C7
C8
T1 — T1
T2
T3
T4
T5
T6
T7
T8
T9
T10
T11
T12
L1 — L1
L2
L3
L4
L5
S1 — S1
S2
S5
Co1

Cervical segments

Thoracic segments

Lumbar segments

Sacral segments

Coccygeal segments

A

Vertebral body: Nerves:

C1 — C1
C2 — C2
C3
C4
C5
C6
C7
C8
T1 — T1
T2
T3
T4
T5
T6
T7
T8
T9
T10
T11
T12
L1 — L1
L2
L3
L4
L5
S1 — S1
S2
S3
S4
S5
Co1 — Co1

Cervical segments

Thoracic segments

Lumbar segments

Sacral segments

Coccygeal segments

Cauda equina

Filum terminale

B

4.70
Subarachnoid space

A. Spinal cord at 12 weeks of gestation. **B.** Spinal cord of an adult. Earlier in development, spinal cord and vertebral (spinal) canal were more equal in length. The canal has grown longer and so spinal nerves have an increasingly longer course to reach the intervertebral foramen at the correct level for their exit. Descending the cord, the spinal nerves become increasingly oblique in the courses. The spinal cord proper terminates at vertebral level L2 and remaining spinal nerves seeking their intervertebral foramen of exit form the cauda equina. At the vertebral level S2, the subarachnoid space ceases, thus spinal taps are usually done between vertebral levels L3 and S2.

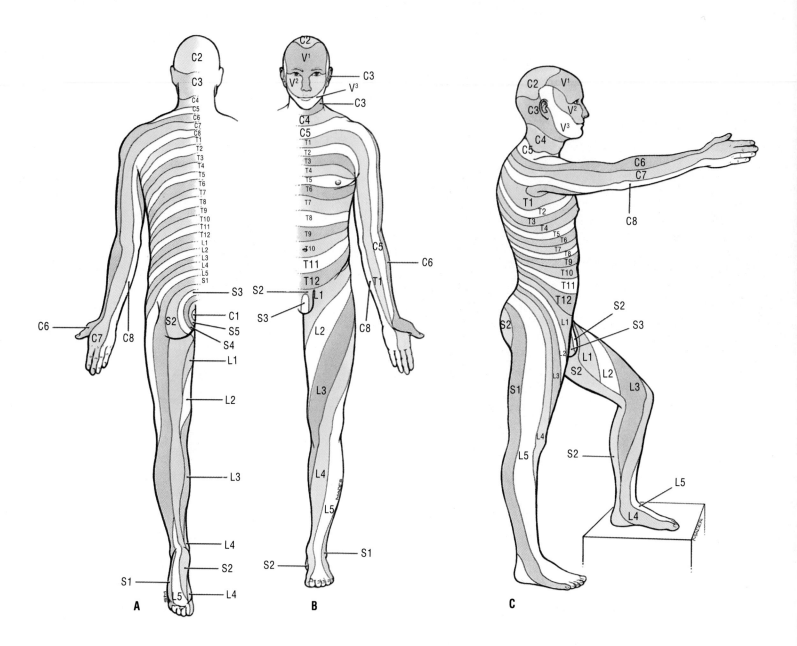

4.71
Dermatomes

A dermatome is an area of skin supplied by the dorsal (sensory) root of a spinal nerve. In the head and trunk, each segment is horizontally disposed, except C1, which has no sensory component. The dermatomes of the limbs from the 5th cervical to the 1st thoracic and from the 3rd lumbar to the 2nd sacral extend as a series of bands from the midline of the trunk posteriorly into the limbs. Note that there is considerable overlapping of adjacent dermatomes; that is to say, each segmental nerve overlaps the territories of its neighbors. As a result, no anesthesia occurs unless two or more consecutive dorsal roots have lost their functions (see Fender FA. *Foerster's scheme of the dermatomes.* Arch Neurol Psychiatr 1939; 41:688; Keegan JJ, Garrett FD. *The segmental distribution of the cutaneous nerves in the limbs of man.* Anat Rec 1948; 102:409).

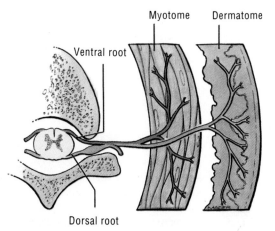

4.72
Segmental innervation: dermatome and myotome

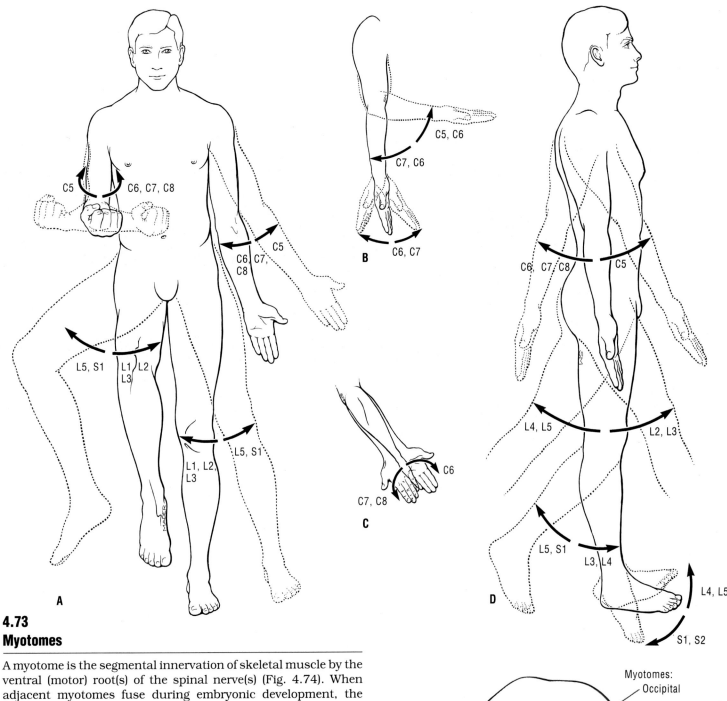

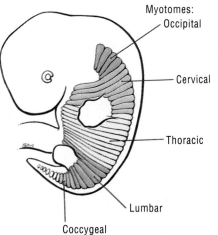

Myotomes:
- Occipital
- Cervical
- Thoracic
- Lumbar
- Coccygeal

4.73
Myotomes

A myotome is the segmental innervation of skeletal muscle by the ventral (motor) root(s) of the spinal nerve(s) (Fig. 4.74). When adjacent myotomes fuse during embryonic development, the resultant muscle may be innervated by one or both of its segmental spinal nerves. In this diagram, the myotomes have been generalized to apply to movements of the joints of the upper and lower extremities (see Hollinshead WH, Markee JE. *The multiple innervation of limb muscles in man.* J Bone Joint Surg 1946; 28:721).

4.74
Myotome region of the somites

Initially, the muscles of the trunk and limbs are segmental, but as development proceeds, various segments fuse and the distinctive segmental pattern is lost (except for the intercostal muscles of the thorax).

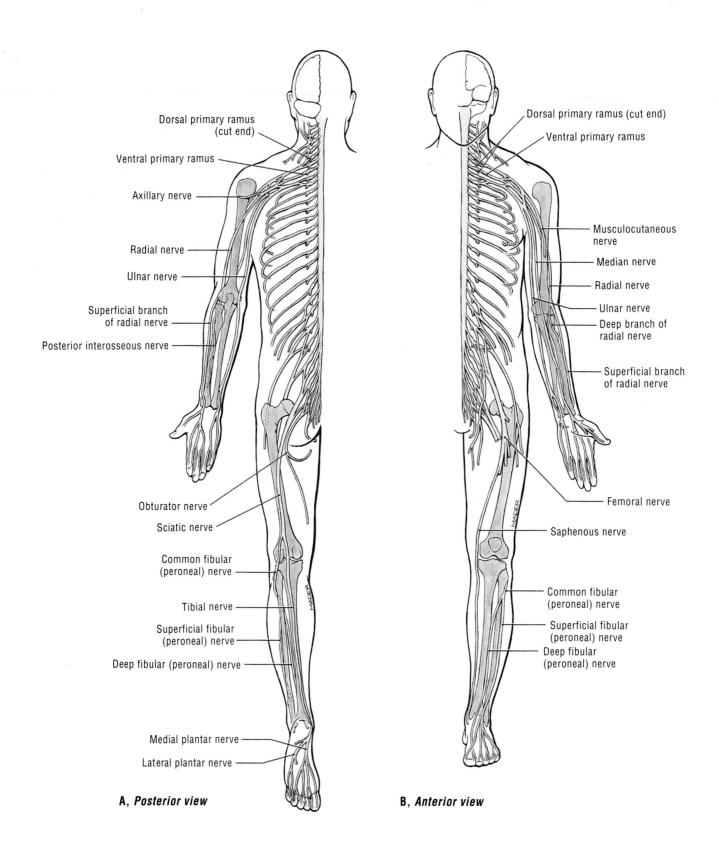

Dorsal primary ramus (cut end)

Ventral primary ramus

Axillary nerve

Radial nerve

Ulnar nerve

Superficial branch of radial nerve

Posterior interosseous nerve

Obturator nerve

Sciatic nerve

Common fibular (peroneal) nerve

Tibial nerve

Superficial fibular (peroneal) nerve

Deep fibular (peroneal) nerve

Medial plantar nerve

Lateral plantar nerve

A, *Posterior view*

Dorsal primary ramus (cut end)

Ventral primary ramus

Musculocutaneous nerve

Median nerve

Radial nerve

Ulnar nerve

Deep branch of radial nerve

Superficial branch of radial nerve

Femoral nerve

Saphenous nerve

Common fibular (peroneal) nerve

Superficial fibular (peroneal) nerve

Deep fibular (peroneal) nerve

B, *Anterior view*

4.75
Overview of the somatic nervous system

5   The Lower Limb

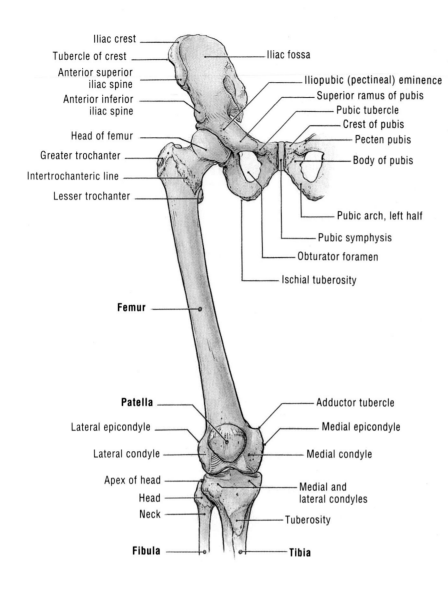

Iliac crest
Tubercle of crest
Anterior superior
iliac spine
Anterior inferior
iliac spine
Head of femur
Greater trochanter
Intertrochanteric line
Lesser trochanter

Iliac fossa
Iliopubic (pectineal) eminence
Superior ramus of pubis
Pubic tubercle
Crest of pubis
Pecten pubis
Body of pubis

Pubic arch, left half
Pubic symphysis
Obturator foramen
Ischial tuberosity

Femur

Patella
Lateral epicondyle
Lateral condyle
Apex of head
Head
Neck
Fibula

Adductor tubercle
Medial epicondyle
Medial condyle
Medial and
lateral condyles
Tuberosity
Tibia

A, *Anterior view*

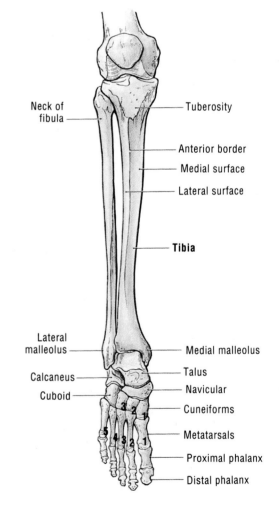

Neck of
fibula
Tuberosity
Anterior border
Medial surface
Lateral surface

Tibia

Lateral
malleolus
Calcaneus
Cuboid
Medial malleolus
Talus
Navicular
Cuneiforms
Metatarsals
Proximal phalanx
Distal phalanx

5.1
Bones of the lower limb

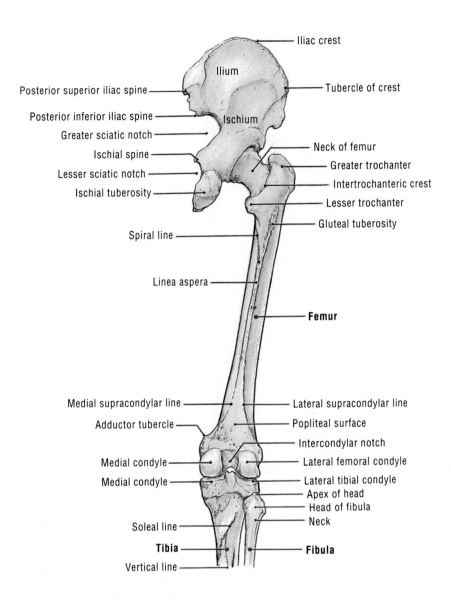

Iliac crest

Ilium

Posterior superior iliac spine

Tubercle of crest

Posterior inferior iliac spine

Ischium

Greater sciatic notch

Neck of femur

Ischial spine

Greater trochanter

Lesser sciatic notch

Intertrochanteric crest

Ischial tuberosity

Lesser trochanter

Gluteal tuberosity

Spiral line

Linea aspera

Femur

Medial supracondylar line

Lateral supracondylar line

Adductor tubercle

Popliteal surface

Intercondylar notch

Medial condyle

Lateral femoral condyle

Medial condyle

Lateral tibial condyle

Apex of head

Head of fibula

Soleal line

Neck

Tibia

Fibula

Vertical line

B, *Posterior view*

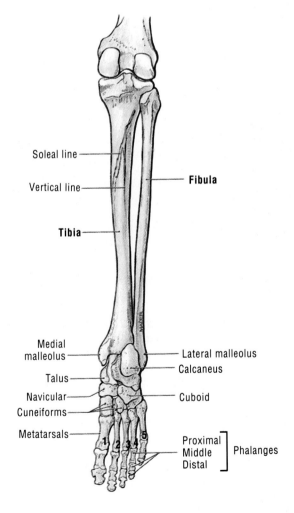

Soleal line

Vertical line

Fibula

Tibia

Medial malleolus

Lateral malleolus

Talus

Calcaneus

Navicular

Cuboid

Cuneiforms

Metatarsals

1 2 3 4 5

Proximal
Middle
Distal

} Phalanges

5.1
Bones of the lower limb *(continued)*

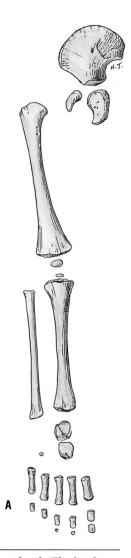

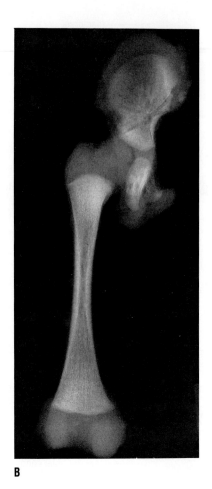

B

5.2
Lower limb

A. Bones of lower limb at birth. The hip bone is in three primary parts: ilium, ischium, and pubis. The diaphyses of the long bones are well ossified. Certain epiphyses and certain tarsal bones have started to ossify: the distal epiphysis of the femur and the proximal epiphysis of the tibia; the calcaneus, talus, and cuboid.

C. Epiphyses at the proximal end of the femur. The epiphysis of the head begins to ossify during the 1st year; that of the greater trochanter before the 5th year; and that of the lesser trochanter before the 14th year. These have in most cases fused completely with the body (shaft) before the end of the 18th year, and in all cases by the 20th.

B and **D**. Radiographs of postmortem specimens shortly after birth showing the bony (white) and cartilaginous (gray) components of the femur and hip bone (os coxae). (Courtesy of Dr. Paul Babyn, Associate Professor of Radiology, University of Toronto, Toronto, Ontario, Canada.)

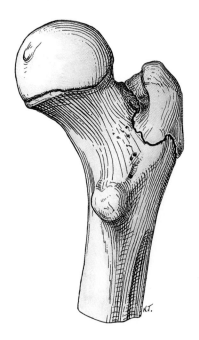

C, *Posterior view*

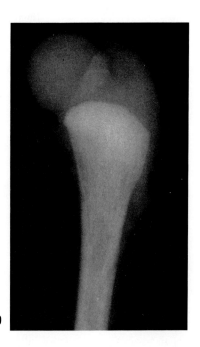

D

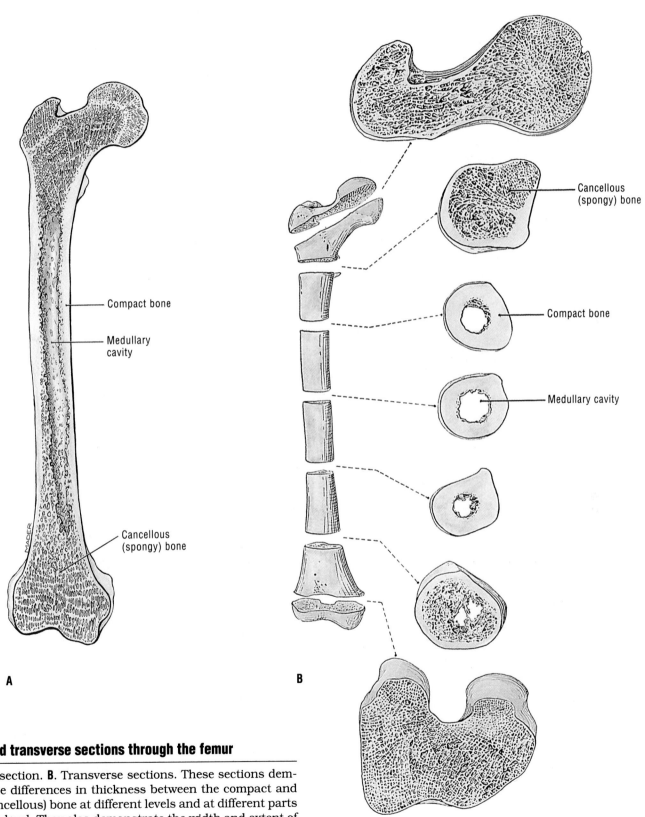

A. Coronal section. **B.** Transverse sections.

A   Compact bone

Medullary cavity

Cancellous (spongy) bone

B

Cancellous (spongy) bone

Compact bone

Medullary cavity

5.3
Coronal and transverse sections through the femur

A. Coronal section. **B.** Transverse sections. These sections demonstrate the differences in thickness between the compact and spongy (cancellous) bone at different levels and at different parts of the same level. They also demonstrate the width and extent of the medullary cavity (canal).

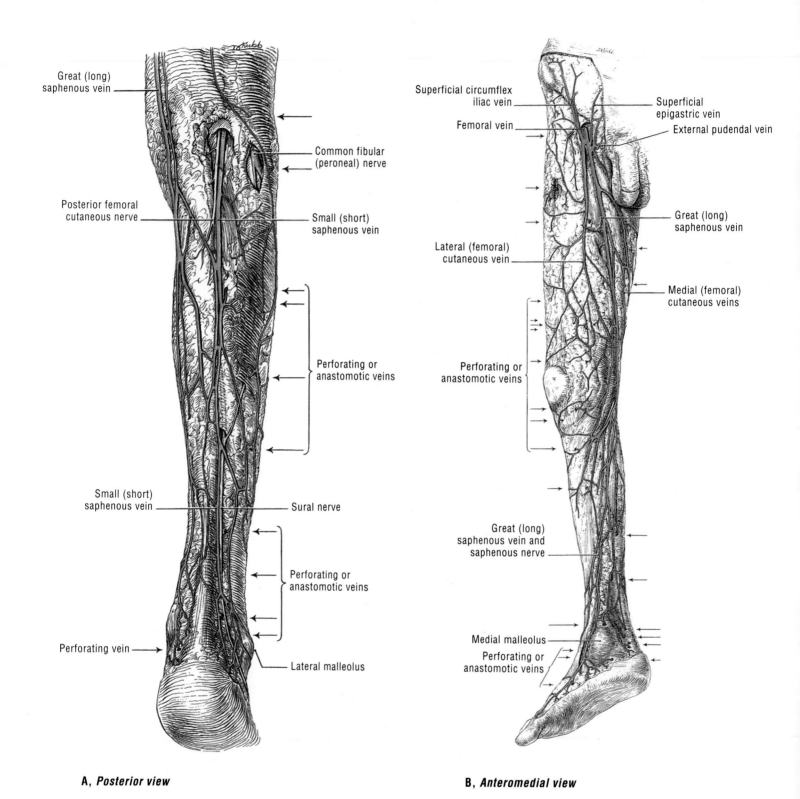

Great (long)
saphenous vein

Common fibular
(peroneal) nerve

Posterior femoral
cutaneous nerve

Small (short)
saphenous vein

Perforating or
anastomotic veins

Small (short)
saphenous vein

Sural nerve

Perforating or
anastomotic veins

Perforating vein

Lateral malleolus

Superficial circumflex
iliac vein

Femoral vein

Superficial
epigastric vein

External pudendal vein

Lateral (femoral)
cutaneous vein

Great (long)
saphenous vein

Medial (femoral)
cutaneous veins

Perforating or
anastomotic veins

Great (long)
saphenous vein and
saphenous nerve

Medial malleolus

Perforating or
anastomotic veins

A, *Posterior view*

B, *Anteromedial view*

5.4
Superficial veins of lower limb

The *arrows* indicate where anastomotic veins perforate the deep
fascia and bring the superficial and deep veins into communication
with each other.

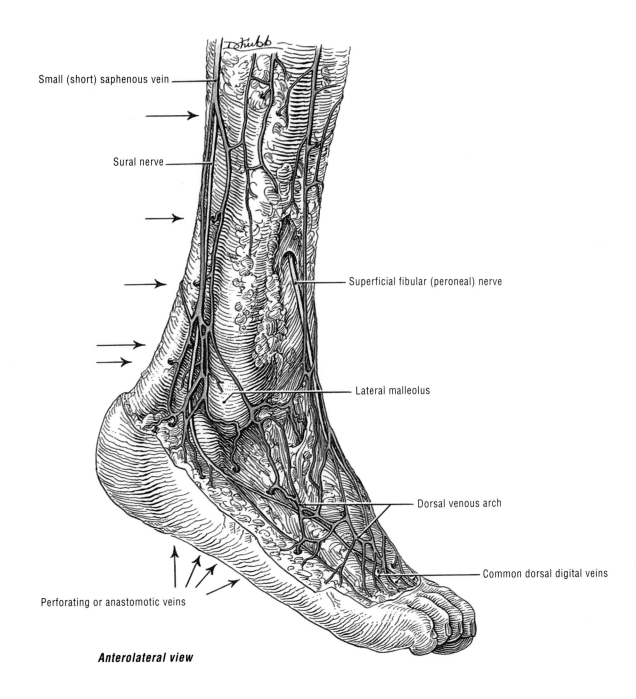

Small (short) saphenous vein

Sural nerve

Superficial fibular (peroneal) nerve

Lateral malleolus

Dorsal venous arch

Common dorsal digital veins

Perforating or anastomotic veins

Anterolateral view

5.5
Superficial veins of the ankle and dorsum of the foot

Figures 5.4 and 5.5 show the superficial veins of the lower limb that lie in the subcutaneous fat. When these veins become enlarged and tortuous, their valves become incompetent and they are termed varicose veins. *Arrows* as in Figure 5.4.

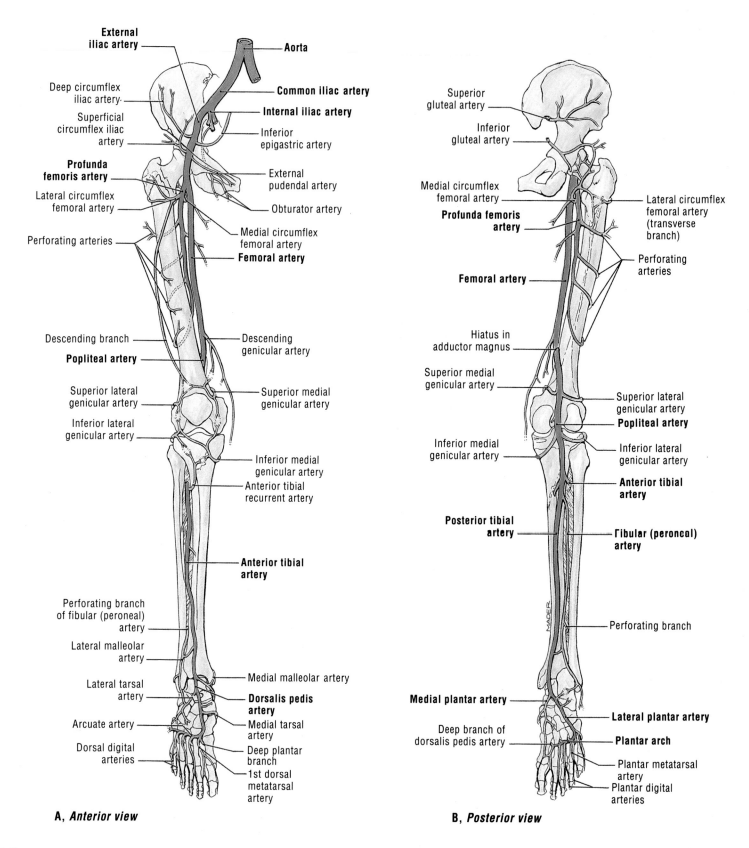

External iliac artery

Aorta

Deep circumflex iliac artery

Common iliac artery

Internal iliac artery

Superficial circumflex iliac artery

Inferior epigastric artery

Profunda femoris artery

External pudendal artery

Lateral circumflex femoral artery

Obturator artery

Perforating arteries

Medial circumflex femoral artery

Femoral artery

Descending branch

Descending genicular artery

Popliteal artery

Superior lateral genicular artery

Superior medial genicular artery

Inferior lateral genicular artery

Inferior medial genicular artery

Anterior tibial recurrent artery

Anterior tibial artery

Perforating branch of fibular (peroneal) artery

Lateral malleolar artery

Medial malleolar artery

Lateral tarsal artery

Dorsalis pedis artery

Arcuate artery

Medial tarsal artery

Dorsal digital arteries

Deep plantar branch

1st dorsal metatarsal artery

A, *Anterior view*

Superior gluteal artery

Inferior gluteal artery

Medial circumflex femoral artery

Lateral circumflex femoral artery (transverse branch)

Profunda femoris artery

Perforating arteries

Femoral artery

Hiatus in adductor magnus

Superior medial genicular artery

Superior lateral genicular artery

Popliteal artery

Inferior medial genicular artery

Inferior lateral genicular artery

Anterior tibial artery

Posterior tibial artery

Fibular (peroneal) artery

Perforating branch

Medial plantar artery

Lateral plantar artery

Deep branch of dorsalis pedis artery

Plantar arch

Plantar metatarsal artery

Plantar digital arteries

B, *Posterior view*

5.6
Diagrams of the arteries of the lower limb

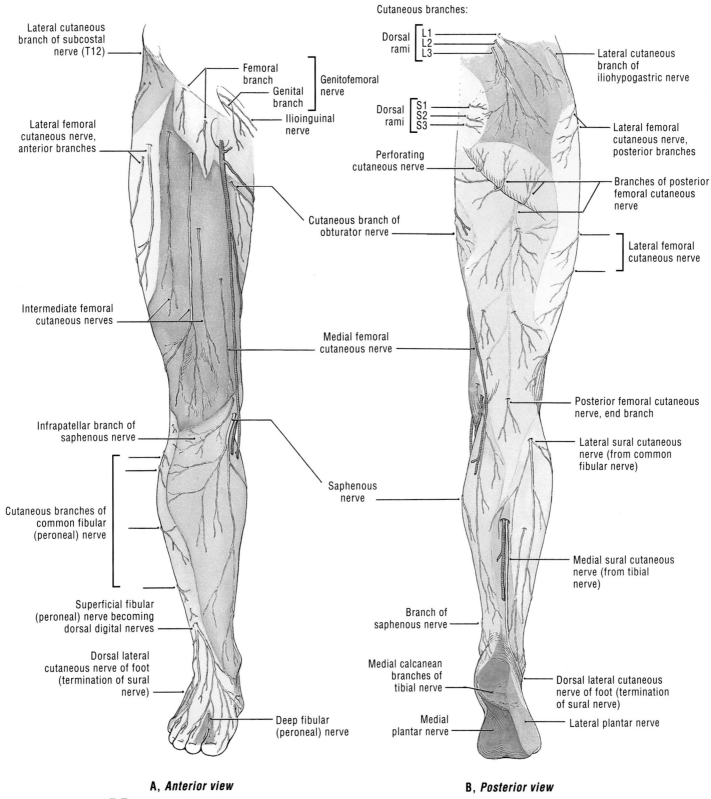

Lateral cutaneous branch of subcostal nerve (T12)

Femoral branch

Genital branch

Genitofemoral nerve

Ilioinguinal nerve

Lateral femoral cutaneous nerve, anterior branches

Intermediate femoral cutaneous nerves

Infrapatellar branch of saphenous nerve

Cutaneous branches of common fibular (peroneal) nerve

Superficial fibular (peroneal) nerve becoming dorsal digital nerves

Dorsal lateral cutaneous nerve of foot (termination of sural nerve)

Cutaneous branch of obturator nerve

Medial femoral cutaneous nerve

Saphenous nerve

Deep fibular (peroneal) nerve

Cutaneous branches:

Dorsal rami L1 L2 L3

Dorsal rami S1 S2 S3

Perforating cutaneous nerve

Lateral cutaneous branch of iliohypogastric nerve

Lateral femoral cutaneous nerve, posterior branches

Branches of posterior femoral cutaneous nerve

Lateral femoral cutaneous nerve

Posterior femoral cutaneous nerve, end branch

Lateral sural cutaneous nerve (from common fibular nerve)

Medial sural cutaneous nerve (from tibial nerve)

Branch of saphenous nerve

Medial calcanean branches of tibial nerve

Medial plantar nerve

Dorsal lateral cutaneous nerve of foot (termination of sural nerve)

Lateral plantar nerve

A, *Anterior view*

B, *Posterior view*

5.7
Cutaneous nerves of the lower limb

Note in **B**: *Sural* is Latin for the calf. The medial sural cutaneous nerve is here joined just proximal to the ankle by a communicating branch (not labeled) of the lateral sural cutaneous nerve to form the sural nerve. The level of the junction is variable, here being very low.

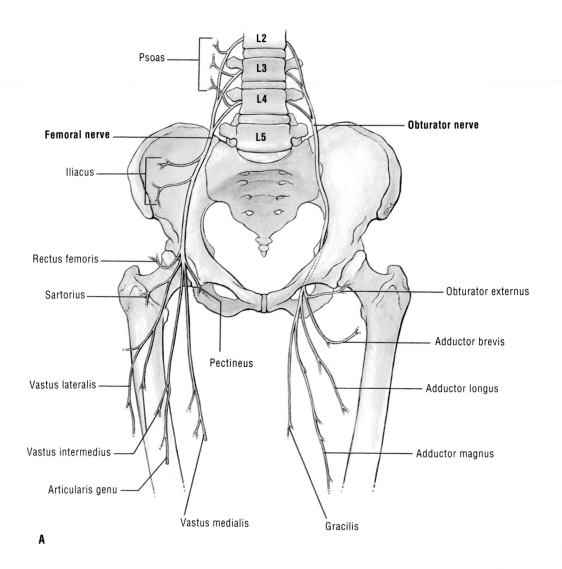

A

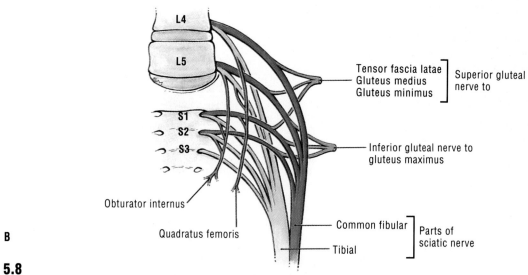

B

5.8
Scheme of the motor distribution of the nerves of the lower limb

A. Femoral and obturator nerves. **B.** Formation of the sciatic nerve in the pelvis. **C.** Common fibular (peroneal) nerve. **D.** Sciatic nerve.

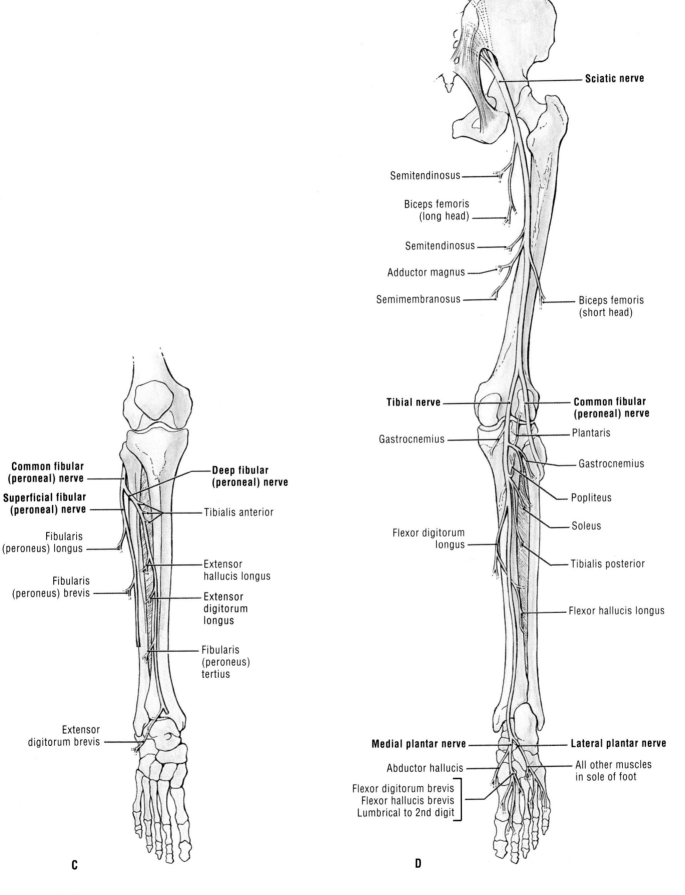

Common fibular (peroneal) nerve

Superficial fibular (peroneal) nerve

Fibularis (peroneus) longus

Fibularis (peroneus) brevis

Extensor digitorum brevis

Deep fibular (peroneal) nerve

Tibialis anterior

Extensor hallucis longus

Extensor digitorum longus

Fibularis (peroneus) tertius

C

Sciatic nerve

Semitendinosus

Biceps femoris (long head)

Semitendinosus

Adductor magnus

Semimembranosus

Biceps femoris (short head)

Tibial nerve

Gastrocnemius

Flexor digitorum longus

Common fibular (peroneal) nerve

Plantaris

Gastrocnemius

Popliteus

Soleus

Tibialis posterior

Flexor hallucis longus

Medial plantar nerve

Abductor hallucis

Flexor digitorum brevis
Flexor hallucis brevis
Lumbrical to 2nd digit

Lateral plantar nerve

All other muscles in sole of foot

D

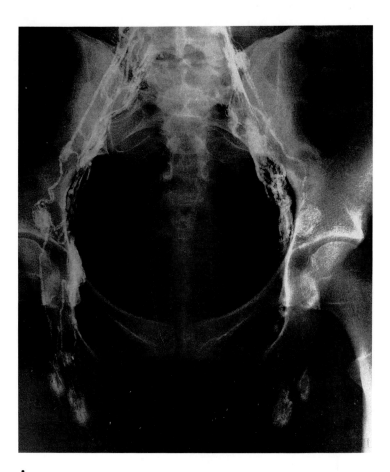

A

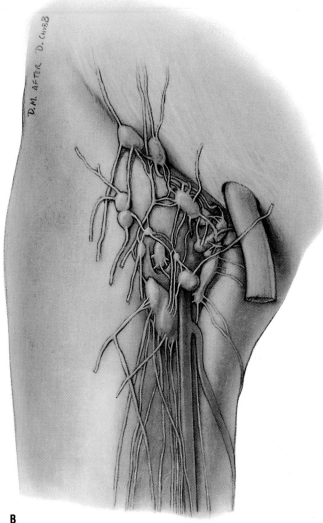

B

5.9
Inguinal lymph nodes

A. Injection. **B.** Dissection. Observe:

1. The arrangement of the nodes: (a) a proximal chain parallel to the inguinal ligament (superficial inguinal nodes); (b) a distal chain on the sides of the great saphenous vein (superficial subinguinal nodes); and, proximal to this, a chain of two or three nodes on the medial side of the femoral vein (deep inguinal nodes), one being inferior to the femoral canal and one or two within it;

2. The free anastomosis between the lymph vessels; about two dozen efferent vessels leave these nodes and, passing deep to the inguinal ligament, enter the external iliac nodes; of these, less than half traverse the femoral canal; the others ascend alongside the femoral artery and vein, some being inside the femoral sheath and some outside it;

3. These nodes receive the superficial and deep lymph vessels of the lower limb; the superficial vessels of the lower part of the abdominal wall; the vessels of the penis, including the glans penis and spongy urethra, and of the scrotum (but not of the testis or ovary); the vessels of the vulva, lower part of the vagina, and some vessels from the uterus that run with the round ligament; and vessels of the lower part of the anal canal;

4. Because of their origin, lymph from the ovary or testis drains through vessels following ovarian and testicular arteries to paraaortic and preaortic nodes, which are considerably less accessible than those in the inguinal region (see Fig. 2.18).

(**A** Courtesy of Dr. E.L. Lansdown, Professor of Radiology, University of Toronto, Toronto, Ontario, Canada.)

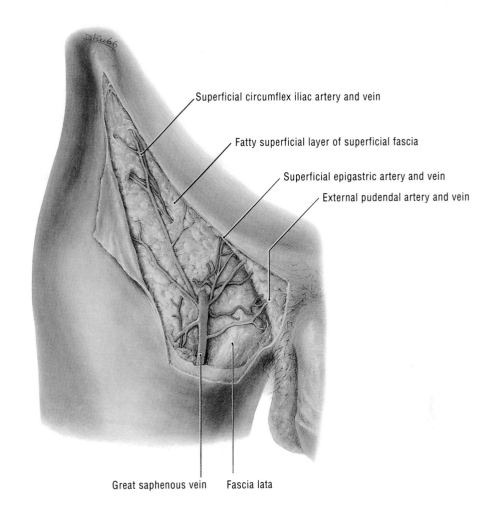

Superficial circumflex iliac artery and vein

Fatty superficial layer of superficial fascia

Superficial epigastric artery and vein

External pudendal artery and vein

Great saphenous vein Fascia lata

5.10
Superficial inguinal arteries and veins

The arteries are branches of the femoral artery but the veins are tributaries of the great saphenous vein.

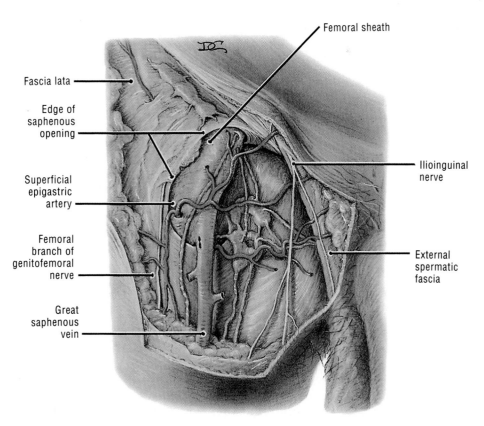

Femoral sheath

Fascia lata

Edge of saphenous opening

Superficial epigastric artery

Femoral branch of genitofemoral nerve

Great saphenous vein

Ilioinguinal nerve

External spermatic fascia

5.11
Saphenous opening

Observe:

1. The oval shape of this hiatus in the fascia lata through which the great (long) saphenous vein passes to join the femoral vein, which lies within the femoral sheath;

2. The sharp superior and inferior free margins of the opening and the less sharply definable lateral margin;

3. The great saphenous vein hooking over the inferior free margin; occasionally it joins the femoral vein 1 or even 2 cm superior to the inferior free margin.

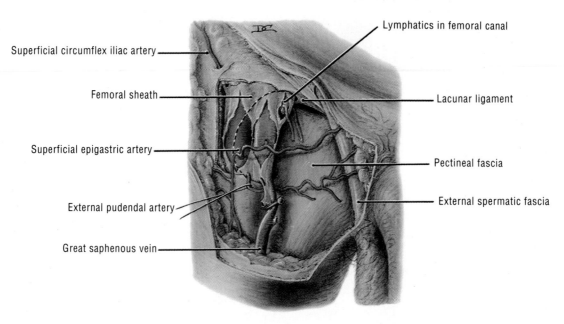

Superficial circumflex iliac artery

Femoral sheath

Superficial epigastric artery

External pudendal artery

Great saphenous vein

Lymphatics in femoral canal

Lacunar ligament

Pectineal fascia

External spermatic fascia

5.12
Femoral sheath, canal, and ring

Observe:

1. The lateral margin of the saphenous opening is cut away;

2. The superior margin of the opening passing toward the pubic tubercle and blending with the inguinal ligament and, in this specimen, with the lacunar ligament also;

3. The medial border of the opening formed by the fascia covering the pectineus muscle and, as such, passing laterally posterior to the femoral sheath;

4. The three compartments of the sheath, each incised longitudinally: (a) the lateral one for the artery, (b) the middle one for the vein, and (c) the medial one, called the femoral canal, for lymph vessels;

5. The proximal end of the femoral canal, called the femoral ring, bounded medially by the lacunar ligament, anteriorly by the inguinal ligament, posteriorly by the pectineus muscle and its fascia, and laterally by the femoral vein.

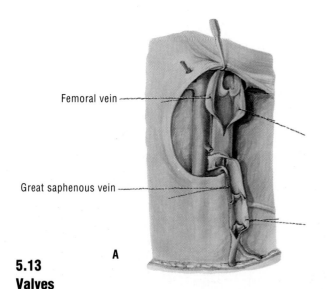

Femoral vein

Great saphenous vein

A

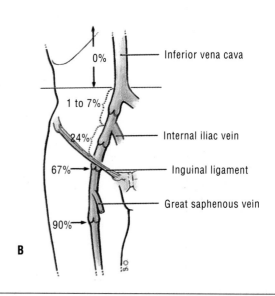

Inferior vena cava

0%

1 to 7%

24%

67%

90%

Internal iliac vein

Inguinal ligament

Great saphenous vein

B

5.13
Valves

A. Valves at the proximal ends of the femoral and great saphenous veins.

B. Percentage incidence of valves between the proximal femoral vein and the inferior vena cava. Between the mouth of the great saphenous vein and the heart, there were no valves in 21% of 506 limbs, one valve in 71%, two in 7%, and three in 1%; valves in the

common iliac vein are rarely competent, but two-thirds of those in the external iliac vein are competent (see Basmajian JV. *The distribution of valves in the femoral, external iliac and common iliac veins and their relationship to varicose veins.* Surg Gynecol Obstet 1952; 95:537).

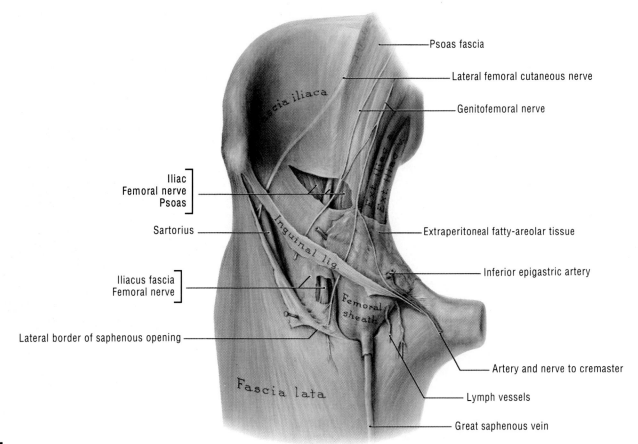

Psoas fascia

Lateral femoral cutaneous nerve

Genitofemoral nerve

Extraperitoneal fatty-areolar tissue

Inferior epigastric artery

Artery and nerve to cremaster

Lymph vessels

Great saphenous vein

Iliac
Femoral nerve
Psoas

Sartorius

Iliacus fascia
Femoral nerve

Lateral border of saphenous opening

5.14
Femoral sheath

The three flat muscles of the abdominal wall are cut away from the superior border of the inguinal ligament, and the fascia lata from the inferior border; the lateral margin of the saphenous opening in the fascia lata is cut and reflected; the inferior epigastric artery is pulled medially; the deep circumflex iliac artery is not labeled.

Observe:
1. The iliacus fascia, continuous medially with the psoas fascia and carried inferiorly, anterior to the iliacus muscle, into the thigh; as it passes posterior to the inguinal ligament, it adheres to it;

2. The extraperitoneal fatty (areolar) tissue, which lines the abdominal cavity and in which the external iliac vessels run, is carried inferiorly around these vessels into the thigh as a delicate funnel-shaped sac, called the femoral sheath; this is loosely adherent to the inguinal ligament anteriorly and to the pecten pubis posteriorly;

3. The femoral sheath containing the femoral artery, vein, and lymph vessels; the femoral nerve, lying posterior to the iliacus fascia, is outside the femoral sheath;

4. The lateral margin of the saphenous opening (part of the fascia lata) lying anterior to the femoral sheath; medially, the fascia passes posterior to the femoral sheath as the pectinal fascia;

5. The genitofemoral nerve pierces the psoas fascia proximally in one or two branches; the lateral femoral cutaneous nerve pierces the iliacus fascia at a variable point, commonly, as here, near the anterior superior iliac spine.

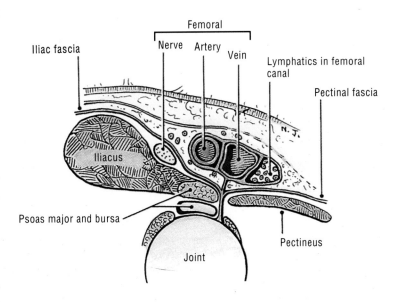

Iliac fascia

Femoral

Nerve   Artery   Vein

Lymphatics in femoral canal

Pectinal fascia

Iliacus

Psoas major and bursa

Pectineus

Joint

5.15
Relation of femoral structures, transverse section

The tough psoas tendon separates the femoral artery from the hip joint.

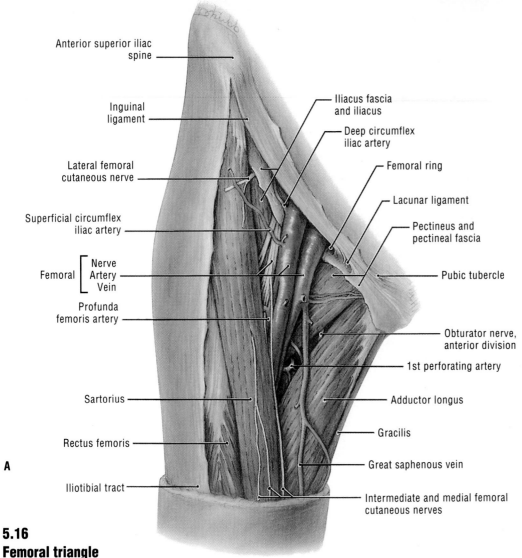

Anterior superior iliac spine

Inguinal ligament

Lateral femoral cutaneous nerve

Superficial circumflex iliac artery

Femoral { Nerve / Artery / Vein }

Profunda femoris artery

Sartorius

Rectus femoris

A

Iliotibial tract

Iliacus fascia and iliacus

Deep circumflex iliac artery

Femoral ring

Lacunar ligament

Pectineus and pectineal fascia

Pubic tubercle

Obturator nerve, anterior division

1st perforating artery

Adductor longus

Gracilis

Great saphenous vein

Intermediate and medial femoral cutaneous nerves

5.16
Femoral triangle

Observe in **A** and **B**:

1. The boundaries of the triangle: the inguinal ligament, which curves gently from anterior superior iliac spine to pubic tubercle, being the base; the medial border of the sartorius muscle being the lateral side; the medial border of the adductor longus muscle being the medial side; and the point where the two converging sides meet distally being the apex (some authors regard the lateral border of the adductor longus muscle as the medial side of the triangle);

2. The femoral artery and vein lying anterior to the fascia covering iliopsoas and pectineus muscles, and the femoral nerve lying posterior to the fascia;

3. The femoral artery appearing midway between the anterior superior iliac spine and the pubic tubercle, and disappearing where the medial border of the sartorius muscle crosses the lateral border of the adductor longus muscle; pulsation of the femoral artery can be felt just distal to the inguinal ligament midway between the anterior superior spine and the pubic tubercle;

4. That when the adjacent borders of the pectineus and adductor longus muscles are not contiguous, as here, the anterior branch of the obturator nerve lying anterior to the adductor brevis muscle is visible.

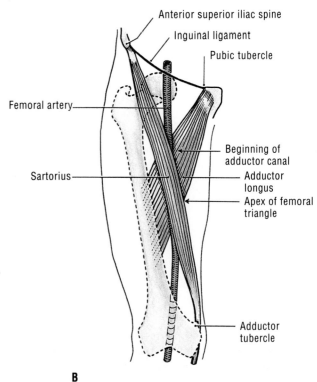

Anterior superior iliac spine

Inguinal ligament

Pubic tubercle

Femoral artery

Sartorius

Beginning of adductor canal

Adductor longus

Apex of femoral triangle

Adductor tubercle

B

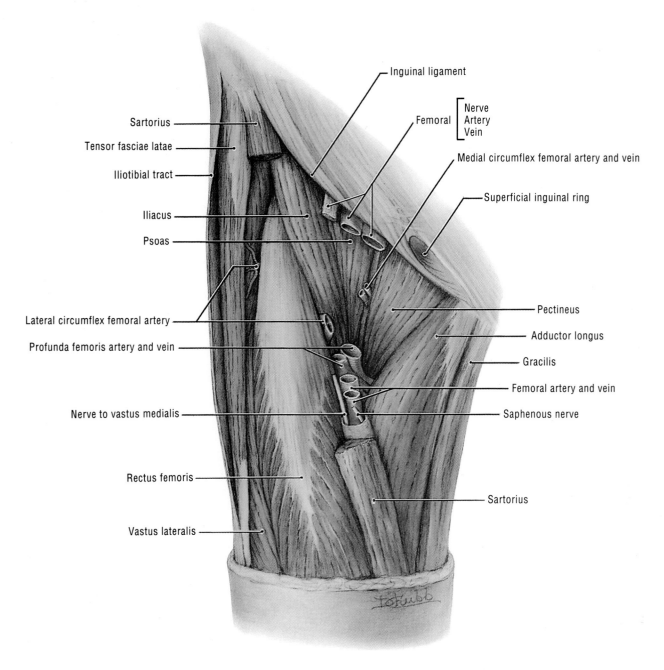

Sartorius

Tensor fasciae latae

Iliotibial tract

Iliacus

Psoas

Lateral circumflex femoral artery

Profunda femoris artery and vein

Nerve to vastus medialis

Rectus femoris

Vastus lateralis

Inguinal ligament

Femoral [Nerve
Artery
Vein

Medial circumflex femoral artery and vein

Superficial inguinal ring

Pectineus

Adductor longus

Gracilis

Femoral artery and vein

Saphenous nerve

Sartorius

5.17
Floor of the femoral triangle

Sections are removed from the sartorius muscle and from the femoral vessels and nerve.

Observe:
1. The floor of the triangle is a trough with sloping lateral and medial walls; this is notably so if the adductor longus muscle is included with the pectineus muscle in the medial wall; the iliopsoas (medial border of rectus femoris) and sartorius muscles form the lateral wall;

2. The trough is shallow at the base and deep at the apex;

3. At the apex of the femoral triangle, four vessels (the femoral artery and vein and the profunda femoris artery and vein) and two nerves (the nerve to vastus medialis and the saphenous nerve) pass into the adductor (subsartorial) canal.

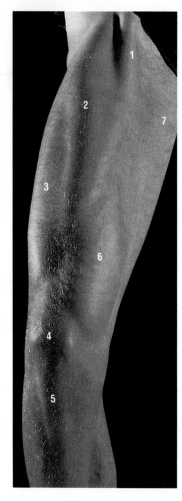

Anterior view

5.18
Surface anatomy of the thigh

Observe:

The quadriceps inserting on the patella and then via the patellar ligament to the tibial tuberosity; the vastus medialis muscle attaching to the base and proximal two-thirds of the medial surface of the patella and the vastus lateralis attaching mainly to the base of the patella and slightly on to the lateral surface.

Numbers refer to structures in Figure 5.20.

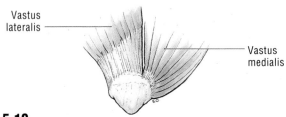

5.19
Patellar attachment of
vastus medialis and lateralis muscles

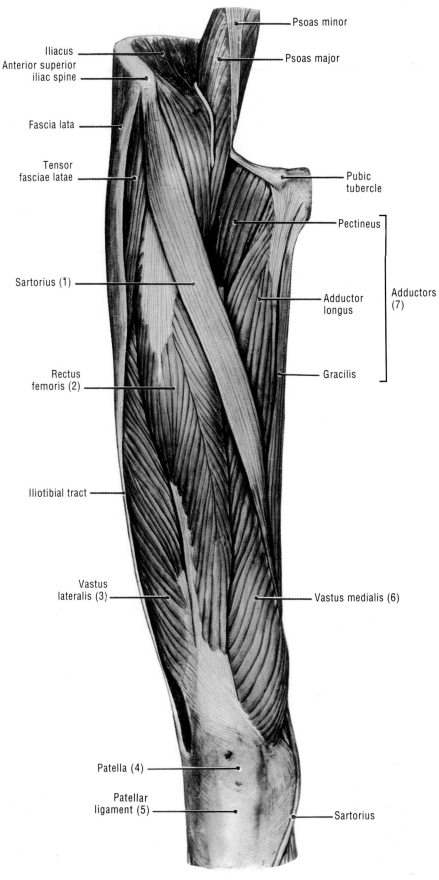

5.20
Muscles, anterior aspect of the thigh–I

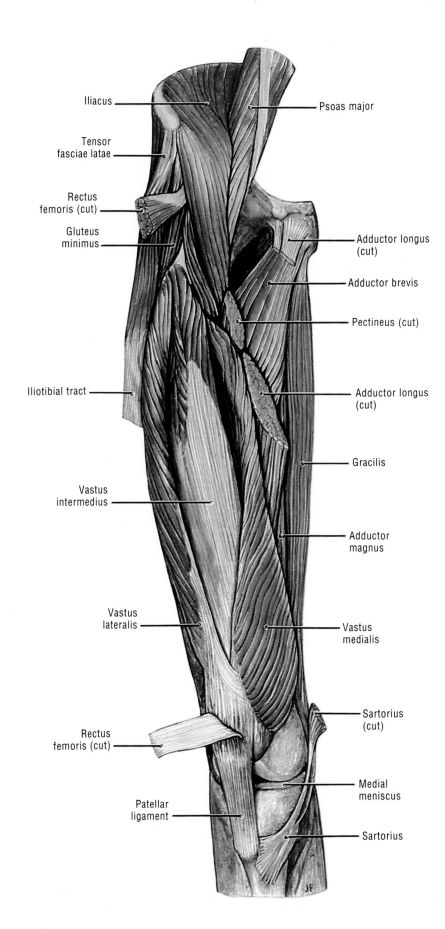

Iliacus

Tensor fasciae latae

Rectus femoris (cut)

Gluteus minimus

Iliotibial tract

Vastus intermedius

Vastus lateralis

Rectus femoris (cut)

Patellar ligament

Psoas major

Adductor longus (cut)

Adductor brevis

Pectineus (cut)

Adductor longus (cut)

Gracilis

Adductor magnus

Vastus medialis

Sartorius (cut)

Medial meniscus

Sartorius

5.21
Muscles, anterior aspect of the thigh–II

The central portion of the muscle bellies of the sartorius, rectus femoris, pectineus, and adductor longus muscles have been removed.

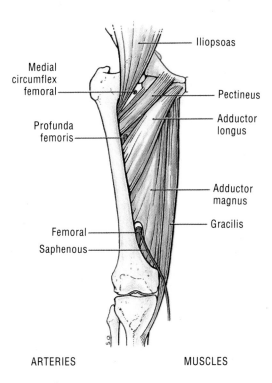

Medial circumflex femoral

Profunda femoris

Femoral

Saphenous

Iliopsoas

Pectineus

Adductor longus

Adductor magnus

Gracilis

ARTERIES   MUSCLES

5.22
Relationship of the adductor muscles to the branches of the femoral artery

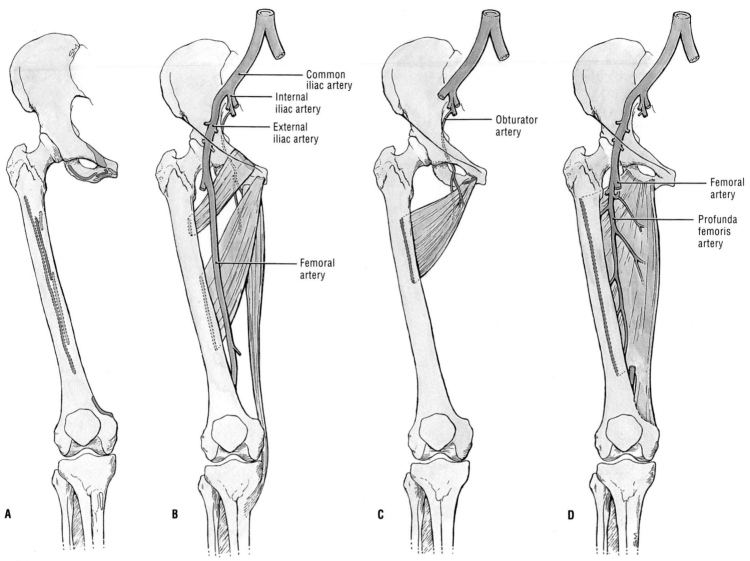

Common
iliac artery

Internal
iliac artery

External
iliac artery

Femoral
artery

Obturator
artery

Femoral
artery

Profunda
femoris
artery

A   B   C   D

5.23
Adductor muscles of the thigh

Each of the adductor group of thigh muscles has a linear attachment to the linea aspera on the posterior surface of the femur. All are adductors of the thigh; their attachments disclose their other actions: the pectineus muscle flexes the thigh; the gracilis muscle flexes the leg and rotates it medially. All contribute to normal gait and posture.

A. The insertions of the adductor muscles are seen from an anterior view as through a transparent femur; most medial (green) are the insertions of the pectineus muscle (more proximal) and the adductor longus muscle (more distal), the adductor brevis muscle (blue) is intermediate, and the adductor magnus muscle (red) is most lateral but swings medially to reach the adductor tubercle.

B. The superficial layer includes: pectineus, adductor longus, and gracilis muscles; the latter alone avoids the femur and inserts on the medial side of the proximal tibia.

C. The adductor brevis muscle attaches to the intermediate area of the linea aspera.

D. The adductor magnus muscle is deepest, attaches most later-

ally on the femur, and has the most extensive origin and insertion; its aponeurosis is punctured by perforating arteries and the femoral artery passes through the hiatus in its insertion (the adductor hiatus).

Blood supply:
C. The obturator artery, a branch of the internal iliac artery, passes through the obturator foramen and divides into anterior and posterior branches that anastomose with each other and with adjacent arteries; the anterior branch supplies the adductor group of thigh muscles; the posterior branch supplies hamstring muscles and sends an acetabular branch to the head of the femur.

D. The femoral artery is a continuation of the external iliac artery, which changes its name to femoral as it passes posterior to the inguinal ligament; it travels first in the femoral triangle then in the adductor canal, supplying thigh muscles of the flexor and adductor groups; as the femoral artery passes into the popliteal fossa through the hiatus in the adductor magnus muscle, it changes its name to the popliteal artery.

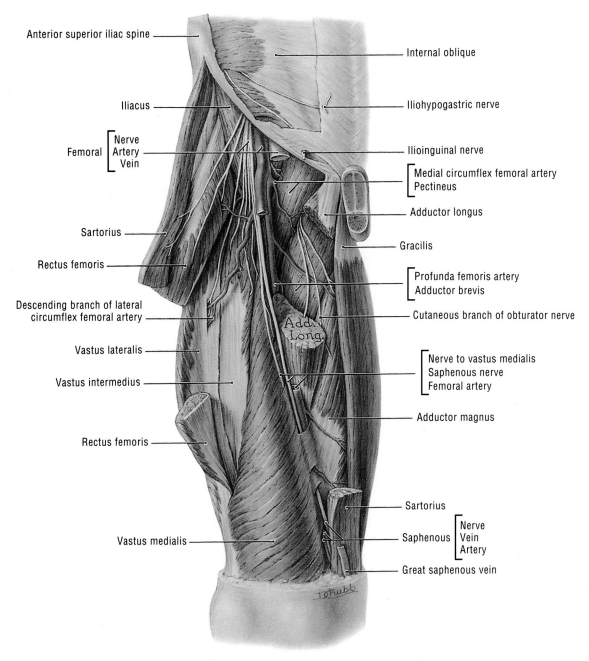

Anterior superior iliac spine

Internal oblique

Iliacus

Iliohypogastric nerve

Femoral ⎡ Nerve
       ⎢ Artery
       ⎣ Vein

Ilioinguinal nerve

⎡ Medial circumflex femoral artery
⎣ Pectineus

Sartorius

Adductor longus

Rectus femoris

Gracilis

⎡ Profunda femoris artery
⎣ Adductor brevis

Descending branch of lateral
circumflex femoral artery

Cutaneous branch of obturator nerve

Vastus lateralis

⎡ Nerve to vastus medialis
⎢ Saphenous nerve
⎣ Femoral artery

Vastus intermedius

Add. Long.

Adductor magnus

Rectus femoris

Sartorius

⎡ Nerve
Saphenous ⎢ Vein
⎣ Artery

Vastus medialis

Great saphenous vein

ToFubb

5.24
Dissection of the anteromedial aspect of the thigh

Observe:

1. The limb is rotated laterally;

2. The femoral nerve breaking up into a leash of nerves on entering the thigh;

3. The femoral artery lying between two motor territories, namely, that of the obturator nerve, which is medial, and that of the femoral nerve, which is lateral; no motor nerve crosses anterior to the femoral artery, but the twig to the pectineus muscle is seen crossing posterior to it;

4. The nerve to the vastus medialis muscle and the saphenous nerve accompanying the femoral artery into the adductor canal; the saphenous nerve and artery and their companion anasto-

motic vein emerging from the canal distally between the sartorius and gracilis muscles;

5. The profunda femoris artery arising 4 cm inferior to the inguinal ligament, lying posterior to the femoral artery, and disappearing posterior to the adductor longus muscle; it supplies the thigh via the medial and lateral circumflex femoral branches and the perforating arteries that pass through the adductor magnus muscle on their way to the posterior aspect of the thigh; both femoral and lateral femoral circumflex arteries have descending genicular branches that contribute to the anastomoses around the knee.

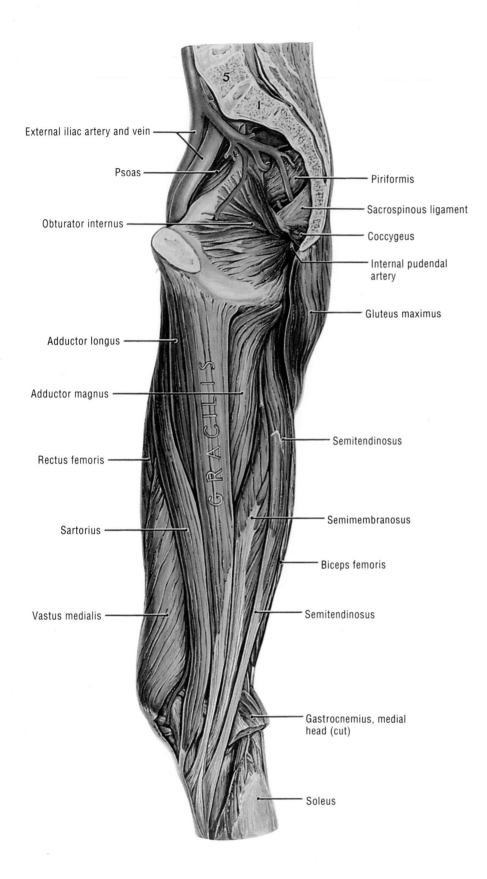

External iliac artery and vein

Psoas

Obturator internus

Adductor longus

Adductor magnus

Rectus femoris

Sartorius

Vastus medialis

GRACILIS

Piriformis

Sacrospinous ligament

Coccygeus

Internal pudendal artery

Gluteus maximus

Semitendinosus

Semimembranosus

Biceps femoris

Semitendinosus

Gastrocnemius, medial head (cut)

Soleus

5.25
Muscles of the medial aspect of the thigh

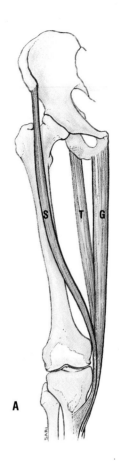

A

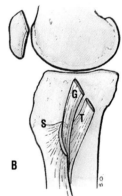

B

5.26
Muscular tripod

A. These three muscles: sartorius *(S)*, gracilis *(G)*, and semitendinosus *(T)*, form an inverted "tripod" with its base separated at the hip bone and its three legs converging to an apex on the medial side of the proximal end of the tibia; examining their attachments, it can be seen that all flex the knee but the sartorius muscle is a lateral rotator and abductor while the gracilis muscle is a medial rotator and adductor.

B. At their insertion to the tibia, all three tendons become thin aponeuroses; the aponeurotic fibers of the sartorius muscle curve posteriorly superior to the insertion of the gracilis muscle.

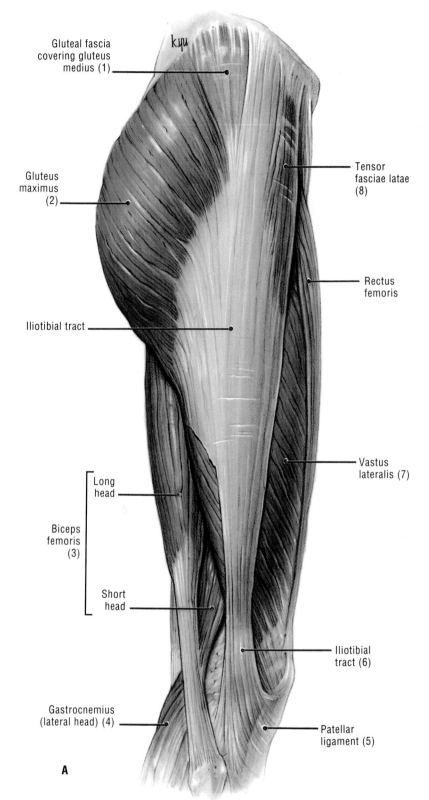

Gluteal fascia covering gluteus medius (1)

Gluteus maximus (2)

Iliotibial tract

Biceps femoris (3)
  Long head
  Short head

Gastrocnemius (lateral head) (4)

Tensor fasciae latae (8)

Rectus femoris

Vastus lateralis (7)

Iliotibial tract (6)

Patellar ligament (5)

A

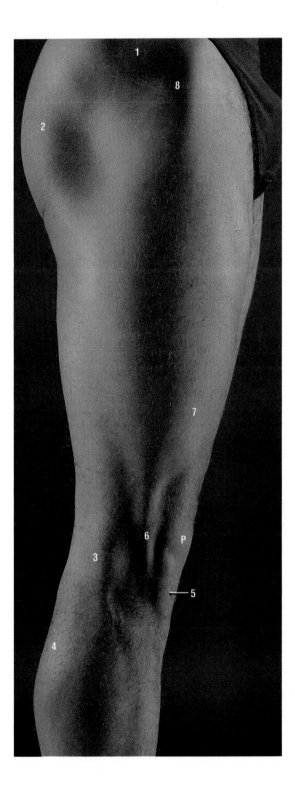

B

5.27
Lateral aspect of the thigh

A. Lateral aspect. **B**. Surface anatomy of the lateral aspect of the thigh. Numbers refer to structures in **A**. Observe the posterior edge of the iliotibial tract (a thickening of the fascia lata) that attaches to the lateral condyle of the tibia; the biceps femoris tendon is inserting on the head of the fibula; the patella *(P)*.

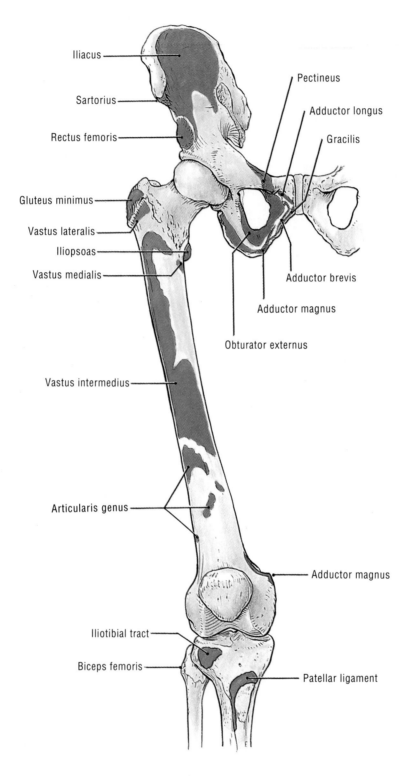

Iliacus

Sartorius

Rectus femoris

Pectineus

Adductor longus

Gracilis

Gluteus minimus

Vastus lateralis

Iliopsoas

Vastus medialis

Adductor brevis

Adductor magnus

Obturator externus

Vastus intermedius

Articularis genus

Adductor magnus

Iliotibial tract

Biceps femoris

Patellar ligament

A, *Anterior view*

5.28
Bones of the lower limb showing attachments of muscles

A. For tibia and fibula, anterior aspect, see Figure 5.74**A**.

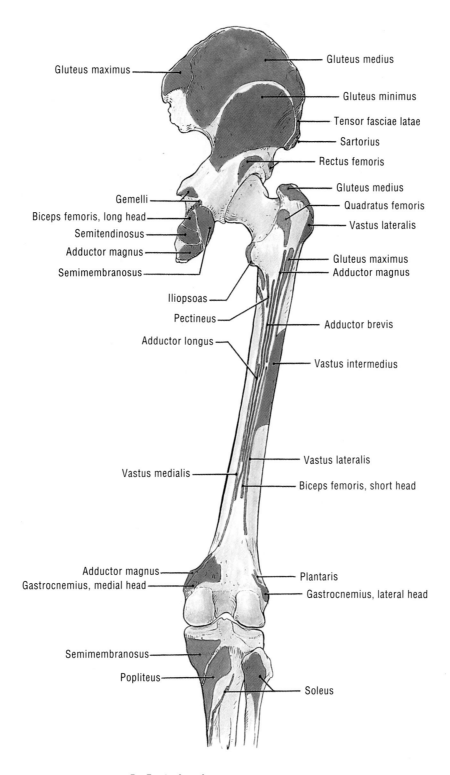

Gluteus maximus

Gluteus medius

Gluteus minimus

Tensor fasciae latae

Sartorius

Rectus femoris

Gemelli

Gluteus medius

Biceps femoris, long head

Quadratus femoris

Semitendinosus

Vastus lateralis

Adductor magnus

Gluteus maximus

Semimembranosus

Adductor magnus

Iliopsoas

Pectineus

Adductor brevis

Adductor longus

Vastus intermedius

Vastus lateralis

Vastus medialis

Biceps femoris, short head

Adductor magnus

Plantaris

Gastrocnemius, medial head

Gastrocnemius, lateral head

Semimembranosus

Popliteus

Soleus

B, *Posterior view*

5.28
Bones of the lower limb showing attachments of muscles *(continued)*

B. For the tibia and fibula, posterior aspect, see Figure 5.90.

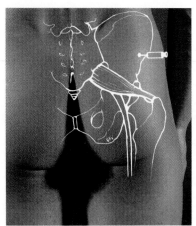

5.29
Surface anatomy of the posterior aspect of the thigh

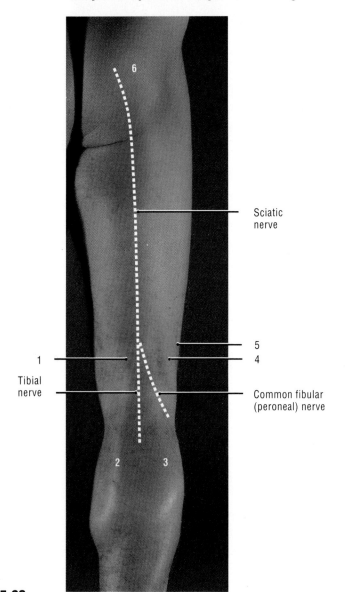

5.30
Surface anatomy of the gluteal region and posterior thigh

Numbers refer to structures in Figure 5.30.

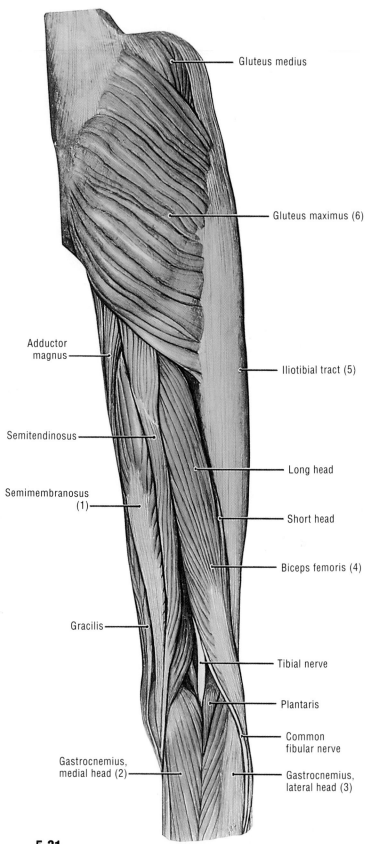

5.31
Muscles of the gluteal region and posterior aspect of the thigh–I

Labels in Figure 5.30:
- Sciatic nerve
- 5
- 4
- 1
- Tibial nerve
- Common fibular (peroneal) nerve
- 6
- 2
- 3

Labels in Figure 5.31:
- Gluteus medius
- Gluteus maximus (6)
- Adductor magnus
- Iliotibial tract (5)
- Semitendinosus
- Long head
- Semimembranosus (1)
- Short head
- Biceps femoris (4)
- Gracilis
- Tibial nerve
- Plantaris
- Common fibular nerve
- Gastrocnemius, medial head (2)
- Gastrocnemius, lateral head (3)

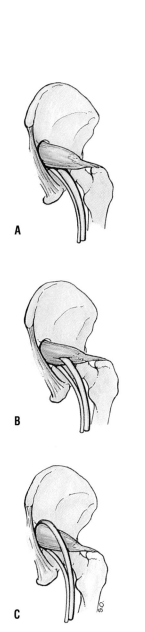

A

B

C

5.32
Relationship of the sciatic nerve to piriformis muscle

Of 640 limbs studied:

A. In 87%, both the tibial and fibular (peroneal) divisions passed inferior to the piriformis muscle;

B. In 12.2%, the fibular (peroneal) division passed through the piriformis muscle;

C. In 0.5%, the fibular (peroneal) division passed superior to the piriformis muscle.

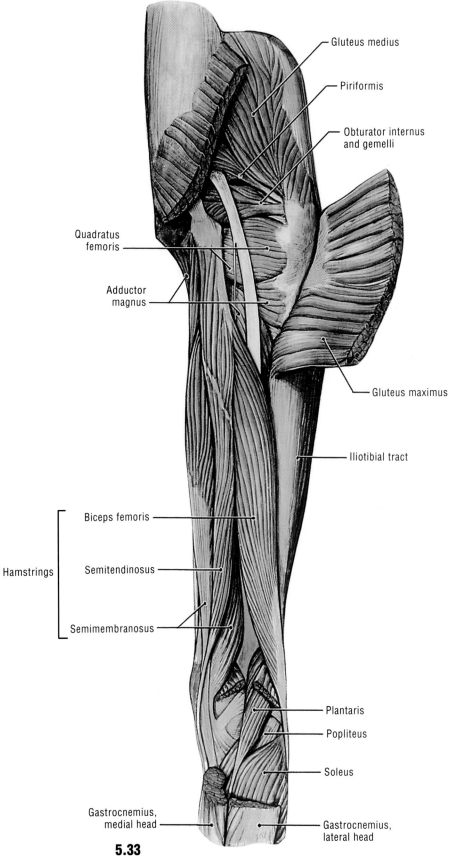

Gluteus medius

Piriformis

Obturator internus and gemelli

Quadratus femoris

Adductor magnus

Gluteus maximus

Iliotibial tract

Biceps femoris

Hamstrings

Semitendinosus

Semimembranosus

Plantaris

Popliteus

Soleus

Gastrocnemius, medial head

Gastrocnemius, lateral head

5.33
Muscles of the gluteal region and posterior aspect of the thigh–II

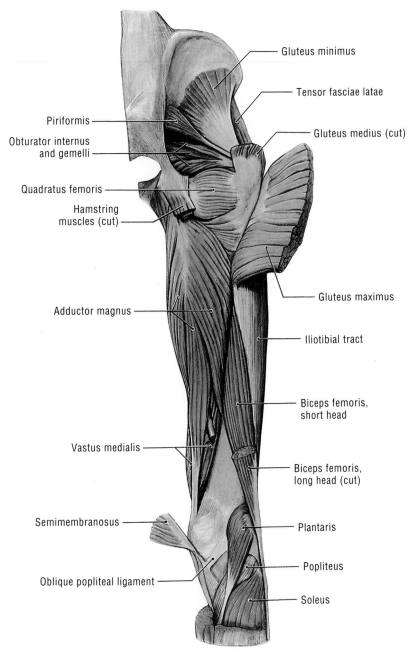

Gluteus minimus

Tensor fasciae latae

Piriformis

Obturator internus and gemelli

Gluteus medius (cut)

Quadratus femoris

Hamstring muscles (cut)

Gluteus maximus

Adductor magnus

Iliotibial tract

Biceps femoris, short head

Vastus medialis

Biceps femoris, long head (cut)

Semimembranosus

Plantaris

Popliteus

Oblique popliteal ligament

Soleus

A, *Posterior view*

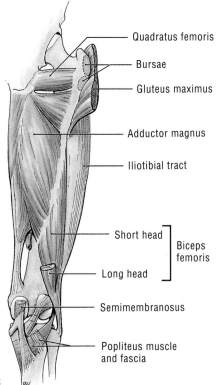

Quadratus femoris

Bursae

Gluteus maximus

Adductor magnus

Iliotibial tract

Short head

Long head

} Biceps femoris

Semimembranosus

Popliteus muscle and fascia

B

5.34
Adductor magnus muscle

A. Muscles of the gluteal region and posterior aspect of the thigh, hamstring muscles removed. **B**. Diagram of the adductor magnus muscle. The adductor magnus is a large muscle with two parts, one belonging to the adductor group and the other to the hamstring group. The portion of adductor magnus muscle that originates from the ischial tuberosity and inserts via a palpable tendon into the adductor tubercle belongs to the hamstring group of muscles and is innervated by the tibial portion of the sciatic nerve. The adductor part of the muscle is innervated by the obturator nerve and originates from the inferior ramus of the ischium and pubis (conjoint ramus) and inserts on the linea aspera and medial supracondylar line of the femur.

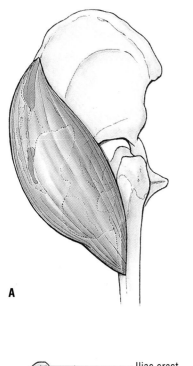

A

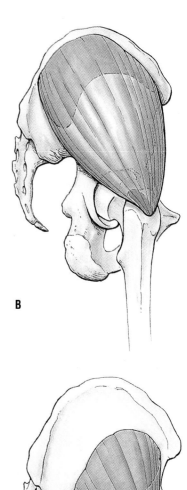

B

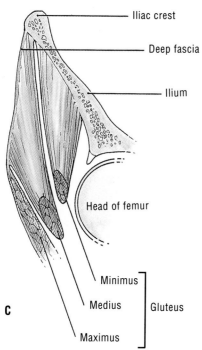

Iliac crest

Deep fascia

Ilium

Head of femur

Minimus

Medius — Gluteus

Maximus

C

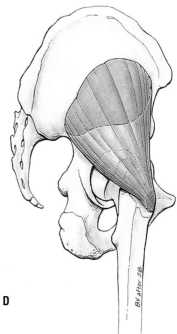

D

BV after JB

5.35
Glutei

The three oblique views and coronal section of the hip region show the bony attachments of the three gluteal muscles. As may be determined by their attachments, all three are extensors and abductors of the thigh. In addition, the maximus muscle is a strong lateral rotator of the thigh, and the minimus muscle (passing anterior to the joint) is a medial rotator. Medius and minimus muscles are crucial in maintaining stability at the hip when the opposite leg is raised in walking.

A. The gluteus maximus muscle is attached proximally to the ilium, sacrum, coccyx, the aponeurosis of the erector spinae, and the sacrotuberous ligament. As well as its attachment to the

femur, shown here, it has a strong attachment to the iliotibial tract.

B. The gluteus medius muscle is attached proximally to the ilium and distally to the greater trochanter.

C. The gluteus medius muscle, the most anterior part, has little bone available to it, so it uses extensively, as an aponeurosis, the deep fascia covering it.

D. The gluteus minimus muscle passes from the ilium to the anterior aspect of the greater trochanter.

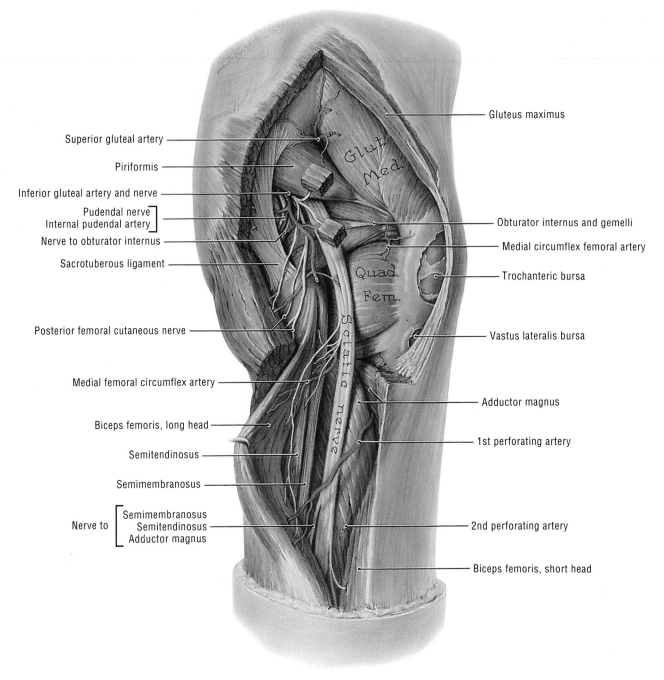

Superior gluteal artery

Piriformis

Inferior gluteal artery and nerve

Pudendal nerve
Internal pudendal artery

Nerve to obturator internus

Sacrotuberous ligament

Posterior femoral cutaneous nerve

Medial femoral circumflex artery

Biceps femoris, long head

Semitendinosus

Semimembranosus

Nerve to [Semimembranosus
Semitendinosus
Adductor magnus]

Gluteus maximus

Glut. Med.

Quad. Fem.

Sciatic nerve

Obturator internus and gemelli

Medial circumflex femoral artery

Trochanteric bursa

Vastus lateralis bursa

Adductor magnus

1st perforating artery

2nd perforating artery

Biceps femoris, short head

5.36
Muscles of the gluteal region and posterior aspect of the thigh–III

The gluteus maximus muscle is split, both superiorly and inferiorly, in the direction of its fibers, and the middle part is excised, but two cubes remain to identify its nerve.

Observe:
1. The gluteus maximus is the only muscle to cover the greater trochanter; it is aponeurotic and has underlying bursae where it glides on the trochanter and on the aponeurosis of the vastus lateralis muscle; a smaller bursa is usually found between the muscle and the ischial tuberosity;

2. The inferior gluteal nerve enters the gluteus maximus muscle in two chief branches near its center;

3. Superior to the piriformis muscle is the gluteus medius muscle, which covers the gluteus minimus muscle;

4. The sciatic nerve appears inferior to the piriformis muscle and crosses in turn: the dorsal surface of the ischium, the obturator internus and gemelli, quadratus femoris, and adductor magnus muscles; its branches spring from its medial side at variable levels to supply the hamstrings and part of the adductor magnus muscles; only the branch to the biceps muscle (short head) springs (usually inferiorly) from its lateral side, which, therefore, is the safer side to dissect on.

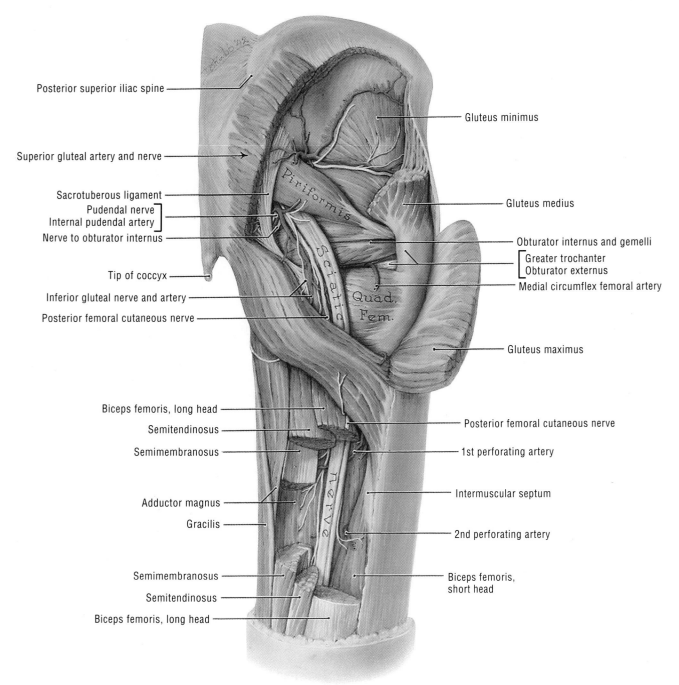

Posterior superior iliac spine

Superior gluteal artery and nerve

Sacrotuberous ligament
Pudendal nerve
Internal pudendal artery
Nerve to obturator internus

Tip of coccyx

Inferior gluteal nerve and artery
Posterior femoral cutaneous nerve

Biceps femoris, long head
Semitendinosus
Semimembranosus

Adductor magnus
Gracilis

Semimembranosus
Semitendinosus
Biceps femoris, long head

Gluteus minimus

Gluteus medius

Obturator internus and gemelli
Greater trochanter
Obturator externus
Medial circumflex femoral artery

Gluteus maximus

Posterior femoral cutaneous nerve

1st perforating artery

Intermuscular septum

2nd perforating artery

Biceps femoris, short head

5.37
Muscles of the gluteal region and the posterior aspect of the thigh–IV

The proximal three-quarters of the gluteus maximus muscle is reflected, and parts of the gluteus medius and the three hamstring muscles are excised.

Observe:
1. The superior gluteal vessels and nerves appearing superior to the piriformis muscle; all other vessels and nerves appearing inferior to it;

2. The superior gluteal artery dividing into superficial and deep branches; the superficial branch supplying the gluteus maximus muscle; the deep branch dividing into a superior ramus that anastomoses with arteries of the region, and an inferior ramus

that supplies the gluteus medius and minimus muscles;

3. The inferior gluteal artery supplying the buttock, proximal part of the thigh, and the sciatic nerve;

4. The horizontal groove (the natal fold) crossing the inferior border of the gluteus maximus muscle indicates the superior limit of the sleeve-like deep fascia of the thigh;

5. The gluteus maximus muscle consisting of bundles of parallel fibers; it is rhomboidal and the deep fascia covering it is thin; the gluteus medius muscle arising, in part, from the covering deep fascia which, therefore, is strong and thick.

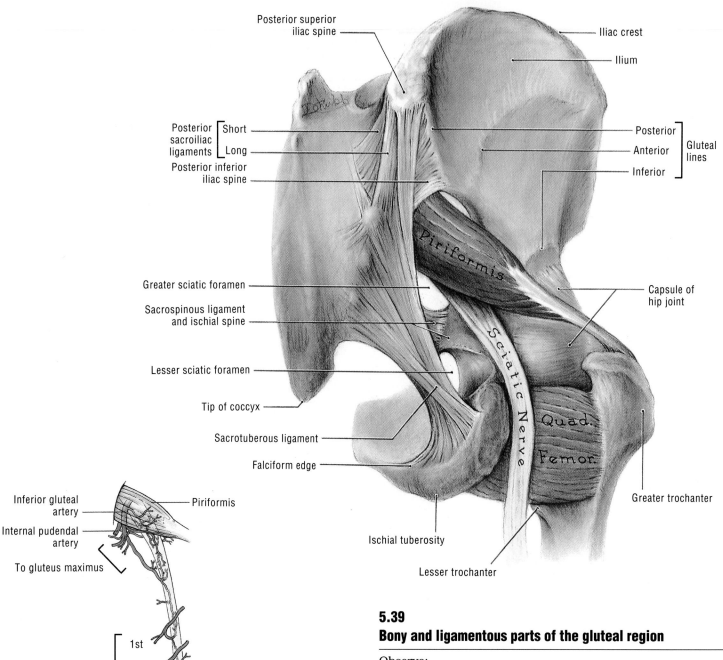

Posterior superior iliac spine

Posterior sacroiliac ligaments — Short — Long

Posterior inferior iliac spine

Greater sciatic foramen

Sacrospinous ligament and ischial spine

Lesser sciatic foramen

Tip of coccyx

Sacrotuberous ligament

Falciform edge

Iliac crest

Ilium

Posterior
Anterior — Gluteal lines
Inferior

Piriformis

Capsule of hip joint

Sciatic Nerve

Quad. Femor.

Greater trochanter

Ischial tuberosity

Lesser trochanter

Inferior gluteal artery

Internal pudendal artery

To gluteus maximus

Piriformis

Perforating arteries

1st

2nd

3rd

4th

Tibial nerve

Common fibular (peroneal) nerve

Popliteal artery

5.38
Blood supply to the sciatic nerve

Observe the continuous anastomotic chain of arteries.

5.39
Bony and ligamentous parts of the gluteal region

Observe:

1. The tip of the coccyx lies superior to the level of the ischial tuberosity and inferior to that of the ischial spine;

2. The inferior border of the piriformis muscle is defined by joining the midpoint between the tip of the coccyx and the posterior superior iliac spine to the greater trochanter;

3. The inferior border of the quadratus femoris muscle is level with the inferior aspect of the ischial tuberosity and it crosses the lesser trochanter;

4. The lateral border of the sciatic nerve lies midway between the lateral surface of the greater trochanter and the medial surface of the ischial tuberosity, provided the body is in the anatomical position.

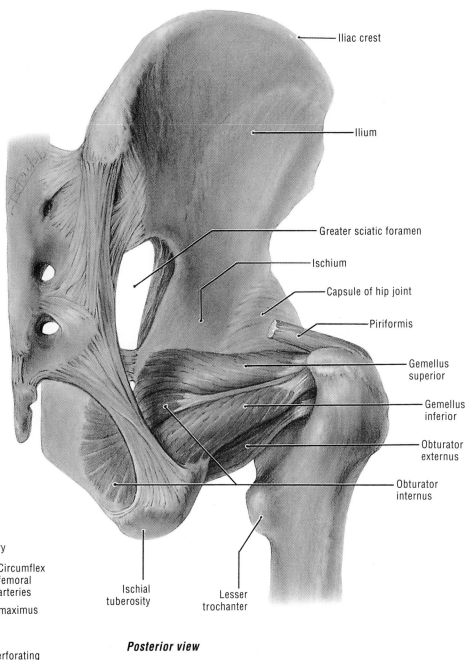

- Iliac crest
- Ilium
- Greater sciatic foramen
- Ischium
- Capsule of hip joint
- Piriformis
- Gemellus superior
- Gemellus inferior
- Obturator externus
- Obturator internus
- Lesser trochanter
- Ischial tuberosity

Posterior view

Psoas
Obturator externus
Pectineus
Adductor longus
Inferior gluteal artery
Medial Circumflex
Lateral femoral arteries
Gluteus maximus
1st
2nd
Perforating branches of profunda femoris artery
3rd
Adductor hiatus
4th
Adductor magnus
Medial and lateral superior genicular arteries
Popliteus
Medial and lateral inferior genicular arteries

5.40
Arteries of the posterior aspect of the hip, thigh, and knee

5.41
Obturator muscles

Observe:

1. The obturator internus and gemelli muscles fill the gap between the piriformis muscle superiorly and the quadratus femoris muscle inferiorly;

2. The obturator externus muscle passing obliquely, inferior to the neck of femur, to its insertion;

3. That the inferior aspect of the ischial tuberosity is on the level of the lesser trochanter.

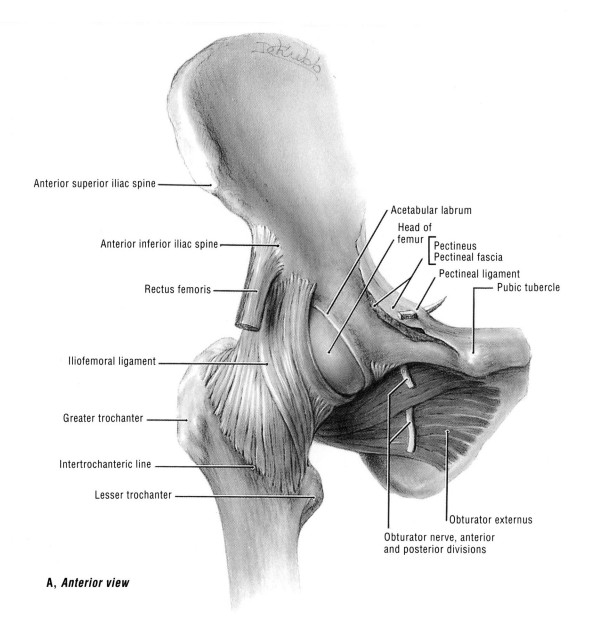

Anterior superior iliac spine

Anterior inferior iliac spine

Rectus femoris

Iliofemoral ligament

Greater trochanter

Intertrochanteric line

Lesser trochanter

Acetabular labrum

Head of femur

Pectineus

Pectineal fascia

Pectineal ligament

Pubic tubercle

Obturator externus

Obturator nerve, anterior and posterior divisions

A, *Anterior view*

5.42
Hip joint

Observe in **A**:

1. The head of the femur exposed just medial to the iliofemoral ligament and facing not only superiorly and medially, but also anteriorly; here, at the site of the psoas bursa, the capsule is weak or, as in this specimen, partially deficient, but it is guarded by the psoas tendon;

2. The iliofemoral ligament, shaped like an inverted "Y", attached superiorly deep to the rectus femoris muscle, and so directed as to become taut on medial rotation of the femur;

3. The obturator externus muscle crossing obliquely inferior to the neck of the femur;

4. The thinness of the pectineus muscle; and its fascia blending with the pectineal ligament along the pecten pubis.

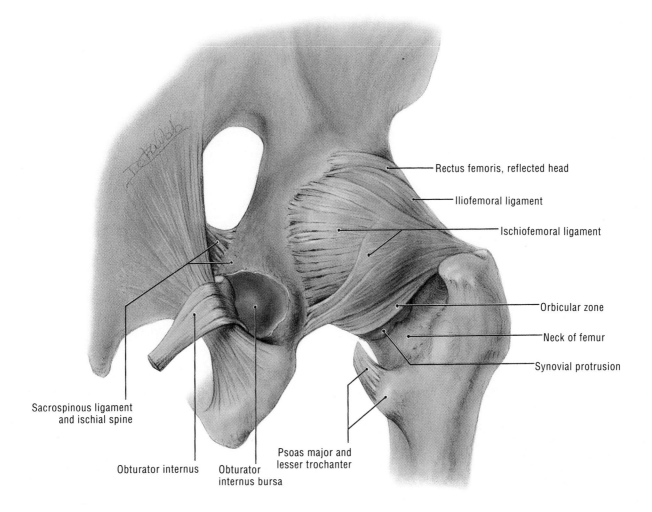

Rectus femoris, reflected head

Iliofemoral ligament

Ischiofemoral ligament

Orbicular zone

Neck of femur

Synovial protrusion

Sacrospinous ligament
and ischial spine

Obturator internus

Obturator
internus bursa

Psoas major and
lesser trochanter

B, *Posterior view*

5.42
Hip joint *(continued)*

Observe in **B**:

1. The fibers of the capsule spiraling as to become taut during extension and medial rotation of the femur;

2. The fibers crossing the neck posteriorly, but not attached to it; the synovial membrane protrudes inferior to the fibrous capsule and there forms a bursa for the tendon of the obturator externus muscle.

5.43
Socket for the head of the femur

Observe:

1. The transverse acetabular ligament converting the acetabular notch into the acetabular foramen;

2. The acetabular labrum, attached to the acetabular rim and to the transverse acetabular ligament; it forms a complete ring around the head of the femur;

3. The lunate ("C"-shaped) articular surface;

4. The synovial membrane attached to the margin of the articular cartilage and covering the pad of fat and the vessels in the acetabular fossa;

5. The ligament of the head of the femur (ligamentum teres), which is a hollow cone of synovial membrane compressed between the head of the femur and its socket; it envelops ligamentous fibers; these are attached superiorly to the pit on the head of the femur, and inferiorly to the transverse acetabular ligament and the margins of the acetabular notch; through it passes the artery to the head of the femur (Fig. 5.44).

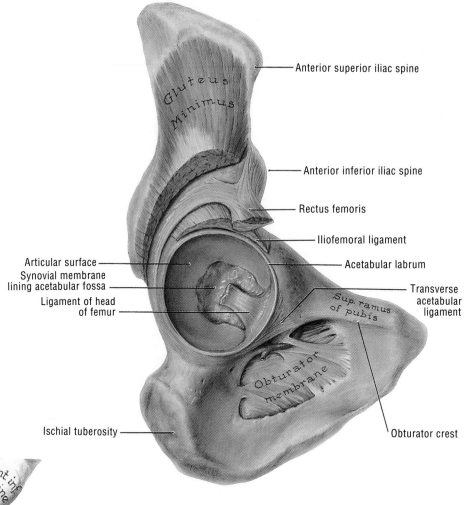

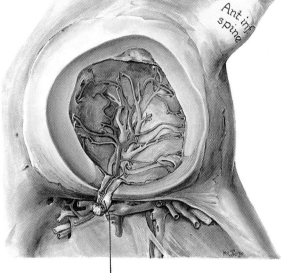

5.44
Blood vessels of the acetabular fossa

The acetabular branches (an artery and a vein) of the posterior division of the obturator vessels pass through the acetabular foramen and enter the acetabular fossa where they ramify in the fatty areolar tissue. The branches radiate to the margin of the fossa where they enter nutrient foramina. A branch of the artery and vein runs through the ligament of the head of the femur to the femoral head.

5.45
Hip bone in youth

The three elements of the hip bone (os coxae) meet in the acetabulum at the triradiate synchondrosis. One or more primary centers of ossification appear in the triradiate cartilage about the 12th year. Secondary centers of ossification appear along the length of the iliac crest, at the anterior inferior iliac spine, at the ischial tuberosity, and at the symphysis pubis at about puberty; fusion is usually complete by age 23.

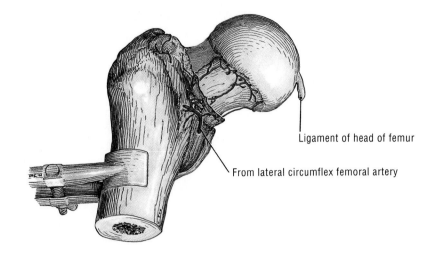

A, *Anterior view*

Ligament of head of femur

From lateral circumflex femoral artery

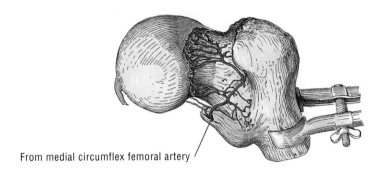

From medial circumflex femoral artery

B, *Posterosuperior view*

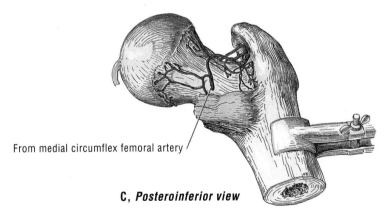

From medial circumflex femoral artery

C, *Posteroinferior view*

5.46
Blood supply to the head of the femur

Observe:

The head receives three sets of arteries: (a) the main set of three or four ascends in the synovial retinacula on the posterosuperior and posteroinferior parts of the neck of the femur, to perforate just distal to the head and anastomose freely with (b) terminal branches of the medullary artery of the shaft, and in 80% of cases, with (c) the artery of the ligament of the head of the femur; this last artery enters the head only when the center of ossification has extended to the pit for the ligament of the head (12th to 14th year);

this anastomosis persists even in advanced age, but in 20% it is never established; the blood supply is in danger in fractures of the neck of the femur (see Wolcott WE. *The evolution of the circulation in the developing femoral head and neck.* Surg Gynecol Obstet 1943; 77:61; and Trueta J, Harrison MHM. *Normal vascular anatomy of the femoral head in adult man.* J Bone Joint Surg 1953; 35B:442).

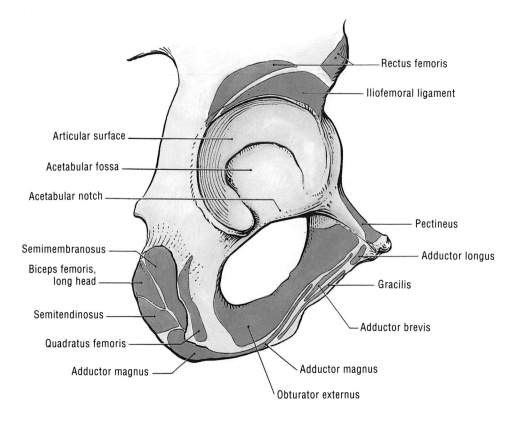

Rectus femoris

Iliofemoral ligament

Articular surface

Acetabular fossa

Acetabular notch

Pectineus

Adductor longus

Semimembranosus

Biceps femoris,
long head

Gracilis

Semitendinosus

Adductor brevis

Quadratus femoris

Adductor magnus

Adductor magnus

Obturator externus

5.47
Acetabular region, muscle attachments

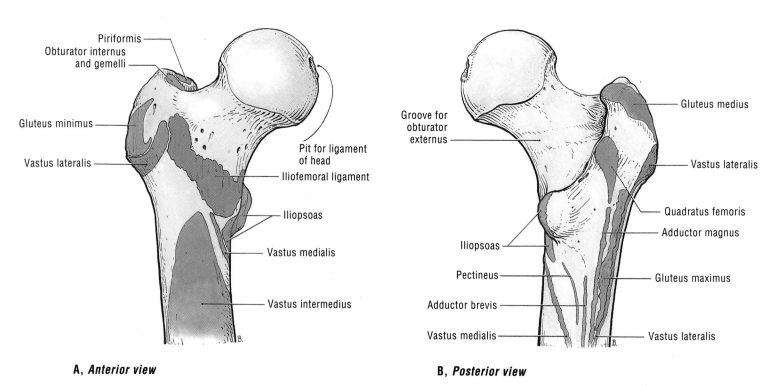

Piriformis
Obturator internus
and gemelli

Gluteus medius

Gluteus minimus

Groove for
obturator
externus

Vastus lateralis

Vastus lateralis

Pit for ligament
of head

Quadratus femoris

Iliofemoral ligament

Adductor magnus

Iliopsoas

Iliopsoas

Vastus medialis

Pectineus

Gluteus maximus

Adductor brevis

Vastus intermedius

Vastus medialis

Vastus lateralis

A, *Anterior view*

B, *Posterior view*

5.48
Proximal femur, muscle attachments

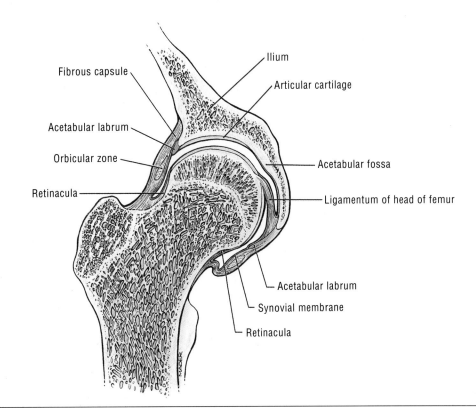

Fibrous capsule

Acetabular labrum

Orbicular zone

Retinacula

Ilium

Articular cartilage

Acetabular fossa

Ligamentum of head of femur

Acetabular labrum

Synovial membrane

Retinacula

5.49
Hip joint, coronal section

Observe:

1. The bony trabeculae of the ilium projected into the head of the femur as lines of pressure and the trabeculae that cross these as lines of tension;

2. The epiphysis of the head of the femur, entirely within the capsule of the joint;

3. The ligament of the head of the femur, as a synovial tube that is fixed superiorly at the pit (fovea) on the head of the femur and

open inferiorly at the acetabular foramen where it is continuous with the synovial membrane covering the fat in the acetabular fossa and also with the synovial membrane covering the transverse acetabular ligament;

4. The ligament of the head becomes taut during adduction of the hip joint, as when crossing the legs.

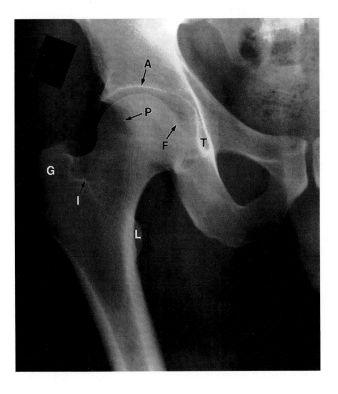

5.50
Radiograph of the hip

Observe:

On the femur: the greater (G) and lesser (L) trochanters, the intertrochanteric crest (I), and the pit or fovea (F) for the ligament of the head.

On the pelvis: the roof (A) and posterior rim (P) of the acetabulum, and the "teardrop" appearance (T) caused by the superimposition of structures at the inferior margin of the acetabulum.

(Courtesy of Dr. E. Becker, Associate Professor of Radiology, University of Toronto, Toronto, Ontario, Canada.)

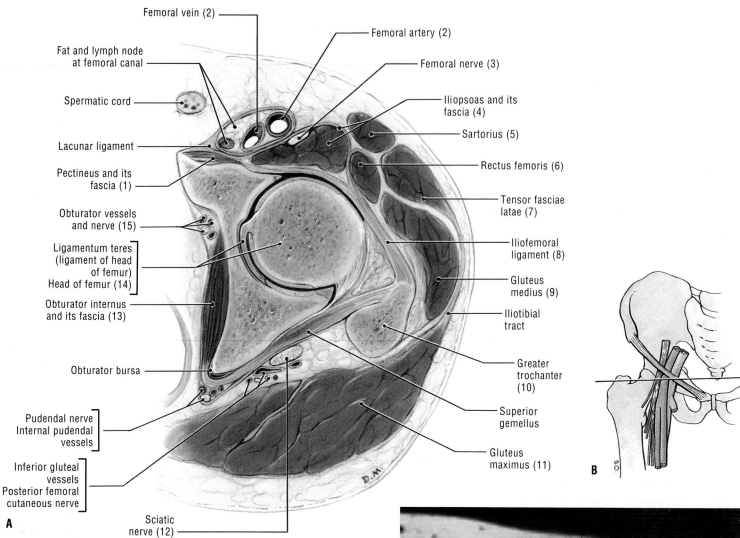

Femoral vein (2)

Femoral artery (2)

Fat and lymph node
at femoral canal

Femoral nerve (3)

Spermatic cord

Iliopsoas and its
fascia (4)

Sartorius (5)

Lacunar ligament

Pectineus and its
fascia (1)

Rectus femoris (6)

Obturator vessels
and nerve (15)

Tensor fasciae
latae (7)

Ligamentum teres
(ligament of head
of femur)
Head of femur (14)

Iliofemoral
ligament (8)

Gluteus
medius (9)

Obturator internus
and its fascia (13)

Iliotibial
tract

Obturator bursa

Greater
trochanter
(10)

Pudendal nerve
Internal pudendal
vessels

Superior
gemellus

Inferior gluteal
vessels
Posterior femoral
cutaneous nerve

Gluteus
maximus (11)

A

B

Sciatic
nerve (12)

D.M

5.51

Transverse section through the thigh at the level of the hip joint

Observe in **A**:

1. The fibrous capsule of the joint is very thick where forming the iliofemoral ligament, and thin posterior to the psoas bursa and tendon;

2. The femoral sheath, which encloses the femoral artery, vein, lymph node, lymph vessels, and fat, is free except posteriorly where, between the psoas and pectineus muscles, it is attached to the capsule of the hip joint;

3. The femoral artery separated from the joint by the tough psoas tendon; the femoral vein at the interval between the psoas and pectineus muscles; the femoral nerve lying between iliacus muscle and fascia.

B. This is an orientation drawing of the level of section shown in **A** and **C**.

C. MRI (magnetic resonance image). Numbers refer to **A**. (Courtesy of Dr. W. Kucharczyk, Clinical Director of Tri-Hospital Magnetic Resonance Centre, Toronto, Ontario, Canada.)

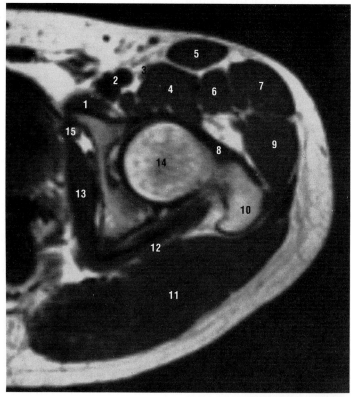

C

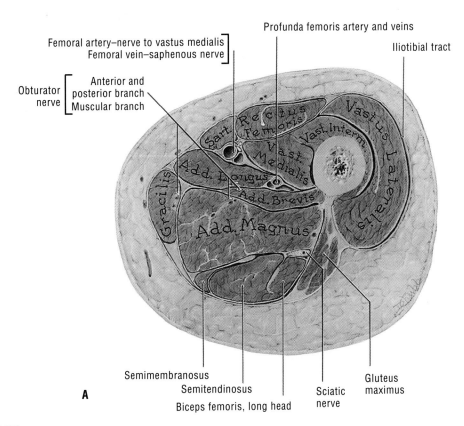

Femoral artery–nerve to vastus medialis
Femoral vein–saphenous nerve

Profunda femoris artery and veins

Iliotibial tract

Obturator nerve
Anterior and posterior branch
Muscular branch

Sart. Rectus Femoris
Vast. Medialis
Vast. Interm.
Vastus Lateralis
Add. Longus
Add. Brevis
Gracilis
Add. Magnus

Semimembranosus
Semitendinosus
Biceps femoris, long head
Sciatic nerve
Gluteus maximus

A

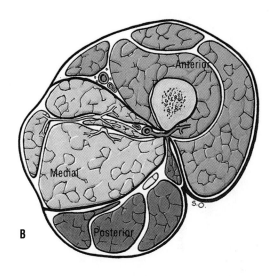

Anterior
Medial
Posterior

B

5.52
Transverse section of the thigh

Observe in **A**:

1. Level of section is just inferior to the apex of the femoral triangle, about 10 to 15 cm down the femur;

2. The gracilis muscle abutting against the free, medial borders of the adductor muscles;

3. The adductor longus muscle intervening between the femoral and the profunda femoris vessels;

4. The adductor brevis muscle intervening between the anterior and the posterior division of the obturator nerve;

5. The aponeurosis of the semimembranosus muscle may be mistaken as the sciatic nerve;

6. The vastus intermedius muscle arising from the anterior and lateral surfaces of the shaft of the femur; the vastus medialis muscle covering the medial surface but not arising from it; that is to say, the vastus intermedius muscle alone arises from the surfaces, the other muscles are relegated to the linea aspera or to its extensions; proximally, the vastus lateralis muscle is large.

B. Diagram. This diagram shows that the muscles of the thigh are in three groups, each with its own nerve supply and primary function:

1. Anterior: femoral nerve – extensors of the knee;

2. Medial: obturator nerve – adductors of the hip;

3. Posterior: sciatic nerve – flexors of the knee.

C. MRI. (Courtesy of Dr. W. Kucharczyk, Clinical Director of Tri-Hospital Magnetic Resonance Centre, Toronto, Ontario, Canada.)

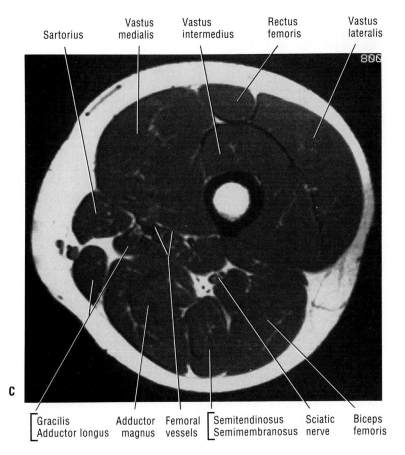

Sartorius
Vastus medialis
Vastus intermedius
Rectus femoris
Vastus lateralis

Gracilis
Adductor longus
Adductor magnus
Femoral vessels
Semitendinosus
Semimembranosus
Sciatic nerve
Biceps femoris

C

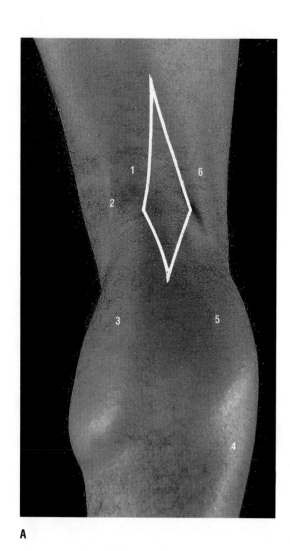

A

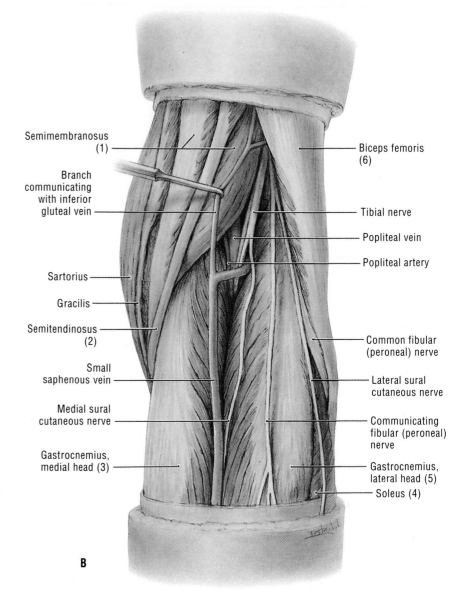

Semimembranosus (1)

Branch communicating with inferior gluteal vein

Sartorius

Gracilis

Semitendinosus (2)

Small saphenous vein

Medial sural cutaneous nerve

Gastrocnemius, medial head (3)

Biceps femoris (6)

Tibial nerve

Popliteal vein

Popliteal artery

Common fibular (peroneal) nerve

Lateral sural cutaneous nerve

Communicating fibular (peroneal) nerve

Gastrocnemius, lateral head (5)

Soleus (4)

B

5.53
Popliteal fossa

A. Surface anatomy. The hamstring muscles, diverge, biceps to the fibula and the two semi-muscles to the tibia; the origins of the medial and lateral heads of gastrocnemius are deep to the hamstrings. The diamond-shaped popliteal fossa is outlined. Numbers refer to structures in **B**. **B**. Superficial dissection.

Observe:

1. The two heads of the gastrocnemius muscle, embraced on the medial side by the semimembranosus muscle, which is overlaid by the semitendinosus muscle, and on the lateral side by the biceps femoris muscle;

2. The small saphenous vein running between the two heads of the gastrocnemius muscle; deep to this vein is the medial sural cutaneous nerve which, followed proximally, leads to the tibial nerve; the tibial nerve is superficial to the popliteal vein, which in turn, is superficial to the popliteal artery;

3. The common fibular (peroneal) nerve following the posterior border of the biceps femoris muscle, and here giving off two cutaneous branches.

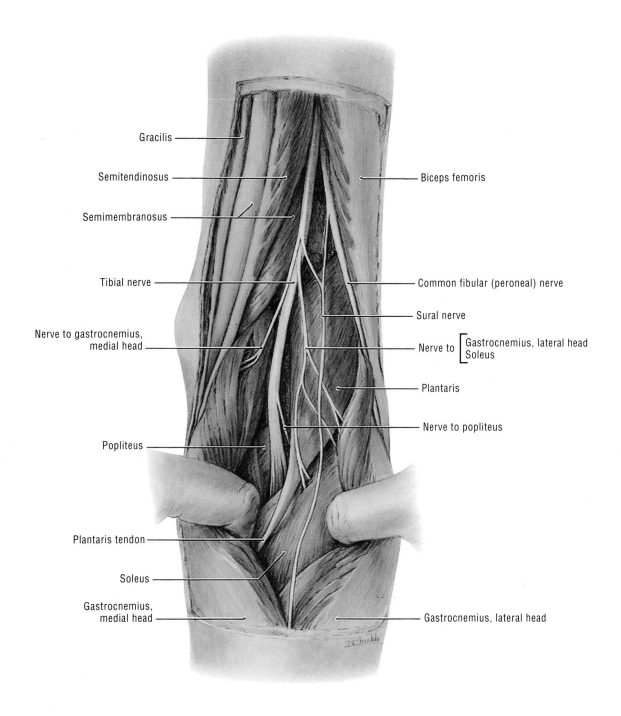

Gracilis

Semitendinosus

Semimembranosus

Tibial nerve

Nerve to gastrocnemius, medial head

Populiteus

Plantaris tendon

Soleus

Gastrocnemius, medial head

Biceps femoris

Common fibular (peroneal) nerve

Sural nerve

Nerve to [Gastrocnemius, lateral head / Soleus]

Plantaris

Nerve to popliteus

Gastrocnemius, lateral head

5.54
Nerves of the popliteal fossa

The two heads of the gastrocnemius muscle are pulled forcibly apart.

Observe:
1. A cutaneous branch of the tibial nerve joining a cutaneous branch of the common fibular (peroneal) nerve to form the sural nerve; here the junction is very high; usually it is 5 to 8 cm proximal to the ankle;

2. All motor branches in this region springing from the tibial nerve, one branch coming from its medial side, the others from its lateral side; hence, it is safer to dissect on the medial side.

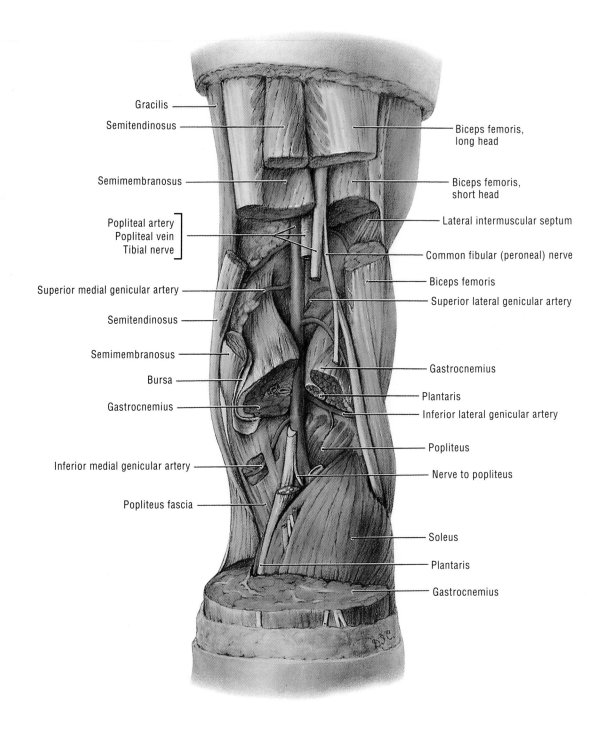

Gracilis

Semitendinosus

Semimembranosus

Popliteal artery
Popliteal vein
Tibial nerve

Superior medial genicular artery

Semitendinosus

Semimembranosus

Bursa

Gastrocnemius

Inferior medial genicular artery

Popliteus fascia

Biceps femoris,
long head

Biceps femoris,
short head

Lateral intermuscular septum

Common fibular (peroneal) nerve

Biceps femoris

Superior lateral genicular artery

Gastrocnemius

Plantaris

Inferior lateral genicular artery

Popliteus

Nerve to popliteus

Soleus

Plantaris

Gastrocnemius

5.55
Step dissection of the popliteal fossa

Observe:

1. The thickness of the various muscles;

2. The popliteal artery lying on the floor of the fossa formed by the femur, the capsule of the knee joint and the popliteus fascia; giving off genicular branches that also lie on the floor, and ending by bifurcating into the anterior and the posterior tibial arteries at the proximal border of the soleus muscle.

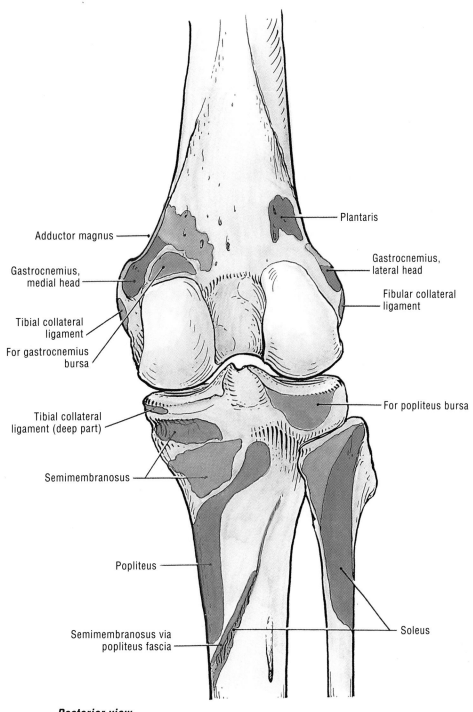

Adductor magnus

Gastrocnemius, medial head

Tibial collateral ligament

For gastrocnemius bursa

Tibial collateral ligament (deep part)

Semimembranosus

Popliteus

Semimembranosus via popliteus fascia

Plantaris

Gastrocnemius, lateral head

Fibular collateral ligament

For popliteus bursa

Soleus

Posterior view

5.56
Bones of the knee joint showing attachments of muscles

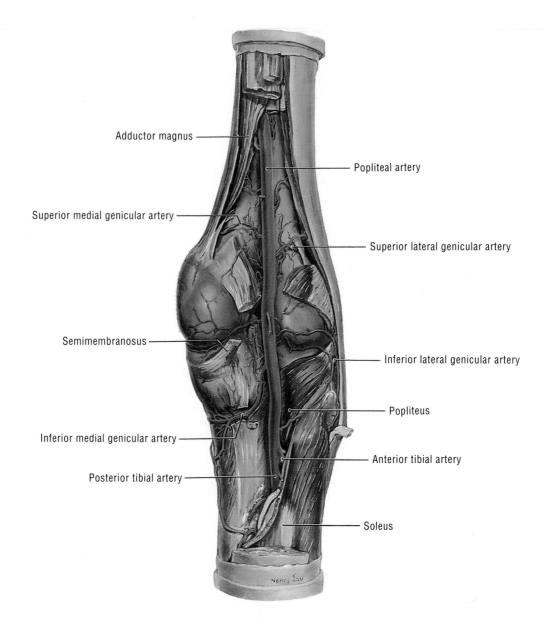

Adductor magnus

Popliteal artery

Superior medial genicular artery

Superior lateral genicular artery

Semimembranosus

Inferior lateral genicular artery

Popliteus

Inferior medial genicular artery

Anterior tibial artery

Posterior tibial artery

Soleus

A, *Posterior view*

5.57
Anastomoses around the knee

Observe in **A**:

1. The popliteal artery (injected with latex) throughout its course, from the hiatus in the adductor magnus muscle proximally to the inferior border of the popliteus muscle distally, where it bifurcates into the anterior and posterior tibial arteries;

2. The three anterior relations of the artery: (a) femur (fat intervening), (b) capsule of the joint, and (c) the popliteus muscle (covered with popliteus fascia);

3. The four named genicular branches that hug the skeletal plane, nothing intervening except the popliteus tendon, which the inferior lateral genicular artery must cross; the median genicular artery is not in view.

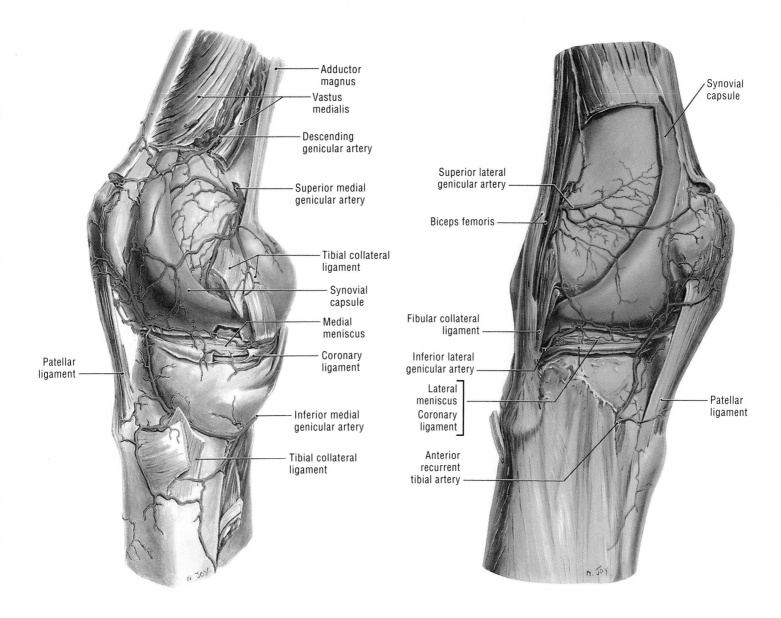

B, *Anteromedial view*

C, *Anterolateral view*

5.57
Anastomoses around the knee *(continued)*

Observe in **B** and **C**:

1. Two named genicular branches of the popliteal artery: on each side, a superior and an inferior;

2. Three supplementary arteries: (a) descending genicular branch of the femoral artery, superomedially; (b) descending branch of lateral femoral circumflex artery, superolaterally; and (c) anterior recurrent branch of anterior tibial artery, inferolaterally;

3. The inferior lateral genicular artery running along the lateral meniscus; an unnamed artery running similarly along the medial meniscus.

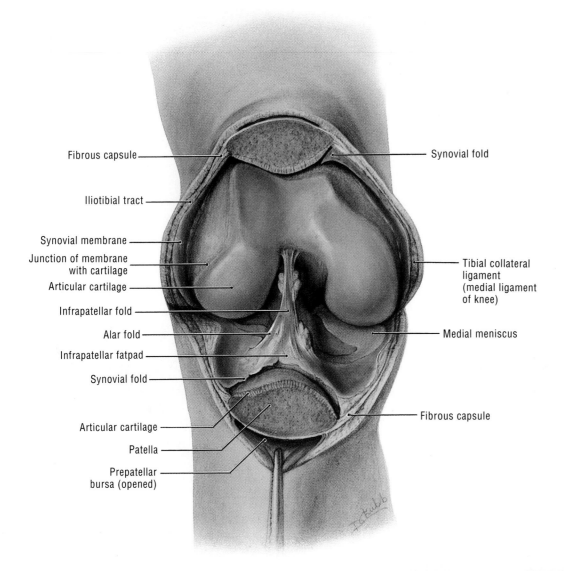

Fibrous capsule

Iliotibial tract

Synovial membrane

Junction of membrane with cartilage

Articular cartilage

Infrapatellar fold

Alar fold

Infrapatellar fatpad

Synovial fold

Articular cartilage

Patella

Prepatellar bursa (opened)

Synovial fold

Tibial collateral ligament (medial ligament of knee)

Medial meniscus

Fibrous capsule

5.58
Knee joint, opened anteriorly

The patella is sawn through; the skin and joint capsule are cut through; and the joint is flexed.

Observe:

1. The articular cartilage of the patella is not of uniform thickness;

2. The infrapatellar synovial fold resembling a partially collapsed bell tent whose apex is attached to the intercondylar notch of the femur and whose base is inferior to the patella;

3. A fracture of the patella would bring the prepatellar bursa into communication with the joint cavity;

4. Articular cartilage and synovial membrane continuous with each other on the lateral aspect of the femoral condyle.

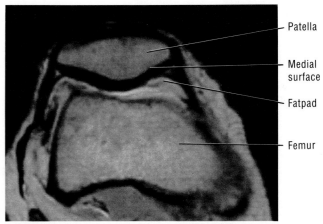

Patella

Medial surface

Fatpad

Femur

5.59
Transverse MRI (magnetic resonance image) of the patellofemoral articulation

(Courtesy of Dr. W. Kucharczyk, Clinical Director of Tri-Hospital Magnetic Resonance Centre, Toronto, Ontario, Canada.)

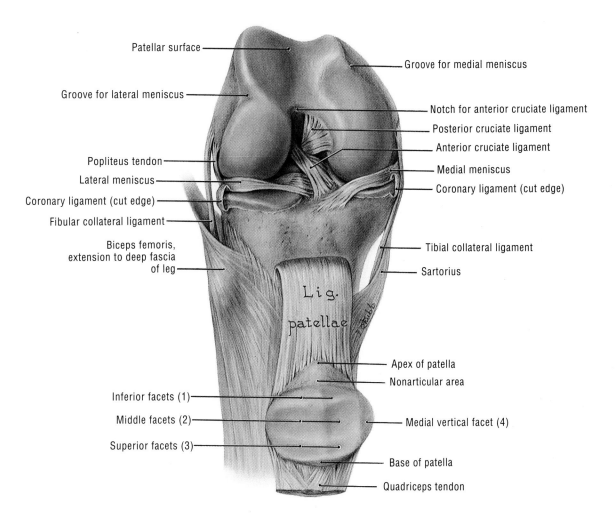

Patellar surface

Groove for medial meniscus

Groove for lateral meniscus

Notch for anterior cruciate ligament

Posterior cruciate ligament

Anterior cruciate ligament

Popliteus tendon

Medial meniscus

Lateral meniscus

Coronary ligament (cut edge)

Coronary ligament (cut edge)

Fibular collateral ligament

Tibial collateral ligament

Biceps femoris, extension to deep fascia of leg

Sartorius

Lig. patellae

Apex of patella

Nonarticular area

Inferior facets (1)

Middle facets (2)

Medial vertical facet (4)

Superior facets (3)

Base of patella

Quadriceps tendon

A, *Anterior view*

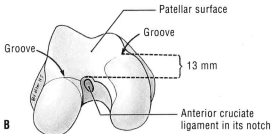

Patellar surface

Groove

Groove

13 mm

B

Anterior cruciate ligament in its notch

5.60
Ligaments of the knee joint

The patella is reflected inferiorly and the joint is fixed.

Observe in **A**, **B**, and **C**:
1. The indentations on the sides of the femoral condyles at the junction of the patellar and tibial articular areas; the lateral tibial articular area, shorter than the medial one;

2. The subsidiary notch, at the anterolateral part of the intercondylar notch, for the reception of the anterior cruciate ligament on full extension.

D. Diagram of the articular surfaces of the patella. The three paired facets on the posterior surface of the patella for articulation with the patellar surface of the femur successively during *(1)* extension, *(2)* slight flexion, *(3)* flexion, and the most medial facet on the patella *(4)* for articulation during full flexion with the crescentic facet that skirts the medial margin of the intercondylar notch of the femur.

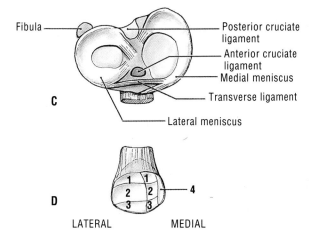

Fibula

Posterior cruciate ligament

Anterior cruciate ligament

Medial meniscus

Transverse ligament

C

Lateral meniscus

D

LATERAL   MEDIAL

5.61
Distended knee joint

Latex was injected into the joint cavity and fixed with acetic acid; the distended synovial capsule was exposed and cleaned; the gastrocnemius muscle is reflected proximally; the biceps femoris muscle and the iliotibial tract are reflected distally; the latex, in this specimen, flowed into the proximal tibiofibular joint cavity.

Observe:

1. The extent of the synovial capsule:
(a) Superiorly, it rises about 2 fingers' breadth superior to the patella and here rests on a layer of fat that allows it to glide freely in movements of the joint; this superior part is called the suprapatellar bursa;
(b) Posteriorly, it rises as high as the origin of the gastrocnemius muscle;
(c) Laterally, it curves inferior to the lateral femoral epicondyle where popliteus tendon and the fibular collateral ligament are attached;
(d) Inferiorly, it bulges inferior to the lateral meniscus, overlapping the tibia; the coronary ligament is removed to show this;

2. The biceps femoris muscle and iliotibial tract protecting the joint laterally;

3. The prepatellar bursa, here more extensive than usual, more than covering the patella.

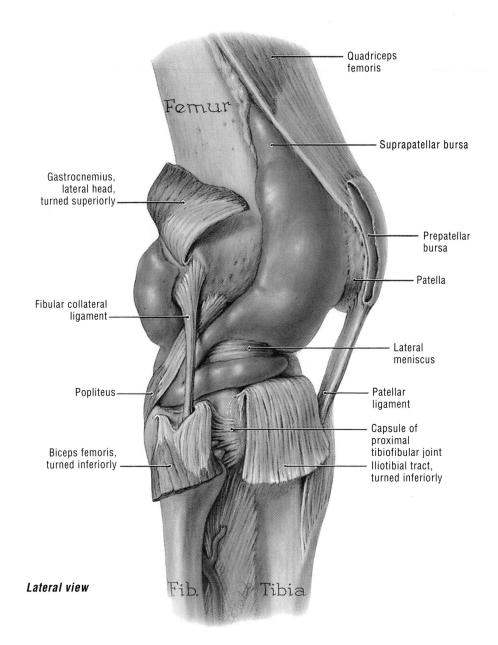

Lateral view

5.62
Proximal tibiofibular joint

The proximal tibiofibular joint has important functions: (a) dissipation of torsional stresses applied at the ankle, (b) dissipation of lateral tibial bending moments, and (c) tensile weight bearing.

The joint exists in two basic forms:
A. Horizontal, with two almost flat surfaces articulating posterior to the lateral edge of the tibia; and

B. Oblique, with joint surfaces inclined at an angle greater than 20 degrees. Generally, the greater the angle, the smaller the surface area of the joint. Rotation at this joint occurs during dorsiflexion of the ankle, especially in horizontal joints. In knee flexion, the fibula moves anteriorly; in extension, posteriorly (see Ogden JA. *The anatomy and function of the proximal tibiofibular joint.* Clin Orthop 1974; 101:186-191).

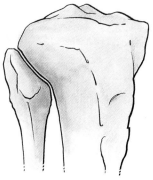

A, *Oblique*

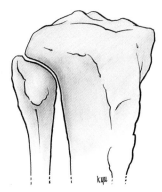

B, *Horizontal*

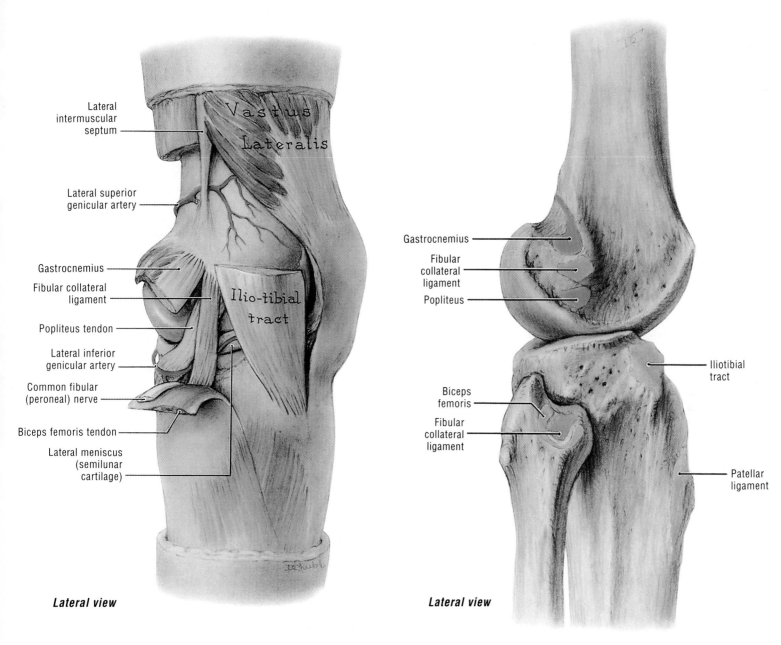

Lateral view

Lateral view

5.63
Dissection of the knee

Observe:

1. The iliotibial tract intervening between the skin and the synovial membrane and which, by virtue of its toughness, protects this exposed aspect of the joint;

2. The three structures that arise from the lateral epicondyle and that are uncovered by reflecting the biceps muscle; of these, the gastrocnemius muscle is posterosuperior; the popliteus muscle is anteroinferior; the fibular collateral ligament is in between, and it crosses superficial to the popliteus muscle;

3. The lateral inferior genicular artery coursing along the lateral meniscus.

5.64
Bones of the knee joint: attachments of muscles and ligaments

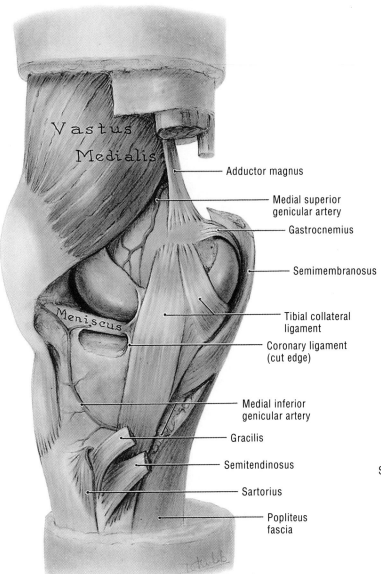

Medial view

5.65
Dissection of the knee

Observe that the band-like part of the tibial collateral ligament attaches to the medial epicondyle of the femur, is almost in line with the tendon of the adductor magnus muscle, bridges superficial to the insertion of the semimembranosus muscle, crosses the medial inferior genicular artery, and is crossed by three tendons (of the sartorius, gracilis, and semitendinosus muscles).

5.67
Articularis genu

The articularis genu muscle, deep to the vastus intermedius muscle, consists of a few fibers arising from the anterior surface of the femur and inserting into the synovial capsule of the knee joint that it retracts during extension.

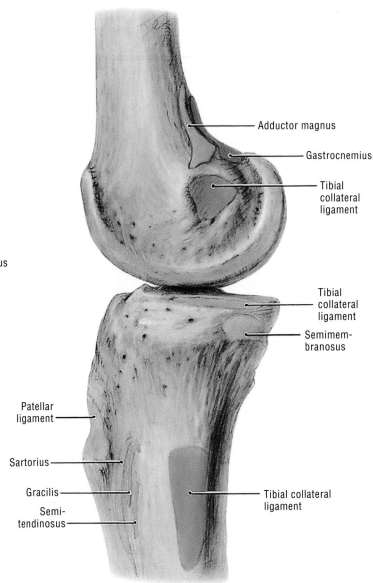

Medial view

5.66
Bones of the knee: muscle and ligament attachments

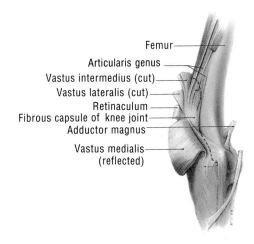

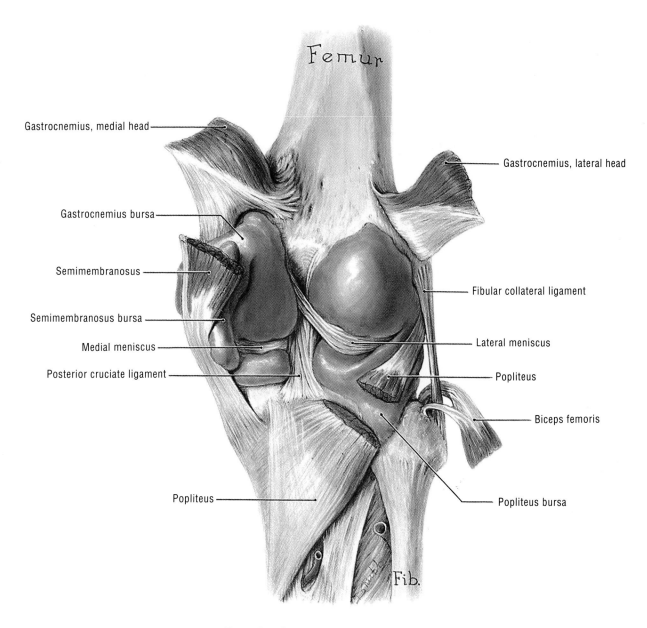

Femur

Gastrocnemius, medial head

Gastrocnemius, lateral head

Gastrocnemius bursa

Semimembranosus

Fibular collateral ligament

Semimembranosus bursa

Medial meniscus

Lateral meniscus

Posterior cruciate ligament

Popliteus

Biceps femoris

Popliteus

Popliteus bursa

Fib.

Posterior view

5.68
Distended knee joint

Both heads of the gastrocnemius muscle are reflected proximally, the biceps muscle is reflected distally, and a section is removed from the popliteus muscle.

Observe:

1. The posterior cruciate ligament exposed posteriorly without opening the synovial capsule (articular cavity);

2. The origins of the gastrocnemius muscle limiting the proximal extent of the synovial capsule;

3. Semimembranosus bursa here communicating with gastrocnemius bursa, which, in turn, communicates with the synovial cavity of the knee joint;

4. The popliteus tendon separated from the lateral meniscus, the proximal end of the tibia, and the proximal tibiofibular joint by an elongated bursa; this popliteus bursa communicates with the synovial cavity of the knee joint both superior and inferior to the meniscus and, in this specimen, it also communicates with the proximal tibiofibular synovial cavity.

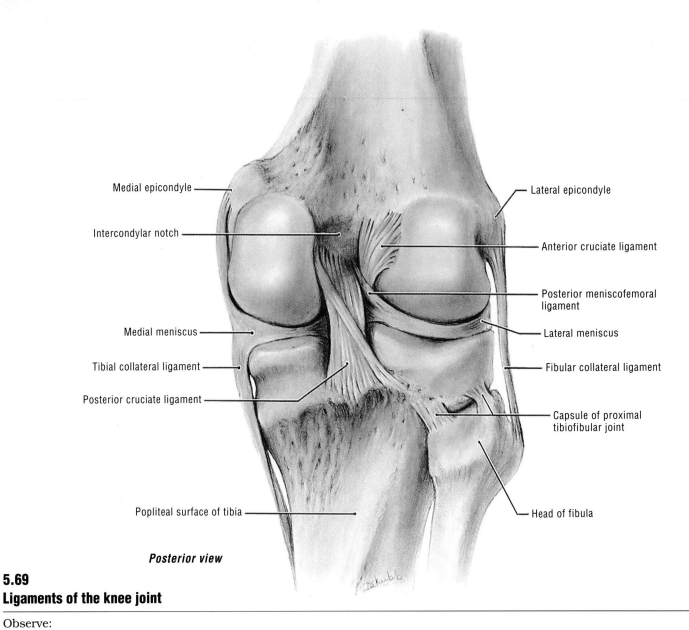

Medial epicondyle

Intercondylar notch

Medial meniscus

Tibial collateral ligament

Posterior cruciate ligament

Popliteal surface of tibia

Lateral epicondyle

Anterior cruciate ligament

Posterior meniscofemoral ligament

Lateral meniscus

Fibular collateral ligament

Capsule of proximal tibiofibular joint

Head of fibula

Posterior view

5.69
Ligaments of the knee joint

Observe:

1. The band-like medial ligament attached to the medial meniscus (semilunar cartilage); the cord-like lateral ligament separated from the lateral meniscus by the width of the popliteus tendon (removed);

2. The posterior cruciate ligament joined by a cord from the lateral meniscus muscle and passing anteriorly to the medial condyle of the femur; the anterior cruciate ligament attached to the lateral condyle posteriorly.

5.70
Cruciate ligaments

In each illustration, one-half of the femur is removed with the proximal part of the corresponding cruciate ligament.

Observe:

A. The posterior cruciate ligament prevents the femur from sliding anteriorly on the tibia, particularly when the knee is flexed;

B. The anterior cruciate ligament prevents the femur from sliding posteriorly on the tibia and hyperextension of the knee and limits medial rotation of the femur when the foot is on the ground, i.e., when the leg is fixed.

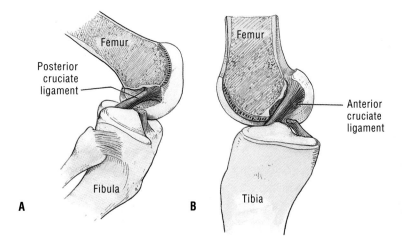

Femur

Posterior cruciate ligament

Fibula

A

Femur

Anterior cruciate ligament

Tibia

B

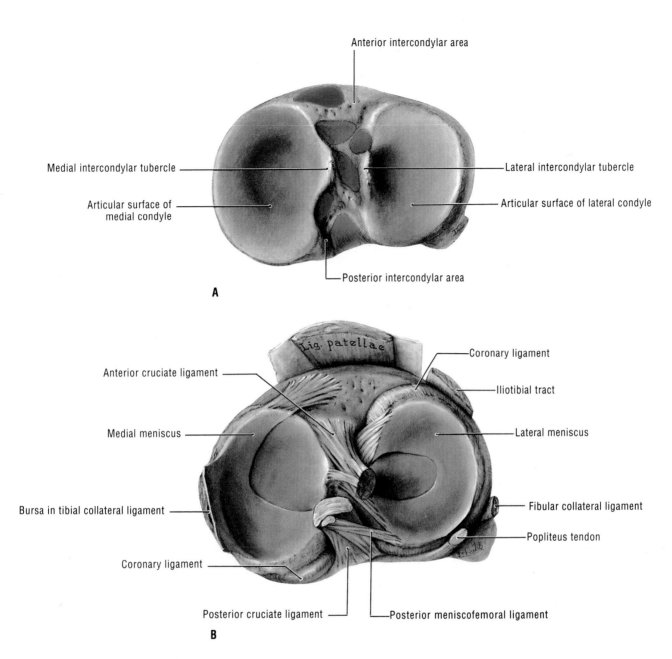

Anterior intercondylar area

Medial intercondylar tubercle

Articular surface of medial condyle

Lateral intercondylar tubercle

Articular surface of lateral condyle

Posterior intercondylar area

A

Lig. patellae

Anterior cruciate ligament

Coronary ligament

Iliotibial tract

Medial meniscus

Lateral meniscus

Bursa in tibial collateral ligament

Fibular collateral ligament

Popliteus tendon

Coronary ligament

Posterior cruciate ligament

Posterior meniscofemoral ligament

B

5.71
Cruciate ligaments and the menisci

Observe in **A** and **B**:

1. The sites of attachment of the cruciate ligaments are colored green; those of the medial meniscus are purple; and those of the lateral meniscus are orange;

2. Of the tibial condyles, the lateral is flatter, shorter from anterior to posterior, and more circular; the medial is concave, longer from anterior to posterior, and more oval;

3. The menisci are cartilaginous and tough where compressed between femur and tibia, but ligamentous and pliable at their attachments, as in the case with other intraarticular fibrocartilages;

4. The menisci conform to the shapes of the surfaces on which they rest; since the horns of the lateral meniscus are attached close together and its coronary ligament is slack, this meniscus can slide anteriorly and posteriorly on the (flat) condyle; since the horns of the medial meniscus are attached far apart, its movements on the (concave) condyle are restricted; the medial meniscus is commonly trapped, injured, and torn;

5. The bursa between the long and short parts of the medial ligament of the knee (see Robichon J, Romero C. *The functional anatomy of the knee joint.* Can J Surg 1968; 11:36; Kennedy JC, Weinberg HW, Wilson AS. *The anatomy and function of the anterior cruciate ligament.* J Bone Joint Surg 1974; 56A:223).

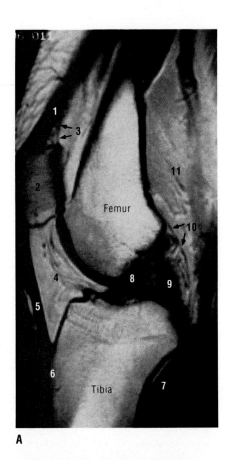

A

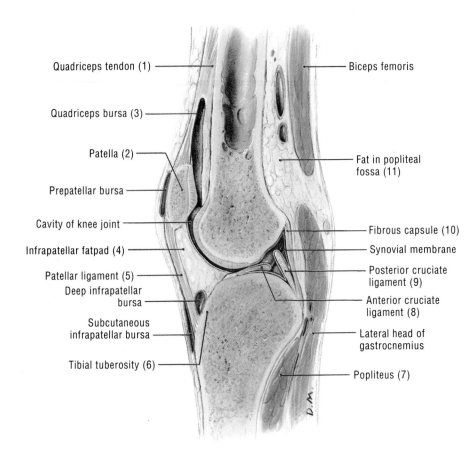

Quadriceps tendon (1) ———————— Biceps femoris

Quadriceps bursa (3) ————————

Patella (2) ———————— ———————— Fat in popliteal fossa (11)

Prepatellar bursa ————————

Cavity of knee joint ———————— ———————— Fibrous capsule (10)

———————— Synovial membrane

Infrapatellar fatpad (4) ———————— ———————— Posterior cruciate ligament (9)

Patellar ligament (5) ————————

Deep infrapatellar bursa ———————— ———————— Anterior cruciate ligament (8)

Subcutaneous infrapatellar bursa ———————— ———————— Lateral head of gastrocnemius

Tibial tuberosity (6) ———————— ———————— Popliteus (7)

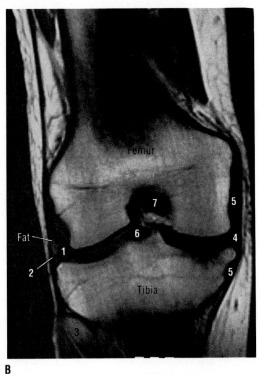

B

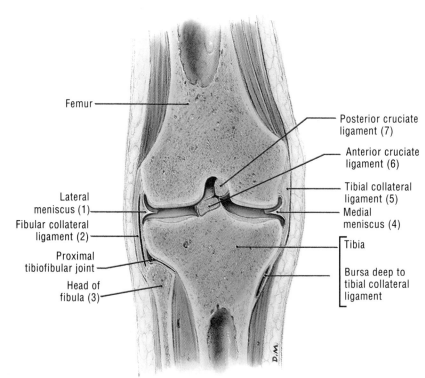

Femur ————————

———————— Posterior cruciate ligament (7)

———————— Anterior cruciate ligament (6)

Lateral meniscus (1) ————————

———————— Tibial collateral ligament (5)

Fibular collateral ligament (2) ————————

———————— Medial meniscus (4)

Proximal tibiofibular joint ———————— ———————— Tibia

Head of fibula (3) ———————— ———————— Bursa deep to tibial collateral ligament

5.72
MRIs (magnetic resonance images) of the knee and orientation drawings

A. Sagittal MRI. **B**. Coronal MRI. Numbers in MRIs refer to structures in the orientation drawings. (Courtesy of Dr. W. Kucharczyk, Clinical Director of Tri-Hospital Magnetic Resonance Centre, Toronto, Ontario, Canada.)

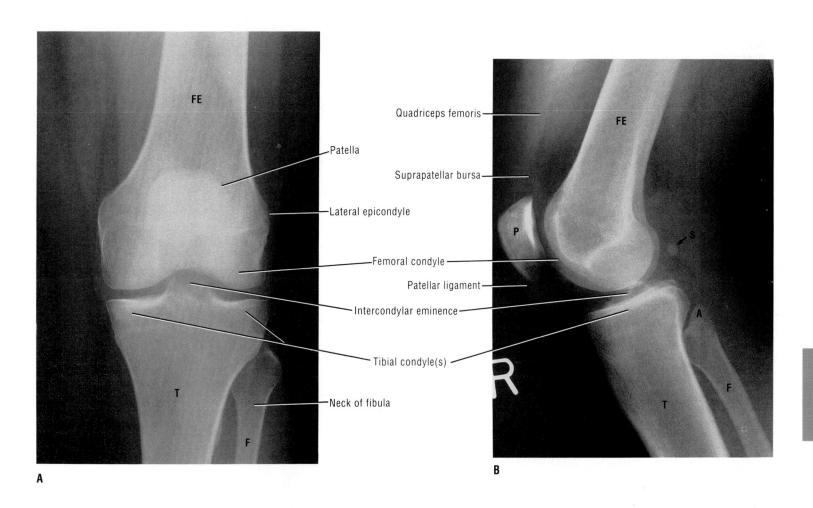

A

B

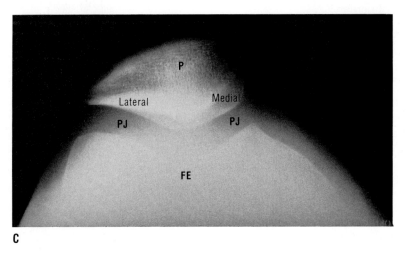

C

5.73
Radiographs of knee

A. Anteroposterior radiograph. **B.** Lateral radiograph of flexed knee. **C.** Skyline view of patella. *FE* - Femur, *T* - Tibia, *F* - Fibula, *A* - Apex of fibula, *S* - Fabella, *P* - Patella, *PJ* - Patellofemoral joint. (Courtesy of Dr. P. Bobechko, Assistant Professor of Radiology, University of Toronto, Toronto, Ontario, Canada.)

5.74

Bones of the leg showing attachments of the muscles in the anterior and lateral compartments

A. Anterior aspect of the tibia and fibula, and dorsum of the foot. **B.** Lateral surface of the fibula. **C.** Tibia and fibula, opposed aspects.

Observe:

1. The lateral (or peroneal) surface of the fibula spiraling slightly so that the proximal end is directed more laterally, the distal end being grooved and facing posteriorly; this allows the lateral malleolus to act as a pulley for the long and short fibularis (peroneal) tendons;

2. The common fibular (peroneal) nerve and its terminal branches having contact with the fibula;

3. On the fibula, two small articular facets for the tibia, one proximally and one distally; inferior to the latter, a large triangular facet for articulation with almost the entire depth of the lateral surface of the body of the talus;

4. The extensor surface of the fibula narrow distally and almost linear proximally;

5. Interosseous borders of the tibia and fibula, for the attachment of the interosseous membrane, separating the anterior or extensor surface from the posterior or flexor surface; each of these borders widening distally into a triangular area for the interosseous ligament; during walking, the fibula moves inferiorly and laterally, stretching the interosseous membrane (see Weinert CR Jr, McMaster JH, Ferguson RJ. *Dynamic function of the human fibula.* Am J Anat 1973; 138:145).

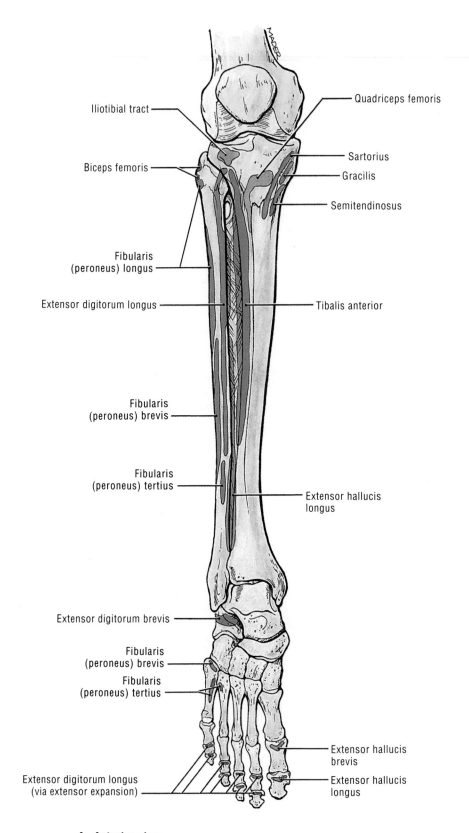

A, *Anterior view*

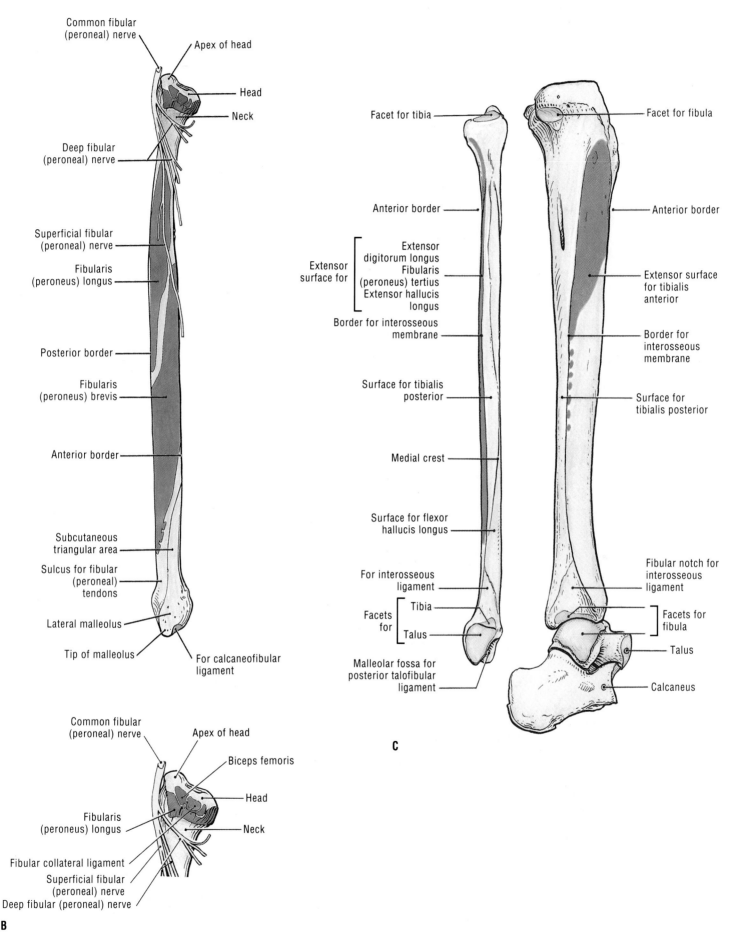

Common fibular (peroneal) nerve

Apex of head

Head

Neck

Deep fibular (peroneal) nerve

Superficial fibular (peroneal) nerve

Fibularis (peroneus) longus

Posterior border

Fibularis (peroneus) brevis

Anterior border

Subcutaneous triangular area

Sulcus for fibular (peroneal) tendons

Lateral malleolus

Tip of malleolus

For calcaneofibular ligament

Common fibular (peroneal) nerve

Apex of head

Biceps femoris

Head

Fibularis (peroneus) longus

Neck

Fibular collateral ligament

Superficial fibular (peroneal) nerve

Deep fibular (peroneal) nerve

B

Facet for tibia

Facet for fibula

Anterior border

Anterior border

Extensor surface for

Extensor digitorum longus
Fibularis (peroneus) tertius
Extensor hallucis longus

Extensor surface for tibialis anterior

Border for interosseous membrane

Border for interosseous membrane

Surface for tibialis posterior

Surface for tibialis posterior

Medial crest

Surface for flexor hallucis longus

Fibular notch for interosseous ligament

For interosseous ligament

Facets for

Tibia

Talus

Facets for fibula

Talus

Malleolar fossa for posterior talofibular ligament

Calcaneus

C

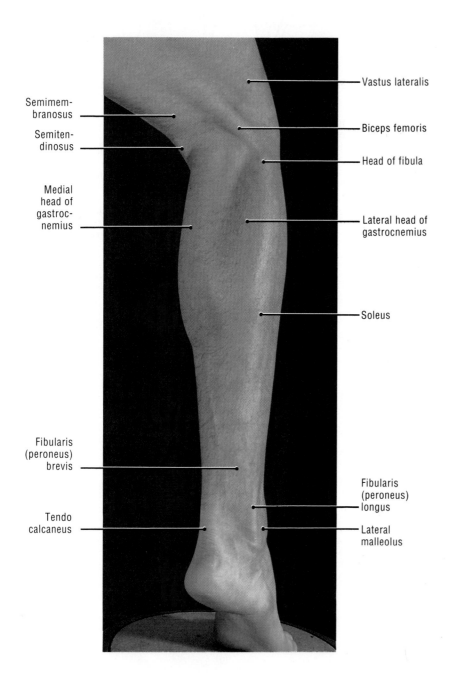

Semimem-
branosus

Semiten-
dinosus

Medial
head of
gastroc-
nemius

Fibularis
(peroneus)
brevis

Tendo
calcaneus

Vastus lateralis

Biceps femoris

Head of fibula

Lateral head of
gastrocnemius

Soleus

Fibularis
(peroneus)
longus

Lateral
malleolus

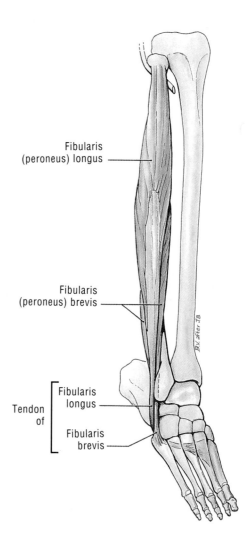

Fibularis
(peroneus) longus

Fibularis
(peroneus) brevis

Tendon
of

Fibularis
longus

Fibularis
brevis

5.75
Surface anatomy of the lateral aspect of the leg and foot

5.76
Diagram of the fibular (peroneal) muscles

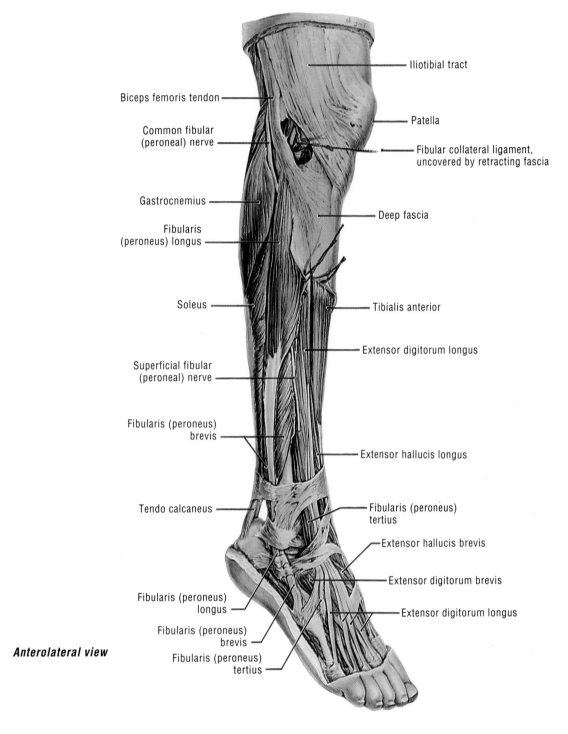

Biceps femoris tendon

Common fibular
(peroneal) nerve

Gastrocnemius

Fibularis
(peroneus) longus

Soleus

Superficial fibular
(peroneal) nerve

Fibularis (peroneus)
brevis

Tendo calcaneus

Fibularis (peroneus)
longus

Fibularis (peroneus)
brevis

Fibularis (peroneus)
tertius

Anterolateral view

Iliotibial tract

Patella

Fibular collateral ligament,
uncovered by retracting fascia

Deep fascia

Tibialis anterior

Extensor digitorum longus

Extensor hallucis longus

Fibularis (peroneus)
tertius

Extensor hallucis brevis

Extensor digitorum brevis

Extensor digitorum longus

5.77
Muscles of the leg and foot

This oblique lateral view of the leg shows the attachment of the two fibular (peroneal) muscles; both attach to two-thirds of the fibula: the fibularis (peroneus) longus muscle to the proximal two-thirds, the fibularis (peroneus) brevis muscle to the distal two-thirds; where they overlap, the fibularis brevis muscle lies anteriorly; the fibularis brevis muscle inserts on the proximal end of the 5th metatarsal; the fibularis (peroneus) longus muscle enters the foot by hooking around the cuboid and traveling medially to the lateral side of the base of the 1st metatarsal and medial cuneiform; note the common fibular (peroneal) nerve in contact with the neck of the fibula deep to the fibularis longus muscle; here it is vulnerable to injury with serious implications as it supplies the extensor group of muscles whose loss results in foot drop.

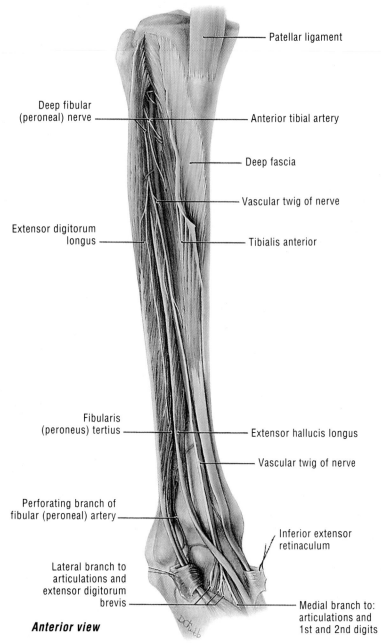

Patellar ligament

Deep fibular
(peroneal) nerve

Anterior tibial artery

Deep fascia

Vascular twig of nerve

Extensor digitorum
longus

Tibialis anterior

Fibularis
(peroneus) tertius

Extensor hallucis longus

Vascular twig of nerve

Perforating branch of
fibular (peroneal) artery

Inferior extensor
retinaculum

Lateral branch to
articulations and
extensor digitorum
brevis

Medial branch to:
articulations and
1st and 2nd digits

Anterior view

5.78
Leg

The muscles are separated in order to display the artery and nerve.

Observe:

1. Tibialis anterior, arising, in part, from the deep fascia, which is strong, has longitudinal fibers, and makes sharp the proximal part of the anterior border of the tibia;

2. The fibularis (peroneus) tertius muscle is merely the inferior part of the extensor digitorum longus muscle; the extensor hallucis longus muscle extends farther proximally than usual; these three muscles are unipennate and arise from the fibula;

3. The vascular and articular branches of the deep fibular (peroneal) nerve.

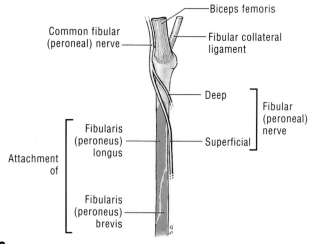

Biceps femoris

Common fibular
(peroneal) nerve

Fibular collateral
ligament

Deep

Fibular
(peroneal)
nerve

Attachment
of

Fibularis
(peroneus)
longus

Superficial

Fibularis
(peroneus)
brevis

5.79
Common fibular (peroneal) nerve

Note the exposed position of the common fibular (peroneal) nerve; it is applied to the posterior aspect of the head of the fibula; its branches are applied directly to the neck and body of the fibula deep to the fibularis (peroneus) longus muscle.

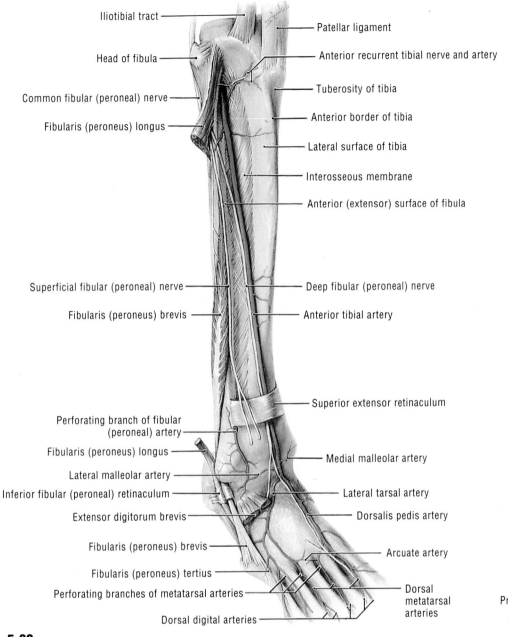

Iliotibial tract

Head of fibula

Common fibular (peroneal) nerve

Fibularis (peroneus) longus

Superficial fibular (peroneal) nerve

Fibularis (peroneus) brevis

Perforating branch of fibular (peroneal) artery

Fibularis (peroneus) longus

Lateral malleolar artery

Inferior fibular (peroneal) retinaculum

Extensor digitorum brevis

Fibularis (peroneus) brevis

Fibularis (peroneus) tertius

Perforating branches of metatarsal arteries

Dorsal digital arteries

Patellar ligament

Anterior recurrent tibial nerve and artery

Tuberosity of tibia

Anterior border of tibia

Lateral surface of tibia

Interosseous membrane

Anterior (extensor) surface of fibula

Deep fibular (peroneal) nerve

Anterior tibial artery

Superior extensor retinaculum

Medial malleolar artery

Lateral tarsal artery

Dorsalis pedis artery

Arcuate artery

Dorsal metatarsal arteries

5.80
Arteries and nerves of the anterior aspect of the leg and dorsum of the foot

The anterior crural muscles (muscles of the anterior compartment) are removed and the fibularis (peroneus) longus muscle is excised.

Observe:

1. The anterior tibial artery entering the region in contact with the medial side of the neck of the fibula; the deep peroneal nerve in contact with the lateral side;

2. The artery and nerve and their named branches lying strictly on the skeletal plane, undisturbed by the removal of the muscles;

3. The superficial fibular (peroneal) nerve following the anterior border of the peroneus brevis muscle, which guides it to the surface to become cutaneous.

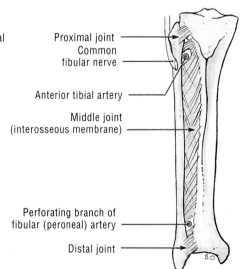

Proximal joint

Common fibular nerve

Anterior tibial artery

Middle joint (interosseous membrane)

Perforating branch of fibular (peroneal) artery

Distal joint

5.81
Diagram of the tibiofibular articulations and their relationship to the arteries of the leg

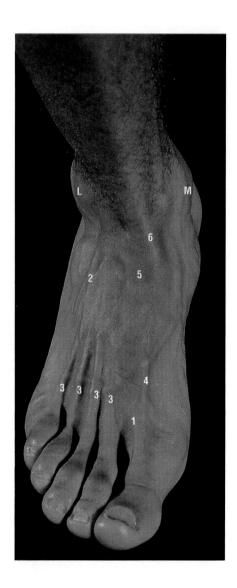

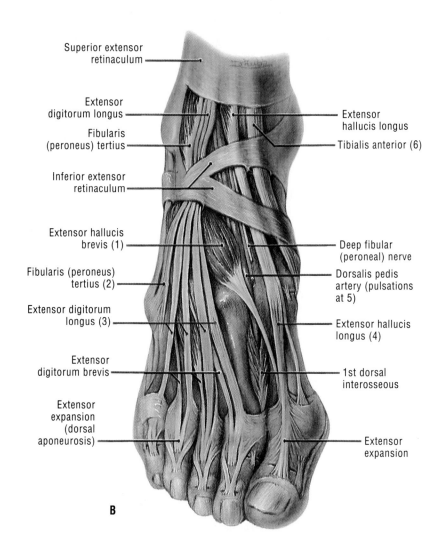

A

B

5.82
Dorsum of the foot

A. Surface anatomy. Follow the tendon of the extensor hallucis longus *(4)* to its insertion into the base of the distal phalanx of the great toe; the tendon of tibialis anterior *(6)* disappears as it moves to its insertion on the medial cuneiform and base of the 1st metatarsal. The pulsations of dorsalis pedis artery *(5)* are palpated on the dorsum of the foot midway between the two malleoli (medial *(M)* and lateral *(L)*), just lateral to the tendon of extensor hallucis longus over the navicular bone.

B. The vessels and nerves are cut short. Observe:
1. At the ankle, the vessels and nerve lying midway between the malleoli and having two tendons on each side;

2. On the dorsum of the foot, the dorsalis pedis artery is crossed by the extensor hallucis brevis muscle and disappears between the two heads of the 1st dorsal interosseous muscle (like the radial artery on the dorsum of the hand);

3. The inferior extensor retinaculum crossing the tendons of the anterior compartment anteromedially.

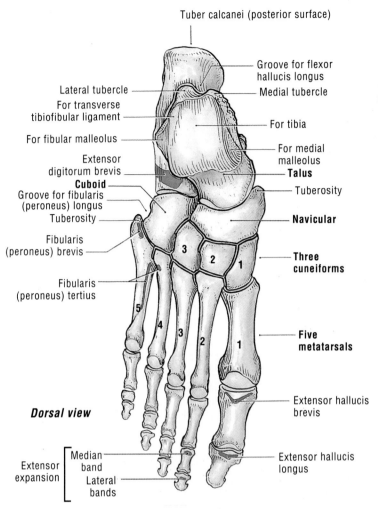

Tuber calcanei (posterior surface)

Lateral tubercle
For transverse tibiofibular ligament
For fibular malleolus
Extensor digitorum brevis
Cuboid
Groove for fibularis (peroneus) longus
Tuberosity
Fibularis (peroneus) brevis
Fibularis (peroneus) tertius

Groove for flexor hallucis longus
Medial tubercle
For tibia
For medial malleolus
Talus
Tuberosity
Navicular
Three cuneiforms
Five metatarsals
Extensor hallucis brevis
Extensor hallucis longus

Dorsal view

Extensor expansion
Median band
Lateral bands

5.83
Bones of the foot

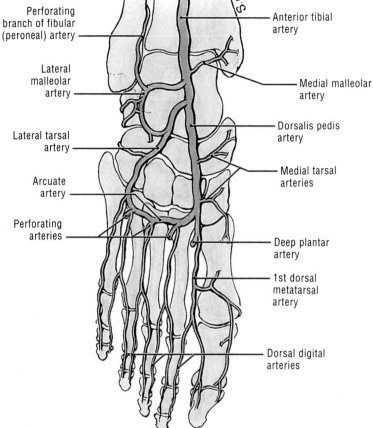

Perforating branch of fibular (peroneal) artery
Lateral malleolar artery
Lateral tarsal artery
Arcuate artery
Perforating arteries

Anterior tibial artery
Medial malleolar artery
Dorsalis pedis artery
Medial tarsal arteries
Deep plantar artery
1st dorsal metatarsal artery
Dorsal digital arteries

5.84
Arterial supply of the dorsum of the foot

Observe the dorsal arterial arch formed by the dorsalis pedis artery that also contributes to the plantar arch formed by the medial and lateral plantar arteries.

5.85
Anomalous dorsalis pedis artery

The dorsalis pedis artery is a continuation of the perforating branch of the fibular (peroneal) artery; when this occurs (3.7% of 592 limbs), the anterior tibial artery either fails to reach the ankle or is a very slender vessel.

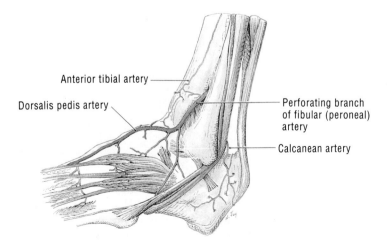

Anterior tibial artery
Dorsalis pedis artery

Perforating branch of fibular (peroneal) artery
Calcanean artery

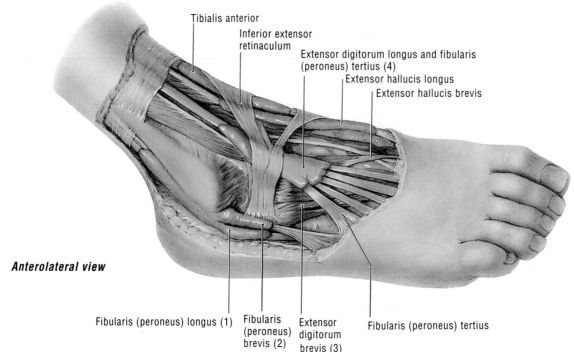

Tibialis anterior

Inferior extensor retinaculum

Extensor digitorum longus and fibularis (peroneus) tertius (4)

Extensor hallucis longus

Extensor hallucis brevis

Anterolateral view

Fibularis (peroneus) longus (1)

Fibularis (peroneus) brevis (2)

Extensor digitorum brevis (3)

Fibularis (peroneus) tertius

5.86
Synovial sheaths of the tendons at the ankle

The tendons of the fibularis (peroneus) longus and fibularis (peroneus) brevis muscle are enclosed in a common synovial sheath posterior to the lateral malleolus; this sheath splits into two, one for each tendon, posterior to the fibular (peroneal) trochlea; the tendon of the fibularis (peroneus) longus has a second sheath (not in view) that accompanies it across the sole of the foot; in almost half of 131 feet studied, the two sheaths of the longus were demonstrated by injection to be in continuity on their deep, or frictional, surface, although not on their superficial surface. Numbers in parentheses refer to Figure 5.87.

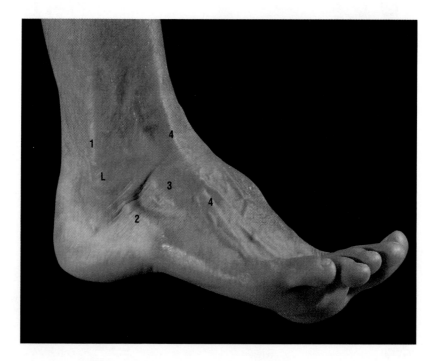

Lateral view

5.87
Surface anatomy of the foot

Observe the soft swelling of the fleshy belly of the extensor digitorum brevis muscle *(3)*; the location of the synovial sheath distal to which the tendons of the extensor digitorum longus muscle *(4)* fan out to reach the digits; the tendons of fibularis (peroneus) longus *(1)* and brevis *(2)* hooking around the lateral malleolus *(L)*.

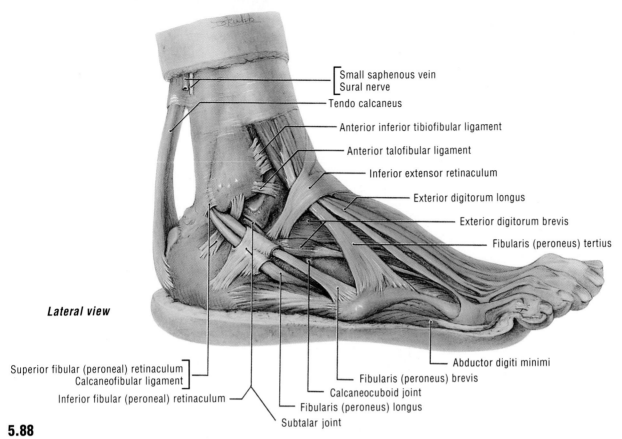

Lateral view

Small saphenous vein
Sural nerve
Tendo calcaneus
Anterior inferior tibiofibular ligament
Anterior talofibular ligament
Inferior extensor retinaculum
Exterior digitorum longus
Exterior digitorum brevis
Fibularis (peroneus) tertius

Abductor digiti minimi
Fibularis (peroneus) brevis
Calcaneocuboid joint
Fibularis (peroneus) longus
Subtalar joint

Superior fibular (peroneal) retinaculum
Calcaneofibular ligament
Inferior fibular (peroneal) retinaculum

5.88
Tendons at the ankle

The ankle, subtalar, and calcaneocuboid joints are exposed in order to reveal their positions.

Observe:

1. The calcaneofibular ligament attached anterior to the tip of the lateral malleolus, thereby allowing the tip of the lateral malleolus to overlap the fibularis (peronei) tendons and so prevent them from slipping anteriorly;

2. The inferior fibular (peroneal) retinaculum, attached to the lateral surface of the calcaneus, is in line with the inferior extensor retinaculum, which is attached to the superior surface of the calcaneus.

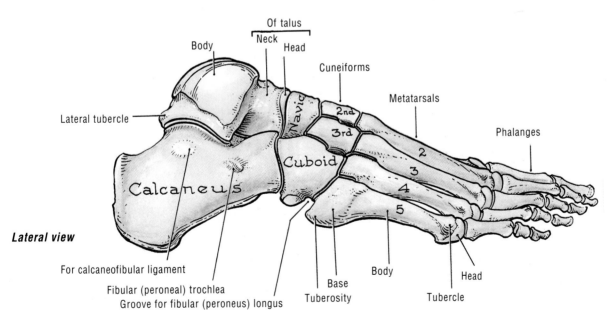

Of talus
Neck
Body
Head
Cuneiforms
Metatarsals
Phalanges

Lateral tubercle
2nd
3rd
Navicular
Cuboid
Calcaneus
2
3
4
5

Lateral view

For calcaneofibular ligament
Fibular (peroneal) trochlea
Groove for fibular (peroneus) longus
Base
Tuberosity
Body
Head
Tubercle

5.89
Bones of the foot

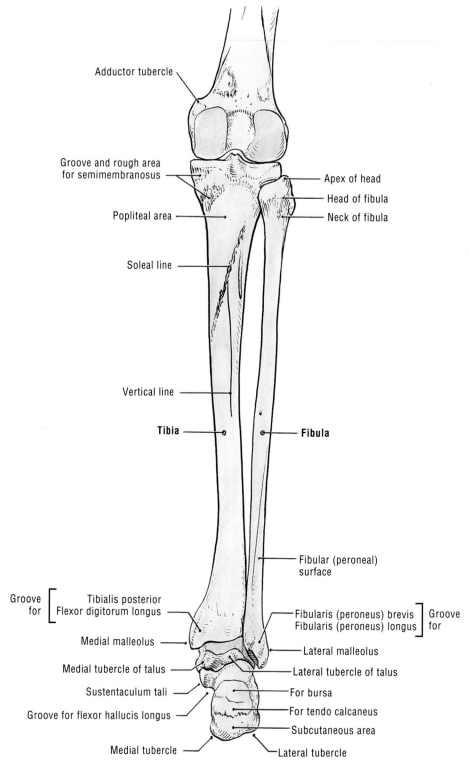

Adductor tubercle

Groove and rough area
for semimembranosus

Popliteal area

Soleal line

Vertical line

Tibia

Apex of head

Head of fibula

Neck of fibula

Fibula

Fibular (peroneal)
surface

Groove
for

Tibialis posterior
Flexor digitorum longus

Medial malleolus

Medial tubercle of talus

Sustentaculum tali

Groove for flexor hallucis longus

Medial tubercle

Fibularis (peroneus) brevis
Fibularis (peroneus) longus

Lateral malleolus

Lateral tubercle of talus

For bursa

For tendo calcaneus

Subcutaneous area

Lateral tubercle

Groove
for

Posterior view

5.90
Bones of the leg

For anterior view, see Figure 5.74**A**.

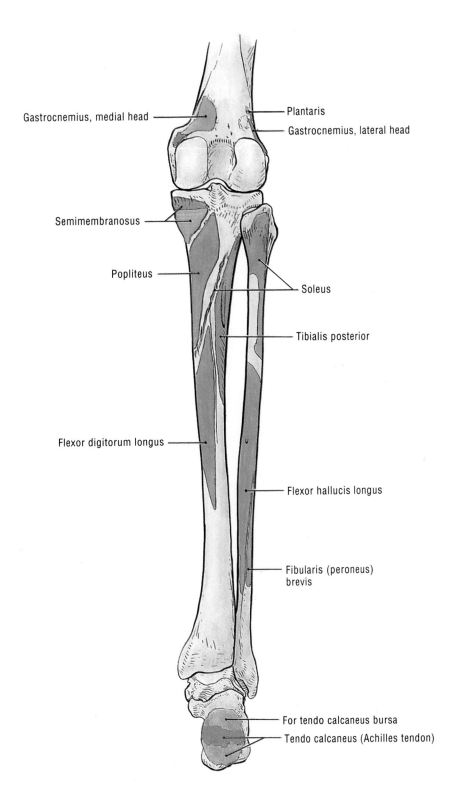

Gastrocnemius, medial head

Plantaris

Gastrocnemius, lateral head

Semimembranosus

Popliteus

Soleus

Tibialis posterior

Flexor digitorum longus

Flexor hallucis longus

Fibularis (peroneus) brevis

For tendo calcaneus bursa

Tendo calcaneus (Achilles tendon)

Posterior view

5.91
Bones of the leg showing attachments of the muscles

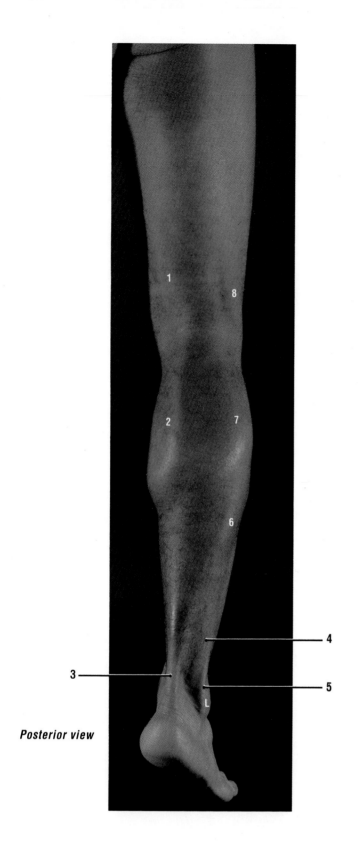

Posterior view

5.92

Surface anatomy of the lower limb

L - Lateral malleolus.

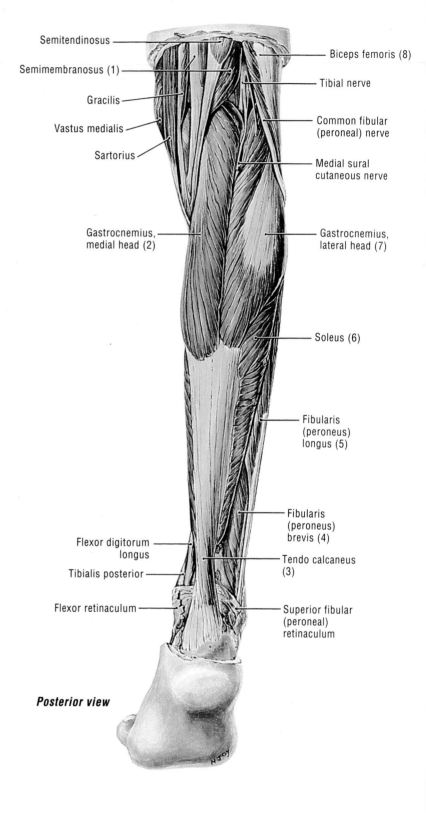

Semitendinosus

Semimembranosus (1)

Gracilis

Vastus medialis

Sartorius

Gastrocnemius, medial head (2)

Flexor digitorum longus

Tibialis posterior

Flexor retinaculum

Biceps femoris (8)

Tibial nerve

Common fibular (peroneal) nerve

Medial sural cutaneous nerve

Gastrocnemius, lateral head (7)

Soleus (6)

Fibularis (peroneus) longus (5)

Fibularis (peroneus) brevis (4)

Tendo calcaneus (3)

Superior fibular (peroneal) retinaculum

Posterior view

5.93

Superficial dissection of the muscles of the leg

Numbers in parentheses refer to Figure 5.92.

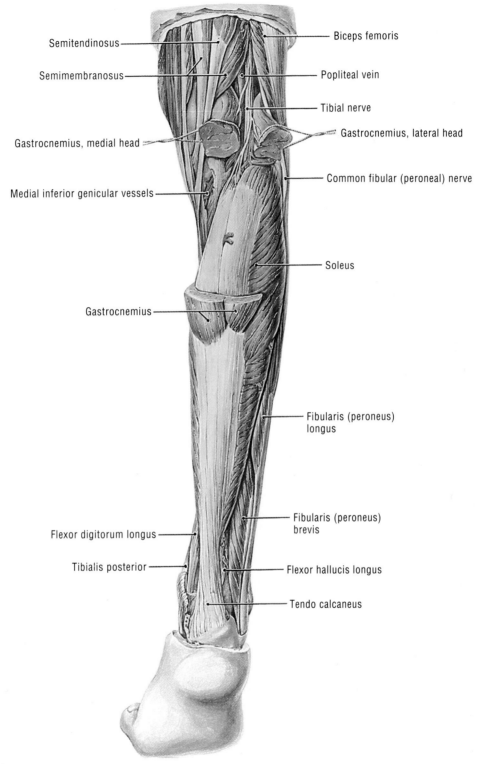

Semitendinosus

Semimembranosus

Gastrocnemius, medial head

Medial inferior genicular vessels

Gastrocnemius

Flexor digitorum longus

Tibialis posterior

Biceps femoris

Popliteal vein

Tibial nerve

Gastrocnemius, lateral head

Common fibular (peroneal) nerve

Soleus

Fibularis (peroneus) longus

Fibularis (peroneus) brevis

Flexor hallucis longus

Tendo calcaneus

5.94
Dissection of the muscles of the superficial posterior crural compartment of the leg

The fleshy bellies of the gastrocnemius muscle are largely excised, and the proximal attachment of the soleus muscle is thereby exposed; the plantaris muscle is absent from this specimen.

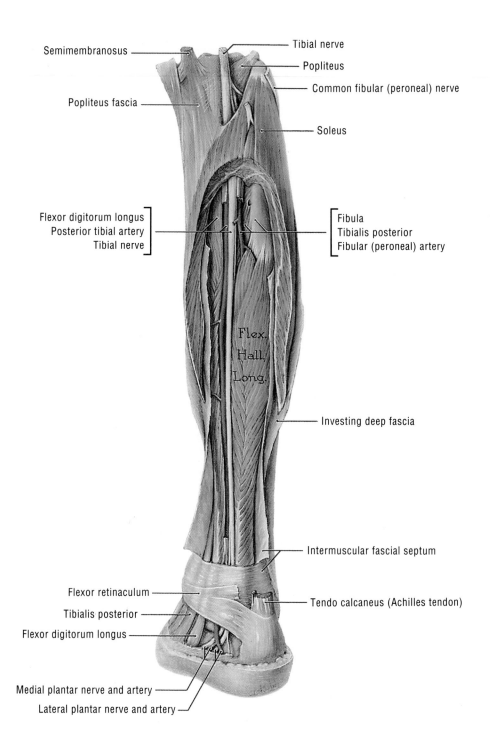

Semimembranosus

Popliteus fascia

Flexor digitorum longus
Posterior tibial artery
Tibial nerve

Flex.
Hall.
Long.

Flexor retinaculum

Tibialis posterior

Flexor digitorum longus

Medial plantar nerve and artery

Lateral plantar nerve and artery

Tibial nerve

Popliteus

Common fibular (peroneal) nerve

Soleus

Fibula
Tibialis posterior
Fibular (peroneal) artery

Investing deep fascia

Intermuscular fascial septum

Tendo calcaneus (Achilles tendon)

5.95

Dissection of the posterior aspect of the leg, deep structures–I

Tendo calcaneus is divided; the gastrocnemius muscle and a horseshoe-shaped section of the soleus muscle are removed.

Observe:
1. The bipennate structure of the large flexor hallucis longus and of the smaller flexor digitorum longus muscles;

2. The posterior tibial artery and the tibial nerve descending

between these two muscles, on a layer of fascia that covers tibialis posterior;

3. The tough, intermuscular fascial septum deep to soleus and tendo calcaneus that acts as a restraining anklet at the ankle and there blends medially with the weaker investing deep fascia to form the flexor retinaculum.

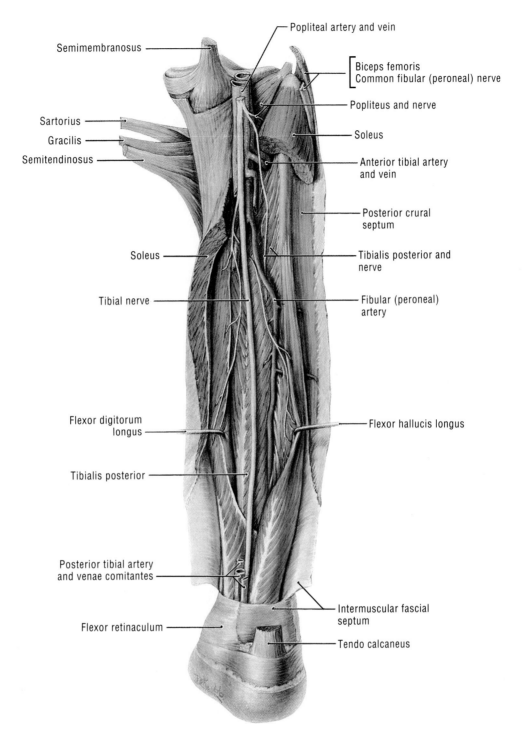

Semimembranosus

Popliteal artery and vein

Biceps femoris
Common fibular (peroneal) nerve

Popliteus and nerve

Sartorius

Gracilis

Semitendinosus

Soleus

Anterior tibial artery
and vein

Posterior crural
septum

Soleus

Tibialis posterior and
nerve

Tibial nerve

Fibular (peroneal)
artery

Flexor digitorum
longus

Flexor hallucis longus

Tibialis posterior

Posterior tibial artery
and venae comitantes

Intermuscular fascial
septum

Flexor retinaculum

Tendo calcaneus

5.96
Dissection of the posterior aspect of the leg, deep structures–II

The soleus muscle is largely cut away; the two long digital flexors are pulled apart; the posterior tibial artery is partly excised.

Observe:

1. Tibialis posterior, bipennate and powerful, lying deep to the two long digital flexors;

2. The fibular (peroneal) artery overlapped by the flexor hallucis longus muscle;

3. The nerve to tibialis posterior arising in conjunction with the nerve to the popliteus muscle, and the nerve to the flexor digitorum longus muscle arising in conjunction with the nerve to the flexor hallucis longus muscle;

4. In the popliteal fossa, the nerve is superficial to the artery; at the ankle, the artery is superficial to the nerve.

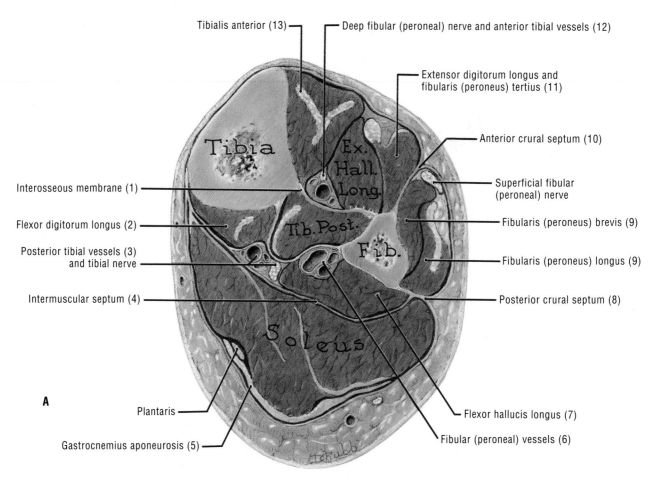

Tibialis anterior (13)

Deep fibular (peroneal) nerve and anterior tibial vessels (12)

Extensor digitorum longus and fibularis (peroneus) tertius (11)

Anterior crural septum (10)

Superficial fibular (peroneal) nerve

Interosseous membrane (1)

Fibularis (peroneus) brevis (9)

Flexor digitorum longus (2)

Fibularis (peroneus) longus (9)

Posterior tibial vessels (3) and tibial nerve

Intermuscular septum (4)

Posterior crural septum (8)

Plantaris

Flexor hallucis longus (7)

Gastrocnemius aponeurosis (5)

Fibular (peroneal) vessels (6)

A

5.97
Transverse section through the leg

Observe in **A**:

1. The gastrocnemius muscle is aponeurotic and the peroneus longus and brevis muscles are both attaching to the fibula;

2. The anterior tibiofibular compartment, bounded by tibia, interosseous membrane, fibula, anterior intermuscular crural septum, and deep fascia, and containing the anterior tibial vessels and deep peroneal nerve; the unyielding walls of this compartment may lead to necrosis of the muscles if pressure increases in the compartment following injury or ischemia (see Waddell JP. *Anterior tibial compartment syndrome.* CMA J 1977; 116:653);

3. The lateral (fibular, peroneal) compartment, bounded by fibula, anterior and posterior intermuscular crural septa, and the deep fascia, and containing the superficial fibular (peroneal) nerve;

4. The posterior tibiofibular compartment, bounded by tibia, interosseous membrane, fibula, posterior intermuscular crural septum, and deep fascia; this compartment is subdivided by two coronal septa into three subcompartments: the deepest contains tibialis posterior; the intermediate contains flexor hallucis longus, flexor digitorum longus, and posterior tibial vessels and tibial nerve; and the most superficial contains the soleus, gastrocnemius, and plantaris muscles.

B. MRI (magnetic resonance image). Numbers refer to structures in **A**. (Courtesy of Dr. W. Kucharczyk, Clinical Director of Tri-Hospital Magnetic Resonance Centre, Toronto, Ontario, Canada.)

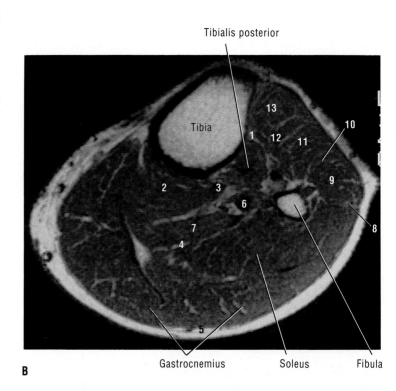

Tibialis posterior

Tibia

Gastrocnemius   Soleus   Fibula

B

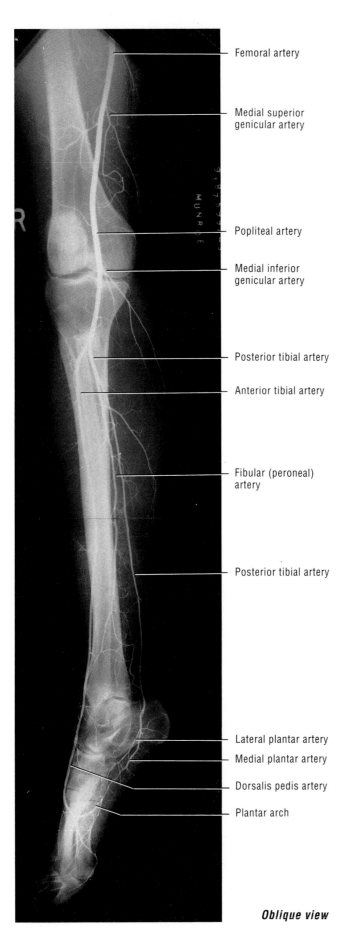

— Femoral artery

— Medial superior
genicular artery

— Popliteal artery

— Medial inferior
genicular artery

— Posterior tibial artery

— Anterior tibial artery

— Fibular (peroneal)
artery

— Posterior tibial artery

— Lateral plantar artery

— Medial plantar artery

— Dorsalis pedis artery

— Plantar arch

Oblique view

5.98
Popliteal arteriogram

Observe:

1. The femoral artery becomes the popliteal artery at the tendinous opening in the adductor magnus muscle, the adductor hiatus;

2. The branches of the popliteal artery supply skin, muscles, and the knee joint; the popliteal artery successively lies on the femur, the capsule of the knee joint, and the popliteus muscle before dividing into anterior and posterior tibial arteries at the inferior angle of the popliteal fossa;

3. The anterior tibial artery supplies the anterior compartment of the leg and the ankle; it continues as the dorsalis pedis artery into the foot;

4. The posterior tibial artery supplies the posterior compartment of the leg and terminates as medial and lateral plantar arteries; its major branch is the fibular (peroneal) artery that supplies the posterior and lateral compartments of the leg. (Courtesy of Dr. K. Sniderman, Associate Professor of Radiology, University of Toronto, Toronto, Ontario, Canada.)

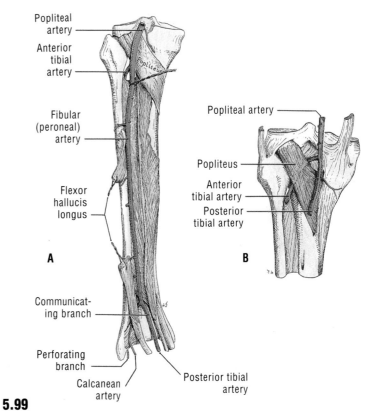

Popliteal artery

Anterior tibial artery

Fibular (peroneal) artery

Flexor hallucis longus

A

Communicating branch

Perforating branch

Calcanean artery

Popliteal artery

Popliteus

Anterior tibial artery

Posterior tibial artery

B

Posterior tibial artery

5.99
Arteries of the posterior aspect of the leg

A and **B**. Arterial anomalies:

1. Absence of posterior tibial artery (**A**), with compensatory enlargement of the fibular (peroneal) artery (**B**), occurs in about 5% of limbs.

2. High division of popliteal artery with the anterior tibial artery descending anterior to the popliteus muscle occurs in about 2% of limbs.

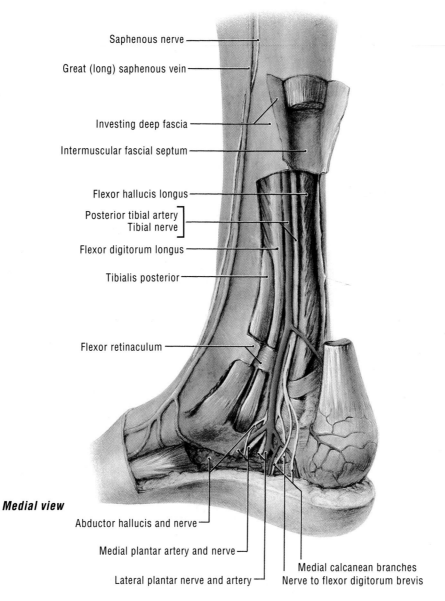

Saphenous nerve

Great (long) saphenous vein

Investing deep fascia

Intermuscular fascial septum

Flexor hallucis longus

Posterior tibial artery
Tibial nerve

Flexor digitorum longus

Tibialis posterior

Flexor retinaculum

Medial view

Abductor hallucis and nerve

Medial plantar artery and nerve

Lateral plantar nerve and artery

Medial calcanean branches
Nerve to flexor digitorum brevis

5.100
Ankle and heel

The posterior part of abductor hallucis is excised.

Observe:

1. The posterior tibial artery and the tibial nerve lying between the flexor digitorum longus and flexor hallucis longus muscles and dividing into medial and lateral plantar branches on the surface of the osseofibrous tunnel of the flexor hallucis longus muscle;

2. Tibialis posterior and flexor digitorum longus occupying separate and individual osseofibrous tunnels posterior to the medial malleolus; the pulsations of the posterior tibial artery are felt just posterior to the medial malleolus and to these two tendons that use the medial malleolus as a pulley;

3. The tendons of tibialis posterior and flexor digitorum longus use the medial malleolus as a pulley; only the flexor hallucis longus muscle uses the sustentaculum tali as a pulley.

4. The medial and lateral plantar nerves lying within the fork of the medial and lateral plantar arteries.

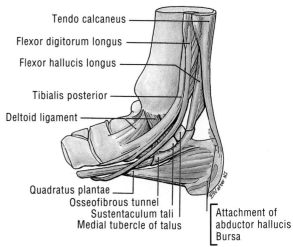

Tendo calcaneus

Flexor digitorum longus

Flexor hallucis longus

Tibialis posterior

Deltoid ligament

Quadratus plantae

Osseofibrous tunnel
Sustentaculum tali
Medial tubercle of talus

Attachment of abductor hallucis
Bursa

5.101
Tendons of the medial aspect of the ankle

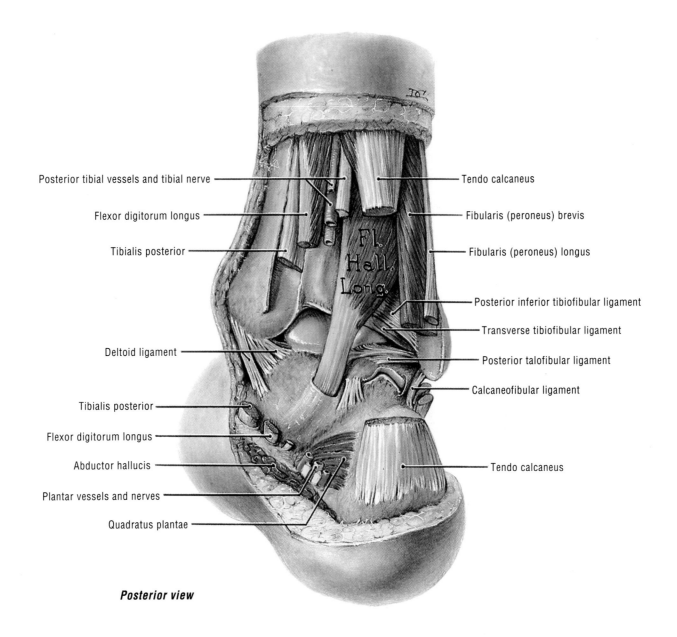

Posterior tibial vessels and tibial nerve — Tendo calcaneus

Flexor digitorum longus — Fibularis (peroneus) brevis

Tibialis posterior — Fibularis (peroneus) longus

Fl. Hall. Long.

Posterior inferior tibiofibular ligament

Transverse tibiofibular ligament

Deltoid ligament — Posterior talofibular ligament

Calcaneofibular ligament

Tibialis posterior —

Flexor digitorum longus —

Abductor hallucis — — Tendo calcaneus

Plantar vessels and nerves —

Quadratus plantae —

Posterior view

5.102
Ankle and heel

Observe:

1. The flexor hallucis longus muscle placed midway between the two malleoli; and having the two tendons (flexor digitorum longus and tibialis posterior) that groove the tibial malleolus medial to it and the two tendons (fibularis longus and brevis) that groove the lateral malleolus lateral to it;

2. The entrance to the sole of the foot lying deep to the abductor hallucis muscle; the plantar vessels and nerves, the two long digital flexors, and part of tibialis posterior enter here; quadratus plantae serves as a soft pad for the vessel and nerves;

3. The posterior tibial artery and the tibial nerve lying medial to the flexor hallucis longus muscle proximally and distally, after bifurcating, posterolateral to it; the crossing takes place where the long flexor is within its osseofibrous tunnel;

4. The strongest parts of the ligaments of the ankle are those that prevent anterior displacement of the leg bones, namely, the posterior part of the deltoid (posterior tibiotalar), the posterior talofibular, the tibiocalcanean, and the calcaneofibular.

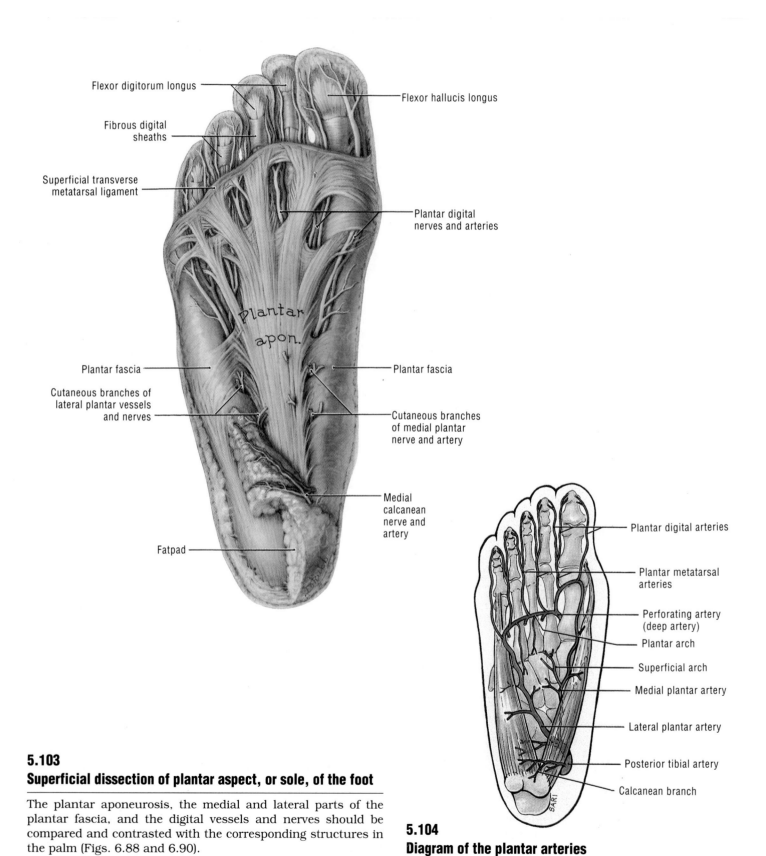

Flexor digitorum longus

Fibrous digital sheaths

Superficial transverse metatarsal ligament

Flexor hallucis longus

Plantar digital nerves and arteries

Plantar apon.

Plantar fascia

Plantar fascia

Cutaneous branches of lateral plantar vessels and nerves

Cutaneous branches of medial plantar nerve and artery

Medial calcanean nerve and artery

Fatpad

5.103

Superficial dissection of plantar aspect, or sole, of the foot

The plantar aponeurosis, the medial and lateral parts of the plantar fascia, and the digital vessels and nerves should be compared and contrasted with the corresponding structures in the palm (Figs. 6.88 and 6.90).

Plantar digital arteries

Plantar metatarsal arteries

Perforating artery (deep artery)

Plantar arch

Superficial arch

Medial plantar artery

Lateral plantar artery

Posterior tibial artery

Calcanean branch

5.104

Diagram of the plantar arteries

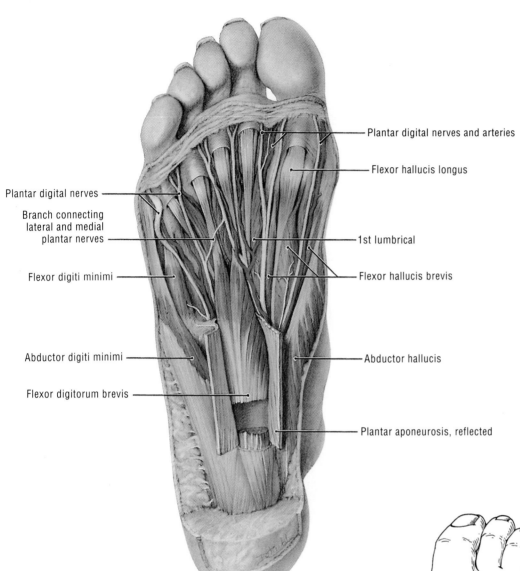

Plantar digital nerves and arteries

Flexor hallucis longus

Plantar digital nerves

Branch connecting lateral and medial plantar nerves

1st lumbrical

Flexor digiti minimi

Flexor hallucis brevis

Abductor digiti minimi

Abductor hallucis

Flexor digitorum brevis

Plantar aponeurosis, reflected

5.105
First layer of plantar muscles, digital nerves, and arteries

Observe:

1. The muscles of this layer are: abductor digiti minimi, flexor digitorum brevis, and abductor hallucis;

2. The plantar aponeurosis and fascia are reflected or removed, and a section is taken from the flexor digitorum brevis muscle in order to show the fibrous tissue encasing it;

3. The lateral and medial plantar digital nerves, like the corresponding palmar digital branches of the ulnar and median nerves, supply 1 1/2 and 3 1/2 digits, respectively, and are united by a connecting (communicating) branch;

4. The lateral nerve to the little toe is thickened here; the flexor digitorum brevis muscle here, as commonly, fails to send a tendon to the little toe.

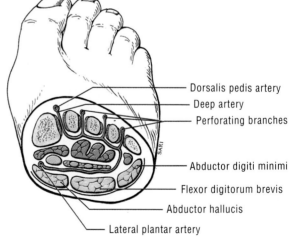

Dorsalis pedis artery

Deep artery

Perforating branches

Abductor digiti minimi

Flexor digitorum brevis

Abductor hallucis

Lateral plantar artery

5.106
Transverse section near the bases of the metatarsals

Layers:
1st
2nd
3rd
4th

5.107
Second layer of plantar muscles

Observe:

1. The muscles of this layer are: flexor hallucis longus, flexor digitorum longus, four lumbricals, and quadratus plantae;

2. The flexor digitorum longus muscle crossing superficial to tibialis posterior to the medial malleolus and superficial to flexor hallucis longus muscle at the tuberosity of the navicular bone;

3. The four lumbrical muscles passing to the hallux (great toe) side of the toes just as, in the hand, they pass to the pollex (thumb) side of the fingers (Fig. 6.83);

4. The flexor hallucis longus muscle sending a strong tendinous slip to the flexor digitorum longus muscle.

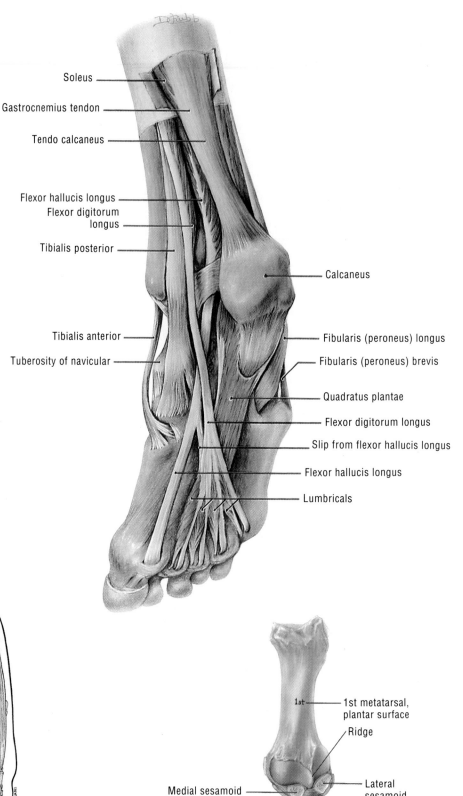

Soleus

Gastrocnemius tendon

Tendo calcaneus

Flexor hallucis longus

Flexor digitorum longus

Tibialis posterior

Tibialis anterior

Tuberosity of navicular

Calcaneus

Fibularis (peroneus) longus

Fibularis (peroneus) brevis

Quadratus plantae

Flexor digitorum longus

Slip from flexor hallucis longus

Flexor hallucis longus

Lumbricals

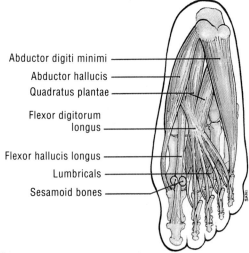

Abductor digiti minimi

Abductor hallucis

Quadratus plantae

Flexor digitorum longus

Flexor hallucis longus

Lumbricals

Sesamoid bones

5.108
Second layer of plantar muscles framed by the abductors of the first layer

1st metatarsal, plantar surface

Ridge

1st

Medial sesamoid

Lateral sesamoid

Sheath of flexor hallucis longus

5.109
Sesamoids of hallux

The sesamoid bones of the hallux are bound together and are located on each side of a bony ridge on the 1st metatarsal.

5.110
Foot raised as in walking

Observe:

1. The heel is raised but the toes remain applied to the ground;

2. The sesamoid bones act as a footstool for the 1st metatarsal, giving it increased height;

3. The quadratus plantae muscle lines the concave medial surface of the calcaneus;

4. By inserting into the flexor digitorum longus muscle, the quadratus plantae muscle acts as a guy line modifying the oblique pull of the flexor tendons;

5. The flexor hallucis longus muscle uses three pulleys: a groove on the posterior aspect of the distal end of the tibia, a groove on the posterior aspect of the talus, and a groove inferior to the sustentaculum tali.

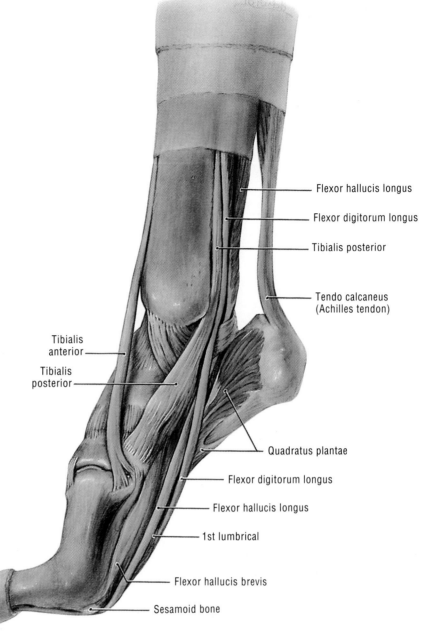

Flexor hallucis longus

Flexor digitorum longus

Tibialis posterior

Tendo calcaneus (Achilles tendon)

Tibialis anterior

Tibialis posterior

Quadratus plantae

Flexor digitorum longus

Flexor hallucis longus

1st lumbrical

Flexor hallucis brevis

Sesamoid bone

Medial view

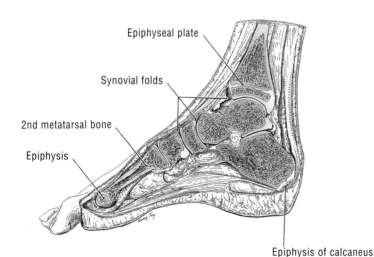

Epiphyseal plate

Synovial folds

2nd metatarsal bone

Epiphysis

Epiphysis of calcaneus

5.111
Longitudinal section through the foot of a 10-year-old child

Observe:

1. Ossification has spread to the dorsal and plantar surfaces of all the tarsal bones in view, and cartilage persists on the articular surfaces only;

2. The traction epiphysis of the calcaneus for the tendo calcaneus and plantar aponeurosis starts to ossify between the ages of 6 and 10 years;

3. The 1st metatarsal bone is similar to a phalanx in that its epiphysis is at the base and not at its head like the 2nd and other metatarsal bones;

4. The tuberosity of the calcaneus and the sesamoid bones of the 1st and the heads of the 2nd to 5th metatarsals (here the 2nd) supporting the longitudinal arch of the foot; the medial part of the longitudinal arch, seen here, is higher and more mobile than the lateral.

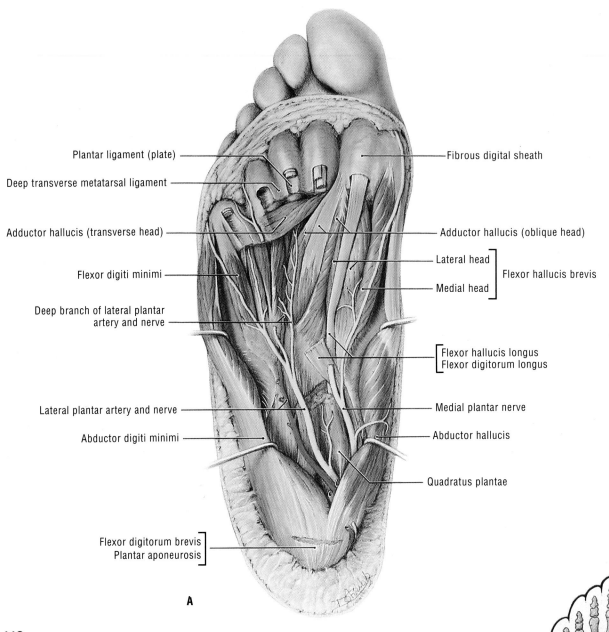

Plantar ligament (plate)

Deep transverse metatarsal ligament

Adductor hallucis (transverse head)

Flexor digiti minimi

Deep branch of lateral plantar artery and nerve

Lateral plantar artery and nerve

Abductor digiti minimi

Flexor digitorum brevis
Plantar aponeurosis

Fibrous digital sheath

Adductor hallucis (oblique head)

Lateral head ⎤
             ⎥ Flexor hallucis brevis
Medial head ⎦

Flexor hallucis longus
Flexor digitorum longus

Medial plantar nerve

Abductor hallucis

Quadratus plantae

A

5.112
Third layer of plantar muscles

Observe in **A**:

1. The muscles of this layer are: flexor digiti minimi, adductor hallucis, and flexor hallucis brevis;

2. Of the first layer, the abductor digiti minimi and abductor hallucis muscles are pulled aside and the flexor digitorum brevis muscle is cut short; of the second layer, the flexor digitorum longus and lumbrical muscles are excised and the quadratus plantae muscle is cut;

3. The lateral interossei muscles are visible;

4. The lateral plantar nerve and artery course laterally between muscles of the first and second layers; their deep branches then course medially between muscles of the third and fourth layers.

B. Diagram.

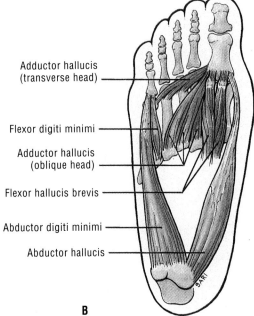

Adductor hallucis (transverse head)

Flexor digiti minimi

Adductor hallucis (oblique head)

Flexor hallucis brevis

Abductor digiti minimi

Abductor hallucis

B

5.113
Fourth layer of plantar muscles

Observe:

1. The muscles of this layer are the three plantar and four dorsal interossei in the anterior half of the foot and the tendon of fibularis (peroneus) longus and of tibialis posterior in the posterior half;

2. Of the first three layers, the abductor and flexor brevis muscles of the 5th toe and the abductor and flexor brevis muscles of the big toe remain for purposes of orientation;

3. Plantar interossei adduct the three lateral toes toward an axial line that passes through the 2nd metatarsal bone and 2nd toe, whereas dorsal interossei abduct from this line.

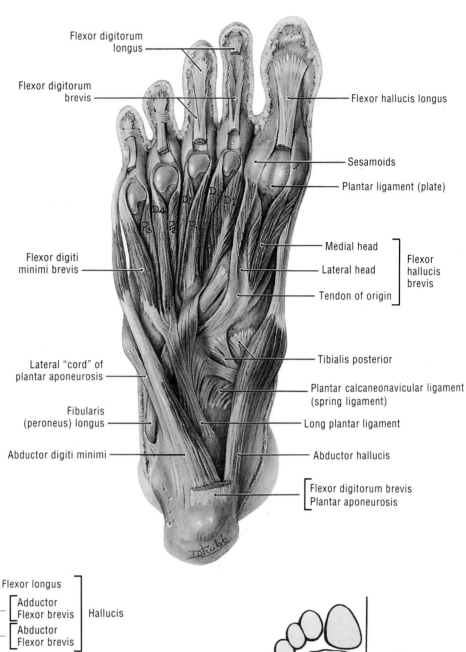

Flexor digitorum longus

Flexor digitorum brevis

Flexor hallucis longus

Sesamoids

Plantar ligament (plate)

Medial head
Lateral head — Flexor hallucis brevis
Tendon of origin

Flexor digiti minimi brevis

Tibialis posterior

Lateral "cord" of plantar aponeurosis

Plantar calcaneonavicular ligament (spring ligament)

Fibularis (peroneus) longus

Long plantar ligament

Abductor digiti minimi

Abductor hallucis

Flexor digitorum brevis
Plantar aponeurosis

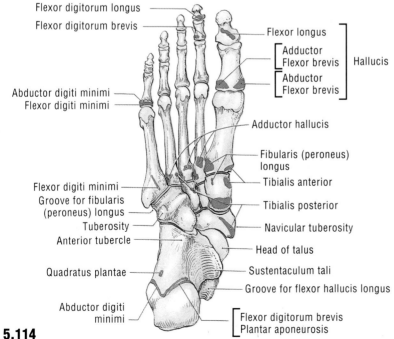

Flexor digitorum longus
Flexor digitorum brevis

Flexor longus

Adductor
Flexor brevis — Hallucis

Abductor
Flexor brevis

Abductor digiti minimi
Flexor digiti minimi

Adductor hallucis

Fibularis (peroneus) longus

Flexor digiti minimi
Groove for fibularis (peroneus) longus
Tuberosity
Anterior tubercle

Tibialis anterior

Tibialis posterior

Navicular tuberosity

Head of talus

Quadratus plantae

Sustentaculum tali

Groove for flexor hallucis longus

Abductor digiti minimi

Flexor digitorum brevis
Plantar aponeurosis

5.114
Bones of the foot, plantar aspect

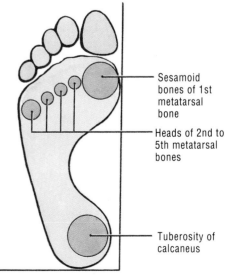

Sesamoid bones of 1st metatarsal bone

Heads of 2nd to 5th metatarsal bones

Tuberosity of calcaneus

5.115
Weight-bearing areas of the foot

5.116
Distended ankle joint

Observe:

1. The extension of the synovial membrane on the neck of the talus;

2. The anterior articular surface of the talus and of the calcaneus, each convex from side to side in order that the foot may be inverted and everted at this, the transverse tarsal joint;

3. The relations of the tendons to the sustentaculum tali: flexor hallucis longus inferior to it, flexor digitorum longus along its medial aspect, and tibialis posterior superior to it and in contact with the deltoid ligament.

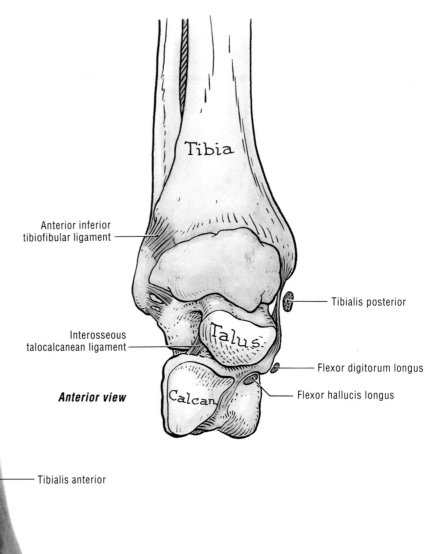

Anterior view

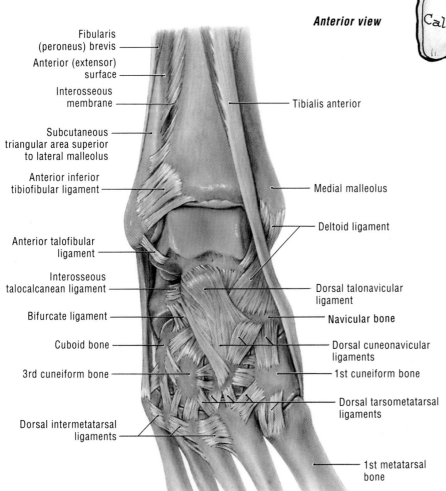

5.117
Ankle joint and the joints of the dorsum of the foot

The ankle joint is plantar flexed; its anterior capsular fibers are removed.

Observe:

1. The fibers of the interosseous membrane and ligaments uniting the fibula to the tibia are so directed as to resist the inferior pull of the muscles, but allow the fibula to be forced superiorly;

2. The anterior talofibular ligament is a weak band, easily torn;

3. The dorsal ligaments of the foot resist the same thrusts as the plantar ligaments, and, therefore, are identically disposed, as reference to Figures 5.129 and 5.130 shows; the plantar ligaments, however, act also as tie beams for the arches of the foot and, therefore, are stronger.

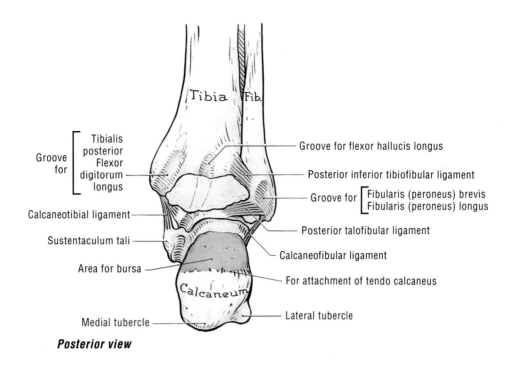

Posterior view

5.118
Distended ankle joint

Observe the groove for:
1. The flexor hallucis longus muscle that crosses the middle of the ankle joint posteriorly;

2. Two tendons posterior to the medial malleolus;

3. Two tendons posterior to the lateral malleolus.

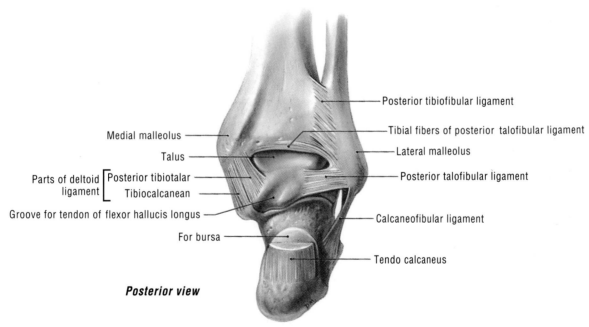

Posterior view

5.119
Ligaments of the ankle joint

Observe:
1. The posterior aspect of the ankle joint is strengthened by the transversely oriented posterior tibiofibular ligament and posterior talofibular ligaments;

2. Laterally the calcaneofibular ligament and medially the posterior tibiotalar and tibiocalcanean parts of the deltoid ligament stabilizing the joint;

3. The groove for the tendon of flexor hallucis longus tendon between the medial and lateral tubercles of the talus and continuing inferior to the sustentaculum tali.

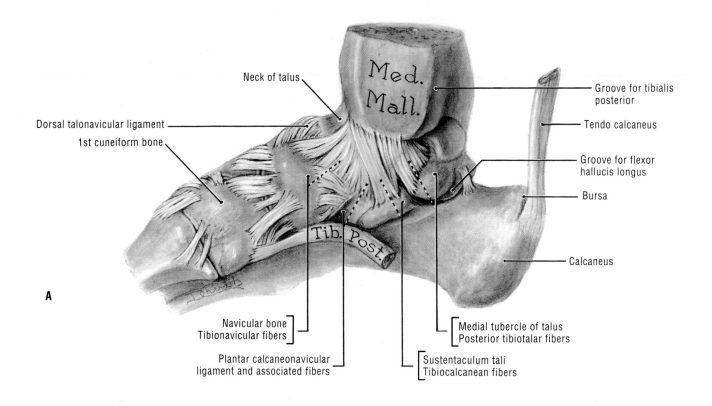

Neck of talus

Dorsal talonavicular ligament

1st cuneiform bone

Med. Mall.

Groove for tibialis posterior

Tendo calcaneus

Groove for flexor hallucis longus

Bursa

Tib. Post.

Calcaneus

A

Navicular bone
Tibionavicular fibers

Plantar calcaneonavicular ligament and associated fibers

Medial tubercle of talus
Posterior tibiotalar fibers

Sustentaculum tali
Tibiocalcanean fibers

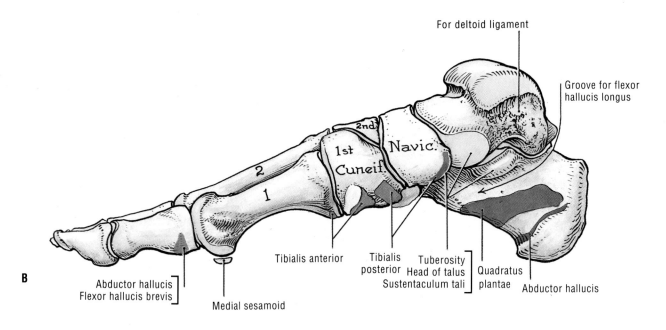

For deltoid ligament

Groove for flexor hallucis longus

2nd

1st

Navic.

Cuneif.

2

1

B

Abductor hallucis
Flexor hallucis brevis

Medial sesamoid

Tibialis anterior

Tibialis posterior
Sustentaculum tali

Tuberosity
Head of talus

Quadratus plantae

Abductor hallucis

5.120
Ankle and foot – medial

A. Ligaments of the ankle joint. Observe:
1. Tibialis posterior displaced from its bed consisting of the medial malleolus, the deltoid ligament, and the plantar calcaneonavicular (spring) ligament;

2. The bed of the flexor hallucis longus muscle consisting of the groove between the two tubercles of the talus and the continuation of that groove inferior to the sustentaculum tali;

3. The chief parts of the medial or deltoid ligament that are attached superiorly to the medial malleolus of the tibia and inferiorly to the talus, the navicular, and the calcaneus.

B. Bones of the foot. Observe that the medial part of the longitudinal arch of the foot consists of the calcaneus, the talus, the navicular, the three cuneiforms, and the 1st, 2nd, and 3rd metatarsals.

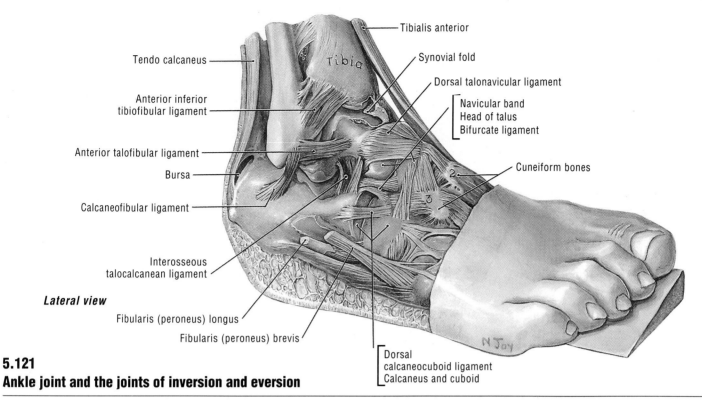

Tibialis anterior

Tendo calcaneus

Synovial fold

Dorsal talonavicular ligament

Anterior inferior
tibiofibular ligament

Navicular band
Head of talus
Bifurcate ligament

Anterior talofibular ligament

Cuneiform bones

Bursa

Calcaneofibular ligament

Interosseous
talocalcanean ligament

Lateral view

Fibularis (peroneus) longus

Fibularis (peroneus) brevis

Dorsal
calcaneocuboid ligament
Calcaneus and cuboid

5.121

Ankle joint and the joints of inversion and eversion

The joints of inversion and eversion are: the subtalar (posterior talocalcanean) joint, the talocalcaneonavicular joint, and the transverse tarsal (i.e., the combined calcaneocuboid and talonavicular) joint. The foot has been inverted in order to demonstrate: the articular surfaces and the ligaments rendered taut, on inverting the foot. Observe:

1. The exposed articular surfaces include: (a) the posterior talar facet of the calcaneus, (b) the anterior surface of the calcaneus, and (c) the head of the talus, all of which are palpable; since inversion of the foot is commonly associated with plantar flexion

of the ankle joint, (d) the superior and lateral articular surfaces of the body of the talus are commonly uncovered too;

2. The ligaments that resist further inversion;

3. The anterior talofibular ligament and the dorsal calcaneocuboid ligament are weak and easily torn; the bifurcate and talonavicular ligaments are under strain; the strong calcaneofibular ligament, not attached to the tip of the malleolus but to a facet anterior to the tip; hence, the projecting tip, being free, helps to retain the fibularis (peroneal) tendons.

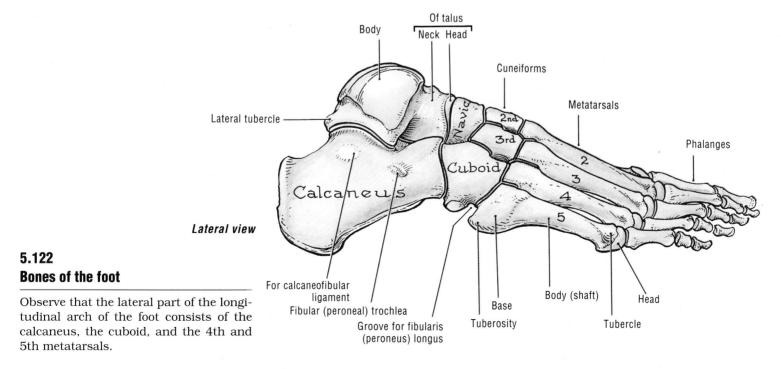

Body

Of talus
Neck Head

Cuneiforms

Metatarsals

Phalanges

Lateral tubercle

Lateral view

5.122

Bones of the foot

Observe that the lateral part of the longitudinal arch of the foot consists of the calcaneus, the cuboid, and the 4th and 5th metatarsals.

For calcaneofibular
ligament
Fibular (peroneal) trochlea

Groove for fibularis
(peroneus) longus

Base

Tuberosity

Body (shaft)

Head

Tubercle

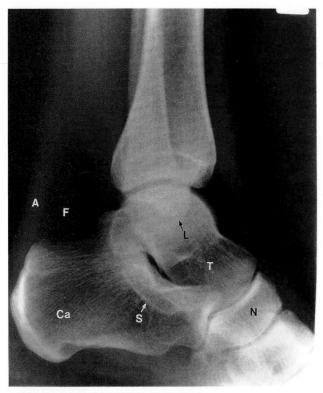

A, *Medial view*

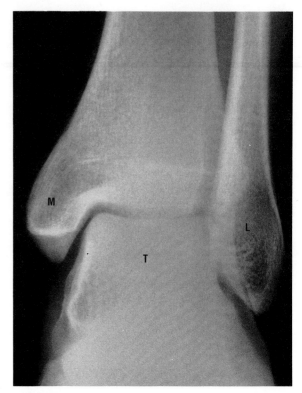

B, *Anterior view*

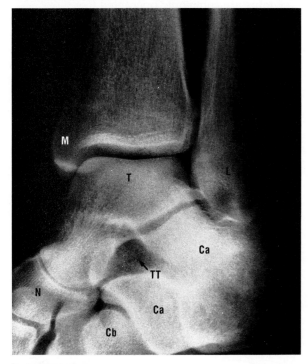

C, *Lateral view*

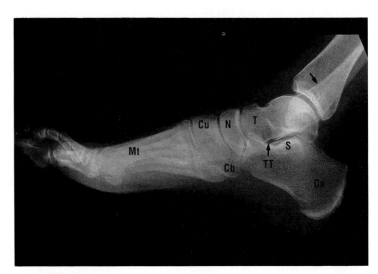

D, *Lateral view*

5.123
Radiographs of the foot and ankle

M - Medial malleolus, *L* - Lateral malleolus, *T* - Talus, *Ca* - Calcaneus, *S* - Sustentaculum tali, *N* - Navicular, *Cu* - Cuneiforms, *Cb* - Cuboid, *Mt* - Metatarsal, *TT* - Tarsal tunnel, *A* - Achilles tendon, *F* - Fat, *Arrowhead* - superimposed tibia and fibula. (**A** and

B Courtesy of Dr. P. Bobechko, Assistant Professor of Radiology, and Dr. E. Becker, Associate Professor of Radiology, University of Toronto, Toronto, Ontario, Canada.)

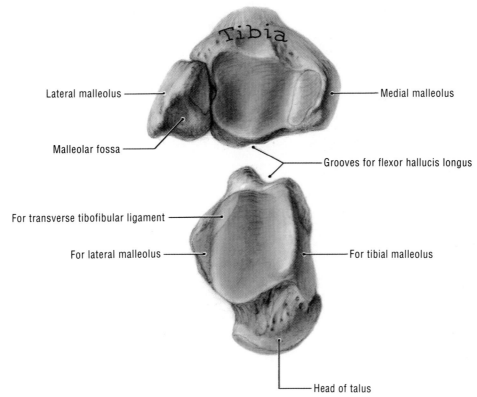

Lateral malleolus

Medial malleolus

Malleolar fossa

Grooves for flexor hallucis longus

For transverse tibofibular ligament

For lateral malleolus

For tibial malleolus

Head of talus

5.124
Articular surfaces of the ankle joint

Observe that the superior articular surface of the talus is broader anteriorly than posteriorly; hence the medial and lateral malleoli, which grasp the sides of the talus tend, in dorsiflexion, to be forced apart; the fully dorsiflexed position is very stable in comparison to the fully plantar flexed position; in plantar flexion, when the tibia and fibula articulate with the narrower posterior part of the superior articular surface of the talus, some side to side movement of the joint is allowed, accounting for the instability of the joint in this position.

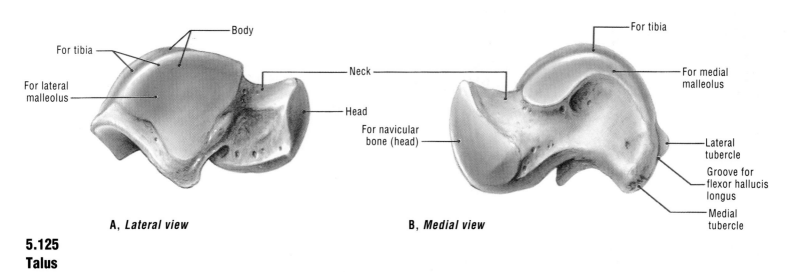

Body

For tibia

For tibia

Neck

For medial malleolus

For lateral malleolus

Head

For navicular bone (head)

Lateral tubercle

Groove for flexor hallucis longus

Medial tubercle

A, *Lateral view*

B, *Medial view*

5.125
Talus

The trochlea of the talus is the part of the body of the talus that articulates with the ankle socket; it has a superior articular area for articulation with the inferior aspects of the tibia and fibula, a medial, comma-shaped area for articulation with the medial malleolus and a lateral, triangular area for articulation with the lateral malleolus.

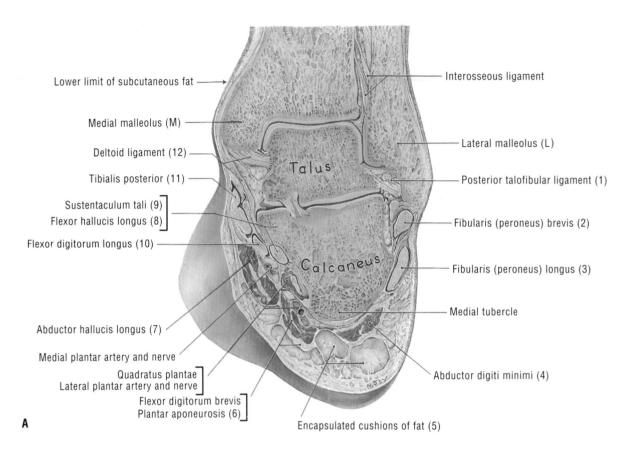

Lower limit of subcutaneous fat

Medial malleolus (M)

Deltoid ligament (12)

Tibialis posterior (11)

Sustentaculum tali (9)
Flexor hallucis longus (8)

Flexor digitorum longus (10)

Abductor hallucis longus (7)

Medial plantar artery and nerve

Quadratus plantae
Lateral plantar artery and nerve

Flexor digitorum brevis
Plantar aponeurosis (6)

Interosseous ligament

Lateral malleolus (L)

Posterior talofibular ligament (1)

Fibularis (peroneus) brevis (2)

Fibularis (peroneus) longus (3)

Medial tubercle

Abductor digiti minimi (4)

Encapsulated cushions of fat (5)

Talus

Calcaneus

A

5.126
Coronal section and coronal MRI (magnetic resonance image) through the ankle region

Observe:

1. Tibia resting on the talus, and the talus resting on the calcaneus; between the calcaneus and the skin, several encapsulated cushions of fat;

2. The lateral malleolus descending much farther inferiorly than the medial malleolus;

3. The weak interosseous tibiofibular ligament;

4. The interosseous band between talus and calcaneus separating the subtalar or posterior talocalcanean joint from the talocalcaneonavicular joint;

5. Sustentaculum tali acting as a pulley for the flexor hallucis longus muscle and giving attachment to the calcaneotibial band of the deltoid ligament.

Numbers in **B** refer to structures in **A**.

(MRI courtesy of Dr. W. Kucharczyk, Clinical Director of Tri-Hospital Magnetic Resonance Centre, Toronto, Ontario, Canada.)

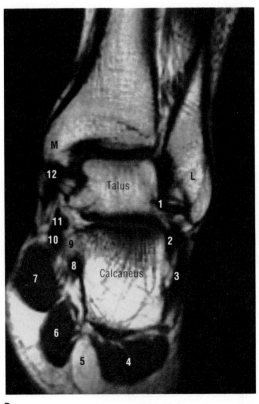

B

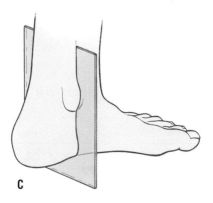

C

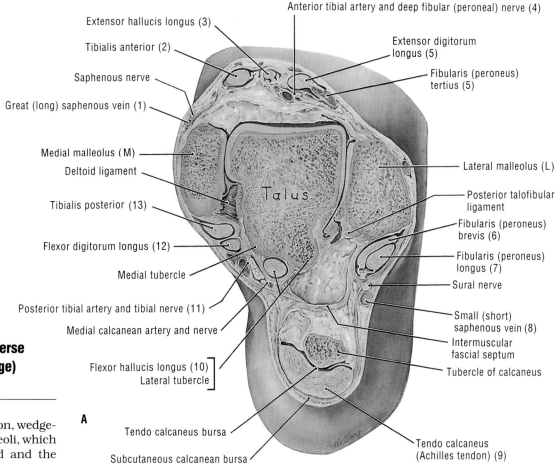

Extensor hallucis longus (3)

Tibialis anterior (2)

Saphenous nerve

Great (long) saphenous vein (1)

Anterior tibial artery and deep fibular (peroneal) nerve (4)

Extensor digitorum longus (5)

Fibularis (peroneus) tertius (5)

Medial malleolus (M)

Deltoid ligament

Tibialis posterior (13)

Flexor digitorum longus (12)

Medial tubercle

Posterior tibial artery and tibial nerve (11)

Medial calcanean artery and nerve

Flexor hallucis longus (10)
Lateral tubercle

Talus

Lateral malleolus (L)

Posterior talofibular ligament

Fibularis (peroneus) brevis (6)

Fibularis (peroneus) longus (7)

Sural nerve

Small (short) saphenous vein (8)

Intermuscular fascial septum

Tubercle of calcaneus

A

Tendo calcaneus bursa

Subcutaneous calcanean bursa

Tendo calcaneus (Achilles tendon) (9)

5.127
Transverse section and transverse MRI (magnetic resonance image) through the ankle joint

Observe:

1. The body of the talus on section, wedge-shaped and grasped by the malleoli, which are bound to it by the deltoid and the posterior talofibular ligament and are thereby prevented from sliding anteriorly;

2. The flexor hallucis longus muscle, within its fibro-osseous sheath, lying between medial and lateral tubercles of talus;

3. Two tendons each within a separate sheath (fibrous and synovial) posterior to the medial malleolus, and two tendons within a common sheath posterior to the lateral malleolus;

4. Because of the intervening fibrous sheath, the posterior tibial vessels and the tibial nerve are not disturbed by the excursions of the flexor hallucis longus muscle;

5. The small inconstant bursa superficial to the tendo calcaneus and the large constant bursa deep to it and containing a long synovial fold;

6. The anterior tibial artery and its companion nerve at the midpoint of the anterior aspect of the ankle, with two tendons medial to it and two tendons lateral to it.

Numbers in **B** refer to structures in **A**.

(MRI courtesy of Dr. W. Kucharczyk, Clinical Director of Tri-Hospital Magnetic Resonance Centre, Toronto, Ontario, Canada.)

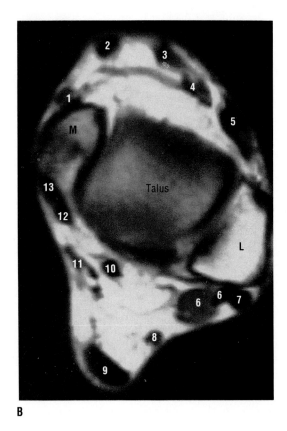

B

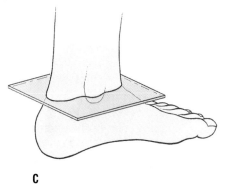

C

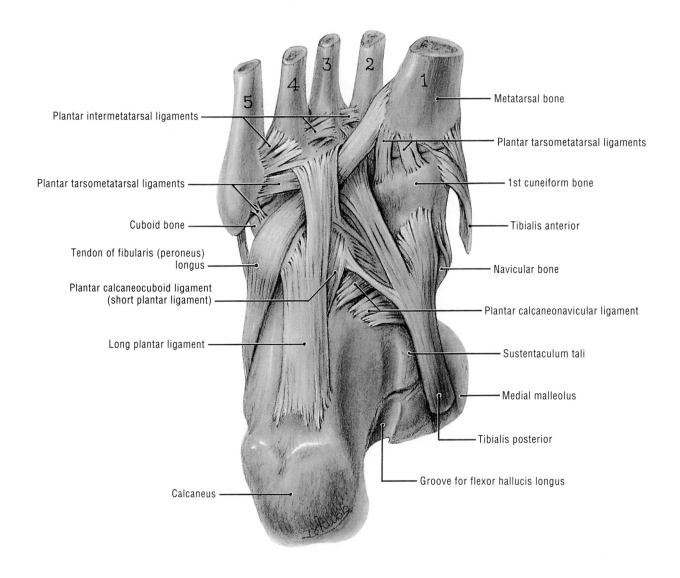

Plantar intermetatarsal ligaments

Plantar tarsometatarsal ligaments

Cuboid bone

Tendon of fibularis (peroneus) longus

Plantar calcaneocuboid ligament (short plantar ligament)

Long plantar ligament

Calcaneus

Metatarsal bone

Plantar tarsometatarsal ligaments

1st cuneiform bone

Tibialis anterior

Navicular bone

Plantar calcaneonavicular ligament

Sustentaculum tali

Medial malleolus

Tibialis posterior

Groove for flexor hallucis longus

5.128
Plantar ligaments–I

Observe:

1. The insertions of three long tendons: fibularis (peroneus) longus, tibialis anterior, and tibialis posterior;

2. The tendon of the fibularis (peroneus) longus muscle crossing the sole of the foot in the groove anterior to the ridge of the cuboid; bridged by some fibers of the long plantar ligament; and inserted into the base of the 1st metatarsal; usually, like tibialis anterior, it is also inserted into the 1st cuneiform; it is an evertor of the foot;

3. Slips of the tendon of tibialis posterior extending like the fingers of an open hand to grasp the bones anterior to the transverse tarsal joint; it is an invertor of the foot.

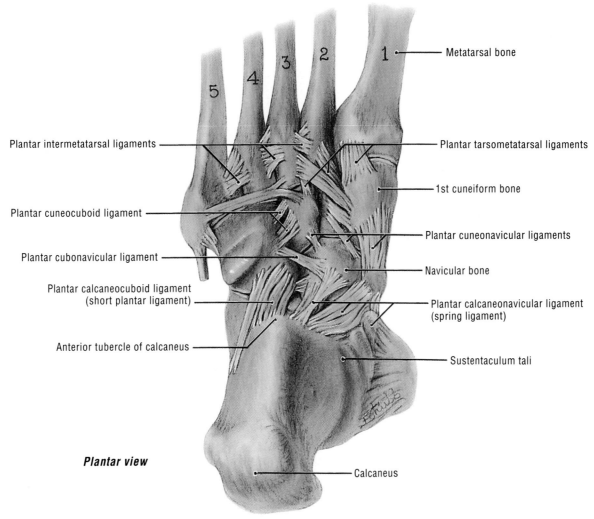

Plantar intermetatarsal ligaments

Plantar cuneocuboid ligament

Plantar cubonavicular ligament

Plantar calcaneocuboid ligament
(short plantar ligament)

Anterior tubercle of calcaneus

Metatarsal bone

Plantar tarsometatarsal ligaments

1st cuneiform bone

Plantar cuneonavicular ligaments

Navicular bone

Plantar calcaneonavicular ligament
(spring ligament)

Sustentaculum tali

Calcaneus

Plantar view

5.129
Plantar ligaments–II

Observe:

1. The plantar calcaneocuboid (short plantar) ligament and the plantar calcaneonavicular (spring) ligament are the inferior ligaments of the transverse tarsal joint;

2. The ligaments in the anterior of the foot diverge posteriorly from each side of the long axis of the 3rd metatarsal and 3rd cuneiform; hence a backward thrust to the 1st metatarsal, as when rising on the big toe in walking, is transmitted directly to the navicular and talus by the 1st cuneiform, and indirectly by the 2nd metatarsal and 2nd cuneiform and also by the 3rd metatarsal and 3rd cuneiform;

3. A posterior thrust to the 4th and 5th metatarsals is transmitted directly to the cuboid and calcaneus; posterior displacement of the bones of the lateral longitudinal arch is prevented by the adjoining ligaments.

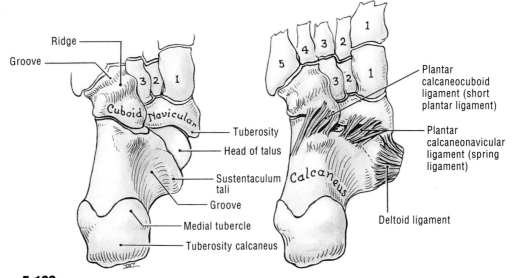

Ridge

Groove

Tuberosity

Head of talus

Sustentaculum tali

Groove

Medial tubercle

Tuberosity calcaneus

Plantar calcaneocuboid ligament (short plantar ligament)

Plantar calcaneonavicular ligament (spring ligament)

Deltoid ligament

5.130
Support for head of talus

The head of the talus is supported by the plantar calcaneonavicular ligaments (spring ligament) and by the tendon of tibialis posterior.

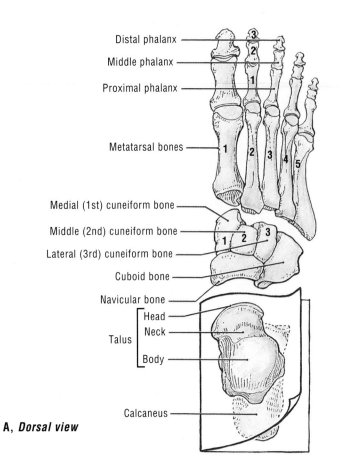

Distal phalanx
Middle phalanx
Proximal phalanx

Metatarsal bones

ANTERIOR PART OF THE FOOT
FIVE METATARSALS AND PHALANGES

Medial (1st) cuneiform bone
Middle (2nd) cuneiform bone
Lateral (3rd) cuneiform bone
Cuboid bone

MIDDLE PART OF FOOT
FIVE SMALL TARSAL BONES

Navicular bone
Head
Neck
Body

Talus

POSTERIOR PART OF THE FOOT
TWO LARGE TARSAL BONES

Calcaneus

A, *Dorsal view*

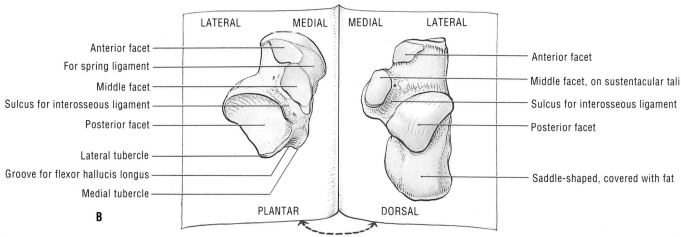

Anterior facet
For spring ligament
Middle facet
Sulcus for interosseous ligament
Posterior facet

Lateral tubercle
Groove for flexor hallucis longus
Medial tubercle

LATERAL   MEDIAL   MEDIAL   LATERAL

Anterior facet
Middle facet, on sustentacular tali
Sulcus for interosseous ligament
Posterior facet

Saddle-shaped, covered with fat

PLANTAR   DORSAL

B

5.131

Bones of foot and talocalcanean joint

A. Bones of the foot. **B.** Bony surfaces of the talocalcanean joints. The plantar surface of the talus and the dorsal surface of the calcaneus are displayed as pages in a book.

Observe in **B**:

1. The joints are synovial gliding joints and, therefore, the apposed or corresponding facets are not exact counterparts of each other, i.e., one being more extensive than the other;

2. The talus takes part in three joints: (a) supratalar joint, i.e., the ankle joint; (b) infratalar joints, the posterior talocalcanean (the subtalar joint) and the anterior talocalcanean; (c) pretalar joint, i.e., the talonavicular;

3. At the supratalar joint, only movements of flexion and extension are normally permitted; at the infratalar and pretalar joints, movements of inversion and eversion take place;

4. The two parts of the infratalar joint are separated from each other by the sulcus tali and the sulcus calcanei, which, when the talus and calcaneus are in articulation, become the tarsal sinus or tunnel;

5. The convex posterior talar facet of the calcaneus, the concave middle and anterior talar facets, and the concave talar facet of the navicular all have their counterparts on the talus.

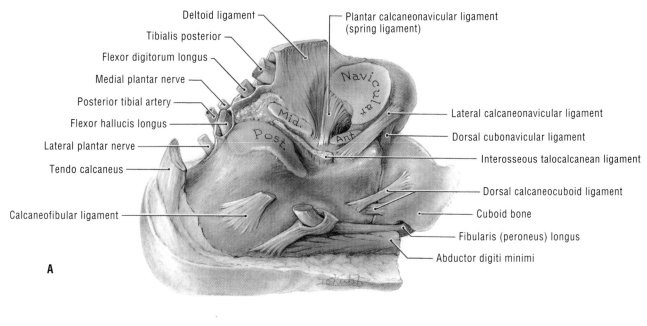

Deltoid ligament

Tibialis posterior

Flexor digitorum longus

Medial plantar nerve

Posterior tibial artery

Flexor hallucis longus

Lateral plantar nerve

Tendo calcaneus

Calcaneofibular ligament

Plantar calcaneonavicular ligament (spring ligament)

Navicular

Mid.

Post.

Ant.

Lateral calcaneonavicular ligament

Dorsal cubonavicular ligament

Interosseous talocalcanean ligament

Dorsal calcaneocuboid ligament

Cuboid bone

Fibularis (peroneus) longus

Abductor digiti minimi

A

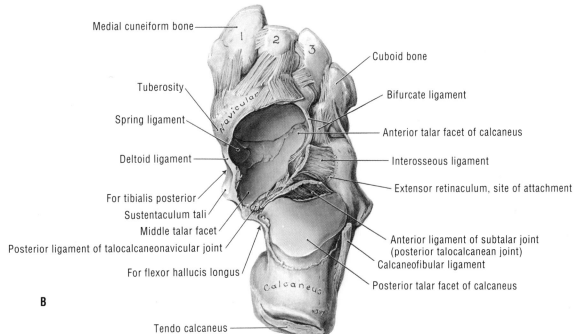

Medial cuneiform bone

Tuberosity

Spring ligament

Deltoid ligament

For tibialis posterior

Sustentaculum tali

Middle talar facet

Posterior ligament of talocalcaneonavicular joint

For flexor hallucis longus

Cuboid bone

Bifurcate ligament

Anterior talar facet of calcaneus

Interosseous ligament

Extensor retinaculum, site of attachment

Anterior ligament of subtalar joint (posterior talocalcanean joint)

Calcaneofibular ligament

Posterior talar facet of calcaneus

Calcaneus

Navicular

Tendo calcaneus

B

5.132
Joints of inversion and eversion

The talus has been removed in these specimens, thereby fully exposing the structures in the tarsal sinus.

Observe:

1. The convex, posterior talar facet separated from the concave, middle, and anterior facets by the ligamentous structures within the tarsal sinus;

2. At the wide lateral end of the sinus: (a) the strong interosseous talocalcanean ligament; and (b) the attachments of the extensor retinaculum, which extend medially between the posterior ligament of the anterior talocalcanean joint and the anterior ligament of the posterior talocalcanean or subtalar joint;

3. The subtalar joint has a synovial cavity to itself, whereas the talonavicular joint and the anterior talocalcanean joint share a common synovial cavity;

4. The angular space between the navicular bone and the middle talar facet, on the sustentaculum tali, to be bridged by the plantar calcaneonavicular ligament, the central part of which is fibrocartilaginous;

5. The socket for the head of the talus to be deepened medially by the part of the deltoid ligament that blends in to the spring ligament, and laterally by the calcaneonavicular part of the bifurcate ligament;

6. Various synovial folds overlying the margins of the articular cartilage, some of these containing fat.

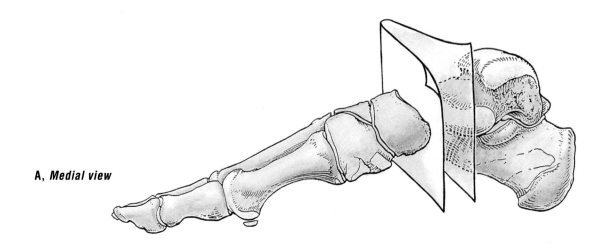

A, *Medial view*

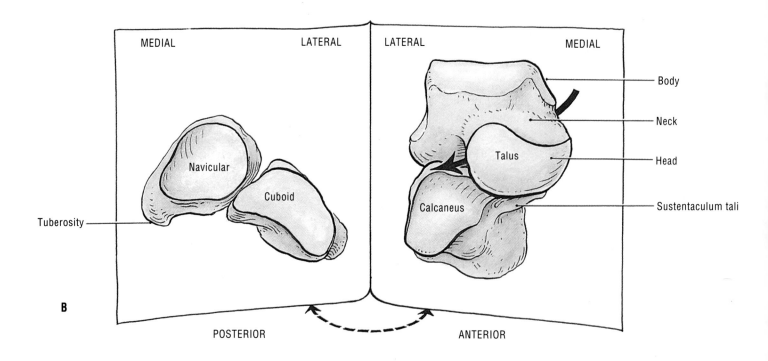

MEDIAL　　　　　　LATERAL

Navicular

Cuboid

Tuberosity

POSTERIOR

LATERAL　　　　　　MEDIAL

Body

Neck

Talus

Head

Calcaneus

Sustentaculum tali

ANTERIOR

B

5.133
Transverse tarsal joint

A. Bones of the foot. **B.** Bony surface of the transverse tarsal joint. This joint includes the talonavicular and the calcaneocuboid articulations. The posterior surfaces of the navicular and cuboid bones and the anterior surfaces of the talus and calcaneus are displayed as pages in a book. The *black arrow* traverses the tarsal sinus (tunnel), in which the interosseous talocalcanean ligament is located.

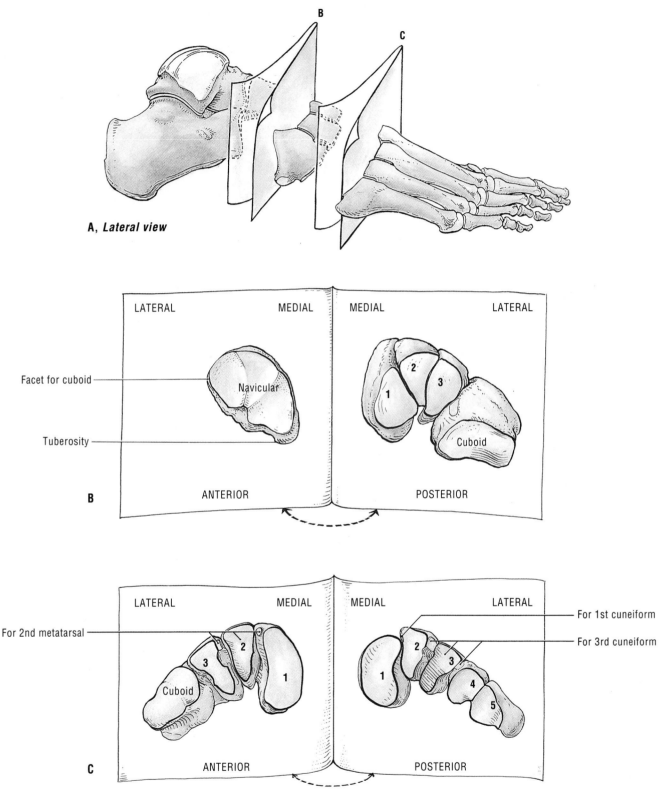

A, *Lateral view*

Facet for cuboid

Navicular

Tuberosity

Cuboid

B

For 2nd metatarsal

Cuboid

For 1st cuneiform

For 3rd cuneiform

C

5.134

Bony surfaces

A. Bones of the foot. **B**. Bony surfaces of the cuneonavicular and cubonavicular joints. The anterior surface of the navicular bone, the posterior surfaces of the three cuneiform bones, and the medial and posterior surfaces of the cuboid bone are displayed as pages in a book. **C**. Bony surfaces of the tarsometatarsal joints. The anterior surfaces of the cuboid and three cuneiform bones and the posterior surfaces of the bases of the five metatarsal bones are displayed as pages in a book.

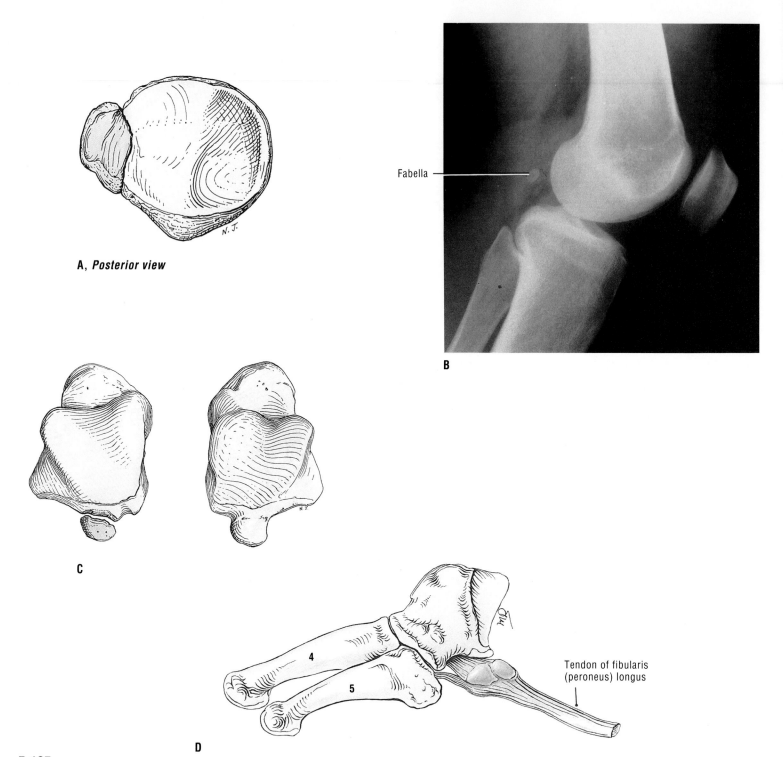

A, *Posterior view*

Fabella

B

C

Tendon of fibularis
(peroneus) longus

4

5

D

5.135
Bony anomalies

A. Bipartite patella. Occasionally, the superolateral angle of the patella ossifies independently and remains discrete.

B. Fabella. A sesamoid bone (fabella) on the lateral head of the gastrocnemius muscle was present in 21.6% of 116 limbs.

C. Os trigonum. The lateral (posterior) tubercle of the talus has a separate center of ossification, which appears between the ages of 7 and 13 years; when this fails to fuse with the body of the talus,

as in the left bone of this pair, it is called an os trigonum. It was found in 7.7% of 558 adult feet; 22 were paired, 21 were unpaired.

D. Sesamoid bone in fibularis (peroneus) longus. A sesamoid bone in fibularis (peroneus) longus tendon was found in 26% of 92 feet. In this specimen, it is bipartite, and the fibularis (peroneus) longus muscle has an additional attachment to the 5th metatarsal bone.

6   The Upper Limb

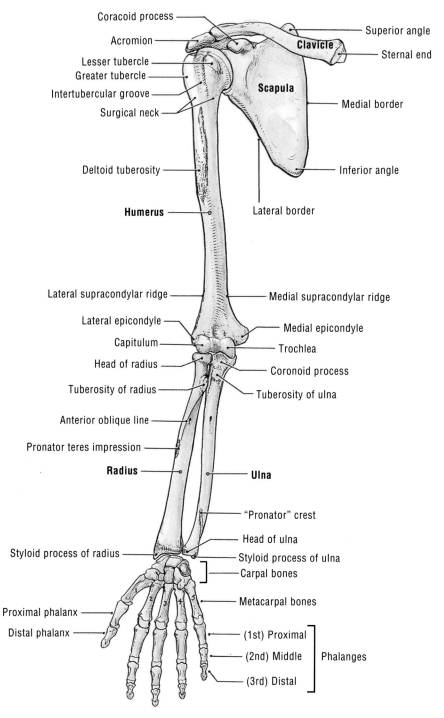

Coracoid process

Acromion

Lesser tubercle

Greater tubercle

Intertubercular groove

Surgical neck

Deltoid tuberosity

Humerus

Lateral supracondylar ridge

Lateral epicondyle

Capitulum

Head of radius

Tuberosity of radius

Anterior oblique line

Pronator teres impression

Radius

Styloid process of radius

Proximal phalanx

Distal phalanx

Superior angle

Clavicle

Sternal end

Scapula

Medial border

Inferior angle

Lateral border

Medial supracondylar ridge

Medial epicondyle

Trochlea

Coronoid process

Tuberosity of ulna

Ulna

"Pronator" crest

Head of ulna

Styloid process of ulna

Carpal bones

Metacarpal bones

(1st) Proximal

(2nd) Middle   Phalanges

(3rd) Distal

A, *Anterior view*

6.1
Bones of the upper limb

For bones of the hand, see Figure 6.130**A** and **B**.

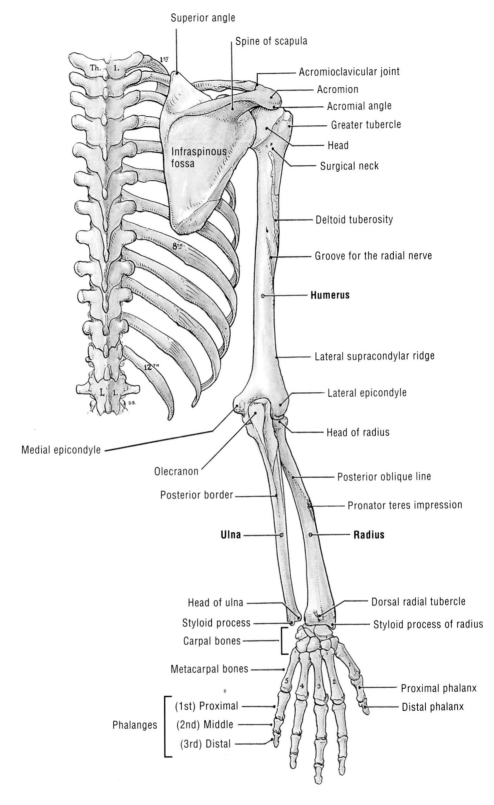

Superior angle

Spine of scapula

Acromioclavicular joint

Acromion

Acromial angle

Greater tubercle

Head

Surgical neck

Infraspinous fossa

Deltoid tuberosity

Groove for the radial nerve

Humerus

Lateral supracondylar ridge

Lateral epicondyle

Head of radius

Medial epicondyle

Olecranon

Posterior oblique line

Posterior border

Pronator teres impression

Ulna

Radius

Head of ulna

Dorsal radial tubercle

Styloid process

Styloid process of radius

Carpal bones

Metacarpal bones

Proximal phalanx

Distal phalanx

Phalanges

(1st) Proximal

(2nd) Middle

(3rd) Distal

B, *Posterior view*

**6.1
Bones of the upper limb (continued)**

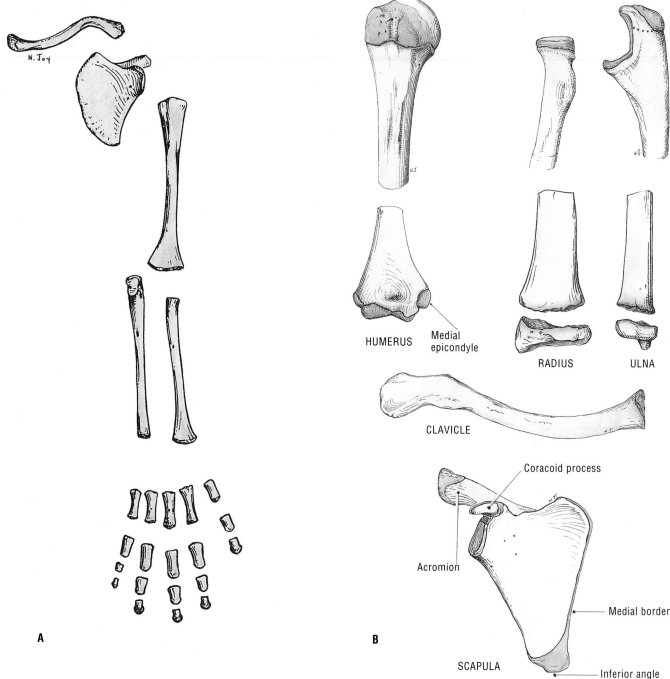

A

B

HUMERUS — Medial epicondyle

RADIUS

ULNA

CLAVICLE

Coracoid process

Acromion

Medial border

SCAPULA — Inferior angle

6.2
Ossification of the bones of the upper limb

A. At birth. The diaphyses of the long bones and the scapula are ossified, but the epiphyses and carpal bones are not. The coracoid process, the medial border of the scapula, and the acromion are cartilaginous (McKern TW, Stewart TD. *Skeletal age changes in young American males.* Natwick, MA. Quartermaster Research & Development Center, 1957; Francis, CC. *The appearance of centers of ossification from 6 to 15 years.* Anat Rec 1940; 27:127).

B. Epiphyses. Observe:
1. The ends of the long bones are ossified by the formation of one or more secondary centers of ossification; these develop from birth to approximately 20 years of age in the clavicle, humerus, radius, ulna, metacarpals and phalanges;

2. When the epiphysis and diaphysis join (fuse), active bone growth stops; sometimes as in the proximal humerus many epiphyses fuse to form a single mass that later fuses with the diaphysis, i.e., three centers of ossification develop (one for the head, the greater tubercle, and the lesser tubercle) and fuse into a single mass by the 7th year and to the diaphysis by the 24th year;

3. The epiphysis of the clavicle is the last of the long bone epiphyses to fuse (by 31 years); the acromial epiphysis of the scapula may also persist into adult life.

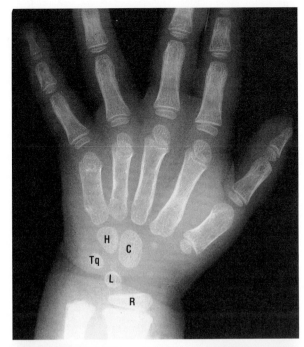

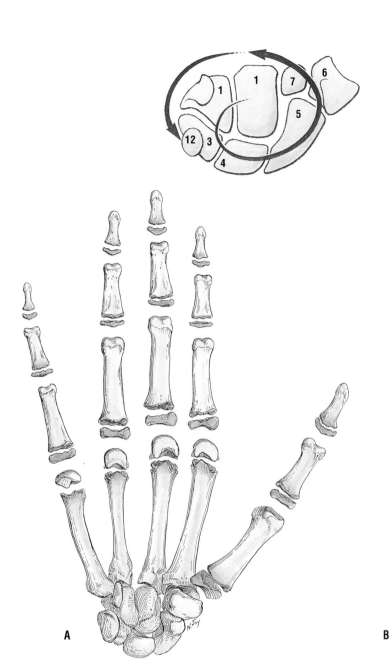

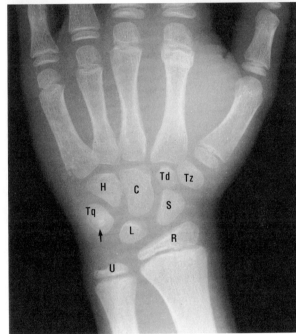

6.3
Epiphyses of hand and wrist

A. Ossification of the bones of the hand. Observe:

1. Phalanges have a single proximal epiphysis;

2. Metacarpals 2, 3, 4, and 5 have single distal epiphyses; the 1st metacarpal behaves as a phalanx by having a proximal epiphysis; Short-lived epiphyses may appear at the other ends of the metacarpals 1 and/or 2;

3. The capitate starts to ossify soon after birth; the *arrows* show the spiral sequence of ossification of the carpals with approximate age in years; there are individual and sex differences in sequence and timing (see Pyle SI, Waterhouse AM, Gruelich WW. *A Radiographic Standard of Reference for the Growing Hand and Wrist.* Chicago, Case Western Reserve University Press, (1971).

B. Radiographs of the hand and wrist are commonly used to assess skeletal age.

1. A 2 1/2-year-old child; *C* - Capitate, *H* - Hamate, *Tq* - Triquetrum, and *L* - Lunate are ossifying; the distal radial epiphysis *(R)* is present.

2. An 11-year-old; all carpal bones are ossified (*S* - Scapnoid, *Td* - Trapezoid, *Tz* - Trapezium, *Arrowhead* - Pisiform); the distal epiphysis of the ulna *(U)* has ossified.

(Courtesy of Dr. D. Armstrong, Associate Professor of Radiology, University of Toronto, Toronto, Ontario, Canada.)

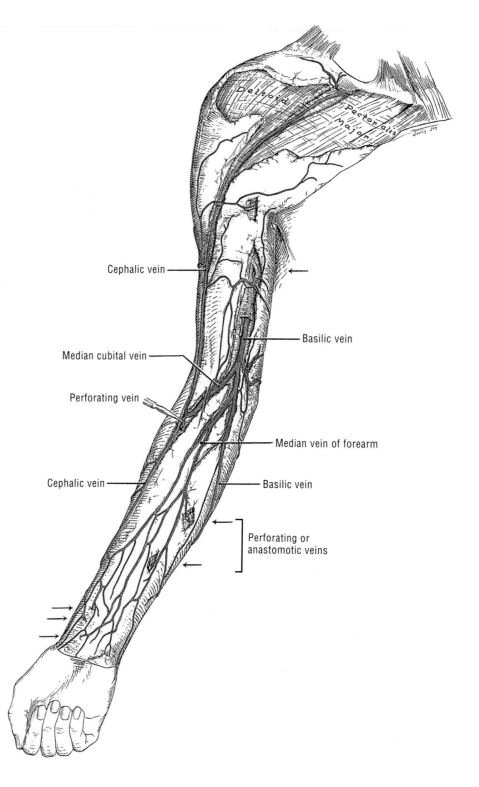

Cephalic vein

Basilic vein

Median cubital vein

Perforating vein

Median vein of forearm

Cephalic vein

Basilic vein

Perforating or anastomotic veins

6.4
Superficial veins of the upper limb

The *arrows* indicate where perforating veins pierce the deep fascia and bring the superficial and deep veins of the limb into communication with each other.

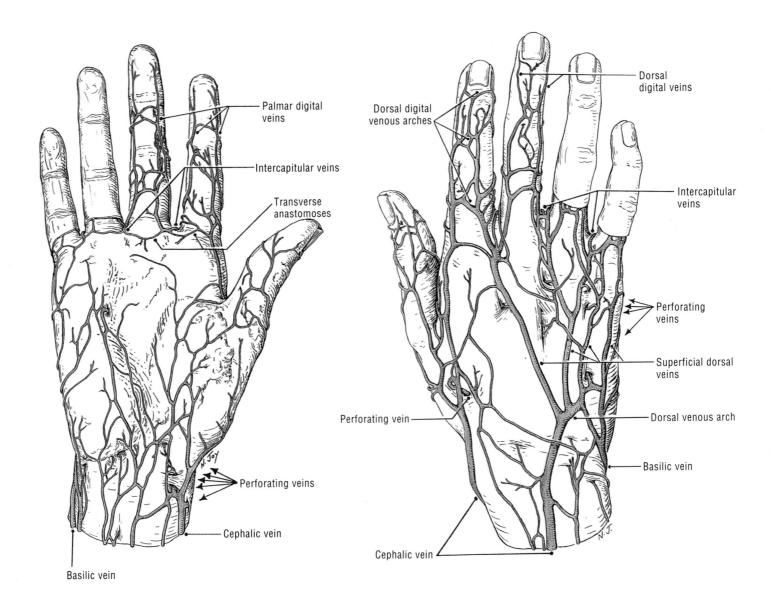

Palmar digital
veins

Intercapitular veins

Transverse
anastomoses

Dorsal digital
venous arches

Dorsal
digital veins

Intercapitular
veins

Perforating
veins

Superficial dorsal
veins

Perforating vein

Dorsal venous arch

Basilic vein

Perforating veins

Cephalic vein

Cephalic vein

Basilic vein

A, *Palmar view*

B, *Dorsal view*

6.5
Superficial veins of the hand

For obvious mechanical reasons, the palmar veins are few and small, and the dorsal veins
are large.

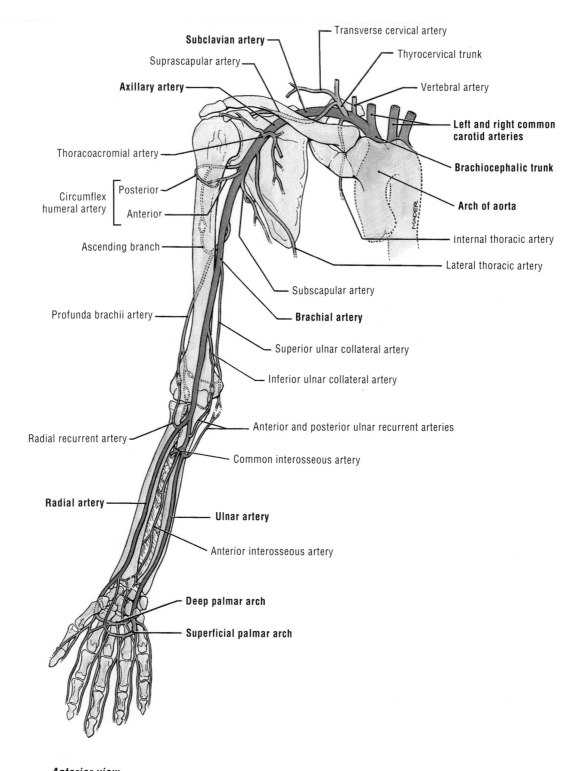

Subclavian artery

Transverse cervical artery

Thyrocervical trunk

Suprascapular artery

Axillary artery

Vertebral artery

Left and right common carotid arteries

Thoracoacromial artery

Brachiocephalic trunk

Circumflex humeral artery
Posterior
Anterior

Arch of aorta

Ascending branch

Internal thoracic artery

Lateral thoracic artery

Subscapular artery

Profunda brachii artery

Brachial artery

Superior ulnar collateral artery

Inferior ulnar collateral artery

Anterior and posterior ulnar recurrent arteries

Radial recurrent artery

Common interosseous artery

Radial artery

Ulnar artery

Anterior interosseous artery

Deep palmar arch

Superficial palmar arch

Anterior view

6.6
Diagram of the arteries of the upper limb

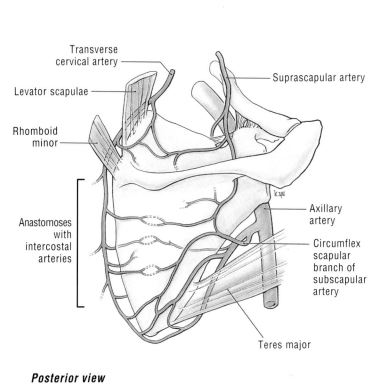

Transverse
cervical artery

Levator scapulae

Rhomboid
minor

Anastomoses
with
intercostal
arteries

Suprascapular artery

Axillary
artery

Circumflex
scapular
branch of
subscapular
artery

Teres major

Posterior view

6.7
Arterial anastomoses around the scapula

Anastomotic
branch

Profunda
brachii artery

Posterior branch
Anterior branch

Ulnar artery

Radial artery

Teres
major

Brachial artery

Superior ulnar
collateral artery

Inferior ulnar
collateral artery

Anterior ⎤ Ulnar
       ⎥ recurrent
Posterior ⎦ arteries

Common ⎤
       ⎥ Interosseous
Anterior ⎥ arteries
       ⎥
Posterior ⎦

6.8
Arterial anastomoses around the elbow

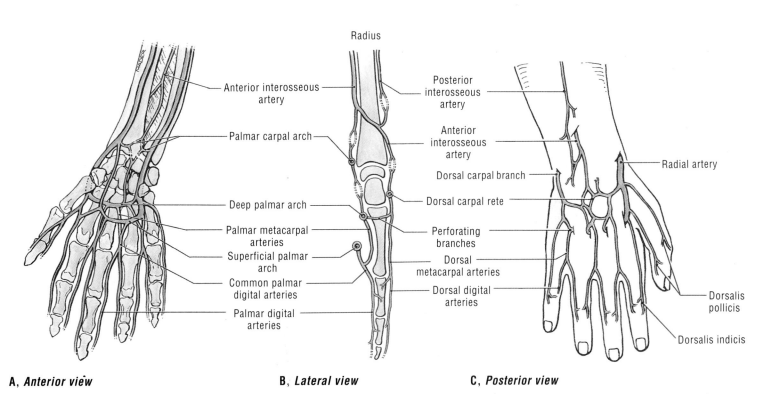

Radius

Anterior interosseous
artery

Palmar carpal arch

Deep palmar arch

Palmar metacarpal
arteries

Superficial palmar
arch

Common palmar
digital arteries

Palmar digital
arteries

Posterior
interosseous
artery

Anterior
interosseous
artery

Dorsal carpal branch

Dorsal carpal rete

Perforating
branches

Dorsal
metacarpal arteries

Dorsal digital
arteries

Radial artery

Dorsalis
pollicis

Dorsalis indicis

A, *Anterior view*   B, *Lateral view*   C, *Posterior view*

6.9
Arterial anastomoses of the hand

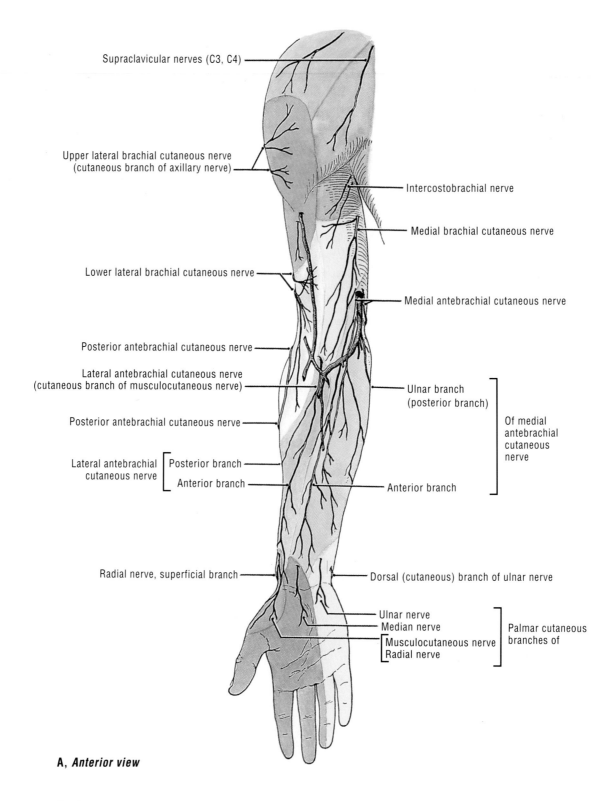

Supraclavicular nerves (C3, C4)

Upper lateral brachial cutaneous nerve
(cutaneous branch of axillary nerve)

Intercostobrachial nerve

Medial brachial cutaneous nerve

Lower lateral brachial cutaneous nerve

Medial antebrachial cutaneous nerve

Posterior antebrachial cutaneous nerve

Lateral antebrachial cutaneous nerve
(cutaneous branch of musculocutaneous nerve)

Ulnar branch
(posterior branch)

Of medial
antebrachial
cutaneous
nerve

Posterior antebrachial cutaneous nerve

Lateral antebrachial
cutaneous nerve { Posterior branch
Anterior branch }

Anterior branch

Radial nerve, superficial branch

Dorsal (cutaneous) branch of ulnar nerve

Ulnar nerve
Median nerve
{ Musculocutaneous nerve
Radial nerve }

Palmar cutaneous
branches of

A, *Anterior view*

6.10
Cutaneous nerves of the upper limb

A. Of the five terminal branches of the brachial plexus – musculocutaneous, median, ulnar, radial, and axillary nerves – the first four contribute cutaneous branches to the hand.

The posterior cord of the plexus is represented by five cutaneous nerves. One of these, the upper lateral brachial cutaneous nerve, is a branch of the axillary nerve.

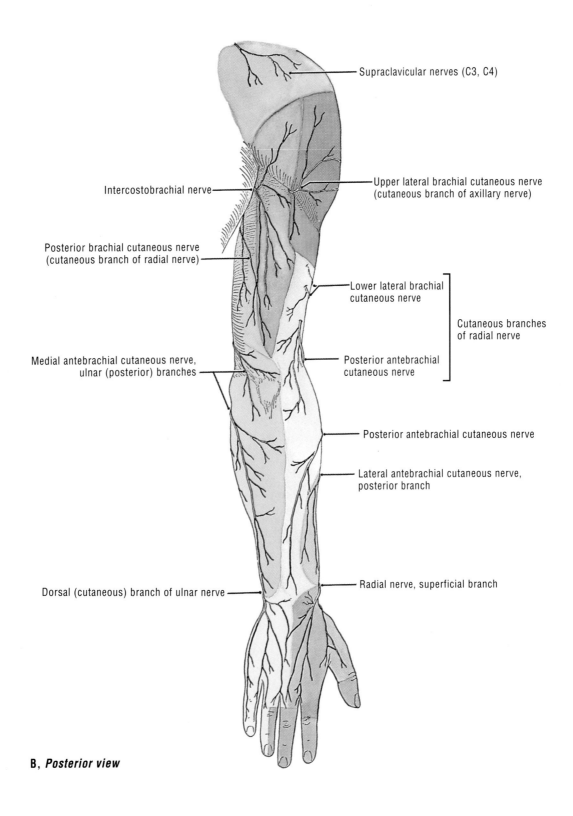

Supraclavicular nerves (C3, C4)

Intercostobrachial nerve

Upper lateral brachial cutaneous nerve
(cutaneous branch of axillary nerve)

Posterior brachial cutaneous nerve
(cutaneous branch of radial nerve)

Lower lateral brachial
cutaneous nerve

Cutaneous branches
of radial nerve

Medial antebrachial cutaneous nerve,
ulnar (posterior) branches

Posterior antebrachial
cutaneous nerve

Posterior antebrachial cutaneous nerve

Lateral antebrachial cutaneous nerve,
posterior branch

Dorsal (cutaneous) branch of ulnar nerve

Radial nerve, superficial branch

B, *Posterior view*

6.10
Cutaneous nerves of the upper limb *(continued)*

B. The other branches of the posterior cord are: the posterior brachial cutaneous nerve, the lower lateral brachial cutaneous nerve, the posterior antebrachial cutaneous nerve, and the superficial branch of the radial nerve.

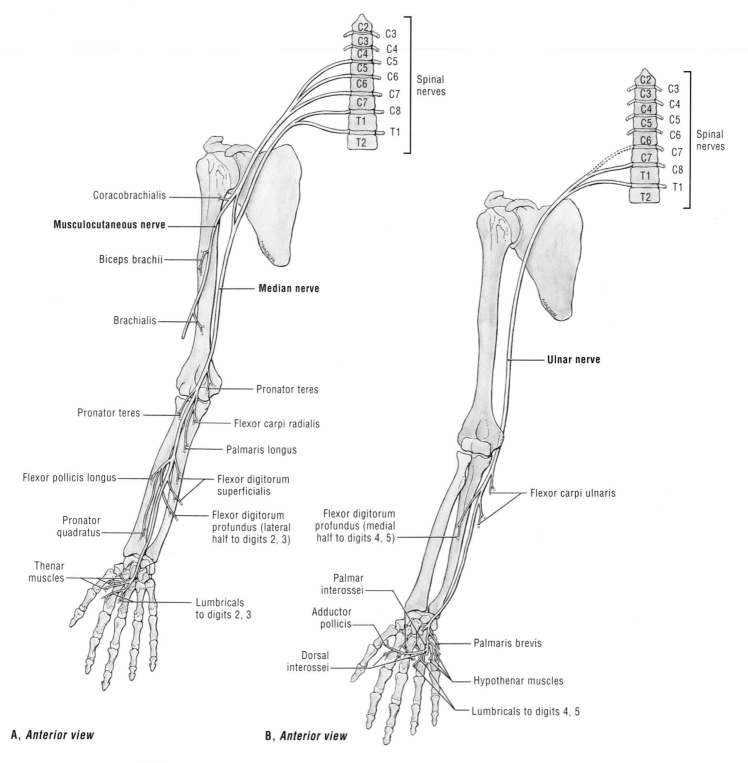

A, *Anterior view*

B, *Anterior view*

Labels in figure A (left):
Coracobrachialis
Musculocutaneous nerve
Biceps brachii
Median nerve
Brachialis
Pronator teres
Pronator teres
Flexor carpi radialis
Palmaris longus
Flexor pollicis longus
Flexor digitorum superficialis
Flexor digitorum profundus (lateral half to digits 2, 3)
Pronator quadratus
Thenar muscles
Lumbricals to digits 2, 3

Spinal nerves
C3 C4 C5 C6 C7 C8 T1
C2 C3 C4 C5 C6 C7 T1 T2

Labels in figure B (right):
Ulnar nerve
Flexor carpi ulnaris
Flexor digitorum profundus (medial half to digits 4, 5)
Palmar interossei
Adductor pollicis
Dorsal interossei
Palmaris brevis
Hypothenar muscles
Lumbricals to digits 4, 5

Spinal nerves
C3 C4 C5 C6 C7 C8 T1
C2 C3 C4 C5 C6 C7 T1 T2

6.11
Summary of the innervation of the muscles of the upper limb

A. Median and musculocutaneous nerves. The average levels at which the motor branches leave the stems of the main nerves are shown.

B. Ulnar nerve. The average levels of origin of the motor branches are shown. There are no fleshy muscle fibers on the dorsum of the hand, and therefore, there are no motor nerves.

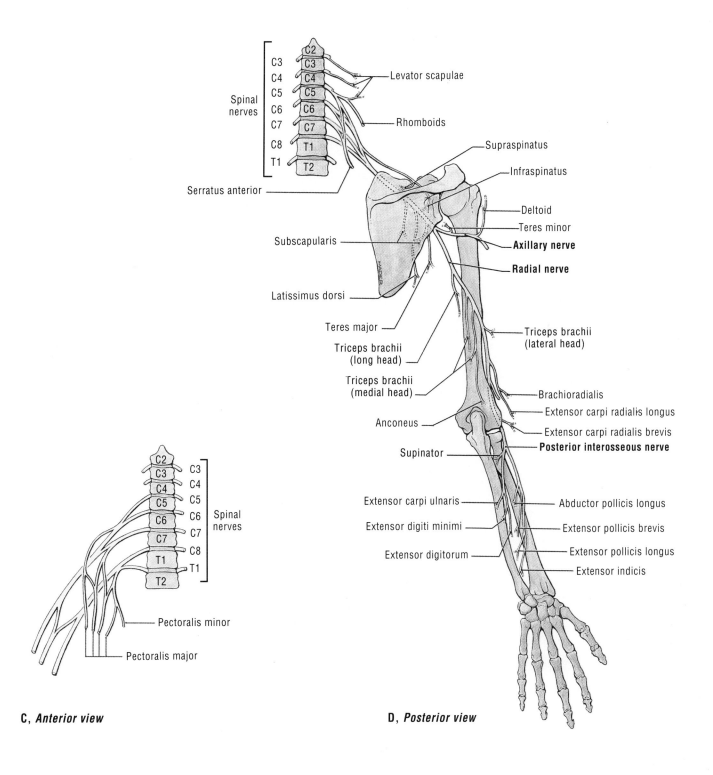

Levator scapulae

Rhomboids

Supraspinatus

Infraspinatus

Deltoid

Teres minor

Axillary nerve

Radial nerve

Triceps brachii
(lateral head)

Brachioradialis

Extensor carpi radialis longus

Extensor carpi radialis brevis

Posterior interosseous nerve

Abductor pollicis longus

Extensor pollicis brevis

Extensor pollicis longus

Extensor indicis

Serratus anterior

Spinal
nerves

Subscapularis

Latissimus dorsi

Teres major

Triceps brachii
(long head)

Triceps brachii
(medial head)

Anconeus

Supinator

Extensor carpi ulnaris

Extensor digiti minimi

Extensor digitorum

Spinal
nerves

Pectoralis minor

Pectoralis major

C, *Anterior view*

D, *Posterior view*

6.11
Summary of the innervation of the muscles of the upper limb *(continued)*

C. Medial and lateral pectoral nerves. **D.** Radial nerve.

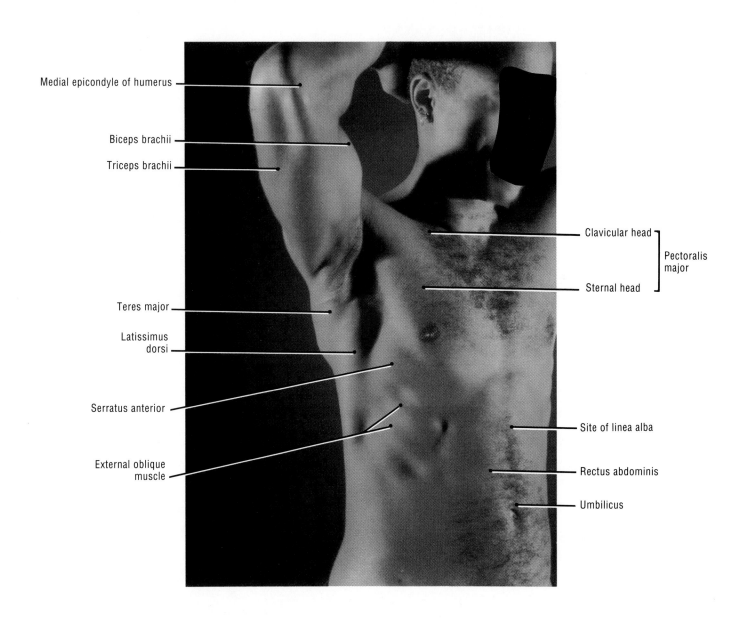

Medial epicondyle of humerus

Biceps brachii

Triceps brachii

Teres major

Latissimus dorsi

Serratus anterior

External oblique muscle

Clavicular head ⎤
                  ⎥ Pectoralis
                  ⎥ major
Sternal head ⎦

Site of linea alba

Rectus abdominis

Umbilicus

6.12
Surface anatomy of the axilla and the anterolateral aspect of the trunk

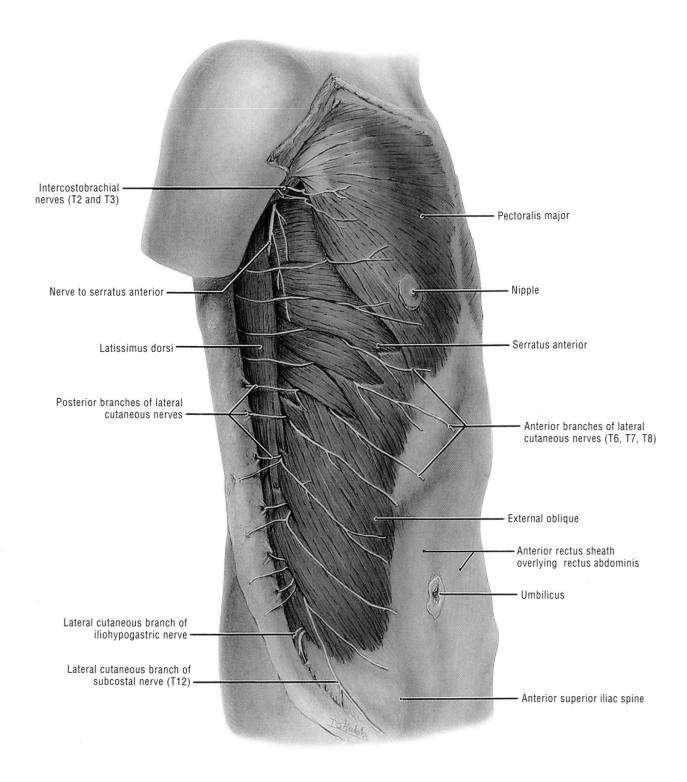

Intercostobrachial nerves (T2 and T3)

Nerve to serratus anterior

Latissimus dorsi

Posterior branches of lateral cutaneous nerves

Lateral cutaneous branch of iliohypogastric nerve

Lateral cutaneous branch of subcostal nerve (T12)

Pectoralis major

Nipple

Serratus anterior

Anterior branches of lateral cutaneous nerves (T6, T7, T8)

External oblique

Anterior rectus sheath overlying rectus abdominis

Umbilicus

Anterior superior iliac spine

Lateral view

6.13
Trunk

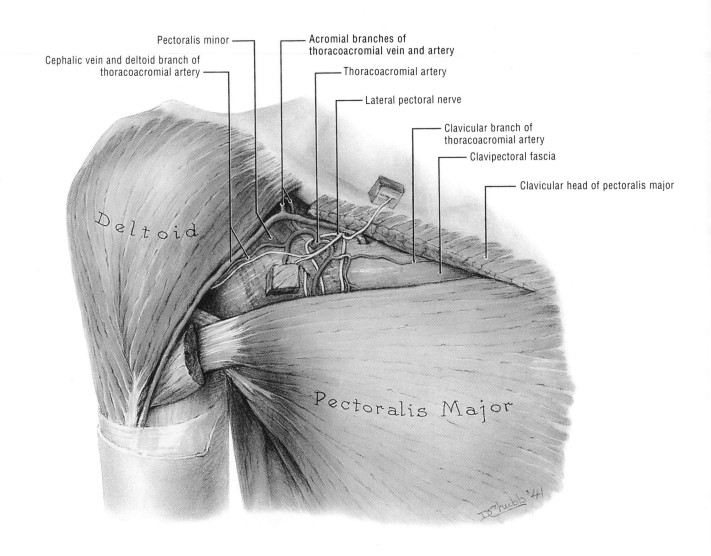

Pectoralis minor

Acromial branches of
thoracoacromial vein and artery

Cephalic vein and deltoid branch of
thoracoacromial artery

Thoracoacromial artery

Lateral pectoral nerve

Clavicular branch of
thoracoacromial artery

Clavipectoral fascia

Clavicular head of pectoralis major

Deltoid

Pectoralis Major

6.14
Anterior wall of axilla, clavipectoral fascia

The clavicular head of pectoralis major is excised except for two cubes that remain to identify its nerves. The thoracoacromial (acromiothoracic) veins, which join the cephalic vein, are removed.

Observe:

1. The part of the clavipectoral fascia superior to pectoralis minor – the costocoracoid membrane pierced by the lateral pectoral nerve and its companion vessels;

2. The part of the fascia enclosing pectoralis minor; here muscle and fascia are pierced by medial pectoral nerve, thoracoacromial artery, and cephalic vein;

3. The trilaminar insertion of pectoralis major;

4. The course of the cephalic vein through the deltopectoral triangle and costocoracoid membrane.

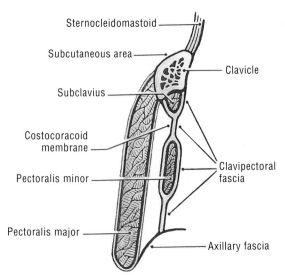

Sternocleidomastoid

Subcutaneous area

Clavicle

Subclavius

Costocoracoid
membrane

Clavipectoral
fascia

Pectoralis minor

Pectoralis major

Axillary fascia

6.15
Pectoral muscles and fascia, sagittal section

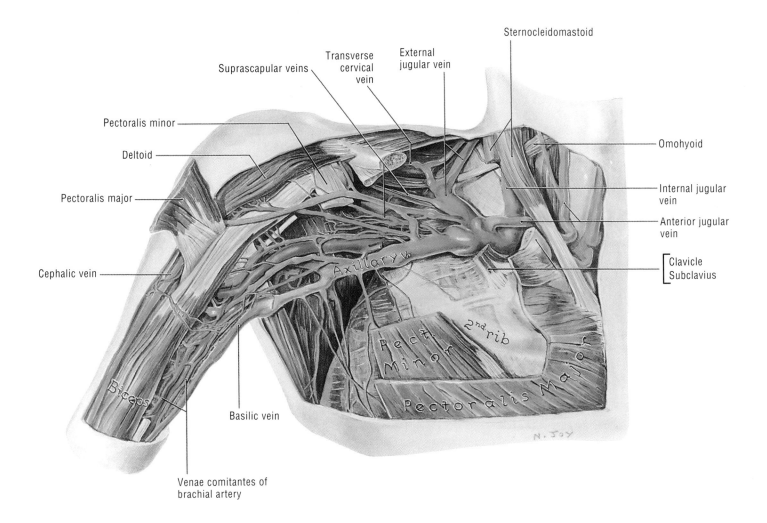

Suprascapular veins

Pectoralis minor

Deltoid

Pectoralis major

Cephalic vein

Transverse cervical vein

External jugular vein

Sternocleidomastoid

Omohyoid

Internal jugular vein

Anterior jugular vein

Clavicle
Subclavius

Axillary v.

2nd rib

Pect. Minor

Pectoralis Major

N. Joy

Biceps

Basilic vein

Venae comitantes of brachial artery

6.16
Veins of the axilla

Observe:

1. The basilic vein becoming the axillary vein at the inferior border of the teres major muscle; the axillary vein becoming the subclavian vein at the 1st rib; and the subclavian joining the internal jugular to become the brachiocephalic vein posterior to the sternal end of the clavicle; over 40 venous valves are shown; note three in the axillary and one in the subclavian, which is the last valve before the heart;

2. Venae comitantes of the brachial artery uniting and joining the axillary vein near the middle of the axilla;

3. The cephalic vein here bifurcating to end both in the axillary and in the external jugular vein;

4. The profunda brachii, posterior humeral circumflex, and cir-

cumflex scapular venae comitantes united and, as one large vein, joining the axillary vein;

5. Three suprascapular veins: one from inferior to the suprascapular ligament to the axillary vein, and two superior to the ligament to the external jugular vein;

6. Anastomotic veins are in view; obviously those on the dorsum of the scapula joining circumflex scapular and suprascapular veins cannot be seen;

7. The large number of veins in the axilla, which should be removed prior to dissection of the nerves and arteries in the region.

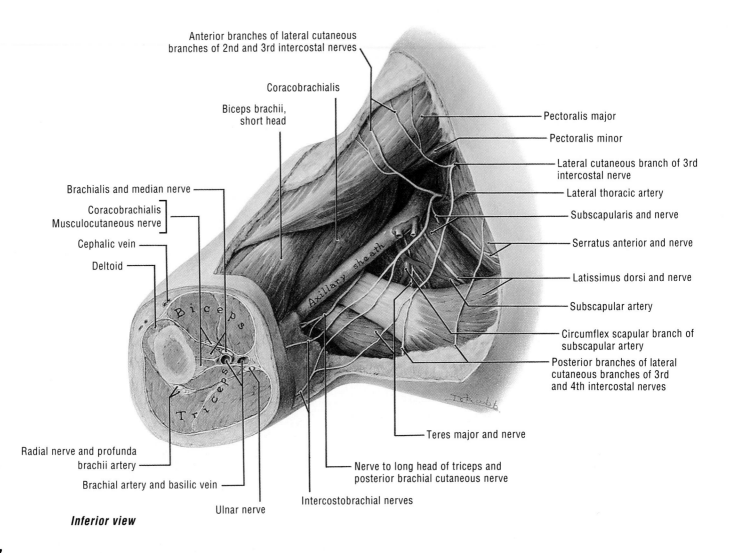

Anterior branches of lateral cutaneous branches of 2nd and 3rd intercostal nerves

Coracobrachialis

Biceps brachii, short head

Brachialis and median nerve

Coracobrachialis
Musculocutaneous nerve

Cephalic vein

Deltoid

Pectoralis major

Pectoralis minor

Lateral cutaneous branch of 3rd intercostal nerve

Lateral thoracic artery

Subscapularis and nerve

Serratus anterior and nerve

Latissimus dorsi and nerve

Subscapular artery

Circumflex scapular branch of subscapular artery

Posterior branches of lateral cutaneous branches of 3rd and 4th intercostal nerves

Teres major and nerve

Radial nerve and profunda brachii artery

Brachial artery and basilic vein

Ulnar nerve

Nerve to long head of triceps and posterior brachial cutaneous nerve

Intercostobrachial nerves

Inferior view

**6.17
Axilla**

**6.18
Walls of the axilla, transverse section**

Observe:

1. The three muscular walls of the axilla: (a) *Anterior wall:* pectoralis major, pectoralis minor, and subclavius muscles, but only the inferior borders of pectoral muscles are in view; (b) *Posterior wall:* subscapularis, latissimus dorsi, and teres major muscles; (c) *Medial wall:* serratus anterior muscle; the lateral or bony wall, the intertubercular (bicipital) groove of the humerus, is concealed by the biceps and coracobrachialis muscles;

2. The axillary sheath and the cutaneous nerves crossing the latissimus dorsi muscle; the most lateral of these nerves is also the sole nerve supply of long head of triceps muscle;

3. The axillary sheath transmits the great nerves and vessels of the limb; it is a neurovascular bundle.

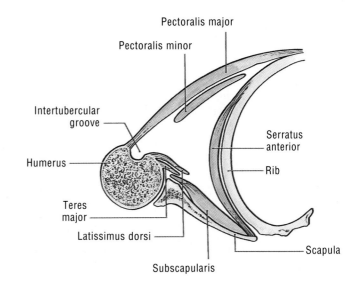

Pectoralis major

Pectoralis minor

Intertubercular groove

Humerus

Teres major

Latissimus dorsi

Subscapularis

Serratus anterior

Rib

Scapula

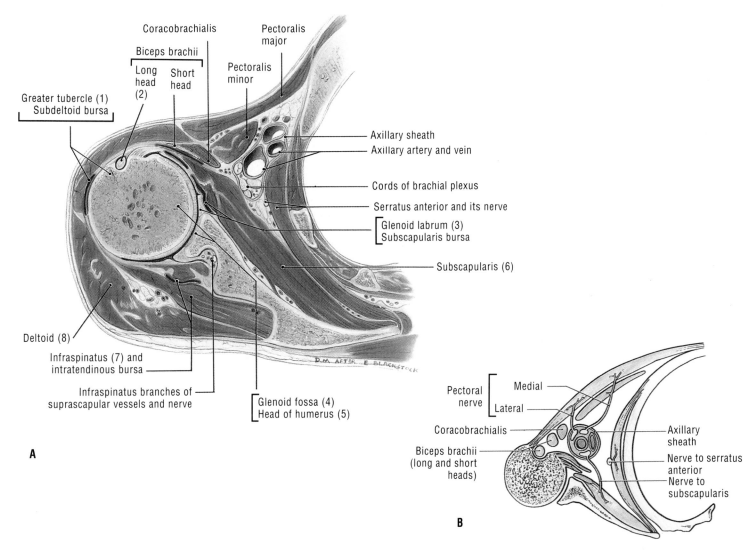

A

Greater tubercle (1)
Subdeltoid bursa

Biceps brachii
Long head (2)   Short head

Coracobrachialis

Pectoralis minor

Pectoralis major

Axillary sheath

Axillary artery and vein

Cords of brachial plexus

Serratus anterior and its nerve

Glenoid labrum (3)
Subscapularis bursa

Subscapularis (6)

Deltoid (8)

Infraspinatus (7) and intratendinous bursa

Infraspinatus branches of suprascapular vessels and nerve

Glenoid fossa (4)
Head of humerus (5)

D.M AFTER E BLACKSTOCK

B

Pectoral nerve
Medial
Lateral

Coracobrachialis

Biceps brachii (long and short heads)

Axillary sheath

Nerve to serratus anterior

Nerve to subscapularis

6.19
Transverse section through the shoulder joint and axilla

Numbers in parentheses refer to Figure 6.20. Observe in **A** and **B**:
1. The tendon of the long head of the biceps brachii muscle, in its synovial sheath, facing anteriorly; the short head of the biceps muscle and the coracobrachialis and pectoralis minor muscles sectioned just inferior to their attachment to the coracoid process;

2. The fibrous capsule, thin posteriorly and partly fused with the tendon of infraspinatus; thicker anteriorly (glenohumeral ligaments); the small glenoid cavity, deepened by the glenoid labrum;

3. Bursae: (a) subdeltoid (subacromial) bursa, between deltoid and greater tubercle; (b) subscapular bursa, between subscapularis tendon and the scapula; (c) coracobrachialis bursa, between coracobrachialis and subscapularis;

4. Walls of the axilla near its apex, formed by subscapularis and scapula posteriorly; serratus anterior, ribs, and intercostals medially; and the pectoralis major and minor muscles anteriorly; there is no bone in the anterior wall;

5. The axillary sheath enclosing the axillary artery and vein and the three cords of the brachial plexus to form a neurovascular bundle, surrounded with axillary fat.

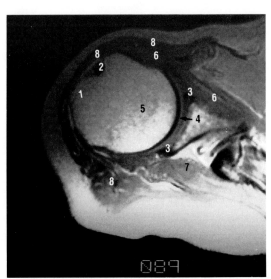

6.20
Transverse MRI (magnetic resonance image) of the shoulder

(Courtesy of Dr. W. Kucharczyk, Clinical Director of Tri-Hospital Magnetic Resonance Centre, Toronto, Ontario, Canada.)

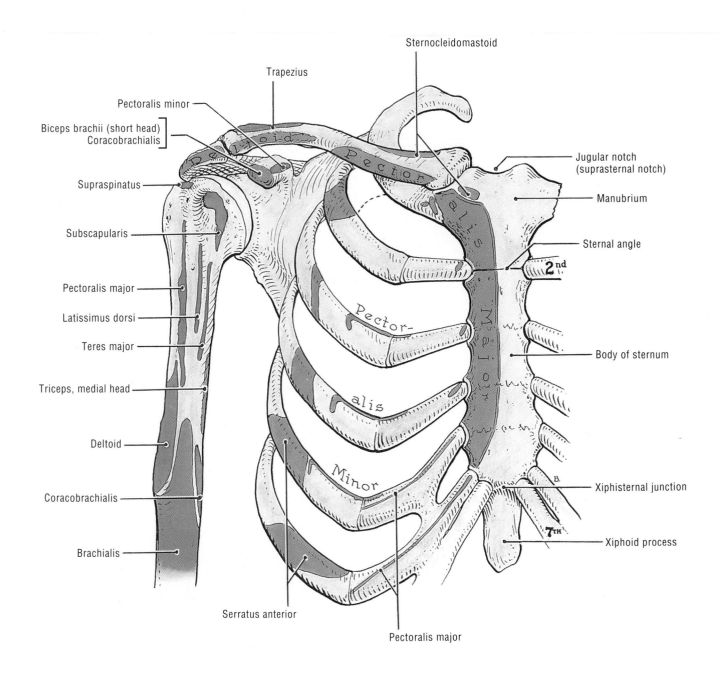

6.21

Bones of the pectoral region and axilla showing attachments of muscles

Observe:

1. The following muscles attached in line with each other: horizontally, on the clavicle: the trapezius and sternocleidomastoid; deltoid and clavicular head of the pectoralis major; longitudinally, on the humerus: supraspinatus, pectoralis major, and anterior fibers of the deltoid; subscapularis and latissimus dorsi and teres major;

2. The pectoralis major muscle has a crescentic attachment from the clavicle, sternum, and the 5th and (or) 6th costal cartilages;

3. The pectoralis minor muscle here attaching to the 3rd, 4th, and 5th ribs; it commonly arises also from either the 2nd or the 6th rib.

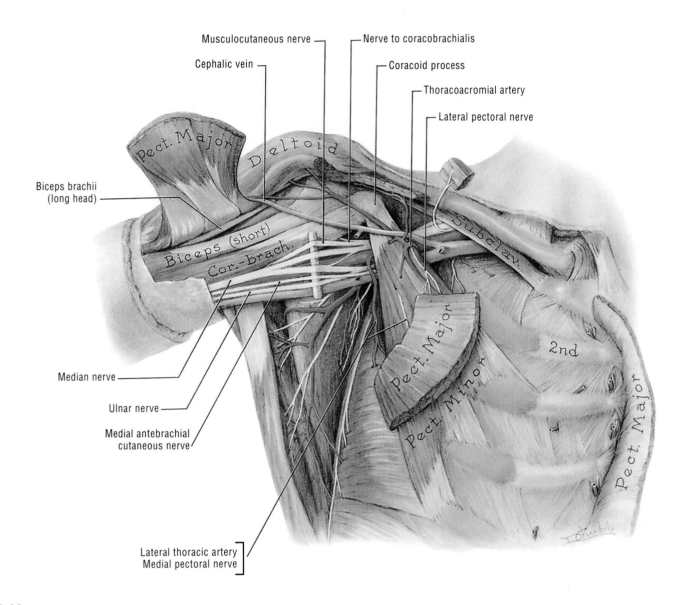

Musculocutaneous nerve

Cephalic vein

Nerve to coracobrachialis

Coracoid process

Thoracoacromial artery

Lateral pectoral nerve

Pect. Major

Deltoid

Biceps brachii (long head)

Subclav.

Biceps (short)

Cor. brach.

Pect. Major

Pect. Minor

2nd

Pect. Major

Median nerve

Ulnar nerve

Medial antebrachial cutaneous nerve

Lateral thoracic artery
Medial pectoral nerve

6.22
Anterior structures of the axilla

The pectoralis major muscle is reflected and the clavipectoral fascia removed.

Observe:

1. Subclavius and pectoralis minor, the two deep muscles of the anterior wall;

2. The axillary artery passing posterior to the pectoralis minor muscle, a finger's breadth from the tip of the coracoid process, and having the lateral cord on its lateral side and the medial cord on its medial side;

3. The axillary vein lying medial to the axillary artery;

4. The median nerve, followed proximally, leading by its lateral root to the lateral cord and the musculocutaneous nerve, and by its medial root to the medial cord and the ulnar nerve; these four nerves and the medial antebrachial cutaneous nerve are raised on a stick; the lateral root of the median nerve may be in several strands;

5. The nerve to coracobrachialis arising within the axilla;

6. The cube of muscle superior to the clavicle is cut from the clavicular head of pectoralis major muscle.

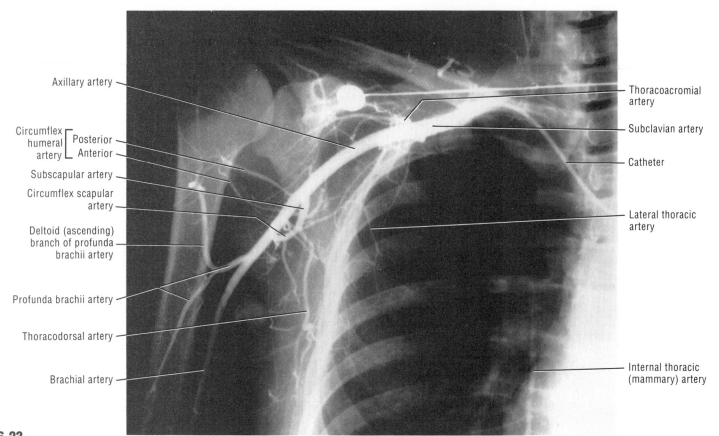

Axillary artery

Circumflex humeral artery [Posterior / Anterior]

Subscapular artery

Circumflex scapular artery

Deltoid (ascending) branch of profunda brachii artery

Profunda brachii artery

Thoracodorsal artery

Brachial artery

Thoracoacromial artery

Subclavian artery

Catheter

Lateral thoracic artery

Internal thoracic (mammary) artery

6.23
Axillary arteriogram

(Courtesy of Dr. D. Armstrong, Associate Professor of Radiology, University of Toronto, Toronto, Ontario, Canada.)

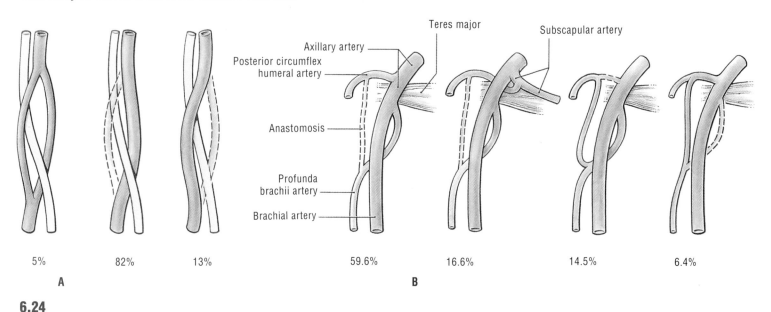

5%   82%   13%

A

Teres major   **Subscapular artery**

Axillary artery

Posterior circumflex humeral artery

Anastomosis

Profunda brachii artery

Brachial artery

59.6%   16.6%   14.5%   6.4%

B

6.24
Arterial anomalies

A. Median nerve and brachial artery. The variable relationship of these two structures may be explained developmentally. In a study of 307 limbs, both primitive brachial arteries persisted in 5%, the posterior in 82%, and the anterior in 13%.

B. Posterior circumflex humeral and profunda brachii arteries. Four types of variations in origin of the posterior humeral circumflex and profunda brachii arteries are shown; in 2.9%, the arteries were otherwise irregular. Percentages are based on 235 specimens.

         Grant's Atlas of Anatomy

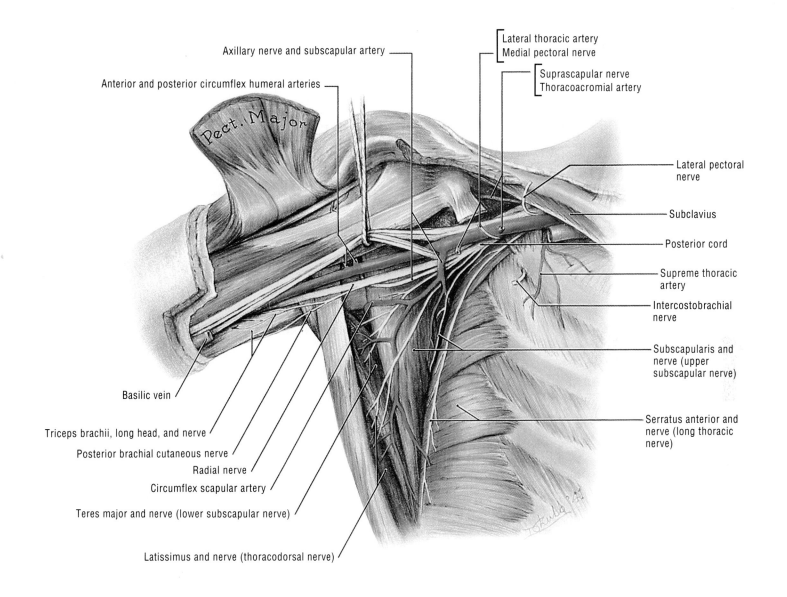

Axillary nerve and subscapular artery

Anterior and posterior circumflex humeral arteries

Pect. Major

Lateral thoracic artery
Medial pectoral nerve

Suprascapular nerve
Thoracoacromial artery

Lateral pectoral nerve

Subclavius

Posterior cord

Supreme thoracic artery

Intercostobrachial nerve

Subscapularis and nerve (upper subscapular nerve)

Serratus anterior and nerve (long thoracic nerve)

Basilic vein

Triceps brachii, long head, and nerve

Posterior brachial cutaneous nerve

Radial nerve

Circumflex scapular artery

Teres major and nerve (lower subscapular nerve)

Latissimus and nerve (thoracodorsal nerve)

6.25
Posterior and medial walls of the axilla

The pectoralis minor muscle is excised; the lateral and medial cords are retracted; the axillary vein is removed.

Observe:
1. The posterior cord and its two terminal branches (the radial and axillary nerves), lying posterior to the axillary artery;

2. The nerves to the three posterior muscles; of these: (a) nerve to the latissimus dorsi muscle enters the deep surface of its muscle 1 cm from its free lateral border at a point midway between the thoracic wall and the abducted arm; (b) upper nerve to subscapularis lies parallel to (a) but superior to it; (c) lower nerve to subscapularis and to teres major muscle lies parallel to (a) but inferior to it;

3. Nerve to serratus anterior clinging to its muscle throughout; superiorly, some fat may intervene;

4. Suprascapular nerve passing toward the base of the coracoid process;

5. Subscapular artery, the largest branch of the axillary artery; here arising more proximally; usually it arises at the inferior border of subscapularis;

6. Posterior circumflex humeral artery accompanying the axillary nerve through the quadrangular space.

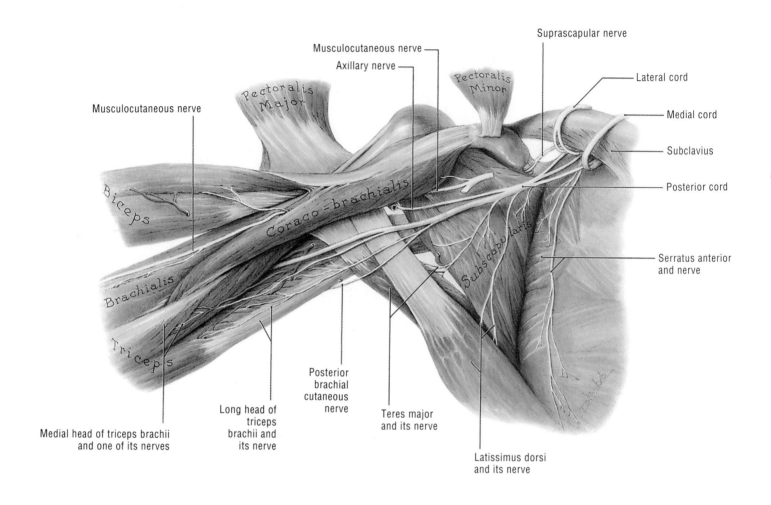

Suprascapular nerve

Musculocutaneous nerve

Axillary nerve

Pectoralis Minor

Pectoralis Major

Lateral cord

Medial cord

Subclavius

Posterior cord

Musculocutaneous nerve

Biceps

Coraco-brachialis

Serratus anterior and nerve

Subscapularis

Brachialis

Triceps

Medial head of triceps brachii and one of its nerves

Long head of triceps brachii and its nerve

Posterior brachial cutaneous nerve

Teres major and its nerve

Latissimus dorsi and its nerve

6.26
Posterior wall of the axilla, musculocutaneous nerve, posterior cord

The pectoralis major and minor muscles are reflected laterally; the lateral and medial cords are reflected superiorly; the arteries, veins, and median and ulnar nerves are removed.

Observe:

1. Coracobrachialis arising with the short head of the biceps brachii muscle from the tip of the coracoid process and attaching halfway down the humerus;

2. The musculocutaneous nerve piercing the coracobrachialis muscle, and supplying it, the biceps, and the brachialis before becoming cutaneous;

3. The posterior cord of the plexus formed by the union of the three posterior divisions, supplying the three muscles of the posterior wall of the axilla, and soon ending as the radial and axillary nerves;

4. The radial nerve giving off, in the axilla, the nerve to the long head of the triceps brachii muscle and a cutaneous branch, and, in this specimen, a branch to the medial head of the triceps; it then enters the radial (spiral) groove of the humerus with the profunda brachii artery;

5. The axillary nerve traversing the quadrangular space with the posterior circumflex humeral artery; the circumflex scapular artery traversing the triangular space.

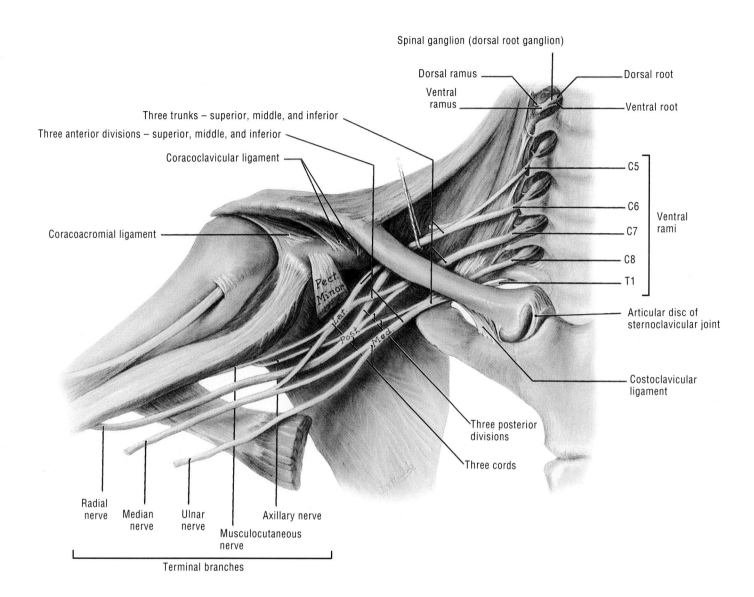

Spinal ganglion (dorsal root ganglion)

Dorsal ramus

Ventral ramus

Three trunks – superior, middle, and inferior

Three anterior divisions – superior, middle, and inferior

Coracoclavicular ligament

Coracoacromial ligament

Dorsal root

Ventral root

C5

C6

C7

C8

T1

Ventral rami

Articular disc of sternoclavicular joint

Costoclavicular ligament

Three posterior divisions

Three cords

Radial nerve

Median nerve

Ulnar nerve

Musculocutaneous nerve

Axillary nerve

Terminal branches

6.27
Brachial plexus, ligaments of the clavicle

Observe:

1. A dorsal (sensory) root of a spinal nerve is larger than a ventral (motor) root;

2. The two roots uniting beyond the ganglion to form a very short mixed spinal nerve;

3. The mixed nerve at once dividing into a small dorsal ramus and a large ventral ramus;

4. The five ventral rami forming the brachial plexus; of these, the middle ramus, C7, is the largest;

5. These five rami uniting to form the three trunks of the plexus;

6. Each trunk dividing into two divisions, an anterior and a posterior;

7. These six divisions becoming three cords – a lateral, a medial, and a posterior;

8. The three cords lying posterior to the pectoralis minor muscle.

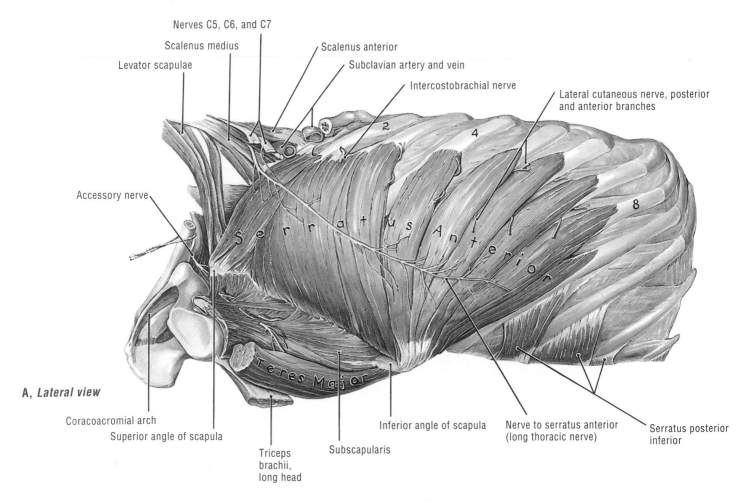

Nerves C5, C6, and C7

Scalenus medius

Levator scapulae

Scalenus anterior

Subclavian artery and vein

Intercostobrachial nerve

Lateral cutaneous nerve, posterior and anterior branches

Accessory nerve

A, *Lateral view*

Coracoacromial arch

Superior angle of scapula

Triceps brachii, long head

Subscapularis

Inferior angle of scapula

Nerve to serratus anterior (long thoracic nerve)

Serratus posterior inferior

6.28
Serratus anterior

A. Supine position. **B.** Distal attachment (insertion). Observe in **A** and **B**:

1. The serratus anterior muscle, which forms the medial wall of the axilla, having an extensive fleshy span from the superior eight (here nine) ribs in the midclavicular line, to the medial border of the scapula (**B**); the fibers from the 1st rib and from the arch between the 1st and 2nd ribs converging on the superior angle of the scapula, those from the 2nd and 3rd ribs diverging to spread thinly along the medial border; and the remainder (from 4th to 9th ribs), which form the bulk of the muscle, converging on the inferior angle and, therefore, having a tendinous insertion;

2. The nerve to serratus anterior, arising from C5, C6, and C7 and applied to the whole length of the muscle; the fibers from C5 and C6 piercing scalenus medius and appearing lateral to the brachial plexus; those from C7 descending posterior to the plexus;

3. The teres major muscle applied to the lateral border of the subscapularis muscle; the nerve to the teres major muscle helping to supply subscapularis;

4. The brachial plexus and the subclavian artery appearing between the scalenus anterior and scalenus medius muscles; the subclavian vein separated from the artery by the scalenus anterior muscle.

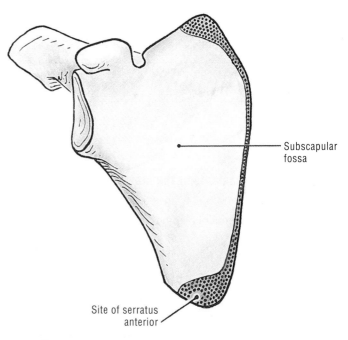

Subscapular fossa

Site of serratus anterior

B

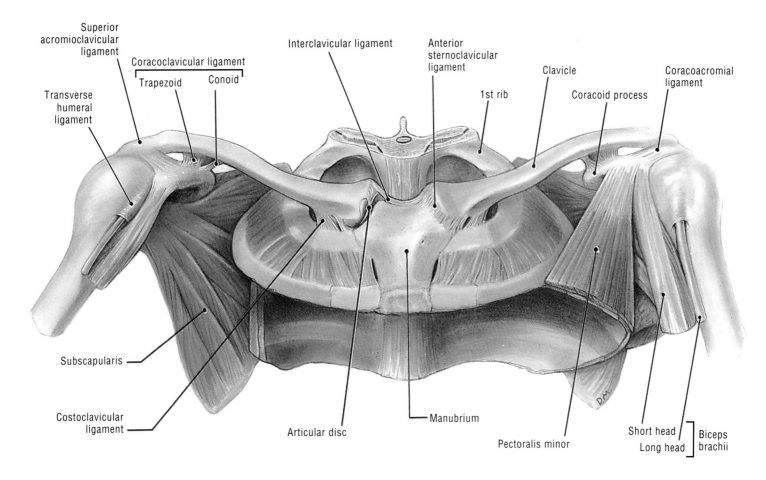

Superior acromioclavicular ligament

Coracoclavicular ligament
Trapezoid   Conoid

Transverse humeral ligament

Interclavicular ligament

Anterior sternoclavicular ligament

Clavicle

Coracoacromial ligament

1st rib

Coracoid process

Subscapularis

Costoclavicular ligament

Articular disc

Manubrium

Pectoralis minor

Short head
Long head

Biceps brachii

Anterosuperior view

6.29
Pectoral girdle

Observe:

1. The pectoral (shoulder) girdle consisting of the sternoclavicular, acromioclavicular, and shoulder (glenohumeral) joints; the mobility of the clavicle is essential for the freedom of movement of the upper limb;

2. The sternoclavicular joint is the only joint connecting the upper limb to the trunk; the articular disc of the sternoclavicular joint dividing the joint cavity into two parts and attaching superiorly to the clavicle and inferiorly to the first costal cartilage; the articular disc resists superior and medial displacement of the clavicle;

3. The strong coracoclavicular ligament, consisting of the conoid and trapezoid ligaments, providing stability to the acromioclavicular joint; the ligament prevents the scapula from being driven medially and the acromion from being driven inferior to the clavicle;

4. The coracoacromial ligament together with the acromion and coracoid process forms a continuous ligamentous and bony structure, the coracoacromial arch; the arch prevents superior displacement of the head of the humerus.

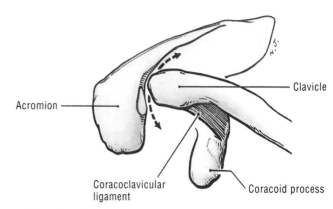

Acromion

Clavicle

Coracoclavicular ligament

Coracoid process

Superior view

6.30
Diagram of the coracoclavicular ligament

Observe that, as long as the coracoclavicular ligament is intact, the acromion cannot be driven inferior to the clavicle. This ligament, however, does not prevent protraction and retraction of the acromion.

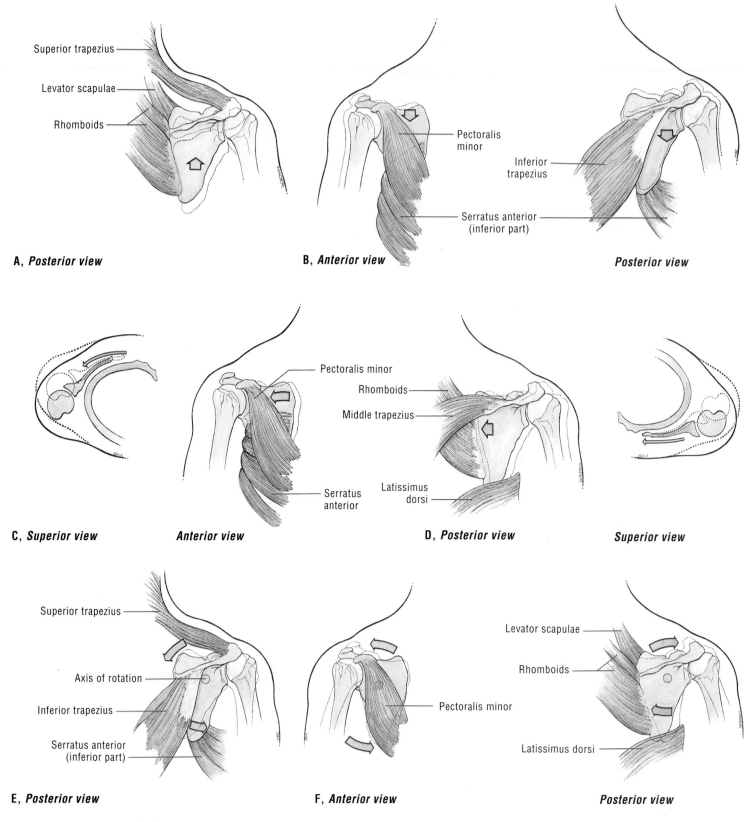

Superior trapezius

Levator scapulae

Rhomboids

A, *Posterior view*

Pectoralis
minor

Inferior
trapezius

Serratus anterior
(inferior part)

B, *Anterior view*

Posterior view

Pectoralis minor

Rhomboids

Middle trapezius

Latissimus
dorsi

Serratus
anterior

C, *Superior view*   *Anterior view*

D, *Posterior view*   *Superior view*

Superior trapezius

Axis of rotation

Inferior trapezius

Serratus anterior
(inferior part)

Pectoralis minor

Levator scapulae

Rhomboids

Latissimus dorsi

E, *Posterior view*

F, *Anterior view*

Posterior view

6.31
Scapular movements

A. Elevation. **B.** Depression. **C.** Protraction. **D.** Retraction. **E.** Elevation with superior (upward) rotation of glenoid fossa. **F.** Depression with inferior (downward) rotation of glenoid fossa. The *dotted outlines* represent the starting position for each of the movements.

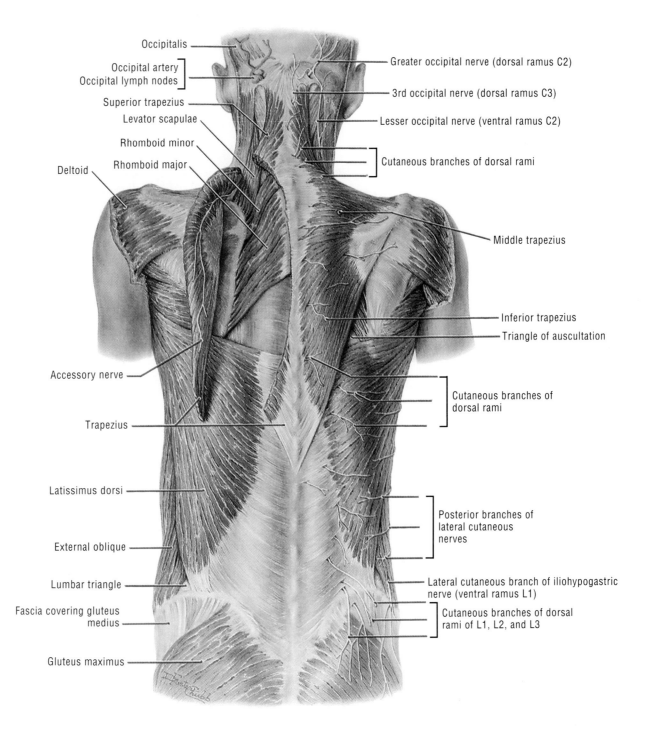

Occipitalis

Occipital artery
Occipital lymph nodes

Superior trapezius

Levator scapulae

Rhomboid minor

Rhomboid major

Deltoid

Accessory nerve

Trapezius

Latissimus dorsi

External oblique

Lumbar triangle

Fascia covering gluteus
medius

Gluteus maximus

Greater occipital nerve (dorsal ramus C2)

3rd occipital nerve (dorsal ramus C3)

Lesser occipital nerve (ventral ramus C2)

Cutaneous branches of dorsal rami

Middle trapezius

Inferior trapezius

Triangle of auscultation

Cutaneous branches of
dorsal rami

Posterior branches of
lateral cutaneous
nerves

Lateral cutaneous branch of iliohypogastric
nerve (ventral ramus L1)

Cutaneous branches of dorsal
rami of L1, L2, and L3

6.32
Cutaneous nerves of the back, the first two layers of muscles

The trapezius muscle is severed and reflected on the left side.

Observe:
1. The cutaneous branches of the dorsal rami;

2. The trapezius and latissimus dorsi muscles of the first layer; levator scapulae and rhomboid muscles of the second layer.

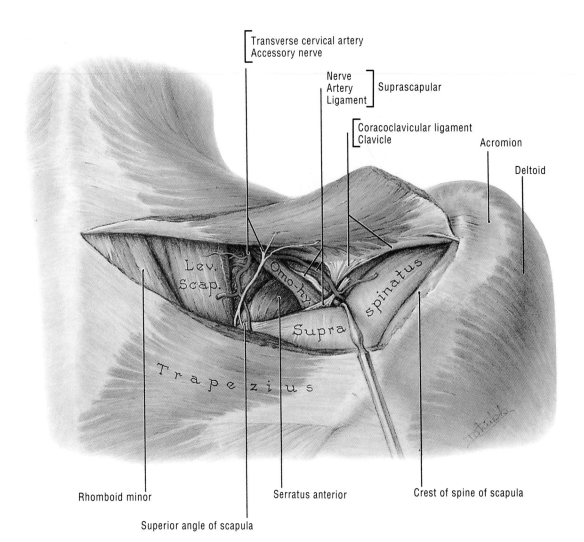

Transverse cervical artery
Accessory nerve

Nerve
Artery } Suprascapular
Ligament

Coracoclavicular ligament
Clavicle

Acromion

Deltoid

Lev.
Scap.

Omo-hy.

Supra   spinatus

T r a p e z i u s

Rhomboid minor

Superior angle of scapula

Serratus anterior

Crest of spine of scapula

6.33
Suprascapular region

The middle fibers of the trapezius muscle, at the level of the superior angle of the scapula, are separated and the incision is carried laterally along the crest of the spine of the scapula.

Observe:

1. The accessory nerve crossing the superior angle of the scapula;

2. The transverse cervical artery split by the levator scapulae muscle into a superficial and a deep branch, one following the accessory nerve, the other (not shown here) following the dorsal scapular nerve (nerve to rhomboid muscles);

3. The suprascapular artery running posterior to the clavicle, before crossing superior to the suprascapular ligament;

4. The suprascapular nerve crossing inferior to the ligament.

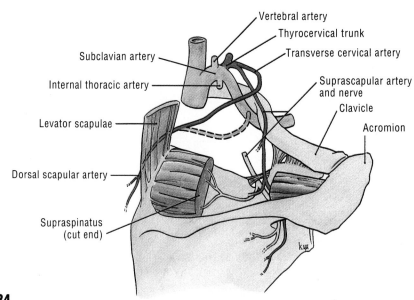

Vertebral artery

Thyrocervical trunk

Transverse cervical artery

Subclavian artery

Internal thoracic artery

Suprascapular artery
and nerve

Clavicle

Acromion

Levator scapulae

Dorsal scapular artery

Supraspinatus
(cut end)

6.34
Suprascapular and dorsal scapular arteries

This diagram shows the source and course of the two arteries. The dorsal scapular artery has alternative origins.

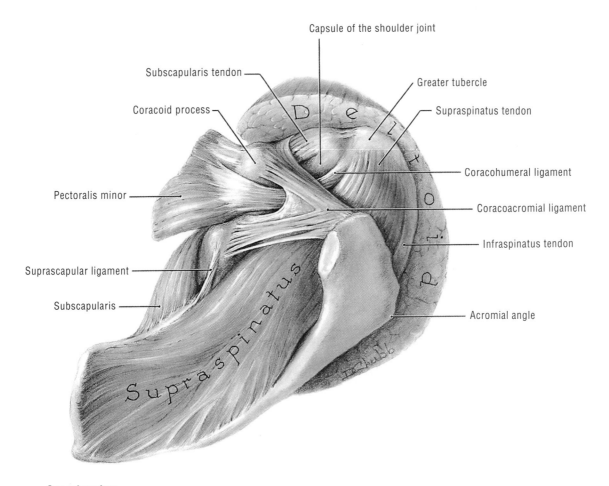

Superior view

6.35
Supraspinous and subdeltoid regions

Observe:

1. The clavicular facet on the acromion; it is small, oval, and obliquely set;

2. The triangular coracoacromial ligament arching from the lateral border of the coracoid process to the acromion between the articular facet and the tip;

3. Part of the pectoralis minor tendon dividing this ligament into two limbs and continuing, as the anterior part of the coracohumeral ligament, to the greater tubercle of the humerus;

4. The supraspinatus muscle passing inferior to the coracoacromial arch, and then lying between the deltoid muscle superiorly and the capsule of the shoulder joint inferiorly; the supraspinatus muscle and the middle fibers of the deltoid muscle are the abductors of the joint; although the middle part of the deltoid muscle is thin, it is multipennate and powerful.

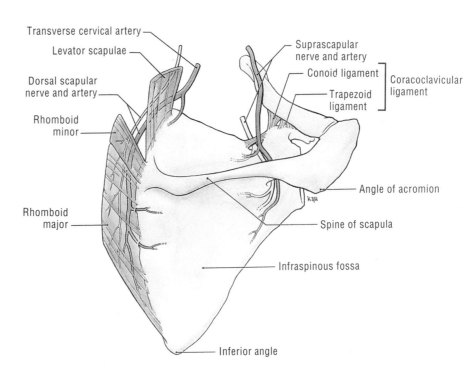

6.36
Suprascapular and dorsal scapular nerves

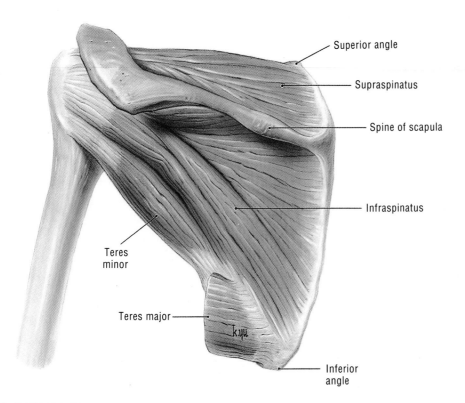

Superior angle

Supraspinatus

Spine of scapula

Infraspinatus

Teres minor

Teres major

Inferior angle

A, *Posterior view*

6.37
Rotator cuff

The four rotator cuff muscles surround the shoulder joint, blend with the capsule, and grasp their four points of attachment to the humerus, thus they maintain the integrity of the joint by acting as "ligaments" as well as moving the humerus.

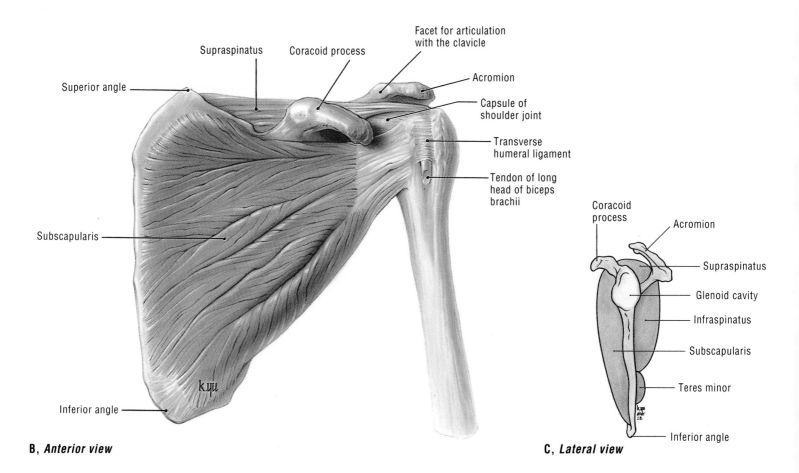

Supraspinatus

Coracoid process

Facet for articulation with the clavicle

Superior angle

Acromion

Capsule of shoulder joint

Transverse humeral ligament

Tendon of long head of biceps brachii

Subscapularis

Inferior angle

B, *Anterior view*

Coracoid process

Acromion

Supraspinatus

Glenoid cavity

Infraspinatus

Subscapularis

Teres minor

Inferior angle

C, *Lateral view*

Grant's Atlas of Anatomy

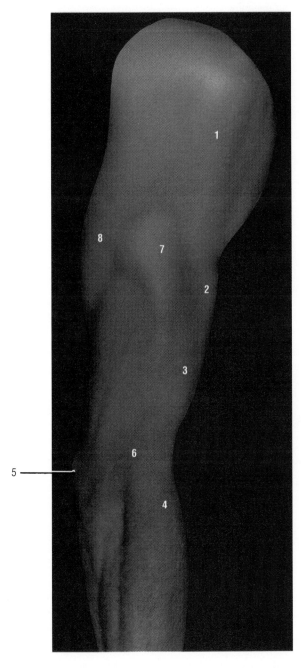

Lateral view

6.38
Surface anatomy of the arm

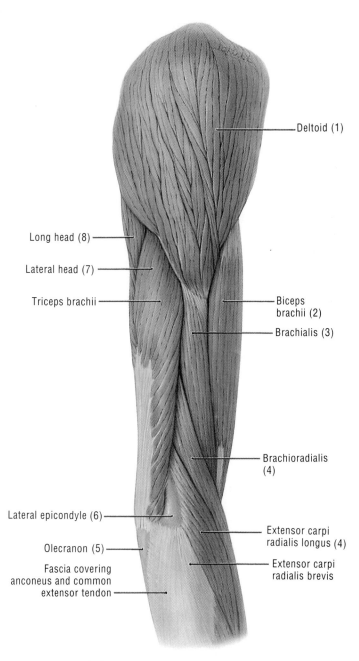

Deltoid (1)

Long head (8)

Lateral head (7)

Triceps brachii

Biceps brachii (2)

Brachialis (3)

Brachioradialis (4)

Lateral epicondyle (6)

Olecranon (5)

Fascia covering anconeus and common extensor tendon

Extensor carpi radialis longus (4)

Extensor carpi radialis brevis

Lateral view

6.39
Muscles of the arm

Numbers in parentheses refer to structures in Figure 6.38.

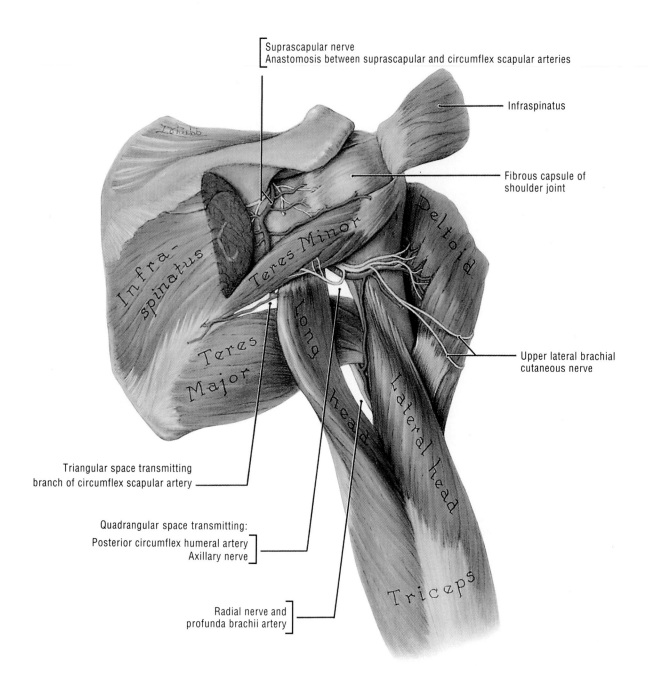

Suprascapular nerve
Anastomosis between suprascapular and circumflex scapular arteries

Infraspinatus

Fibrous capsule of shoulder joint

Upper lateral brachial cutaneous nerve

Triangular space transmitting branch of circumflex scapular artery

Quadrangular space transmitting:
Posterior circumflex humeral artery
Axillary nerve

Radial nerve and profunda brachii artery

6.40
Dorsal scapular and subdeltoid regions

Observe:

1. The thickness of the infraspinatus muscle, which, aided by the teres minor muscle and the posterior fibers of deltoid, rotates the humerus laterally;

2. Long head of the triceps muscle passing between the teres minor (a lateral rotator) and teres major (a medial rotator) muscles;

3. Long head of the triceps muscle separating the quadrangular space from the triangular space;

4. The arterial anastomoses posterior to the scapula;

5. The distribution of the suprascapular and axillary nerves; each comes from C5 and C6; each supplies two muscles; the suprascapular nerve innervates the supraspinatus and infraspinatus, and the axillary nerve innervates the teres minor and deltoid muscles; each supplies the shoulder joint; but only the axillary nerve has cutaneous branches.

6.41
Triceps and its three related nerves

Observe:

1. The long head is most medial and attaches to the infraglenoid tubercle of the scapula; the lateral head is divided and reflected laterally to reveal its attachment to the humerus; the medial head is attached to the deep surface of the triceps tendon, which attaches to the olecranon and the deep fascia of the forearm;

2. The radial nerve travels in the gap between the origins of the lateral and medial heads of the triceps muscle;

3. The axillary nerve, passing through the quadrangular space, supplies the deltoid and teres minor muscles;

4. The ulnar nerve, following the medial border of triceps.

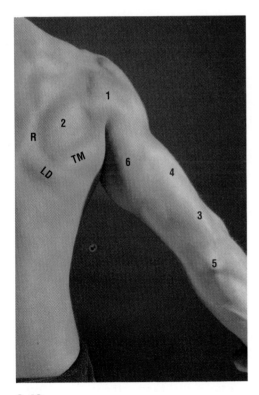

6.42
Surface anatomy of the dorsal scapular region and posterior aspect of the arm

R - Rhomboids, *TM* - Teres major, *LD* - Latissimus dorsi. Numbers refer to structures in Figure 6.41.

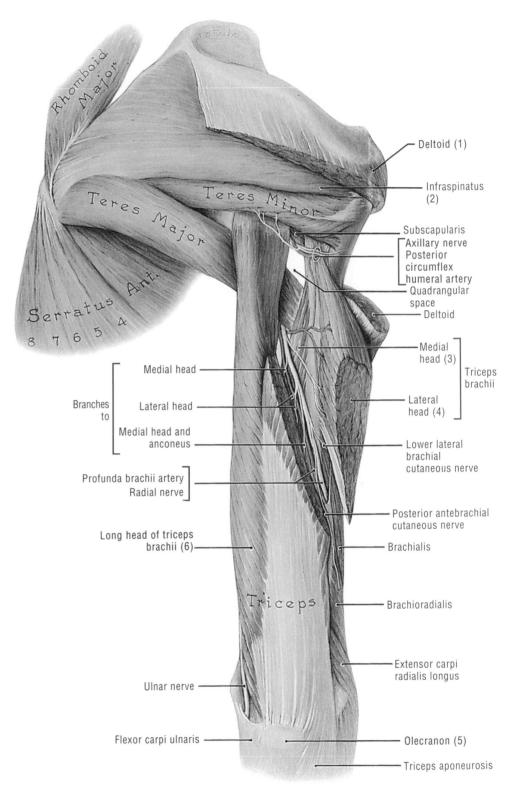

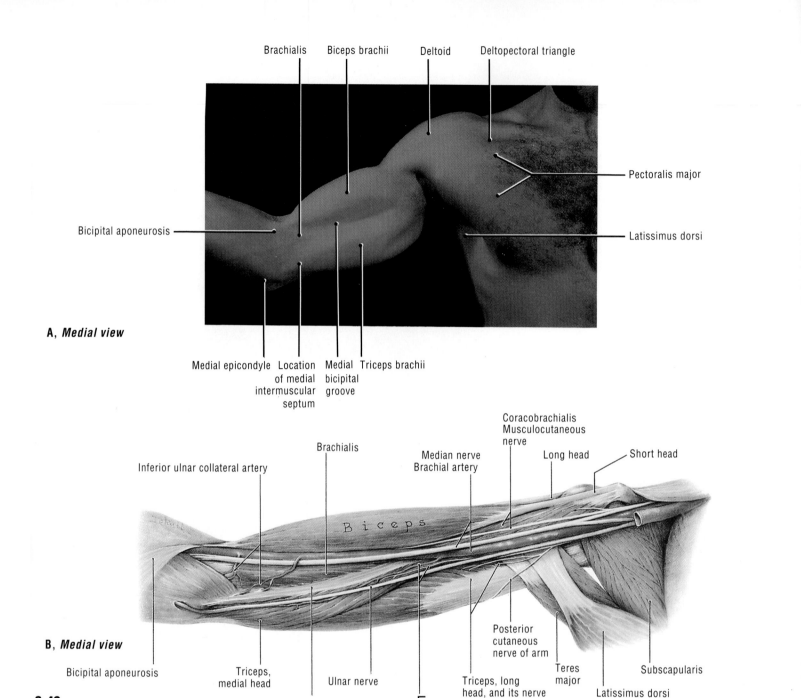

Brachialis　Biceps brachii　Deltoid　Deltopectoral triangle

Pectoralis major

Bicipital aponeurosis

Latissimus dorsi

A, *Medial view*

Medial epicondyle　Location　Medial　Triceps brachii
of medial　bicipital
intermuscular　groove
septum

Coracobrachialis
Musculocutaneous
nerve

Brachialis

Median nerve
Brachial artery

Long head

Short head

Inferior ulnar collateral artery

Biceps

B, *Medial view*

Posterior
cutaneous
nerve of arm

Teres
major

Subscapularis

Bicipital aponeurosis

Triceps,
medial head

Ulnar nerve

Triceps, long
head, and its nerve

Latissimus dorsi

Medial
intermuscular septum

Ulnar collateral nerve
Superior ulnar collateral artery

6.43
Arm

A. Surface anatomy. **B**. Dissection.

Observe in **B**:

1. Three muscles: biceps, brachialis, and coracobrachialis lying in the anterior compartment of the arm; triceps brachii lying in the posterior compartment; the medial intermuscular septum separating these two muscle groups in the distal two-thirds of the arm;

2. The great artery of the limb (axillary/brachial) passing a finger's breadth medial to the tip of the coracoid process, and applied to the medial side of coracobrachialis proximally and to the anterior aspect of brachialis distally;

3. The median nerve adjacent to the artery throughout and crossing the artery from lateral to medial;

4. The ulnar nerve adjacent to the medial side of the artery, then passing posterior to the medial intermuscular septum, and descending on the medial head of triceps, to pass posterior to the medial epicondyle, where it is palpable;

5. The superior ulnar collateral artery and the ulnar collateral branch of the radial nerve (to medial head of the triceps) accompanying the ulnar nerve;

6. The musculocutaneous nerve supplying the coracobrachialis muscle, following the lateral side of the brachial artery, and disappearing between the biceps and brachialis, accompanied by an arterial branch to these two muscles; more commonly, it pierces the coracobrachialis muscle.

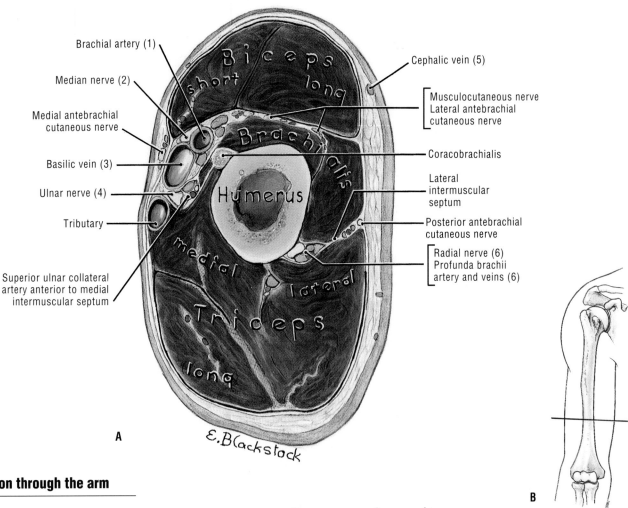

Brachial artery (1)

Median nerve (2)

Medial antebrachial cutaneous nerve

Basilic vein (3)

Ulnar nerve (4)

Tributary

Superior ulnar collateral artery anterior to medial intermuscular septum

Cephalic vein (5)

Musculocutaneous nerve
Lateral antebrachial cutaneous nerve

Coracobrachialis

Lateral intermuscular septum

Posterior antebrachial cutaneous nerve

Radial nerve (6)
Profunda brachii artery and veins (6)

Biceps short long

Brachialis

Humerus

medial

lateral

Triceps

long

A

E. Blackstock

B

6.44
Transverse section through the arm

Observe in **A**:

1. The body (shaft) of the humerus is nearly circular, its cortex being thickest at this level;

2. The three heads of the triceps muscle, in the posterior compartment of the arm;

3. The radial nerve and its companion vessels in contact with the bone;

4. The musculocutaneous nerve and its companion vessels in the septum between the biceps and brachialis muscles;

5. The median nerve crossing to the medial side of the brachial artery and its venae comitantes; the ulnar nerve moving posteriorly onto the medial side of the triceps muscle; the basilic vein (here as two vessels) has pierced the deep fascia;

B. Diagram showing the level of section illustrated in **A**.

C. Transverse MRI (magnetic resonance image). (Courtesy of Dr. W. Kucharczyk, Clinical Director of Tri-Hospital Resonance Centre, Toronto, Ontario, Canada.)

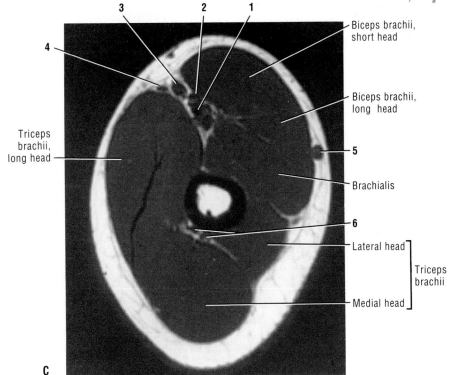

Biceps brachii, short head

Biceps brachii, long head

Brachialis

Lateral head ⎱
                 ⎰ Triceps brachii
Medial head ⎱

Triceps brachii, long head

C

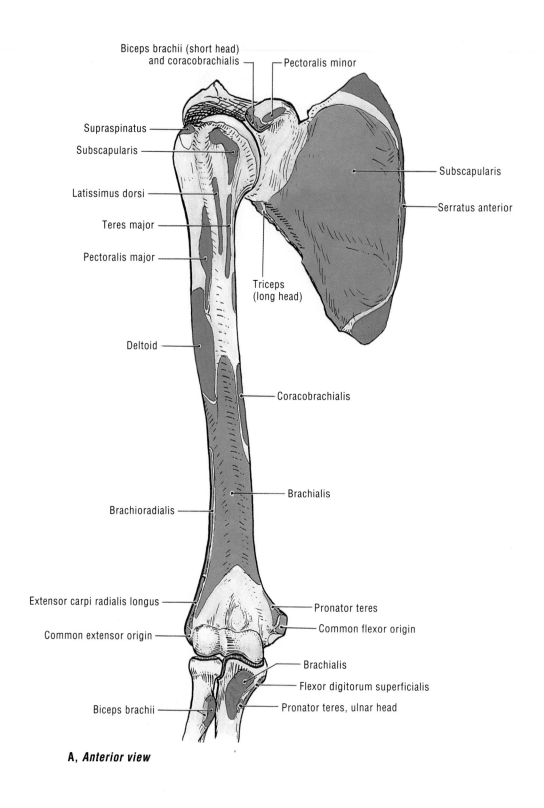

Biceps brachii (short head)
and coracobrachialis
Pectoralis minor
Supraspinatus
Subscapularis
Latissimus dorsi
Teres major
Pectoralis major
Deltoid
Brachioradialis
Extensor carpi radialis longus
Common extensor origin
Biceps brachii
Subscapularis
Serratus anterior
Triceps
(long head)
Coracobrachialis
Brachialis
Pronator teres
Common flexor origin
Brachialis
Flexor digitorum superficialis
Pronator teres, ulnar head

A, Anterior view

6.45
Bones of the upper limb showing attachments of muscles

A. For anterior view of bones of the forearm, see Figure 6.77.

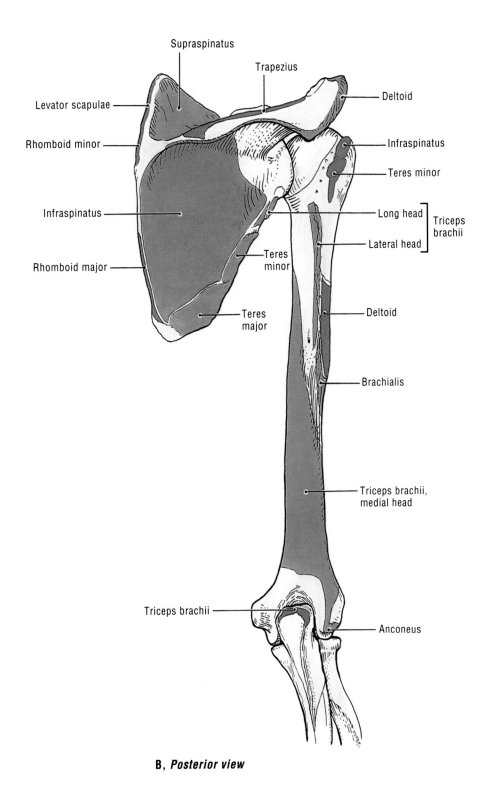

Supraspinatus

Trapezius

Deltoid

Levator scapulae

Rhomboid minor

Infraspinatus

Teres minor

Infraspinatus

Long head ⎤ **Triceps**
Lateral head ⎦ **brachii**

Teres minor

Rhomboid major

Teres major

Deltoid

Brachialis

Triceps brachii, medial head

Triceps brachii

Anconeus

B, *Posterior view*

6.45
Bones of the upper limb showing attachments of muscles *(continued)*

B. For posterior view of bones of the forearm, see Figure 6.101.

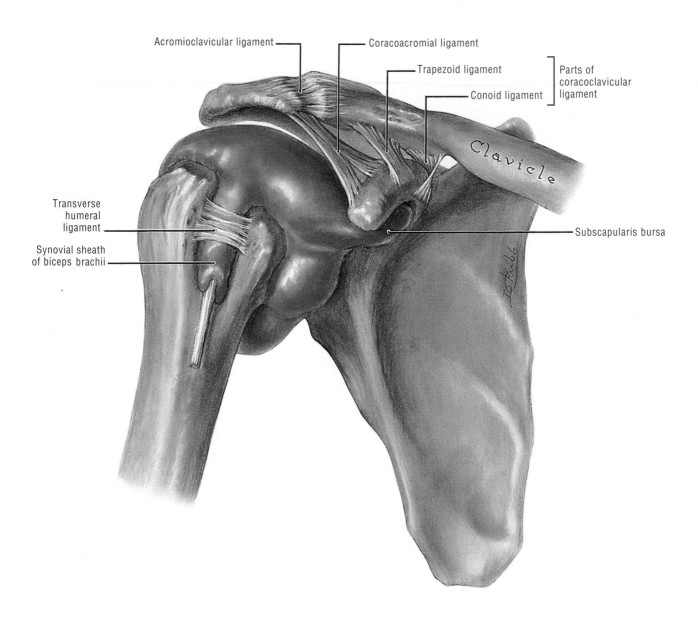

Acromioclavicular ligament ——   —— Coracoacromial ligament

—— Trapezoid ligament   ⎤ Parts of
                                    ⎥ coracoclavicular
—— Conoid ligament   ⎦ ligament

Clavicle

Transverse
humeral
ligament ——

Synovial sheath
of biceps brachii ——

—— Subscapularis bursa

6.46

Synovial capsule of the shoulder joint, ligaments at the lateral end of the clavicle

Observe:

1. The capsule cannot extend onto the lesser and greater tubercles of the humerus, due to the attachments of the four rotator cuff muscles, but it does extend inferiorly onto the surgical neck of the humerus;

2. The capsule has two prolongations: (a) where it forms a synovial sheath for the tendon of the long head of the biceps muscle in its osseofibrous tunnel, and (b) inferior to the coracoid process where it forms a bursa between subscapularis tendon and the margin of the glenoid cavity.

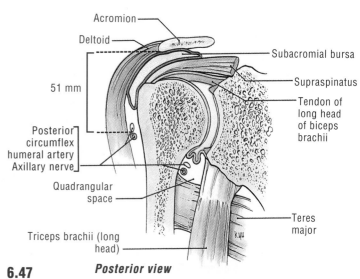

Acromion ——

Deltoid ——

—— Subacromial bursa

51 mm

—— Supraspinatus

—— Tendon of
long head
of biceps
brachii

Posterior
circumflex
humeral artery
Axillary nerve

Quadrangular
space

—— Teres
major

Triceps brachii (long
head)

Posterior view

6.47

Subacromial bursa, coronal section of the shoulder region

6.48
Subacromial bursa

Observe:

1. The bursa has been injected with purple latex;

2. The term "subacromial bursa" is usually understood to include the subdeltoid bursa, for the two bursae are usually combined;

3. Superficial to the bursa are parts of deltoid, acromion, and coracoacromial ligament and the acromioclavicular joint;

4. Deep to the bursa are the greater tubercle of the humerus and supraspinatus tendon;

5. The bursa may extend more widely under the acromion, and it may, through attrition, communicate with the shoulder joint and also with the acromioclavicular joint (Fig. 6.49);

6. The acromial branches of the thoracoacromial (acromiothoracic) and suprascapular arteries are seen contributing to the acromial rete network; the branches of the circumflex artery (not shown) also contribute to the anastomosis.

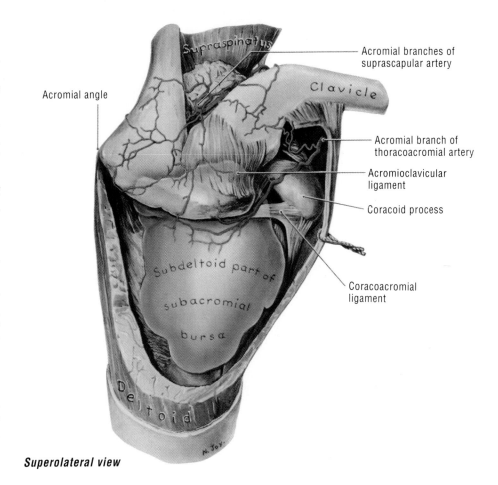

Acromial angle

Supraspinatus

Clavicle

Acromial branches of suprascapular artery

Acromial branch of thoracoacromial artery

Acromioclavicular ligament

Coracoid process

Subdeltoid part of subacromial bursa

Coracoacromial ligament

Deltoid

Superolateral view

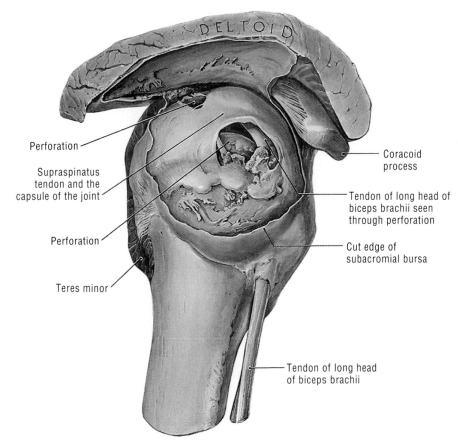

DELTOID

Perforation

Supraspinatus tendon and the capsule of the joint

Perforation

Teres minor

Coracoid process

Tendon of long head of biceps brachii seen through perforation

Cut edge of subacromial bursa

Tendon of long head of biceps brachii

6.49
Attrition of supraspinatus tendon

As a result of wearing away of the supraspinatus tendon and underlying capsule, the subacromial bursa and the shoulder joint come into wide open communication; the intracapsular part of the long tendon of the biceps muscle becomes frayed – even worn away – leaving it adherent to the intertubercular groove;

Of 95 dissecting room subjects of proved age, none of the 18 under 50 years of age had a perforation, but 4 of the 19 between 50 and 60 years and 23 of the 57 over 60 years had perforations. The perforation was bilateral in 11 subjects and unilateral in 14.

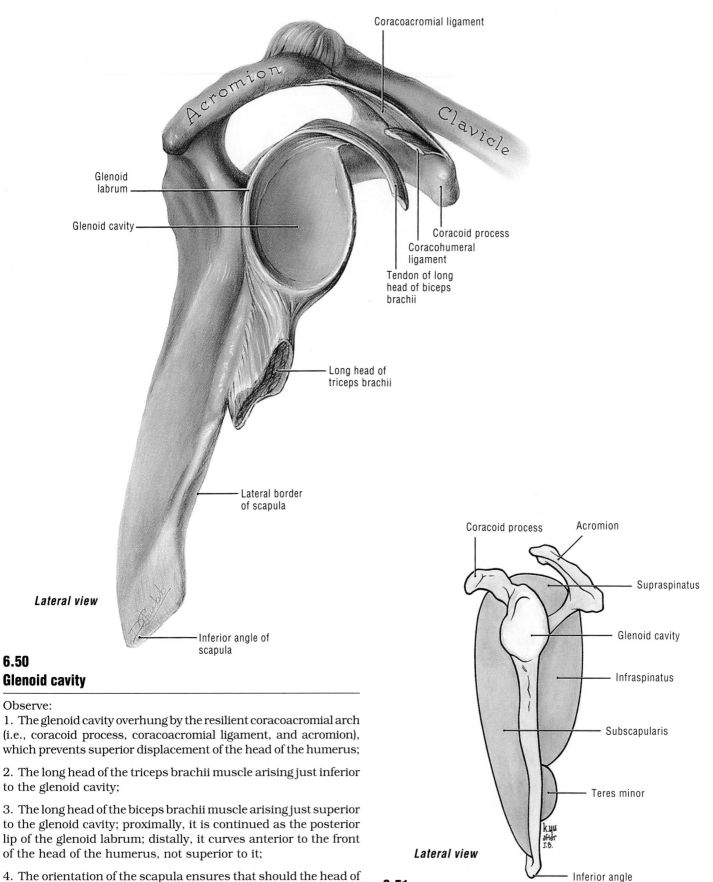

Coracoacromial ligament

Acromion

Clavicle

Glenoid labrum

Glenoid cavity

Coracoid process

Coracohumeral ligament

Tendon of long head of biceps brachii

Long head of triceps brachii

Lateral border of scapula

Lateral view

Inferior angle of scapula

6.50
Glenoid cavity

Observe:

1. The glenoid cavity overhung by the resilient coracoacromial arch (i.e., coracoid process, coracoacromial ligament, and acromion), which prevents superior displacement of the head of the humerus;

2. The long head of the triceps brachii muscle arising just inferior to the glenoid cavity;

3. The long head of the biceps brachii muscle arising just superior to the glenoid cavity; proximally, it is continued as the posterior lip of the glenoid labrum; distally, it curves anterior to the front of the head of the humerus, not superior to it;

4. The orientation of the scapula ensures that should the head of the humerus be dislocated inferiorly it would pass onto the costal surface of the scapula.

Coracoid process   Acromion

Supraspinatus

Glenoid cavity

Infraspinatus

Subscapularis

Teres minor

Lateral view

Inferior angle

6.51
Diagram of the rotator cuff

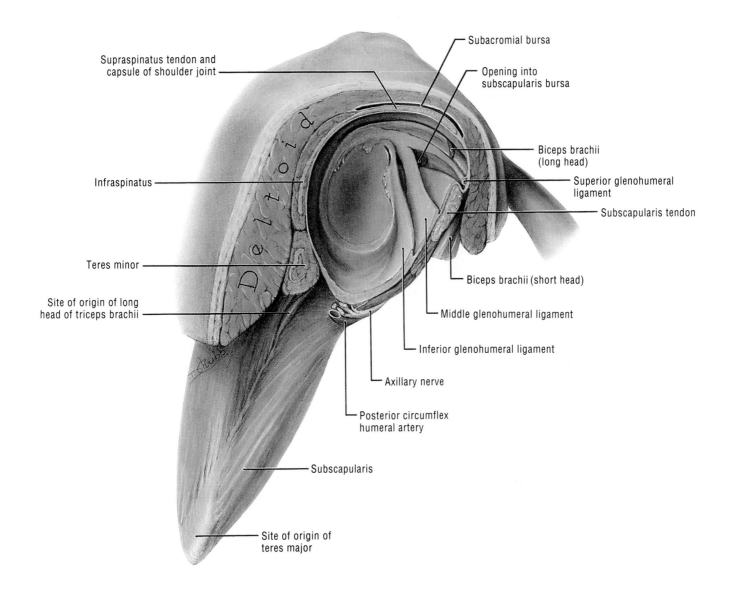

Supraspinatus tendon and
capsule of shoulder joint

Subacromial bursa

Opening into
subscapularis bursa

Infraspinatus

Teres minor

Site of origin of long
head of triceps brachii

Biceps brachii
(long head)

Superior glenohumeral
ligament

Subscapularis tendon

Biceps brachii (short head)

Middle glenohumeral ligament

Inferior glenohumeral ligament

Axillary nerve

Posterior circumflex
humeral artery

Subscapularis

Site of origin of
teres major

6.52
Humerus view of the glenoid cavity

Observe:

1. The fibrous capsule of the joint thickened anteriorly by the three glenohumeral ligaments that converge from the humerus to attach with the long tendon of the biceps brachii muscle to the supraglenoid tubercle;

2. The subacromial bursa between the acromion and deltoid superiorly and the tendon of supraspinatus inferiorly;

3. The four short rotator cuff muscles (supraspinatus, infraspinatus, teres minor, and subscapularis) crossing the joint,

blending with the capsule and retaining the head of the humerus in its socket;

4. In contact with the capsule inferiorly, the axillary nerve and the posterior circumflex humeral artery;

5. The subscapularis bursa opening superior and inferior to the middle glenohumeral ligament; several synovial folds overlapping the glenoid cavity.

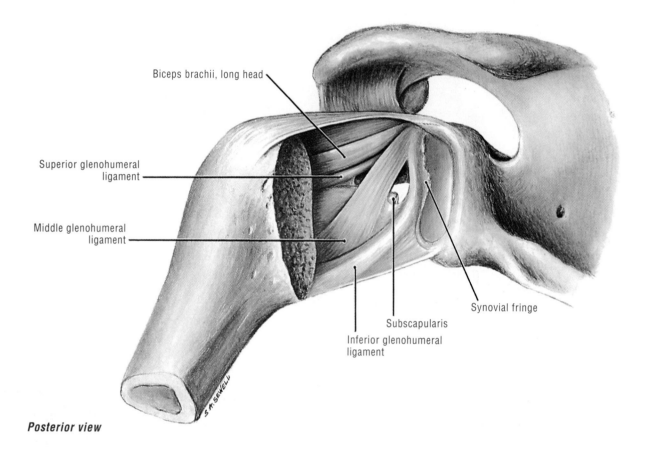

Biceps brachii, long head

Superior glenohumeral
ligament

Middle glenohumeral
ligament

Inferior glenohumeral
ligament

Subscapularis

Synovial fringe

Posterior view

6.53
Interior of the shoulder joint

Exposed from the posterior aspect by cutting away the posterior part of the capsule and sawing off the head of the humerus.

Observe:
1. The three thickenings of the anterior part of the fibrous capsule, called the glenohumeral ligaments, which are visible from within the joint, but not easily seen from the outside of the joint;

2. How these three ligaments and the long tendon of the biceps brachii muscle converge on the supraglenoid tubercle;

3. The slender superior glenohumeral ligament parallel to the biceps tendon; the middle ligament free medially due to the fact that the subscapularis bursa communicates with the joint cavity both superior and inferior to this ligament; the inferior ligament contributing largely to the anterior lip of the glenoid labrum;

4. The synovial fringe (membrane) that overlies the anterior part of the glenoid cavity.

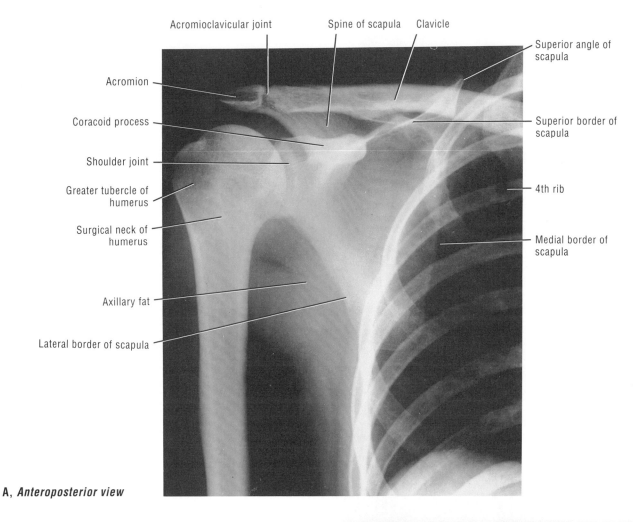

Acromioclavicular joint — Spine of scapula — Clavicle

Acromion

Coracoid process

Shoulder joint

Greater tubercle of humerus

Surgical neck of humerus

Axillary fat

Lateral border of scapula

Superior angle of scapula

Superior border of scapula

4th rib

Medial border of scapula

A, *Anteroposterior view*

6.54
Shoulder

A. Radiograph. (Courtesy of Dr. E.L. Lansdown, Professor of Radiology, University of Toronto, Toronto, Ontario, Canada.) **B.** Coronal MRI (magnetic resonance image). *A* - Acromion, *C* - Clavicle, *Cp* - Coracoid process, *Gr* - Greater tubercle, *N* - Surgical neck of humerus, *G* - Glenoid cavity, *H* - Head of humerus. (Courtesy of Dr. W. Kucharczyk, Clinical Director of Tri-Hospital Magnetic Resonance Centre, Toronto, Ontario, Canada.)

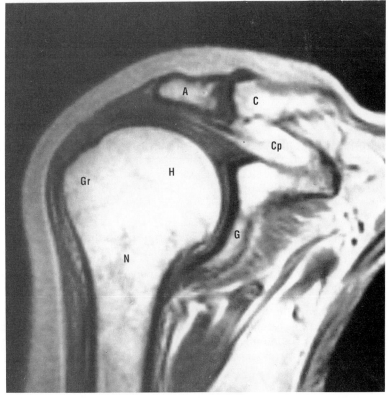

B

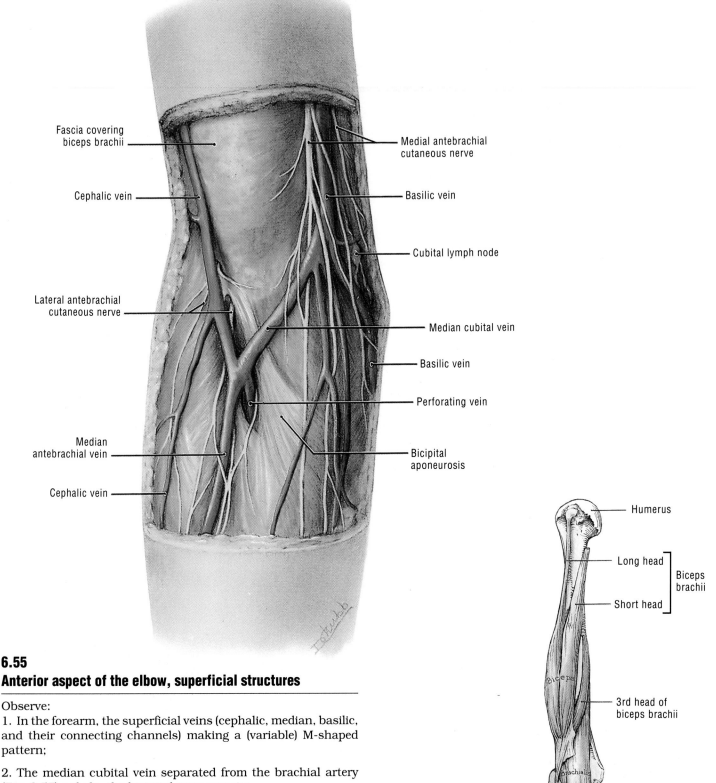

Fascia covering biceps brachii

Cephalic vein

Lateral antebrachial cutaneous nerve

Median antebrachial vein

Cephalic vein

Medial antebrachial cutaneous nerve

Basilic vein

Cubital lymph node

Median cubital vein

Basilic vein

Perforating vein

Bicipital aponeurosis

Humerus

Long head

Biceps brachii

Short head

3rd head of biceps brachii

6.55
Anterior aspect of the elbow, superficial structures

Observe:

1. In the forearm, the superficial veins (cephalic, median, basilic, and their connecting channels) making a (variable) M-shaped pattern;

2. The median cubital vein separated from the brachial artery (Fig. 6.57) only by the bicipital aponeurosis;

3. A perforating vein, lateral to the bicipital aponeurosis, connecting the deep veins to the median cubital vein;

4. In the arm, the cephalic and basilic veins occupying the bicipital furrows, one on each side of biceps brachii; in the lateral bicipital furrow, the lateral antebrachial cutaneous nerve appearing just superior to the elbow crease; in the medial bicipital furrow, the medial antebrachial cutaneous nerve becoming cutaneous about the midpoint of the arm.

6.56
Third head of biceps brachii

A third or humeral head occurs in about 5% of limbs. In this case, there is also attrition of the biceps tendon.

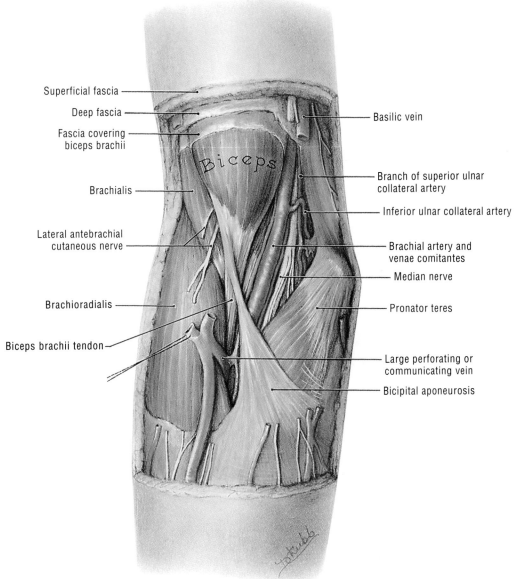

Superficial fascia

Deep fascia

Fascia covering
biceps brachii

Brachialis

Lateral antebrachial
cutaneous nerve

Brachioradialis

Biceps brachii tendon

Biceps

Basilic vein

Branch of superior ulnar
collateral artery

Inferior ulnar collateral artery

Brachial artery and
venae comitantes

Median nerve

Pronator teres

Large perforating or
communicating vein

Bicipital aponeurosis

6.57
Anterior aspect of the elbow, cubital fossa

The cubital fossa is the triangular space inferior to the elbow
crease. It is bounded laterally by the extensor muscles (represented here by the brachioradialis) and medially by the flexor
muscles (represented here by the pronator teres). The apex is
where these two muscles meet distally.

Observe:

1. The large perforating vein piercing the deep fascia at the apex
of the fossa;

2. The three chief contents: biceps brachii tendon, brachial
artery, and median nerve;

3. Biceps brachii tendon, on approaching its insertion, rotating
through a right angle, and the bicipital aponeurosis springing
from the tendon.

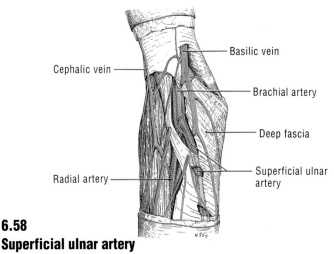

Cephalic vein

Basilic vein

Brachial artery

Deep fascia

Radial artery

Superficial ulnar
artery

6.58
Superficial ulnar artery

The ulnar artery descends superficial to the flexor muscles in
about 3% of limbs. This must be kept in mind when doing
intravenous injections in the cubital area (see Hazlett JW. *The
superficial ulnar artery with references to accidental intra-arterial
injection*. Can Med Assoc J 1949; 61:289).

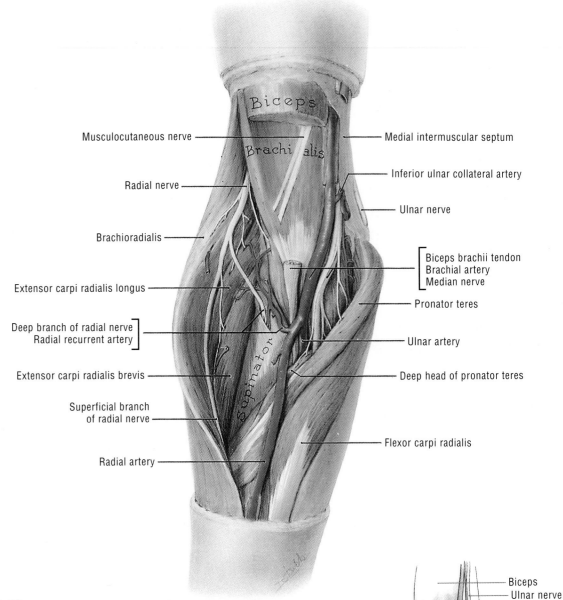

Musculocutaneous nerve

Radial nerve

Brachioradialis

Extensor carpi radialis longus

Deep branch of radial nerve
Radial recurrent artery

Extensor carpi radialis brevis

Superficial branch
of radial nerve

Radial artery

Biceps

Brachialis

Supinator

Medial intermuscular septum

Inferior ulnar collateral artery

Ulnar nerve

Biceps brachii tendon
Brachial artery
Median nerve

Pronator teres

Ulnar artery

Deep head of pronator teres

Flexor carpi radialis

6.59
Anterior aspect of the elbow, deep structures

Observe:

1. Part of the biceps muscle is excised and the cubital fossa is opened widely, exposing the brachialis and supinator muscles in the floor of the fossa; the deep branch of the radial nerve piercing supinator;

2. The brachial artery lying between biceps tendon and median nerve, and dividing into two nearly equal branches, the ulnar and radial arteries;

3. The median nerve supplying the flexor muscles; hence its motor branches arise from its medial side, the twig to the deep head of pronator teres excepted;

4. The radial nerve supplying extensor muscles; hence its motor branches arise from its lateral side, the twig to brachialis excepted; the radial nerve has been displaced laterally, so its lateral branches appear in the drawing to run medially.

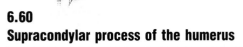

Biceps
Ulnar nerve
Superior ulnar
collateral artery

Supracondylar process
Brachial artery
Median nerve
Pronator teres

6.60
Supracondylar process of the humerus

A fibrous band joins this supracondylar process to the medial epicondyle; the median nerve passes through the foramen so-formed, the brachial artery may go with it; a process was found in 7 of 1000 living subjects (see Terry RJ. *A study of the supracondyloid process in the living*. Am J Phys Anthropol 1921; 4:129).

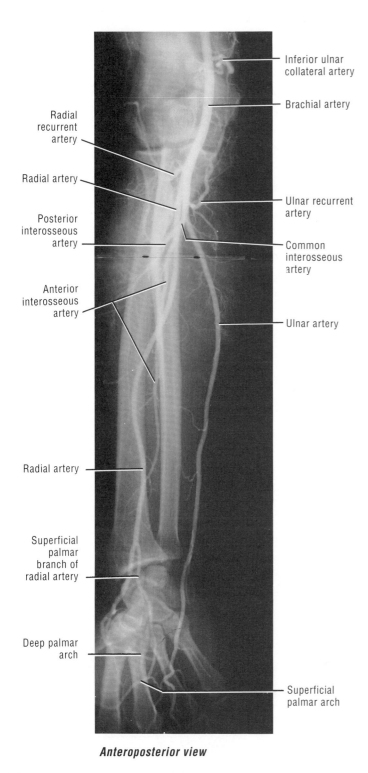

Anteroposterior view

Inferior ulnar collateral artery

Brachial artery

Radial recurrent artery

Radial artery

Posterior interosseous artery

Anterior interosseous artery

Ulnar recurrent artery

Common interosseous artery

Ulnar artery

Radial artery

Superficial palmar branch of radial artery

Deep palmar arch

Superficial palmar arch

6.61
Brachial arteriogram

Note the vessels that supply the elbow, forearm, wrist, and hand. (Courtesy of Dr. K. Sniderman, Associate Professor of Radiology, University of Toronto, Toronto, Ontario, Canada.)

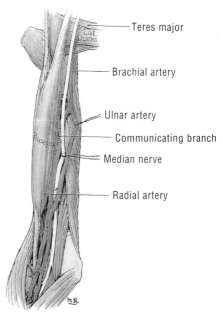

Teres major

Brachial artery

Ulnar artery

Communicating branch

Median nerve

Radial artery

6.62
Anomalous division of the brachial artery

In this case, the median nerve passes between the radial and ulnar arteries, which arise high in the arm. The musculocutaneous and median nerves commonly communicate, as shown here.

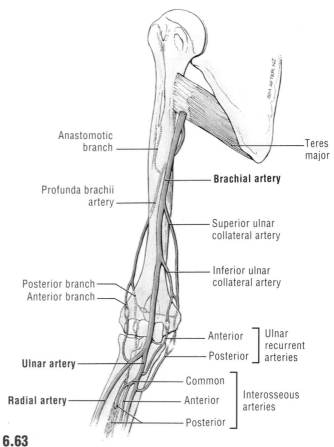

Anastomotic branch

Profunda brachii artery

Posterior branch
Anterior branch

Ulnar artery

Radial artery

Teres major

Brachial artery

Superior ulnar collateral artery

Inferior ulnar collateral artery

Anterior ⎤
Posterior ⎦ Ulnar recurrent arteries

Common ⎤
Anterior ⎥ Interosseous arteries
Posterior ⎦

6.63
Anastomoses of the elbow region

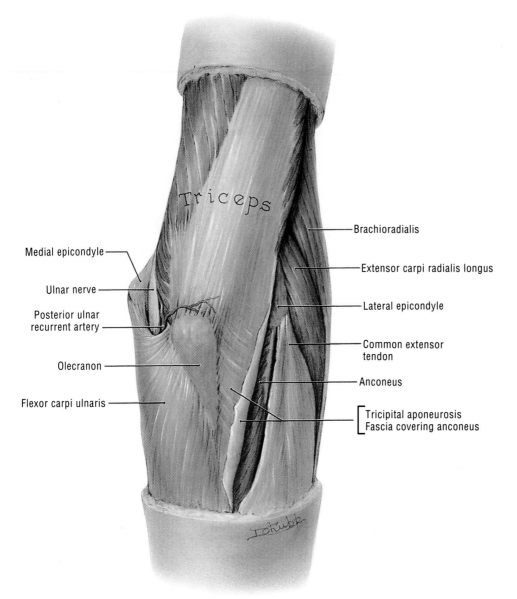

Triceps

Medial epicondyle

Ulnar nerve

Posterior ulnar
recurrent artery

Olecranon

Flexor carpi ulnaris

Brachioradialis

Extensor carpi radialis longus

Lateral epicondyle

Common extensor
tendon

Anconeus

Tricipital aponeurosis
Fascia covering anconeus

6.64
Posterior aspect of the elbow, superficial structures

Observe:

1. The triceps brachii is inserted not only into the superior surface of the olecranon but also via the deep fascia covering anconeus, tricipital aponeurosis, into lateral border of olecranon;

2. The subcutaneous and palpable posterior surfaces of the medial epicondyle, lateral epicondyle, and olecranon;

3. The ulnar nerve, also palpable, running subfascially posterior to the medial epicondyle; distal to this point, it disappears deep to the two heads of flexor carpi ulnaris;

4. The two heads of flexor carpi ulnaris; one arising from the common flexor tendon, the other from the medial border of the olecranon and posterior border of the shaft of the ulna;

5. The continuous linear origin from the humerus of the superficial extensor muscles; these are brachioradialis, extensor carpi radialis longus, common extensor tendon, and anconeus (Fig. 6.77).

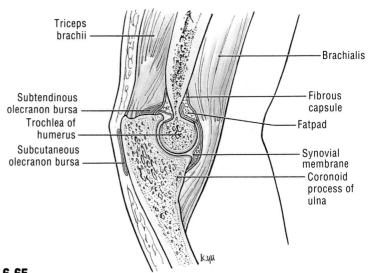

Triceps
brachii

Subtendinous
olecranon bursa
Trochlea of
humerus
Subcutaneous
olecranon bursa

Brachialis

Fibrous
capsule

Fatpad

Synovial
membrane
Coronoid
process of
ulna

6.65
Olecranon bursa, sagittal section of the elbow

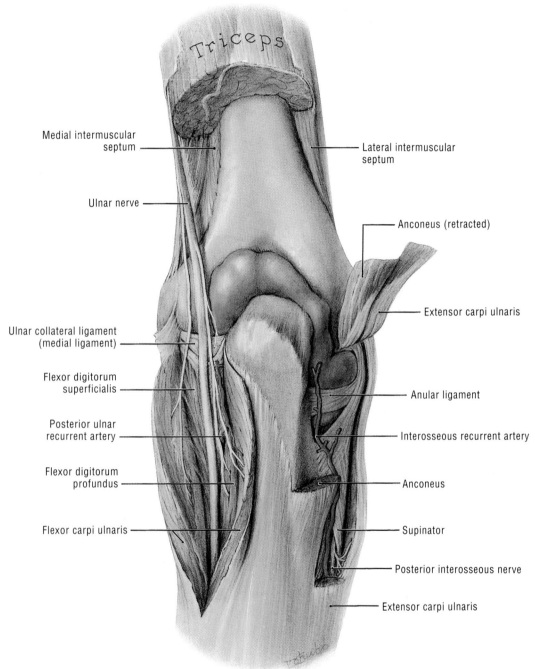

Medial intermuscular septum

Ulnar nerve

Ulnar collateral ligament (medial ligament)

Flexor digitorum superficialis

Posterior ulnar recurrent artery

Flexor digitorum profundus

Flexor carpi ulnaris

Triceps

Lateral intermuscular septum

Anconeus (retracted)

Extensor carpi ulnaris

Anular ligament

Interosseous recurrent artery

Anconeus

Supinator

Posterior interosseous nerve

Extensor carpi ulnaris

6.66
Posterior aspect of the elbow

The distal portion of the triceps brachii muscle is removed.

Observe:

1. The ulnar nerve descending: subfascially, within the posterior compartment of the arm, applied to the medial head of the triceps muscle, and posterior to the medial epicondyle; then applied to the ulnar collateral ligament of the elbow joint; and finally between the flexor carpi ulnaris and flexor digitorum profundus muscles;

2. The proximal branches of the ulnar nerve distributed to the flexor carpi ulnaris muscle, half of the profundus, and the elbow joint;

3. Laterally, the synovial membrane protruding inferior to the anular ligament; the joint is here covered with anconeus and the common extensor tendon, including extensor carpi ulnaris;

4. The posterior interosseous nerve (continuation of the deep branch of the radial nerve), appearing through supinator inferior to the head of the radius.

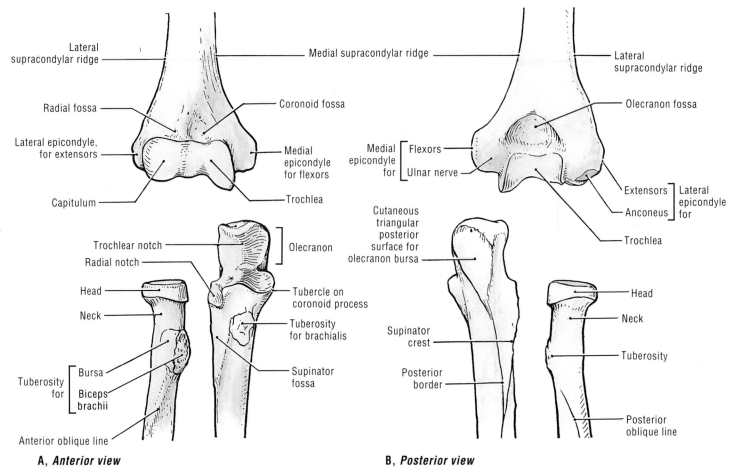

A, **Anterior view**

B, **Posterior view**

6.67
Bones of the elbow region

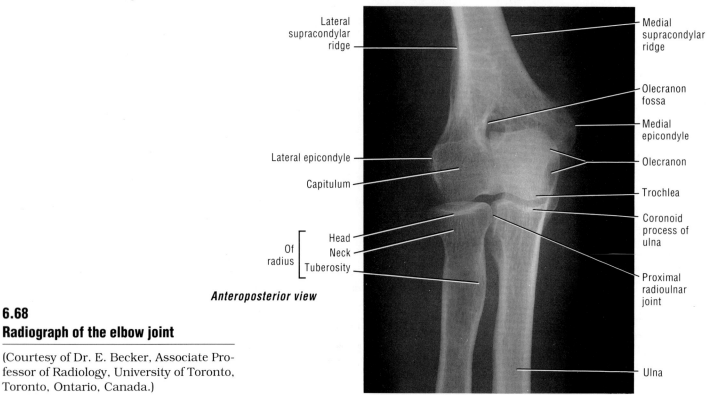

Anteroposterior view

6.68
Radiograph of the elbow joint

(Courtesy of Dr. E. Becker, Associate Professor of Radiology, University of Toronto, Toronto, Ontario, Canada.)

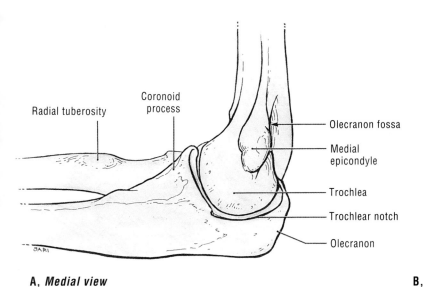

Radial tuberosity — Coronoid process — Olecranon fossa — Medial epicondyle — Trochlea — Trochlear notch — Olecranon

A, *Medial view*

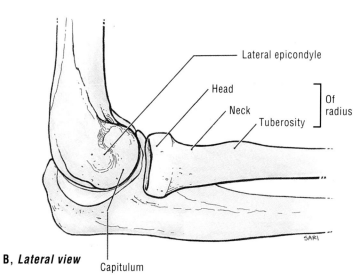

Lateral epicondyle — Head — Neck — Tuberosity } Of radius — Capitulum

B, *Lateral view*

6.69
Bones of the elbow region

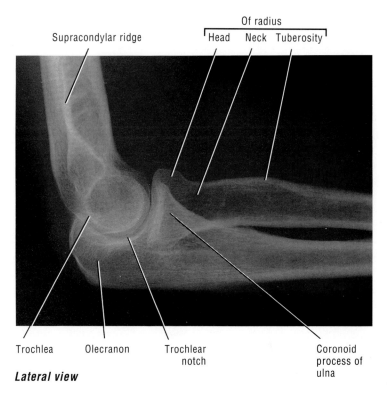

Supracondylar ridge — Of radius [Head — Neck — Tuberosity] — Trochlea — Olecranon — Trochlear notch — Coronoid process of ulna

Lateral view

6.70
Radiograph of the elbow joint

(Courtesy of Dr. E. Becker, Associate Professor of Radiology, University of Toronto, Toronto, Ontario, Canada.)

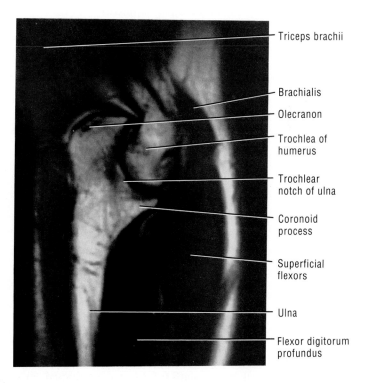

Triceps brachii — Brachialis — Olecranon — Trochlea of humerus — Trochlear notch of ulna — Coronoid process — Superficial flexors — Ulna — Flexor digitorum profundus

6.71
Sagittal MRI (magnetic resonance image) of the elbow

(Courtesy of Dr. W. Kucharczyk, Clinical Director of Tri-Hospital Magnetic Resonance Centre, Toronto, Ontario, Canada.)

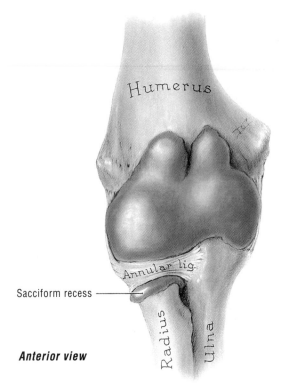

Humerus

Annular lig.

Sacciform recess

Radius

Ulna

Anterior view

6.72
Articular cavity of the elbow and proximal radioulnar joints

The cavity of the elbow was injected with wax. The fibrous capsule has been removed; the synovial capsule remains.

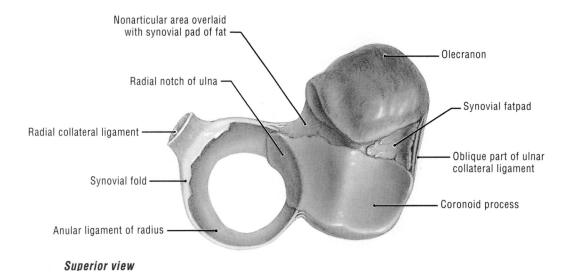

Nonarticular area overlaid with synovial pad of fat

Olecranon

Radial notch of ulna

Synovial fatpad

Radial collateral ligament

Oblique part of ulnar collateral ligament

Synovial fold

Coronoid process

Anular ligament of radius

Superior view

6.73
Socket for head of radius and trochlea of humerus

The anular ligament keeps the head of the radius applied to the radial notch of the ulna, and with it forms a cup-shaped socket (i.e., wide superiorly, narrow inferiorly). The anular ligament is bound to the humerus by the radial collateral ligament of the elbow.

A common injury in childhood is displacement of the head of the radius following traction on a pronated forearm. Part of the anular ligament becomes trapped between the radial head and the capitulum.

A crescentic synovial fold occupies the angular space between the head of the radius and the capitulum of the humerus. Similarly, synovial folds containing fat occupy the two angular nonarticular areas between the coronoid process and the olecranon.

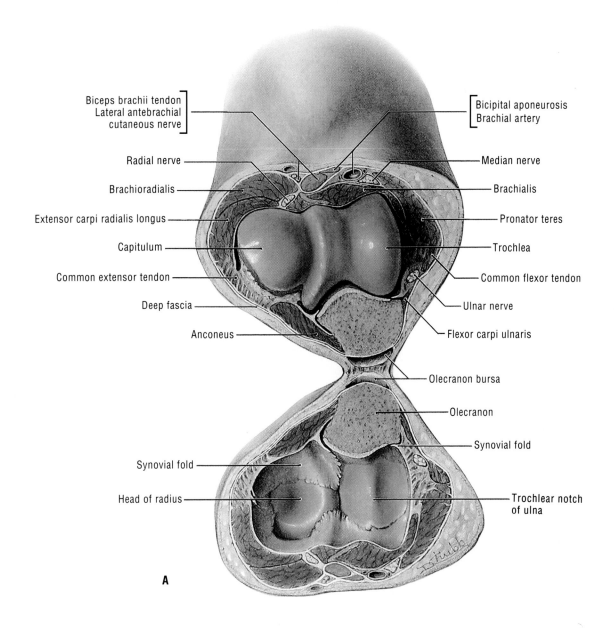

Biceps brachii tendon
Lateral antebrachial cutaneous nerve

Bicipital aponeurosis
Brachial artery

Radial nerve

Median nerve

Brachioradialis

Brachialis

Extensor carpi radialis longus

Pronator teres

Capitulum

Trochlea

Common extensor tendon

Common flexor tendon

Deep fascia

Ulnar nerve

Anconeus

Flexor carpi ulnaris

Olecranon bursa

Olecranon

Synovial fold

Synovial fold

Head of radius

Trochlear notch of ulna

A

6.74
Transverse section through the elbow joint

Observe in **A**:

1. The radial nerve is in contact with the joint capsule; the ulnar nerve is in contact with the ulnar collateral ligament; the median nerve is separated from the joint capsule by the brachialis muscle;

2. Synovial folds, containing fat, overlie the periphery of the head of the radius and the nonarticular indentations on the trochlear notch of the ulna;

3. The olecranon bursa lying between the olecranon process and the skin.

B shows the level of section illustrated in **A**.

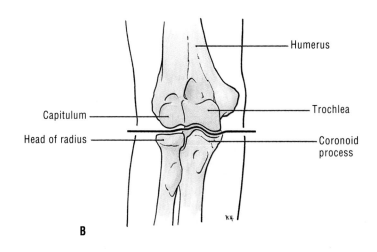

Humerus

Capitulum

Trochlea

Head of radius

Coronoid process

B

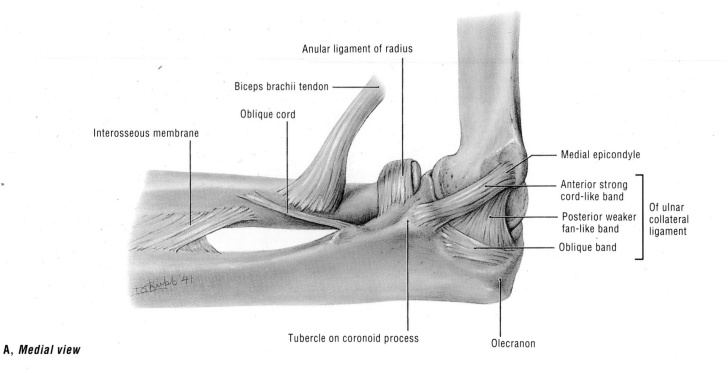

Anular ligament of radius

Biceps brachii tendon

Oblique cord

Interosseous membrane

Medial epicondyle

Anterior strong cord-like band

Posterior weaker fan-like band

Oblique band

Of ulnar collateral ligament

Tubercle on coronoid process

Olecranon

A, Medial view

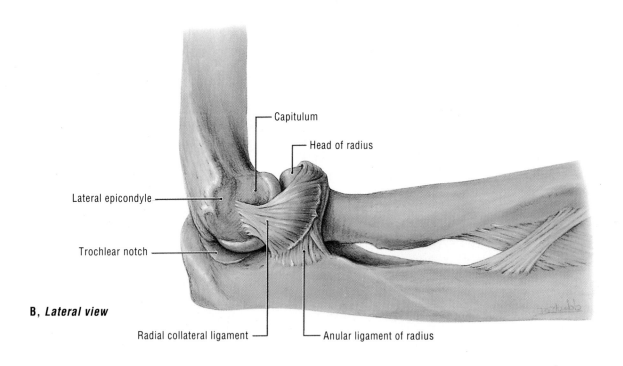

Capitulum

Head of radius

Lateral epicondyle

Trochlear notch

B, Lateral view

Radial collateral ligament

Anular ligament of radius

6.75
Collateral ligaments of the elbow

A. Ulnar (medial) collateral ligament. The anterior band (part) is a strong, round cord, taut when the elbow joint is extended; the posterior band is a weak fan, taut in flexion of the joint; the oblique fibers merely deepen the socket for the trochlea of the humerus.

B. Radial (lateral) collateral ligament. The fan-shaped lateral ligament is attached to the anular ligament of radius, but its superficial fibers are continued on to the radius; the supinator blends with the radial collateral ligament and the anular ligament and attaches to the supinator crest of the ulna.

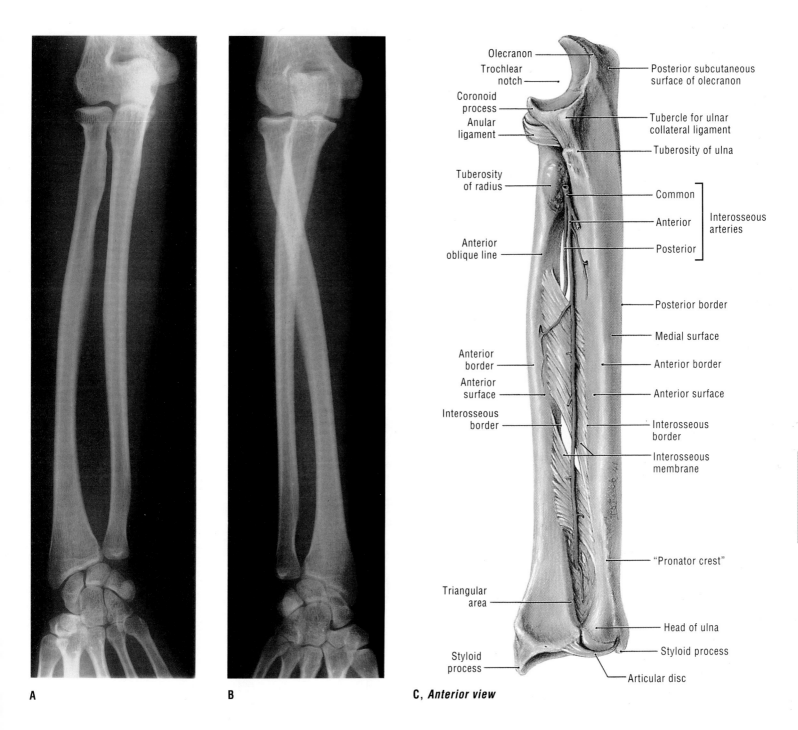

Olecranon —
Trochlear notch —
Coronoid process —
Anular ligament —
Tuberosity of radius —
Anterior oblique line —
Anterior border —
Anterior surface —
Interosseous border —
Triangular area —
Styloid process —

— **Posterior subcutaneous surface of olecranon**
— **Tubercle for ulnar collateral ligament**
— **Tuberosity of ulna**
— **Common**
— **Anterior** } **Interosseous arteries**
— **Posterior**
— **Posterior border**
— **Medial surface**
— **Anterior border**
— **Anterior surface**
— **Interosseous border**
— **Interosseous membrane**
— **"Pronator crest"**
— **Head of ulna**
— **Styloid process**
— **Articular disc**

A   B   **C**, *Anterior view*

6.76
Radioulnar joints

Anterior radiograph of the forearm in supination (**A**) and in pronation (**B**). Note that the radius crosses the ulna when the forearm is pronated. (Courtesy of Dr. J. Heslin, Assistant Professor of Anatomy, University of Toronto, Toronto, Ontario, Canada.)

C. Radioulnar ligaments and interosseous arteries. The ligament of the proximal radioulnar joint is the anular ligament; that of the

distal joint is the articular disc; that of the middle joint is the interosseous membrane. The general direction of the fibers of the membrane is such that a superior thrust to the hand is received by the radius, and is transmitted to the ulna. The membrane is attached to the interosseous borders of the radius and ulna, but it also spreads onto their surfaces.

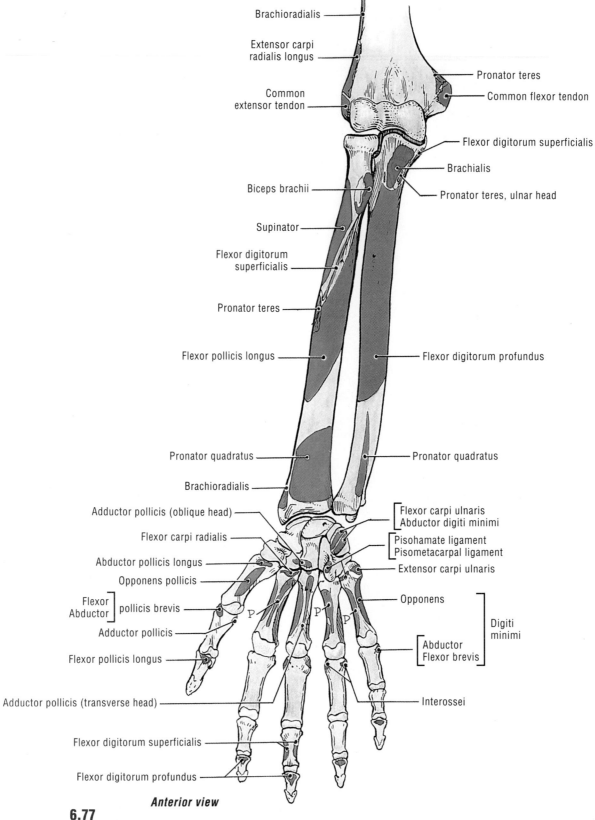

Brachioradialis

Extensor carpi
radialis longus

Common
extensor tendon

Biceps brachii

Supinator

Flexor digitorum
superficialis

Pronator teres

Flexor pollicis longus

Pronator quadratus

Brachioradialis

Adductor pollicis (oblique head)

Flexor carpi radialis

Abductor pollicis longus

Opponens pollicis

Flexor ⎤ pollicis brevis
Abductor ⎦

Adductor pollicis

Flexor pollicis longus

Adductor pollicis (transverse head)

Flexor digitorum superficialis

Flexor digitorum profundus

Pronator teres

Common flexor tendon

Flexor digitorum superficialis

Brachialis

Pronator teres, ulnar head

Flexor digitorum profundus

Pronator quadratus

Flexor carpi ulnaris
Abductor digiti minimi

Pisohamate ligament
Pisometacarpal ligament

Extensor carpi ulnaris

Opponens ⎤
⎦ Digiti
minimi
Abductor ⎤
Flexor brevis ⎦

Interossei

P   P   P

Anterior view

6.77

Bones of the forearm and hand showing attachments of muscles

Observe that the proximal attachments of the three palmar interossei are indicated by
the letters *P, P, P;* those of the four dorsal interossei by color only; proximal attachments
of the three thenar and two of the hypothenar muscles are omitted.

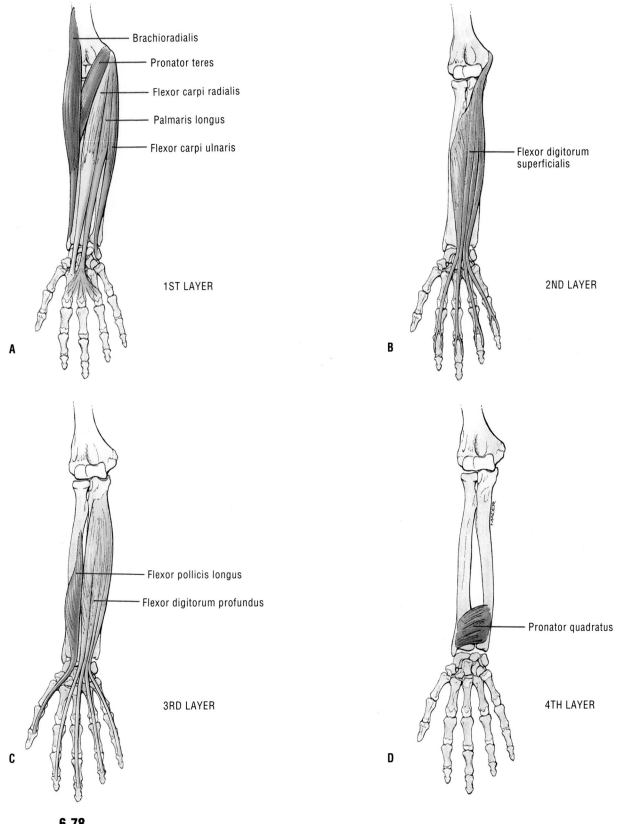

Brachioradialis

Pronator teres

Flexor carpi radialis

Palmaris longus

Flexor carpi ulnaris

1ST LAYER

A

Flexor digitorum
superficialis

2ND LAYER

B

Flexor pollicis longus

Flexor digitorum profundus

3RD LAYER

C

Pronator quadratus

4TH LAYER

D

6.78

Four layers of anterior forearm muscles

Examine these four diagrams arranged sequentially from superficial to deep, in relation to the origins and insertions shown in Figure 6.77. **A**. First (most superficial) layer. **B**. Second layer. **C**. Third layer. **D**. Fourth (deepest) layer.

6.79
Superficial muscles of the forearm and palmar aponeurosis *(at right)*

Observe:

1. At the elbow, the brachial artery lying between the biceps tendon and the median nerve, and then bifurcating into the radial and ulnar arteries;

2. At the wrist, the radial artery lateral to flexor carpi radialis tendon and the ulnar artery lateral to flexor carpi ulnaris tendon;

3. In the forearm, the radial artery lying between two muscle groups or two motor territories; the muscles lateral to the artery are supplied by the radial nerve; those medial to it, by the median and ulnar nerves; thus, no motor nerve crosses the radial artery;

4. The lateral group of muscles, represented by the brachioradialis muscle, slightly overlapping the radial artery that, otherwise, is superficial;

5. The four superficial muscles (pronator teres, flexor carpi radialis, palmaris longus, and flexor carpi ulnaris) radiating from the medial epicondyle; the muscle of the second layer, the flexor digitorum superficialis, is partially in view;

6. The palmaris longus muscle continued into the palm as the palmar aponeurosis.

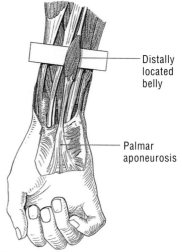

Distally located belly

Palmar aponeurosis

6.80
Palmaris longus muscle *(above)*

This muscle is absent in about 14% of limbs. It usually has a small belly at the common flexor origin and a long tendon, which is continued into the palm as the palmar aponeurosis.

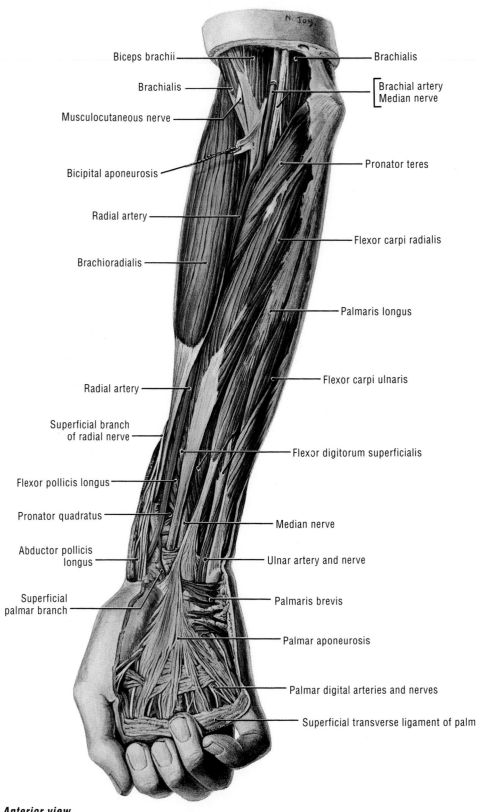

Biceps brachii — Brachialis

Brachialis — Brachial artery / Median nerve

Musculocutaneous nerve — Pronator teres

Bicipital aponeurosis

Radial artery — Flexor carpi radialis

Brachioradialis

Palmaris longus

Radial artery — Flexor carpi ulnaris

Superficial branch of radial nerve — Flexor digitorum superficialis

Flexor pollicis longus

Pronator quadratus — Median nerve

Abductor pollicis longus — Ulnar artery and nerve

Superficial palmar branch — Palmaris brevis

Palmar aponeurosis

Palmar digital arteries and nerves

Superficial transverse ligament of palm

Anterior view

6.81
Flexor digitorum superficialis and related structures *(at right)*

Observe:

1. The oblique attachment of the flexor digitorum superficialis muscle from (a) the medial epicondyle of the humerus, (b) the ulnar collateral ligament of the elbow, (c) the coronoid process, (d) the anterior oblique line of the radius;

2. The ulnar artery descending obliquely posterior to superficialis to meet and accompany the ulnar nerve;

3. The ulnar nerve descending vertically near the medial border of superficialis; it is exposed by splitting the septum between superficialis and flexor carpi ulnaris muscles;

4. The median nerve descending vertically posterior to superficialis, supplying the muscle as it clings to its posterior surface, and appearing distally at its lateral border;

5. The tendons of the superficialis to the 3rd and 4th digits lying superficially side by side and the tendons to the 5th and 2nd digits lying deeply.

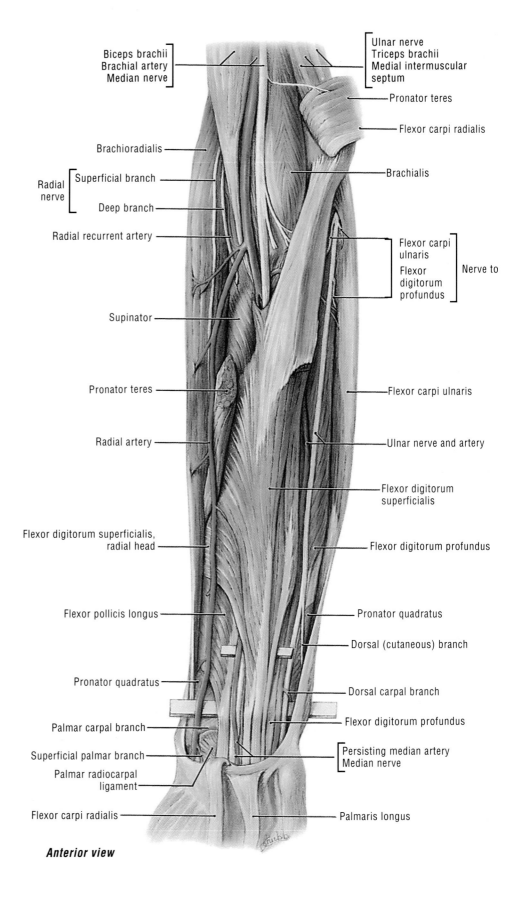

Biceps brachii
Brachial artery
Median nerve

Ulnar nerve
Triceps brachii
Medial intermuscular septum

Pronator teres

Flexor carpi radialis

Brachioradialis

Brachialis

Radial nerve — Superficial branch
Deep branch

Radial recurrent artery

Flexor carpi ulnaris
Flexor digitorum profundus — Nerve to

Supinator

Pronator teres

Flexor carpi ulnaris

Radial artery

Ulnar nerve and artery

Flexor digitorum superficialis

Flexor digitorum superficialis, radial head

Flexor digitorum profundus

Flexor pollicis longus

Pronator quadratus

Dorsal (cutaneous) branch

Pronator quadratus

Dorsal carpal branch

Flexor digitorum profundus

Palmar carpal branch

Persisting median artery
Median nerve

Superficial palmar branch

Palmar radiocarpal ligament

Flexor carpi radialis

Palmaris longus

Anterior view

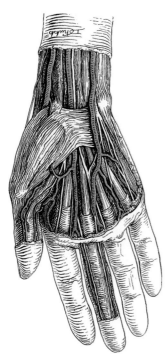

6.82
Persisting median artery *(above)*

6.83

Deep flexors of the digits and the related structures

Observe:

1. The two deep digital flexor muscles, flexor pollicis longus and flexor digitorum profundus, that arise from the flexor aspects of radius, interosseous membrane, and ulna between the origin of superficialis proximally and pronator quadratus distally;

2. The median nerve crossing anterior to the ulnar artery at the elbow and posterior to the flexor retinaculum at the wrist;

3. The ulnar nerve is sheltered by the medial epicondyle at the elbow and by the pisiform bone at the wrist;

4. The ulnar nerve entering the forearm posterior to the medial epicondyle, descending on profundus, joined by the ulnar artery, continuing on profundus to the wrist, and there passing anterior to the flexor retinaculum and lateral to the pisiform as it enters the palm; at the elbow, it supplies the flexor carpi ulnaris and the medial half of profundus muscles; superior to the wrist, it gives off its dorsal branch;

5. The recurrent, common interosseous, and dorsal carpal branches as well as muscular branches of the ulnar artery;

6. The four lumbricals arising from the profundus tendons.

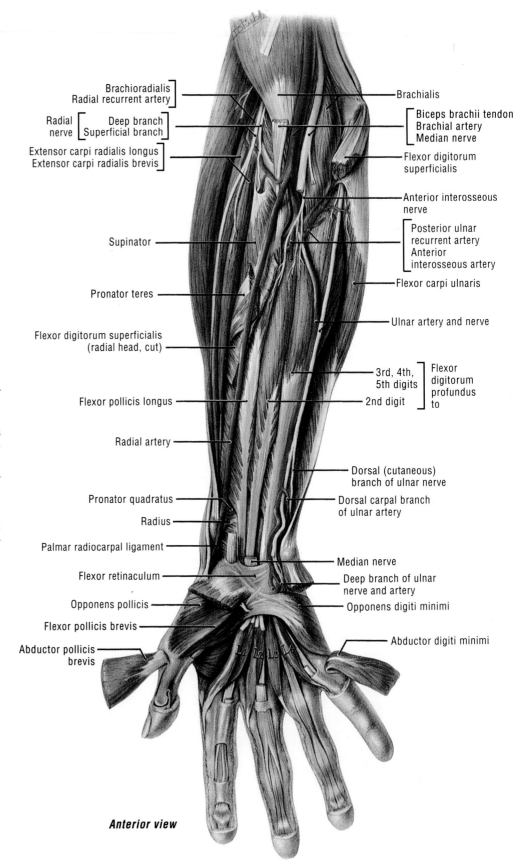

Brachioradialis
Radial recurrent artery
Brachialis
Biceps brachii tendon
Brachial artery
Median nerve
Radial nerve — Deep branch / Superficial branch
Extensor carpi radialis longus
Extensor carpi radialis brevis
Flexor digitorum superficialis
Anterior interosseous nerve
Supinator
Posterior ulnar recurrent artery
Anterior interosseous artery
Flexor carpi ulnaris
Pronator teres
Ulnar artery and nerve
Flexor digitorum superficialis (radial head, cut)
3rd, 4th, 5th digits / 2nd digit — Flexor digitorum profundus to
Flexor pollicis longus
Radial artery
Dorsal (cutaneous) branch of ulnar nerve
Pronator quadratus
Dorsal carpal branch of ulnar artery
Radius
Palmar radiocarpal ligament
Median nerve
Flexor retinaculum
Deep branch of ulnar nerve and artery
Opponens pollicis
Opponens digiti minimi
Flexor pollicis brevis
Abductor pollicis brevis
Abductor digiti minimi

Anterior view

414

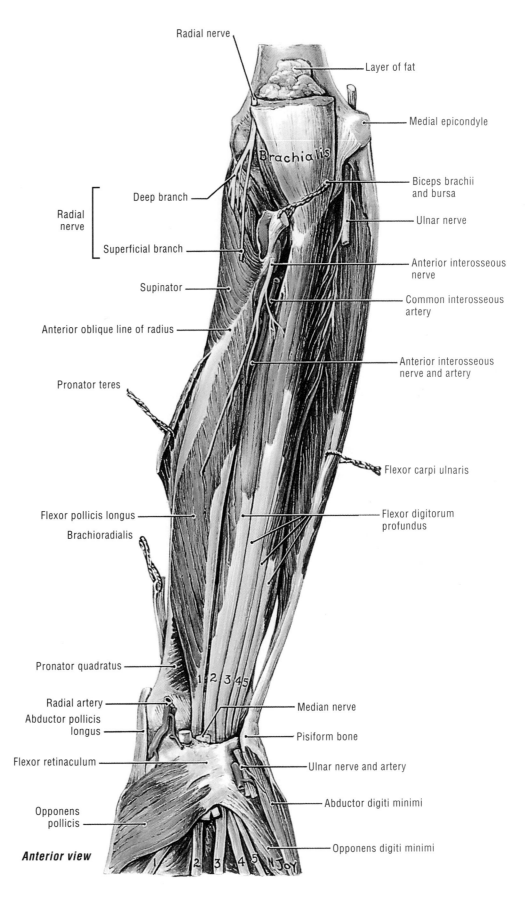

Radial nerve

Layer of fat

Medial epicondyle

Brachialis

Deep branch

Biceps brachii
and bursa

Radial
nerve

Ulnar nerve

Superficial branch

Anterior interosseous
nerve

Supinator

Common interosseous
artery

Anterior oblique line of radius

Anterior interosseous
nerve and artery

Pronator teres

Flexor carpi ulnaris

Flexor pollicis longus

Flexor digitorum
profundus

Brachioradialis

Pronator quadratus

1 2 3 4 5

Radial artery

Median nerve

Abductor pollicis
longus

Pisiform bone

Flexor retinaculum

Ulnar nerve and artery

Opponens
pollicis

Abductor digiti minimi

Opponens digiti minimi

Anterior view

1   2   3   4 5   N Joy

6.84
Deep flexors of the digits

Observe:

1. The five tendons of the deep digital flexors, side by side, converging on the carpal tunnel, and, having traversed it, diverging to the distal phalanges of the digits;

2. The biceps brachii muscle attaching the medial aspect of radius, hence it can rotate laterally, i.e., supinate, whereas the pronator teres muscle by attaching to the lateral surface can rotate medially, i.e., pronate;

3. The deep branch of the radial nerve piercing the supinator muscle;

4. The anterior interosseous nerve and artery disappearing between the flexor pollicis longus and flexor digitorum profundus muscles to lie on the interosseous membrane.

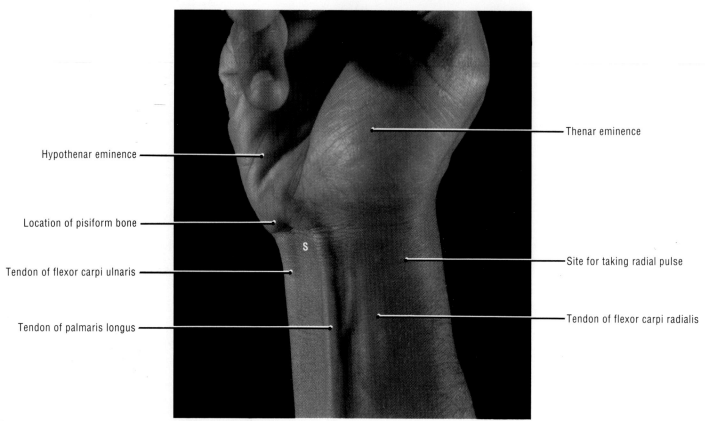

6.85
Surface anatomy of the distal forearm and wrist

S - Location of tendons of flexor digitorum superficialis.

Hypothenar eminence

Location of pisiform bone

Tendon of flexor carpi ulnaris

Tendon of palmaris longus

Thenar eminence

Site for taking radial pulse

Tendon of flexor carpi radialis

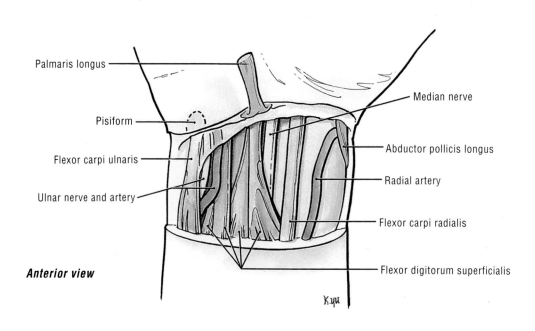

Palmaris longus

Pisiform

Flexor carpi ulnaris

Ulnar nerve and artery

Median nerve

Abductor pollicis longus

Radial artery

Flexor carpi radialis

Flexor digitorum superficialis

Anterior view

6.86
Diagram of the superficial structures at the wrist

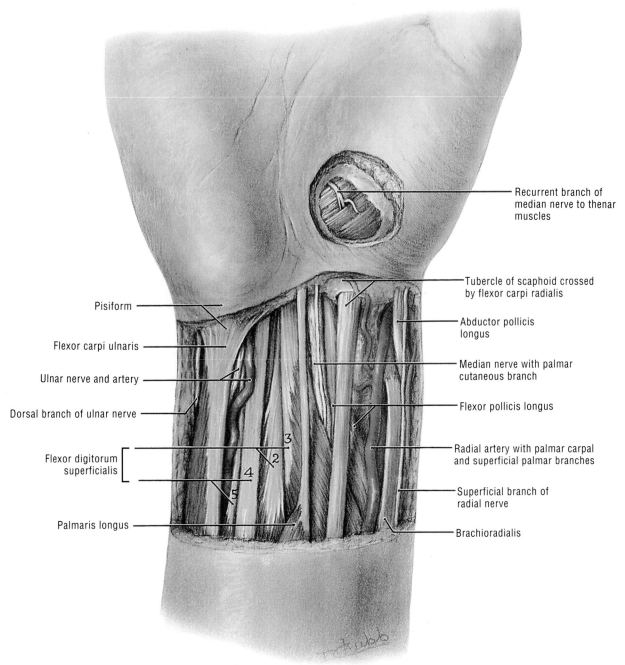

Pisiform

Flexor carpi ulnaris

Ulnar nerve and artery

Dorsal branch of ulnar nerve

Flexor digitorum superficialis

Palmaris longus

Recurrent branch of median nerve to thenar muscles

Tubercle of scaphoid crossed by flexor carpi radialis

Abductor pollicis longus

Median nerve with palmar cutaneous branch

Flexor pollicis longus

Radial artery with palmar carpal and superficial palmar branches

Superficial branch of radial nerve

Brachioradialis

6.87
Structures of the anterior aspect of the wrist

Observe:

1. The distal skin incision follows the transverse skin crease at the wrist crossing the pisiform, to which the flexor carpi ulnaris muscle is a guide, and the tubercle of the scaphoid, to which the tendon of flexor carpi radialis is a guide;

2. Palmaris longus tendon bisects the crease; deep to its lateral margin is the median nerve;

3. The radial artery disappearing deep to the abductor pollicis longus muscle;

4. The ulnar nerve and artery sheltered by flexor carpi ulnaris tendon and by the expansion this gives to the flexor retinaculum;

5. Flexor digitorum superficialis tendons to the 3rd and 4th digits somewhat anterior to those to the 2nd and 5th digits;

6. The recurrent branch of the median nerve to the thenar muscles lying within a circle whose center is from 2.5 to 4 cm inferior to the tubercle of the scaphoid.

6.88
Attachments of the palmar aponeurosis, digital vessels, and nerves

Observe:

1. From the palmar aponeurosis a few longitudinal fibers enter the fingers; the other fibers, forming extensive fibroareolar septa, pass posteriorly, to the palmar ligaments (Fig. 6.99), and also, more proximally, to the fascia covering the interossei; thus, two sets of tunnels exist in the distal half of the palm: (a) tunnels for long flexor tendons, and (b) tunnels for lumbricals, digital vessels, and digital nerves;

2. The absence of fat deep to the skin creases of the fingers;

3. The three compartments of the palm: (a) the thenar, posterior to the thenar fascia; (b) the hypothenar, posterior to the hypothenar fascia; between these (c), the middle, posterior to the palmar aponeurosis (Fig. 6.89);

4. The middle compartment contains superficialis and profundus tendons, lumbricals, and digital vessels and nerves; it is bounded posteriorly by the fascia covering the interossei and adductor pollicis muscles, the palmar ligaments, and the deep transverse metacarpal ligaments of the palm;

5. The plane between the fascia covering the 1st dorsal interosseous muscle and that covering the adductor pollicis muscle (Fig. 6.89).

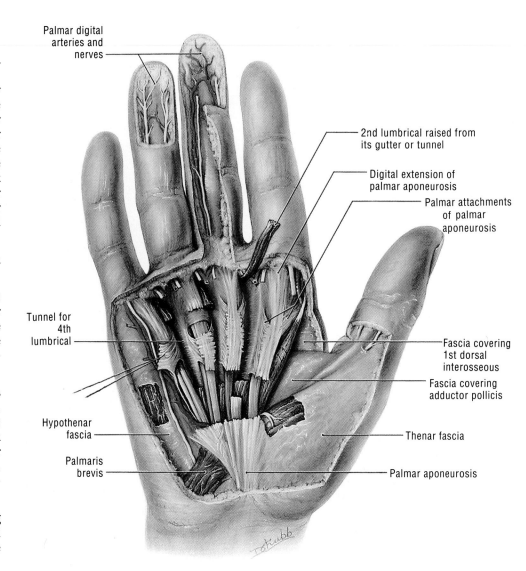

Palmar digital arteries and nerves

2nd lumbrical raised from its gutter or tunnel

Digital extension of palmar aponeurosis

Palmar attachments of palmar aponeurosis

Tunnel for 4th lumbrical

Fascia covering 1st dorsal interosseous

Fascia covering adductor pollicis

Hypothenar fascia

Thenar fascia

Palmaris brevis

Palmar aponeurosis

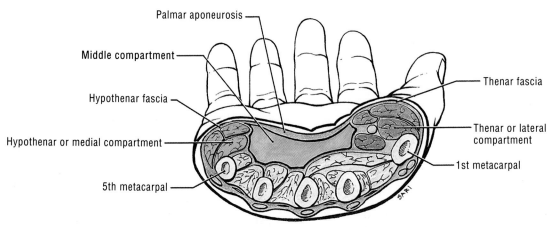

Palmar aponeurosis

Middle compartment

Thenar fascia

Hypothenar fascia

Thenar or lateral compartment

Hypothenar or medial compartment

1st metacarpal

5th metacarpal

6.89
Compartments of the palm of the hand

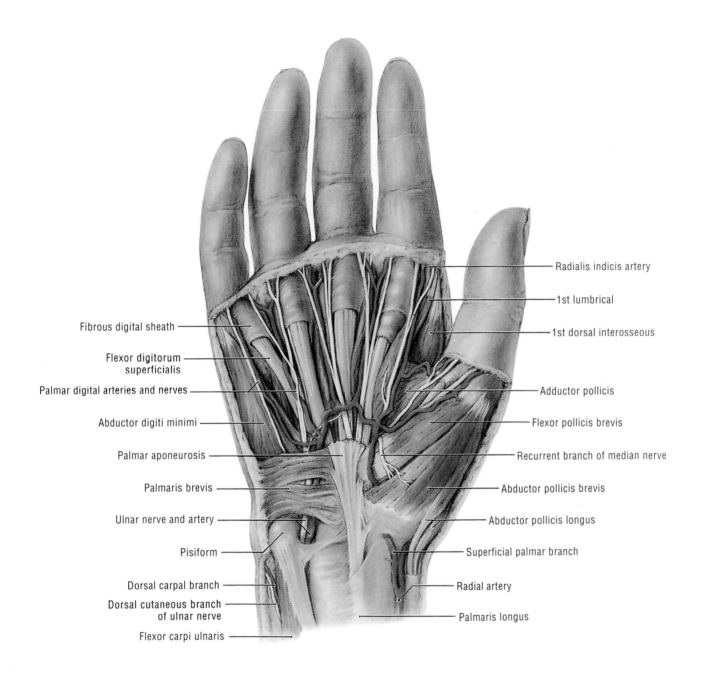

Fibrous digital sheath

Flexor digitorum superficialis

Palmar digital arteries and nerves

Abductor digiti minimi

Palmar aponeurosis

Palmaris brevis

Ulnar nerve and artery

Pisiform

Dorsal carpal branch

Dorsal cutaneous branch of ulnar nerve

Flexor carpi ulnaris

Radialis indicis artery

1st lumbrical

1st dorsal interosseous

Adductor pollicis

Flexor pollicis brevis

Recurrent branch of median nerve

Abductor pollicis brevis

Abductor pollicis longus

Superficial palmar branch

Radial artery

Palmaris longus

6.90
Superficial dissection of the palm

Observe:

1. Dissection has removed skin, superficial fascia, the palmar aponeurosis, and the thenar and hypothenar fasciae;

2. The superficial palmar arch is formed by the ulnar artery and is completed by the superficial palmar branch of the radial artery; only the structures removed from dissection and palmaris brevis cover the arch; it is truly superficial; so are the digital vessels and nerves and the recurrent branch of the median nerve;

3. The four lumbricals lie posterior to the digital vessels and nerves;

4. The prominent pisiform shelters the ulnar nerve and artery as they pass into the palm;

5. In the digits, a digital artery and nerve lying on the medial and lateral sides of the fibrous digital sheath.

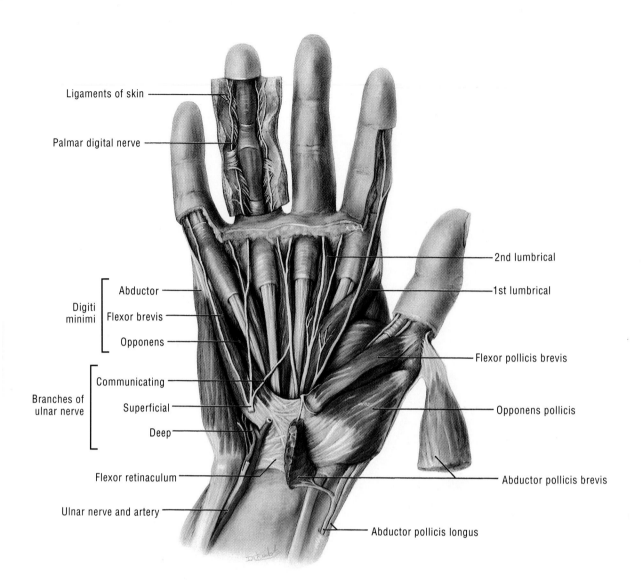

Ligaments of skin

Palmar digital nerve

Digiti minimi
- Abductor
- Flexor brevis
- Opponens

Branches of ulnar nerve
- Communicating
- Superficial
- Deep

Flexor retinaculum

Ulnar nerve and artery

2nd lumbrical

1st lumbrical

Flexor pollicis brevis

Opponens pollicis

Abductor pollicis brevis

Abductor pollicis longus

6.91
Superficial dissection of the palm, ulnar and median nerves

Observe:

1. The three thenar and three hypothenar muscles attaching to the flexor retinaculum and to the four marginal carpal bones united by the retinaculum;

2. The four lumbricals arise from the lateral sides of the profundus tendons, and are inserted into the lateral sides of the dorsal expansions (Fig. 6.112) of the corresponding digits; the medial two lumbricals, however, also arise from the medial sides of adjacent profundus tendons; and the 3rd lumbrical is commonly inserted into two extensor expansions, as here;

3. The median nerve is distributed in the hand to five muscles (three thenar and two lumbrical) and provides cutaneous branches to three digits;

4. The ulnar nerve supplies all other short (intrinsic) muscles in the hand and provides cutaneous branches to 1 1/2 digits; the communicating branch joining the ulnar and median nerves.

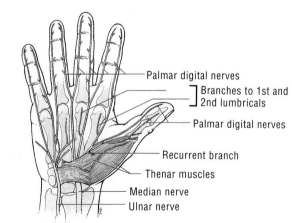

Palmar digital nerves

Branches to 1st and 2nd lumbricals

Palmar digital nerves

Recurrent branch

Thenar muscles

Median nerve

Ulnar nerve

6.92
Nerve supply of the hand

Observe that the recurrent branch (motor branch) of the median nerve arises from the lateral side of the nerve at the distal border of the flexor retinaculum muscle. The recurrent branch lies superficially and can easily be severed.

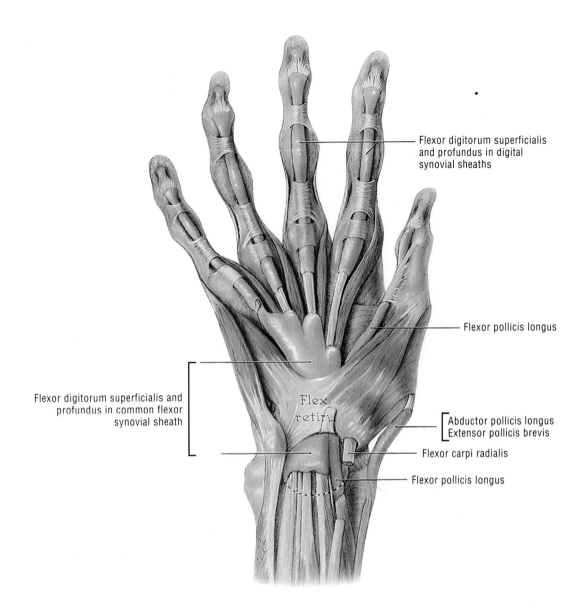

Flexor digitorum superficialis and profundus in digital synovial sheaths

Flexor pollicis longus

Flexor digitorum superficialis and profundus in common flexor synovial sheath

Flex. retin.

Abductor pollicis longus
Extensor pollicis brevis

Flexor carpi radialis

Flexor pollicis longus

6.93
Synovial sheaths of the long flexor tendons of the digits

Observe:

1. There are two sets: (a) proximal or carpal, posterior to the flexor retinaculum; (b) distal or digital, posterior to the fibrous sheaths of the digital flexors;

2. The carpal synovial sheaths, although developmentally separate, unite with one another to form a common flexor sheath, and the carpal sheath of the thumb tendon usually communicates with it; this common flexor sheath extends 1 to 2.5 cm proximal to the flexor retinaculum and distally farthest on the thumb and little finger where it is continuous with the distal sheaths;

3. Each digital sheath extends from the proximal end of the palmar ligament or plate to the base of a distal phalanx;

4. The flexor tendons glide across the very prominent anterior border of the inferior articular surface of the radius; hence the common flexor sheath extends further posteriorly *(broken line)* than anteriorly.

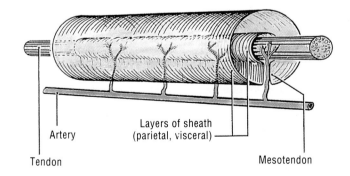

Layers of sheath
(parietal, visceral)

Artery

Tendon

Mesotendon

6.94
Synovial sheaths

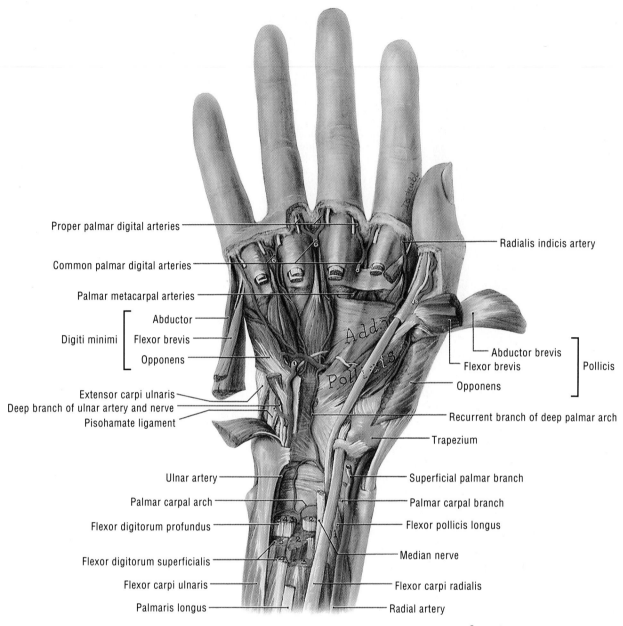

Proper palmar digital arteries

Common palmar digital arteries

Palmar metacarpal arteries

Radialis indicis artery

Digiti minimi — { Abductor / Flexor brevis / Opponens

Add
Pollicis

Abductor brevis
Flexor brevis   } Pollicis
Opponens

Extensor carpi ulnaris

Deep branch of ulnar artery and nerve

Pisohamate ligament

Recurrent branch of deep palmar arch

Trapezium

Ulnar artery

Palmar carpal arch

Flexor digitorum profundus

Superficial palmar branch

Palmar carpal branch

Flexor pollicis longus

Flexor digitorum superficialis

Median nerve

Flexor carpi ulnaris

Flexor carpi radialis

Palmaris longus

Radial artery

6.95
Deep dissection of the palm

Observe:

1. Flexor pollicis longus tendon making a spiral turn around the flexor carpi radialis muscle;

2. The deep branch of the ulnar artery joining the radial artery to form the deep palmar arch;

3. The transverse and oblique heads of the adductor pollicis muscle attaching to the medial side of the proximal phalanx of the thumb; there is usually a sesamoid bone contained in the tendon of insertion; the radial artery emerges on the palmar surface of the hand between the two heads of adductor pollicis muscle.

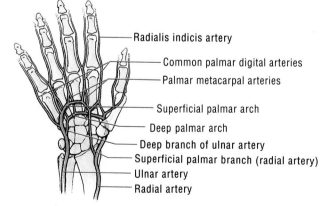

Radialis indicis artery

Common palmar digital arteries

Palmar metacarpal arteries

Superficial palmar arch

Deep palmar arch

Deep branch of ulnar artery

Superficial palmar branch (radial artery)

Ulnar artery

Radial artery

6.96
Diagram of the palmar arterial arches

Observe that the deep palmar arch lies at the level of the bases of the metacarpals and that the superficial palmar arch is more distally located.

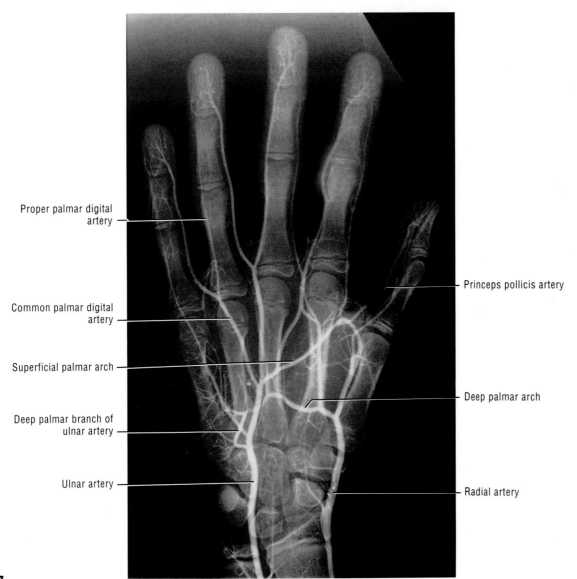

Proper palmar digital artery

Common palmar digital artery

Superficial palmar arch

Deep palmar branch of ulnar artery

Ulnar artery

Princeps pollicis artery

Deep palmar arch

Radial artery

6.97
Arteriogram of the hand

(Courtesy of Dr. D. Armstrong, Associate Professor of Radiology, University of Toronto, Toronto, Ontario, Canada.)

6.98
Dissection of the palmar arterial arches

The superficial palmar arch is formed primarily by the ulnar artery and is usually completed by the superficial palmar branch of the radial artery (Fig. 6.96). Here the dorsalis pollicis artery completes the arch. The deep palmar arch is formed by the radial artery that enters the palmar surface of the hand passing between the bases of the 1st and 2nd metacarpals and between the two heads of the 1st dorsal interosseous and adductor pollicis muscles. The deep branch of the ulnar artery completes the arch.

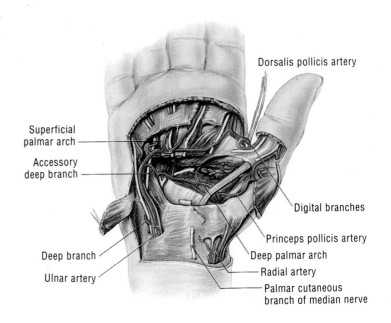

Dorsalis pollicis artery

Superficial palmar arch

Accessory deep branch

Digital branches

Princeps pollicis artery

Deep palmar arch

Radial artery

Deep branch

Ulnar artery

Palmar cutaneous branch of median nerve

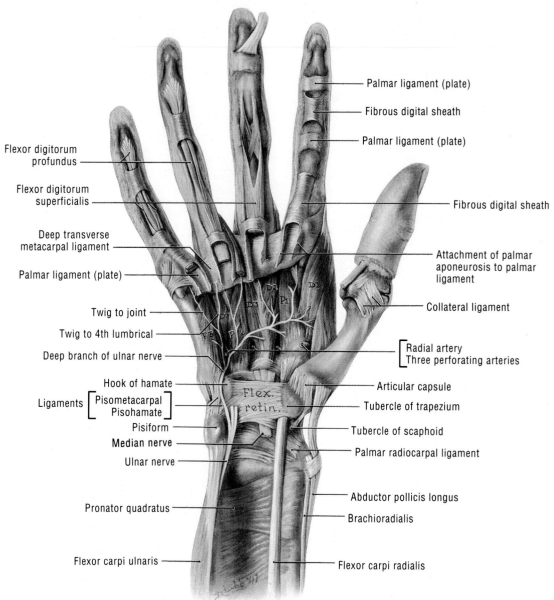

Flexor digitorum profundus

Flexor digitorum superficialis

Deep transverse metacarpal ligament

Palmar ligament (plate)

Twig to joint

Twig to 4th lumbrical

Deep branch of ulnar nerve

Hook of hamate

Ligaments [Pisometacarpal / Pisohamate]

Pisiform

Median nerve

Ulnar nerve

Pronator quadratus

Flexor carpi ulnaris

Palmar ligament (plate)

Fibrous digital sheath

Palmar ligament (plate)

Fibrous digital sheath

Attachment of palmar aponeurosis to palmar ligament

Collateral ligament

Radial artery / Three perforating arteries

Articular capsule

Tubercle of trapezium

Tubercle of scaphoid

Palmar radiocarpal ligament

Abductor pollicis longus

Brachioradialis

Flexor carpi radialis

Flex. retin.

6.99
Deep dissection of the palm and digits, ulnar nerve

Observe:

1. The flexor retinaculum uniting the four marginal carpal bones; the ulnar nerve lying anterior and the median nerve lying posterior to the retinaculum;

2. The flexor carpi radialis muscle descending vertically anterior to the tubercle of the scaphoid and along the groove on the trapezium to the 2nd metacarpal;

3. The flexor carpi ulnaris muscle continuing beyond the pisiform as the pisohamate and the pisometacarpal ligament;

4. The loose capsule of the carpometacarpal joint of the thumb and the strong collateral ligament of its metacarpophalangeal joint;

5. Four dorsal and three palmar interossei muscles;

6. The ulnar nerve crossing the hook of the hamate to be distributed by its deep branch to the three hypothenar muscles, all seven interossei, two lumbricals, the adductor pollicis, and several joints; the superficial branch supplies the palmaris brevis muscle and sensation to 1 1/2 digits;

7. The palmar ligaments, with the deep transverse metacarpal ligaments uniting them, and the septa from the palmar aponeurosis attached to them;

8. Lumbricals passing anterior to the deep transverse metacarpal ligament, and interossei passing posterior to the ligament;

9. On the index finger, a proximal and distal osseofibrous tunnel; on the middle finger, a superficialis tendon spreading like a "V" and then decussating like an "X"; on the ring finger, a profundus tendon; and on the little finger, both superficialis and profundus tendons.

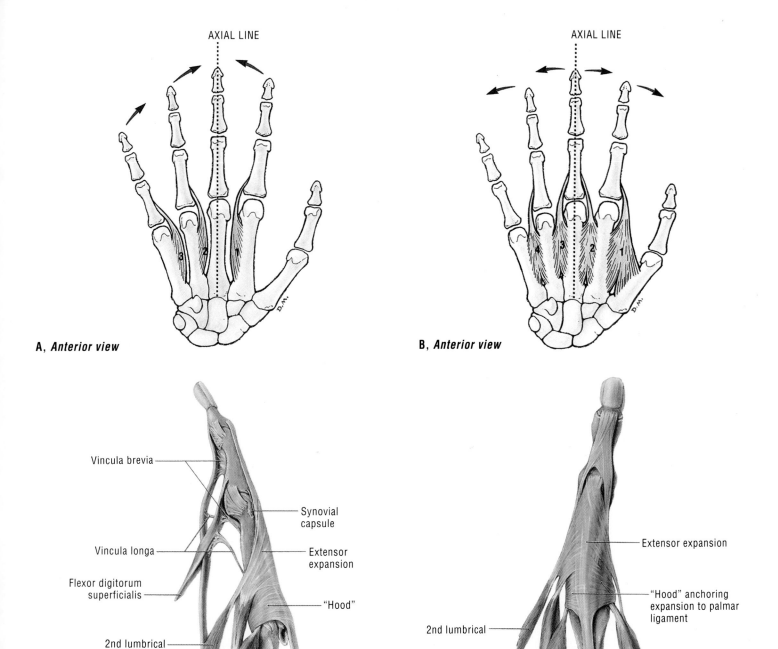

A, *Anterior view*

B, *Anterior view*

Vincula brevia

Synovial capsule

Vincula longa

Extensor expansion

Flexor digitorum superficialis

"Hood"

2nd lumbrical

2nd dorsal interosseous

Extensor digitorum

Flexor digitorum profundus

3rd

C, *Lateral view*

Extensor expansion

"Hood" anchoring expansion to palmar ligament

2nd lumbrical

3rd dorsal interosseous

2nd dorsal interosseous

Extensor digitorum

D, *Dorsal view*

6.100
Interossei

A. Palmar interossei. **B.** Dorsal interossei. **C.** and **D.** Extensor expansion of the 3rd (middle) digit.

Observe:

1. Three, unipennate palmar and four, bipennate dorsal interosseous muscles; the palmar interossei adduct the fingers and the dorsal interossei abduct the fingers in relation to the axial line, an imaginary line drawn through the long axis of the 3rd digit (**A** and **B**);

2. The palmar and dorsal interossei pass posterior to the deep transverse metacarpal ligament (Fig. 6.99) and insert into the base of the proximal phalanx and into the extensor expansion (**C**) and (**D**); the part of the muscle attaching to the base of the proximal phalanx functions in abduction and adduction of the fingers and the part attaching to the extensor expansion functions in flexion of the metacarpophalangeal joints and extension of the interphalangeal joints of the fingers.

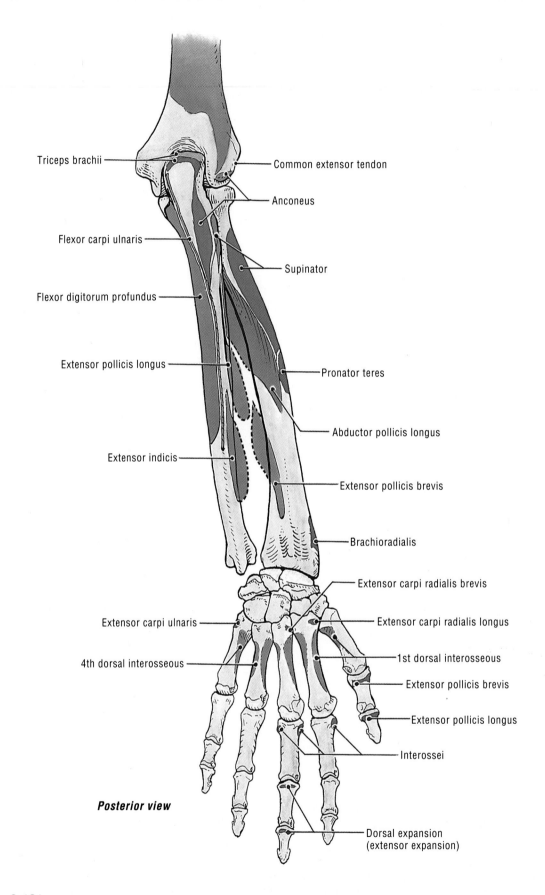

Triceps brachii

Flexor carpi ulnaris

Flexor digitorum profundus

Extensor pollicis longus

Extensor indicis

Extensor carpi ulnaris

4th dorsal interosseous

Common extensor tendon

Anconeus

Supinator

Pronator teres

Abductor pollicis longus

Extensor pollicis brevis

Brachioradialis

Extensor carpi radialis brevis

Extensor carpi radialis longus

1st dorsal interosseous

Extensor pollicis brevis

Extensor pollicis longus

Interossei

Dorsal expansion
(extensor expansion)

Posterior view

6.101
Bones of forearm and hand showing attachments of muscles

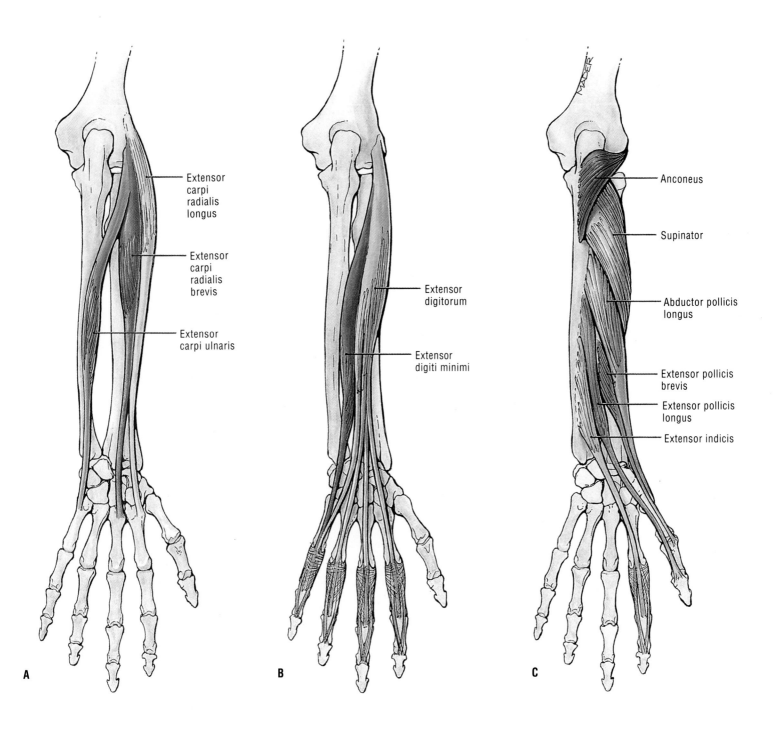

A

Extensor carpi radialis longus

Extensor carpi radialis brevis

Extensor carpi ulnaris

B

Extensor digitorum

Extensor digiti minimi

C

Anconeus

Supinator

Abductor pollicis longus

Extensor pollicis brevis

Extensor pollicis longus

Extensor indicis

6.102
Superficial and deep (outcropping) posterior forearm muscles

Examine the diagrams in relation to the origins and insertions shown in Fig. 6.101. **A** and **B** show the superficial layer of muscle (brachioradialis is not shown). **C** shows the supinator muscle and the deep (outcropping) muscles attaching to the thumb and index finger. Note the tendons of extensor digitorum, extensor digiti minimi, and extensor indicis forming the extensor (dorsal) expansion. The lumbricals and interossei also contribute to the expansion.

6.103
Muscles of the extensor region of the forearm

Observe:

1. The digital extensors have been reflected without disturbing the arteries since they lie on the skeletal plane;

2. No muscle is attached to the posterior surface of a carpal bone;

3. The radial artery disappearing between the two heads of the 1st dorsal interosseous muscle.

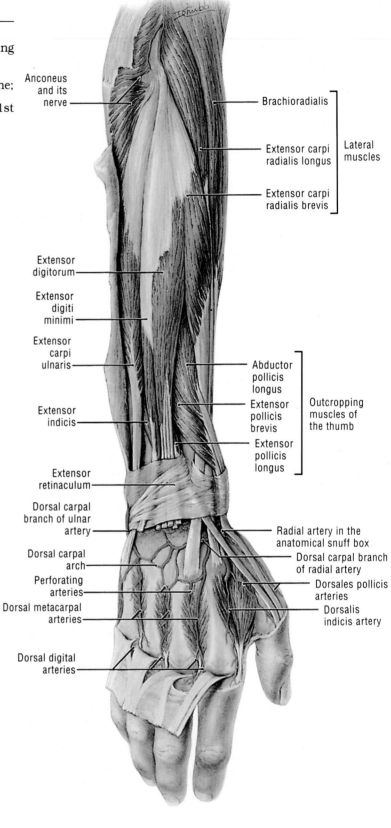

Anconeus and its nerve

Brachioradialis

Extensor carpi radialis longus — Lateral muscles

Extensor carpi radialis brevis

Extensor digitorum

Extensor digiti minimi

Extensor carpi ulnaris

Abductor pollicis longus

Extensor pollicis brevis — Outcropping muscles of the thumb

Extensor indicis

Extensor pollicis longus

Extensor retinaculum

Dorsal carpal branch of ulnar artery

Radial artery in the anatomical snuff box

Dorsal carpal arch

Dorsal carpal branch of radial artery

Perforating arteries

Dorsales pollicis arteries

Dorsal metacarpal arteries

Dorsalis indicis artery

Dorsal digital arteries

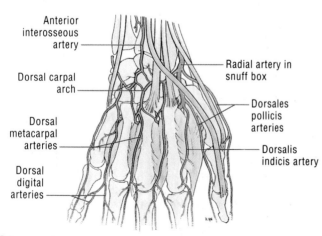

Anterior interosseous artery

Radial artery in snuff box

Dorsal carpal arch

Dorsal metacarpal arteries

Dorsales pollicis arteries

Dorsal digital arteries

Dorsalis indicis artery

6.104
Branches of the radial artery on the dorsum of the hand

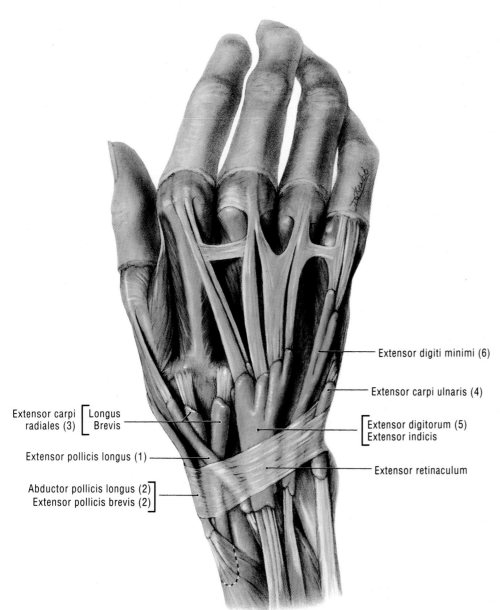

Extensor digiti minimi (6)

Extensor carpi ulnaris (4)

Extensor carpi radiales (3) [Longus / Brevis]

Extensor digitorum (5)
Extensor indicis

Extensor pollicis longus (1)

Extensor retinaculum

Abductor pollicis longus (2)
Extensor pollicis brevis (2)

6.105
Synovial sheaths on the dorsum of the wrist

Observe:

1. These six sheaths occupy the six osseofibrous tunnels deep to the extensor retinaculum and contain nine tendons: tendons for the thumb in sheaths 1 and 2; tendons for the extensors of wrist in sheaths 3 and 4; tendons for the extensors of the wrist and fingers in sheaths 5 and 6;

2. The band of thickened deep fascia, the extensor retinaculum.

3. The tendon of the extensor pollicis longus hooking around the dorsal radial tubercle to pass obliquely across the tendons of extensor carpi radialis longus and brevis muscles to the thumb.

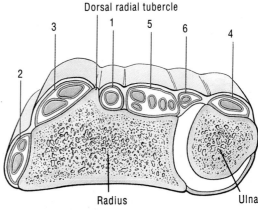

Dorsal radial tubercle

3 1 5 6 4

2

Radius   Ulna

6.106
Tendons on dorsum of the wrist, transverse section

Numbers refer to structures in Figure 6.105.

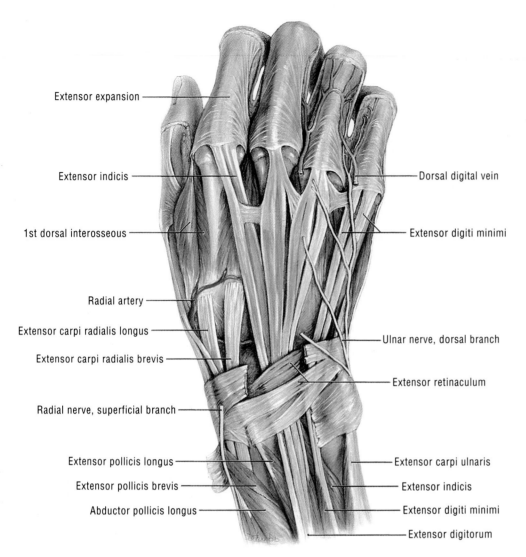

Extensor expansion

Extensor indicis

1st dorsal interosseous

Radial artery

Extensor carpi radialis longus

Extensor carpi radialis brevis

Radial nerve, superficial branch

Extensor pollicis longus

Extensor pollicis brevis

Abductor pollicis longus

Dorsal digital vein

Extensor digiti minimi

Ulnar nerve, dorsal branch

Extensor retinaculum

Extensor carpi ulnaris

Extensor indicis

Extensor digiti minimi

Extensor digitorum

6.107
Tendons on the dorsum of the hand, extensor retinaculum muscle

Observe:

1. The disposition of the tendons of the muscles on the dorsum of the wrist and hand;

2. The deep fascia, here thickened and called the extensor retinaculum, stretching obliquely from one ridge on the radius to another; medially, it passes distal to the ulna to attach to the pisiform and triquetrum bones, as depicted in Figure 6.119**B**;

3. The bands, proximal to the knuckles, that connect the tendons of the digital extensors and thereby restrict the independent action of the fingers;

4. The digital veins passing to the dorsum of the hand where they are not subjected to pressure;

5. The body (shaft) of the 2nd metacarpal is not covered with an extensor tendon.

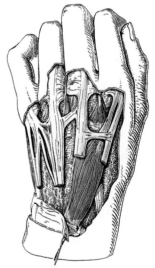

6.108
Extensor digitorum brevis muscle

This muscle, constant on the dorsum of the foot, is found occasionally on the dorsum of the hand, usually as a single bundle.

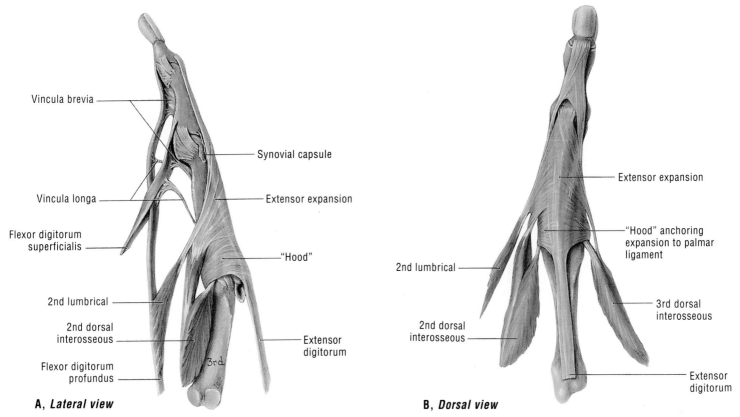

Vincula brevia

Synovial capsule

Vincula longa

Extensor expansion

Flexor digitorum superficialis

"Hood"

2nd lumbrical

2nd dorsal interosseous

Extensor digitorum

Flexor digitorum profundus

A, *Lateral view*

Extensor expansion

"Hood" anchoring expansion to palmar ligament

2nd lumbrical

3rd dorsal interosseous

2nd dorsal interosseous

Extensor digitorum

B, *Dorsal view*

6.109
Extensor (dorsal) expansion of the 3rd digit

Observe:

1. Interossei, in part, inserted into the bases of the proximal phalanges and, in part, into the extensor expansion;

2. Lumbrical inserted wholly into the radial side of the expansion;

3. The hood covering the head of the metacarpal; it is attached to the palmar ligament; hence medial and lateral bowstringing of the extensor tendon and expansion is prevented;

4. The expansion extending to the bases of the middle and distal phalanges, and giving a strong areolar band to the base of the proximal phalanx, here not in view;

5. The vincula longa and brevia are all that remain of the primitive mesotendons.

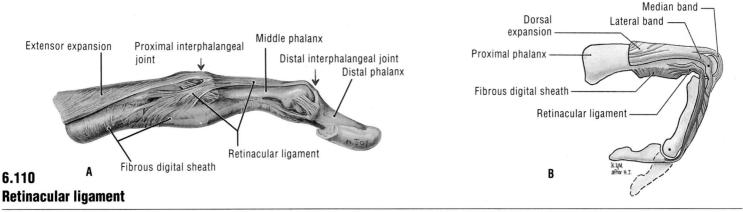

Extensor expansion

Proximal interphalangeal joint

Middle phalanx

Distal interphalangeal joint

Distal phalanx

Retinacular ligament

Fibrous digital sheath

A

Median band

Dorsal expansion

Lateral band

Proximal phalanx

Fibrous digital sheath

Retinacular ligament

B

6.110
Retinacular ligament

Observe in **A** and **B**:

1. The retinacular ligament is a delicate fibrous band that runs from the proximal phalanx and the fibrous digital sheath obliquely across the middle phalanx and the two interphalangeal joints to join the dorsal expansion, and so to the distal phalanx;

2. On flexing the distal interphalangeal joint, the retinacular ligament becomes taut and pulls the proximal joint into flexion;

3. Similarly, on extending the proximal joint, the distal joint is pulled by the retinacular ligament into nearly complete extension (see Landsmeer JMF. *The anatomy of the dorsal aponeurosis of the human finger and its functional significance.* Anat Rec 1949; 104:31).

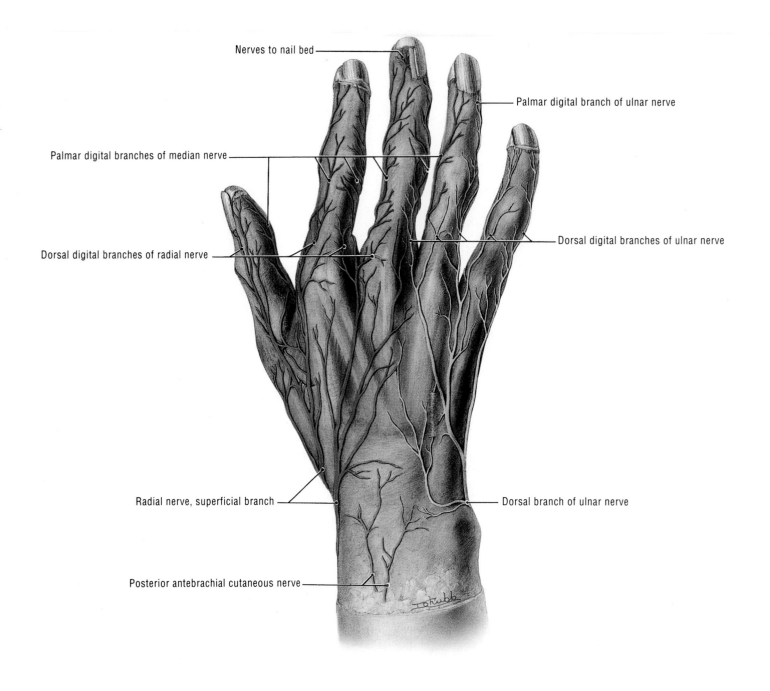

Nerves to nail bed

Palmar digital branch of ulnar nerve

Palmar digital branches of median nerve

Dorsal digital branches of ulnar nerve

Dorsal digital branches of radial nerve

Radial nerve, superficial branch

Dorsal branch of ulnar nerve

Posterior antebrachial cutaneous nerve

6.111
Cutaneous nerves of the dorsum of the hand

Observe:

1. The radial nerve and the dorsal branch of the ulnar nerve distributed nearly equally and symmetrically on the dorsum of the hand and digits; the radial nerve supplies the radial half of the dorsum of the hand and the lateral 2 1/2 digits (all the way along the 1st digit); the dorsal branch of the ulnar nerve behaves similarly on the ulnar half of the hand;

2. The palmar digital branches of the median and ulnar nerves alone supply the distal halves of the three middle digits, including the nail beds;

3. Communications between adjacent nerves are numerous.

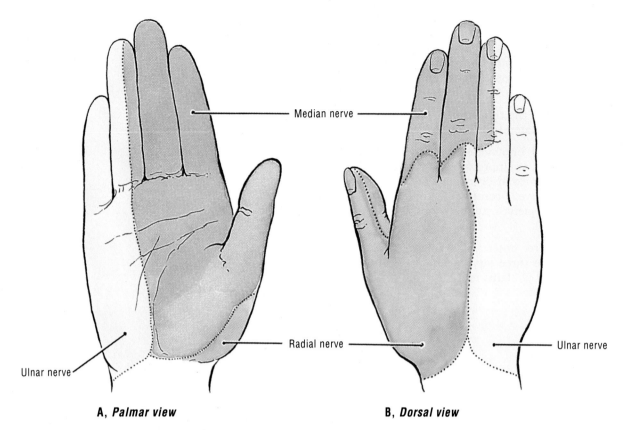

A, *Palmar view*

B, *Dorsal view*

6.112
Distribution of cutaneous nerves to palm and dorsum of the hand

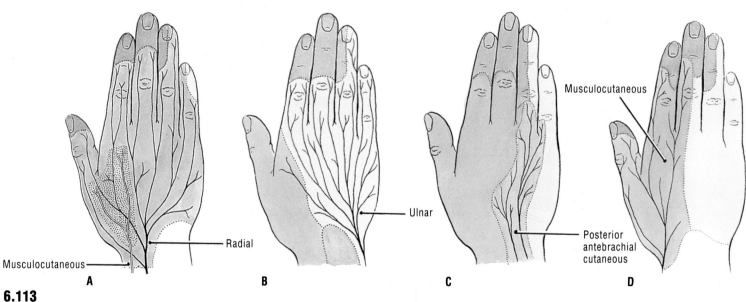

A

B

C

D

6.113
Variations in pattern of cutaneous nerves in the dorsum of the hand

(See Appleton AB. *A case of abnormal distribution of the musculocutaneous nerve.* J Anat Physiol 1911; 46:89; Hutton WR. *Remarks on the innervation of the dorsus manus with special reference to certain rare abnormalities.* J Anat Physiol 1906; 40:326; Learmonth JR. *A variation in the distribution of the "radial nerve."* J Anat 1919; 53:371; and Stopford JSB. *The variation in distribution of the cutaneous nerves of the hand and digits.* J Anat 1918; 53:14.)

6.114
Deep structures on the posterior aspect of the forearm

Observe:

1. Three muscles of the thumb outcropping between extensor carpi radialis brevis and extensor digitorum: abductor pollicis longus, extensor pollicis brevis, and extensor pollicis longus;

2. The furrow from which the three muscles outcrop has been opened proximally to the lateral epicondyle exposing supinator;

3. The laterally retracted brachioradialis and extensor carpi radialis longus and brevis are innervated by the deep branch of the radial nerve, the other extensor muscles are supplied by the posterior interosseous nerve (a continuation of the deep branch of the radial nerve after it pierces supinator and emerges inferior to the head of the radius);

4. The tendons of the three outcropping muscles of the thumb pass to the bases of the three long bones of the thumb, the metacarpal, the proximal phalanx, and the distal phalanx.

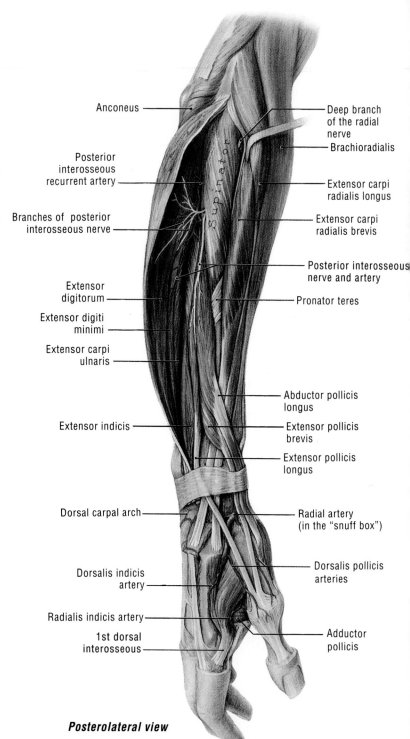

Posterolateral view

6.115
Transverse section of forearm showing nerve supply

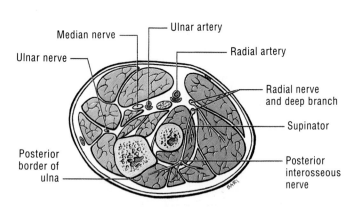

The flexor territory (orange), supplied by ulnar and median nerves, is separated from extensor territory (red) supplied by the radial nerve, by the radial artery laterally, and by the posterior, sharp, palpable border of the ulna posteromedially. No motor nerve crosses either line.

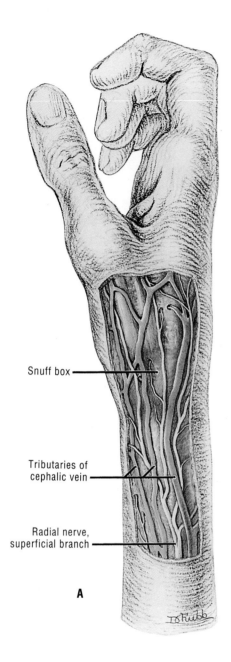

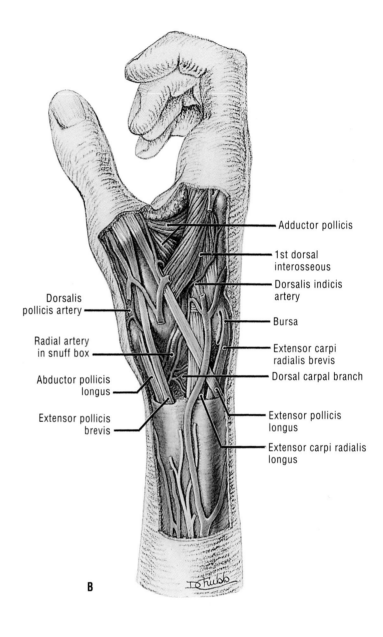

Snuff box

Tributaries of
cephalic vein

Radial nerve,
superficial branch

A

Dorsalis
pollicis artery

Radial artery
in snuff box

Abductor pollicis
longus

Extensor pollicis
brevis

Adductor pollicis

1st dorsal
interosseous

Dorsalis indicis
artery

Bursa

Extensor carpi
radialis brevis

Dorsal carpal branch

Extensor pollicis
longus

Extensor carpi radialis
longus

B

6.116
Lateral aspect of the wrist

Observe in **A**:

1. The depression at the base of the thumb: the "anatomical snuff box," retaining its name from an archaic habit;

2. Superficial veins, including the cephalic vein and/or its tributaries, and cutaneous nerves crossing the snuff box;

3. Perforating veins and articular nerves piercing the deep fascia.

Observe in **B**:

1. Three long tendons of the thumb forming the boundaries of the snuff box;

2. The radial artery and its venae comitantes crossing the floor of the snuff box and disappearing between the two heads of the 1st dorsal interosseous;

3. Adductor pollicis and 1st dorsal interosseous, proximal to the web between the pollex and index digits; both are supplied by the ulnar nerve.

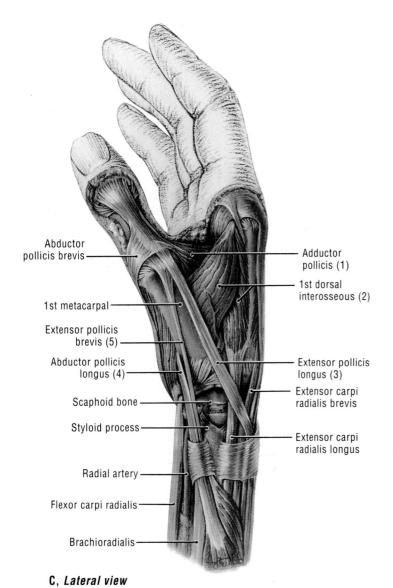

Abductor
pollicis brevis

1st metacarpal

Extensor pollicis
brevis (5)

Abductor pollicis
longus (4)

Scaphoid bone

Styloid process

Radial artery

Flexor carpi radialis

Brachioradialis

Adductor
pollicis (1)

1st dorsal
interosseous (2)

Extensor pollicis
longus (3)

Extensor carpi
radialis brevis

Extensor carpi
radialis longus

C, *Lateral view*

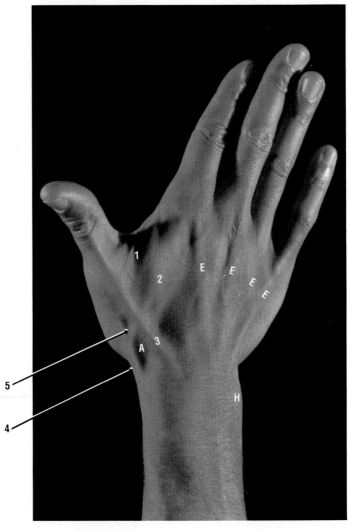

6.116
Lateral aspect of the wrist *(continued)*

Observe in **C**:

1. The scaphoid bone; the wrist joint (and radius) proximal to the scaphoid; and the midcarpal joint (and trapezium and trapezoid) distal to it;

2. The capsule of the 1st carpometacarpal joint;

3. The abductor pollicis brevis and adductor pollicis muscles partly inserted into the dorsal (extensor) expansion.

6.117
Surface anatomy of the wrist and hand

H - Head of ulna, *E* - Tendons of extensor digitorum longus, *A* - Anatomical snuff box. Numbers refer to structures in Figure 6.116**C**.

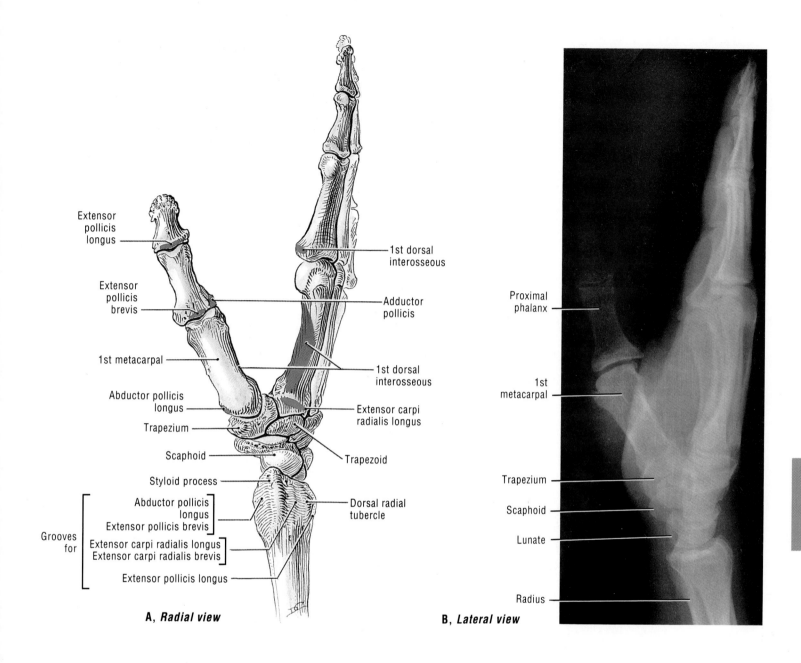

A, Radial view

Extensor pollicis longus

Extensor pollicis brevis

1st metacarpal

Abductor pollicis longus

Trapezium

Scaphoid

Styloid process

Grooves for
{
Abductor pollicis longus
Extensor pollicis brevis
}
{
Extensor carpi radialis longus
Extensor carpi radialis brevis
}
Extensor pollicis longus

1st dorsal interosseous

Adductor pollicis

1st dorsal interosseous

Extensor carpi radialis longus

Trapezoid

Dorsal radial tubercle

B, Lateral view

Proximal phalanx

1st metacarpal

Trapezium

Scaphoid

Lunate

Radius

6.118
Wrist and hand

Observe in **A**:

1. The attachments of muscles to bone;

2. Articular surfaces (pale blue);

3. The anatomical snuff box, limited proximally by the styloid process of the radius and distally by the base of the 1st metacarpal;

4. The two lateral marginal bones of the carpus (scaphoid and trapezium) forming the floor of the snuff box.

B. Radiograph. (Courtesy of Dr. E.L. Lansdown, Professor of Radiology, University of Toronto, Toronto, Ontario, Canada.)

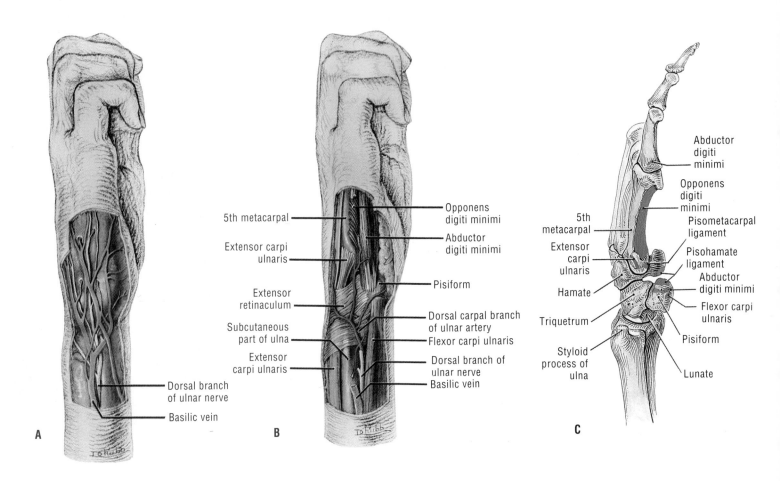

6.119
Serial dissection of the medial border of the wrist from superficial to deep

Observe in **A**:

1. The superficial veins and their perforating branches;

2. The cutaneous nerve appearing from deep to the flexor carpi ulnaris.

Observe in **B**: A vertical incision made along the medial subcutaneous surface of the ulna and along the medial border of the hand passes between two motor territories (flexor carpi ulnaris, abductor digiti minimi, and opponens digiti minimi, supplied by the ulnar nerve; and extensor carpi ulnaris by the posterior interosseous nerve); superficial veins, nerves, and arteries will be divided, but no motor nerves will be touched.

Observe in **C**:

1. Attachments of muscles to bone;

2. Extensor carpi ulnaris is inserted directly into the base of the 5th metacarpal;

3. Flexor carpi ulnaris is inserted indirectly through the medium of the pisiform bone and the pisometacarpal ligament to the base of the 5th metacarpal.

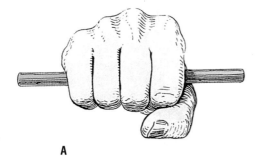
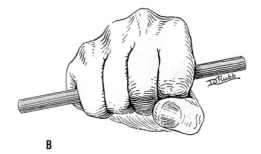

A

B

6.120
Grasping hand

A. Loosely held.

B. Firmly gripped. The 2nd and 3rd carpometacarpal joints are rigid and stable; but the 4th and 5th are hinge joints permitting flexion and extension; this is apparent on inspection of the skeleton and on grasping a cylindrical structure; it is a forward movement, or flexion, of the 4th and 5th metacarpals that gives tenacity to the grip on a rod, such as the handle of a rake or wheelbarrow.

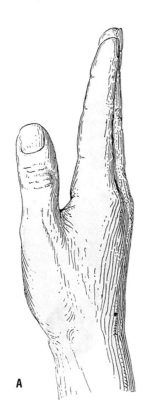
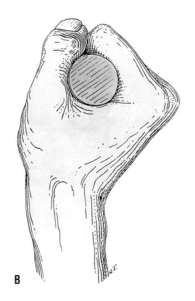

A

B

6.121
Wrist extension of the grasping hand

A. The extended hand.

B. When grasping an object, the metacarpophalangeal and the interphalangeal joints are flexed, but the radiocarpal (wrist) and transverse carpal joints are extended; the grasping hand requires an extended wrist; without this extension, the grip is feeble and insecure; the extensor carpi radialis longus and brevis and extensor carpi ulnaris muscles, as synergists, are essential to the digital flexors when grasping, hence their strength.

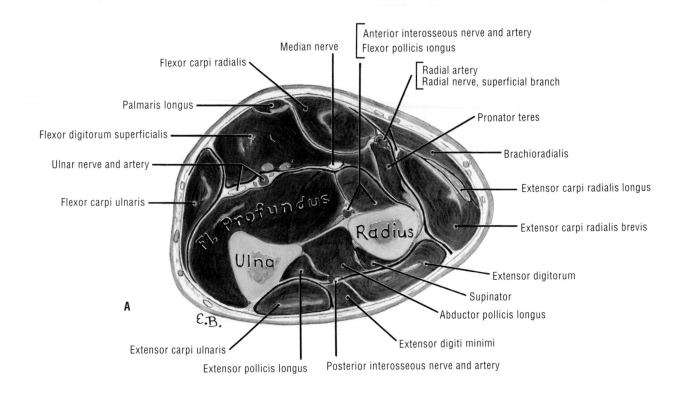

Median nerve

Flexor carpi radialis

Palmaris longus

Flexor digitorum superficialis

Ulnar nerve and artery

Flexor carpi ulnaris

Anterior interosseous nerve and artery
Flexor pollicis longus

Radial artery
Radial nerve, superficial branch

Pronator teres

Brachioradialis

Extensor carpi radialis longus

Extensor carpi radialis brevis

Fl. Profundus

Radius

Ulna

Extensor digitorum

Supinator

Abductor pollicis longus

E.B.

A

Extensor carpi ulnaris

Extensor pollicis longus

Extensor digiti minimi

Posterior interosseous nerve and artery

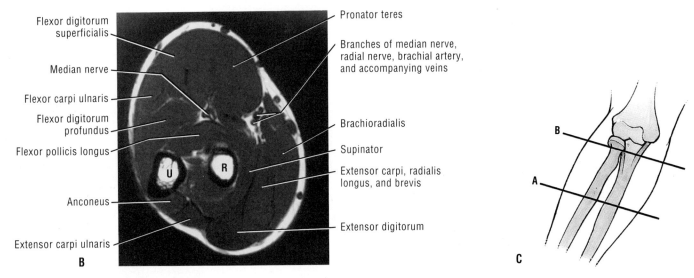

Flexor digitorum superficialis

Median nerve

Flexor carpi ulnaris

Flexor digitorum profundus

Flexor pollicis longus

Anconeus

Extensor carpi ulnaris

B

Pronator teres

Branches of median nerve, radial nerve, brachial artery, and accompanying veins

Brachioradialis

Supinator

Extensor carpi, radialis longus, and brevis

Extensor digitorum

U

R

B

A

C

6.122
Transverse section through the midforearm

Observe in **A**:

1. The interosseous membrane spanning from the interosseous (lateral) border of the ulna to a fibrocartilaginous labrum along the interosseous (medial) border of the radius;

2. The ulnar nerve and artery and the median nerve lying in the areolar septum between the superficial and deep digital flexors, i.e., between flexor digitorum superficialis and flexor digitorum profundus and flexor pollicis longus; the ulnar nerve clinging to profundus and supplying its medial part; the median nerve clinging to superficialis and supplying it; the anterior interosseous branch of the median nerve, placed on the skeletal plane;

3. The radial artery overlapped by the brachioradialis muscle;

4. The superficial branch of the radial nerve following the anterior border of extensor carpi radialis brevis; the posterior interosseous nerve lying between the superficial and deep layers of digital extensors;

5. Flexor digitorum profundus and flexor pollicis longus muscles wrapped around the medial and anterior surfaces of the ulna and the anterior surface of the radius; the pronator teres muscle inserted into the lateral surface of the radius, hence its ability to pronate;

6. The fascial planes between the muscle(s).

B. Transverse MRI (magnetic resonance image) of the proximal forearm. *U* - Ulna, *R* - Radius. (Courtesy of Dr. W. Kucharczyk, Clinical Director of Tri-Hospital Resonance Centre, Toronto, Ontario, Canada.)

C shows the level of section in **A** and **B**.

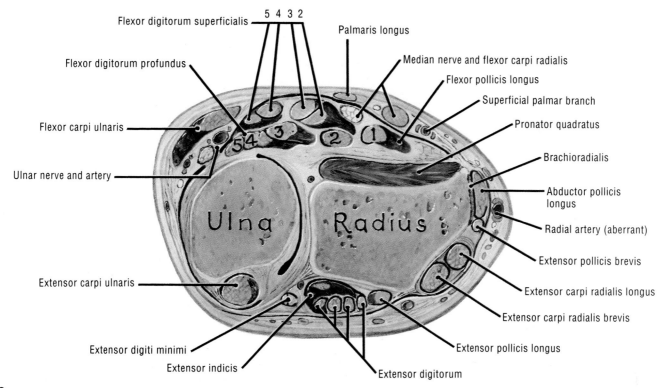

Flexor digitorum superficialis 5 4 3 2

Flexor digitorum profundus

Palmaris longus

Median nerve and flexor carpi radialis

Flexor pollicis longus

Superficial palmar branch

Flexor carpi ulnaris

Pronator quadratus

Ulnar nerve and artery

Brachioradialis

Abductor pollicis longus

Radial artery (aberrant)

Extensor pollicis brevis

Extensor carpi ulnaris

Extensor carpi radialis longus

Extensor carpi radialis brevis

Extensor digiti minimi

Extensor pollicis longus

Extensor indicis

Extensor digitorum

6.123
Transverse section through the distal forearm

Observe:

1. The synovial cavity of the distal radioulnar joint;

2. Flexor carpi radialis, palmaris longus, and flexor carpi ulnaris constituting a surface layer of flexors of the wrist;

3. Deep to these, the long flexors of the digits: (a) the four tendons of the flexor digitorum superficialis lying two deep, those to the middle and ring fingers being anterior to those to the index and little fingers; (b) the five tendons of the deep digital flexors, lying side by side, those to the thumb and index being free;

4. The ulnar nerve and artery under cover of flexor carpi ulnaris where the pulse of the artery could not be felt; the median nerve at the midpoint on the front of the wrist, deep to palmaris longus, and at the lateral border of flexus digitorum superficialis; the radial artery is here aberrant, so its pulse might be missed;

5. Four tendons on the dorsum of the wrist, large, because, being inserted into metacarpal bones, they work as synergists with the powerful flexors of the digits, whereas the remaining tendons, being extensors of the digits, are slender.

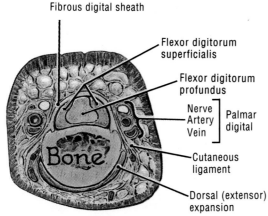

Fibrous digital sheath

Flexor digitorum superficialis

Flexor digitorum profundus

Nerve
Artery } Palmar
Vein   digital

Cutaneous ligament

Dorsal (extensor) expansion

6.124
Transverse section of proximal phalanx

Observe that the palmar digital nerve and vessels are applied to the fibrous sheath, not to bone. The skin is thickest on the palmar surface.

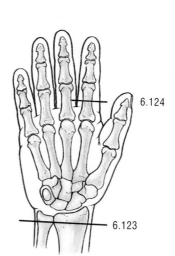

6.124

6.123

6.125
Level of section

Diagram shows the level of section in Figures 6.123 and 6.124.

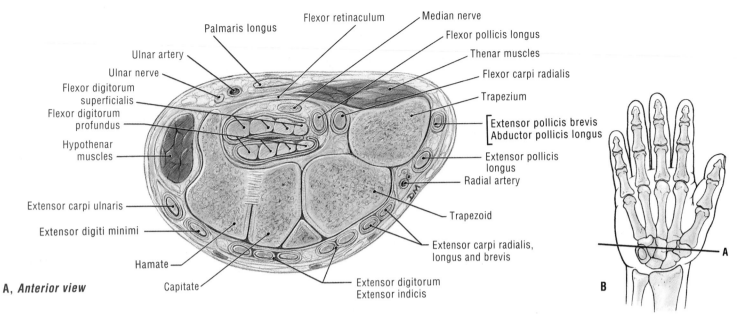

A, Anterior view

6.126
Transverse section of the wrist, carpal tunnel

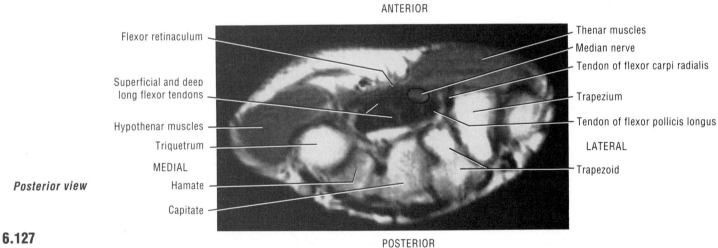

6.127
Transverse MRI (magnetic resonance image) of the wrist, carpal tunnel

(Courtesy of Dr. W. Kucharczyk, Clinical Director of Tri-Hospital Resonance Centre, Toronto, Ontario, Canada.)

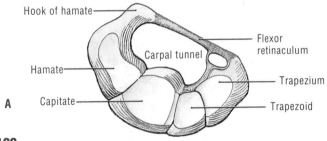

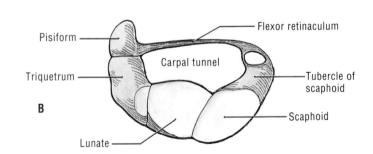

6.128
Diagram of transverse section through the carpal tunnel

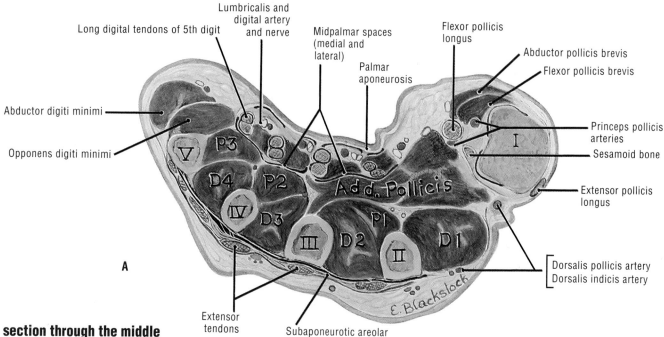

6.129

Transverse section through the middle of the palm

Observe in **A**:

1. The section passes through the head of the 1st metacarpal and is, therefore, distal to the opponens pollicis muscle;

2. The four dorsal interosseous muscles (abductors) fill the spaces between the five metacarpal bones;

3. The three palmar interosseous muscles (adductors) arise from the palmar aspects of the 2nd, 4th, and 5th metacarpal bones, and the adductor pollicis muscle from the palmar aspects of the 3rd;

4. All interossei and the adductor muscle are supplied by the ulnar nerve;

5. Between the foregoing muscles and the palmar aponeurosis lie the long flexor tendons (superficial and deep) of the four fingers, and four lumbricals, and the palmar digital nerves and arteries;

6. Flexor pollicis longus tendon, in its synovial sheath, accompanied by its palmar digital arteries and nerves, and passing anterior to the palmar ligament (palmar plate) of the metacarpophalangeal joint;

7. The flattened tendons of the extensor digitorum muscle.

B. Diagram shows level of section in **A**.

C. Coronal MRI (magnetic resonance image) of the wrist and hand. (Courtesy of Dr. W. Kucharczyk, Clinical Director of Tri-Hospital Resonance Centre, Toronto, Ontario, Canada.)

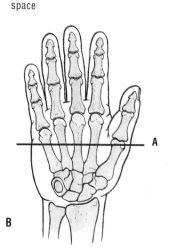

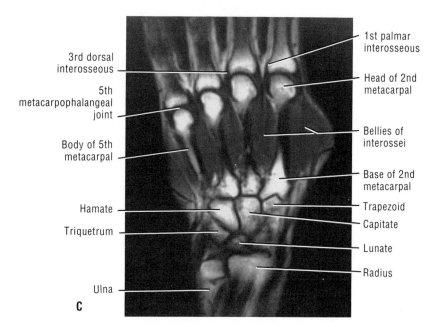

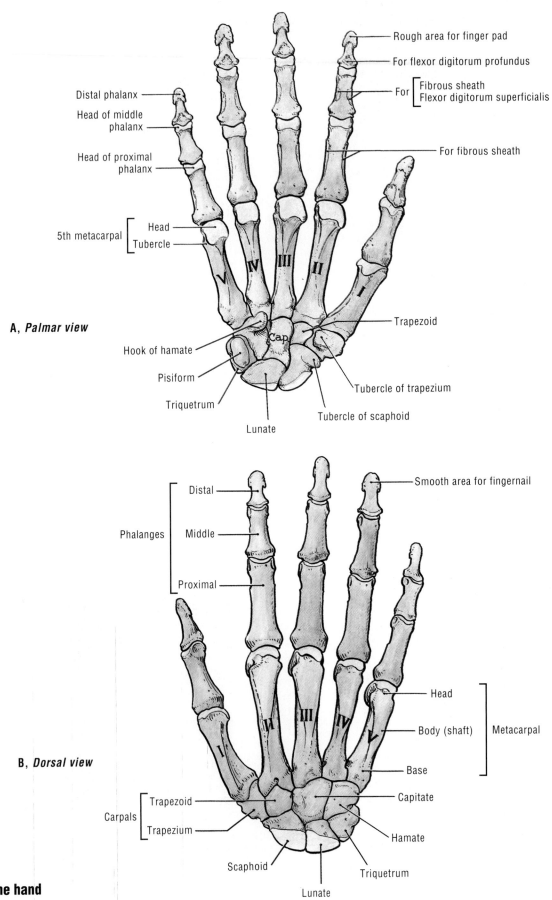

A, *Palmar view*

Rough area for finger pad

For flexor digitorum profundus

For [Fibrous sheath
Flexor digitorum superficialis

Distal phalanx

Head of middle phalanx

Head of proximal phalanx

For fibrous sheath

5th metacarpal [Head
Tubercle

Trapezoid

Hook of hamate

Cap.

Pisiform

Triquetrum

Lunate

Tubercle of trapezium

Tubercle of scaphoid

B, *Dorsal view*

Distal

Smooth area for fingernail

Phalanges

Middle

Proximal

Head

Body (shaft) Metacarpal

Base

Capitate

Carpals [Trapezoid
Trapezium

Hamate

Scaphoid

Triquetrum

Lunate

6.130
Bones of the hand

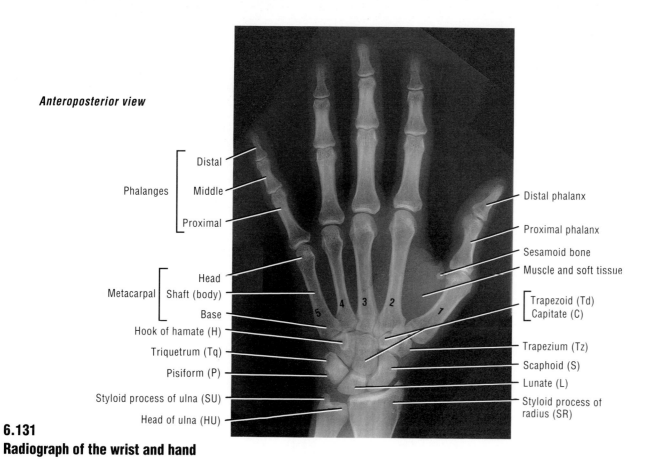

Anteroposterior view

Phalanges
- Distal
- Middle
- Proximal

Metacarpal
- Head
- Shaft (body)
- Base

Hook of hamate (H)
Triquetrum (Tq)
Pisiform (P)
Styloid process of ulna (SU)
Head of ulna (HU)

Distal phalanx
Proximal phalanx
Sesamoid bone
Muscle and soft tissue
Trapezoid (Td)
Capitate (C)
Trapezium (Tz)
Scaphoid (S)
Lunate (L)
Styloid process of radius (SR)

6.131
Radiograph of the wrist and hand

Observe:

1. The eight carpal bones in two rows; in the distal row: hamate capitate, trapezoid, and trapezium, which forms a saddle-shaped joint with metacarpal; in the proximal row: scaphoid, lunate, and pisiform superimposed on triquetrum;

2. The ulnar styloid process; the apex of the articular disc attaches to a pit at the root of the styloid and its base attaches to the ulnar notch of the radius; thus, the disc separates the distal radioulnar joint from the radiocarpal joint. (Courtesy of Dr. E.L. Lansdown, Professor of Radiology, University of Toronto, Toronto, Ontario, Canada.)

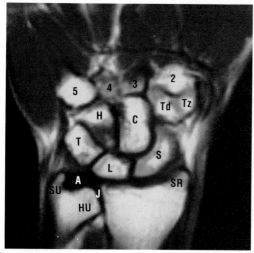

A

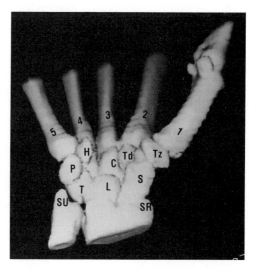

B, *Anterior view*

6.132
Scans of the wrist

A. Coronal MRI (magnetic resonance image) of the wrist. A - Articular disc, J - Distal radioulnar joint. (Courtesy of Dr. W. Kucharczyk, Clinical Director of Tri-Hospital Magnetic Resonance Centre, Toronto, Ontario, Canada.)

B. Three-dimensional computer-generated image of the wrist and hand. (Courtesy of Dr. D. Armstrong, Associate Professor of Radiology, University of Toronto, Toronto, Ontario, Canada.)

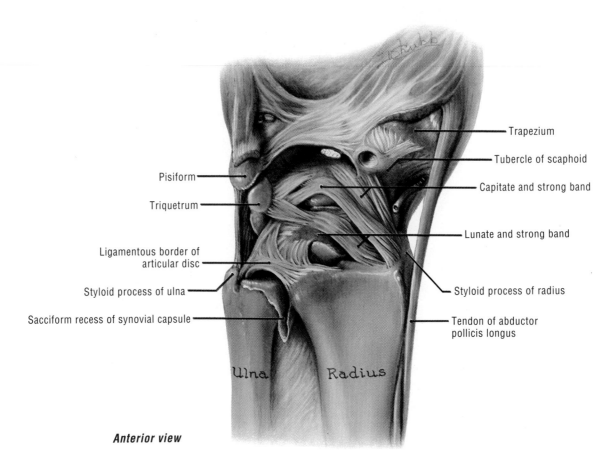

Trapezium

Tubercle of scaphoid

Pisiform

Capitate and strong band

Triquetrum

Lunate and strong band

Ligamentous border of
articular disc

Styloid process of ulna

Styloid process of radius

Sacciform recess of synovial capsule

Tendon of abductor
pollicis longus

Ulna   Radius

Anterior view

6.133
Ligaments of the distal radioulnar, radiocarpal, and intercarpal joints

The hand is forcibly extended. Observe the anterior or palmar ligaments, passing from the radius to the two rows of carpal bones; they are strong, and so directed that the hand shall follow the radius during supination; the dorsal ligaments take the same direction; hence the hand is obedient during pronation also.

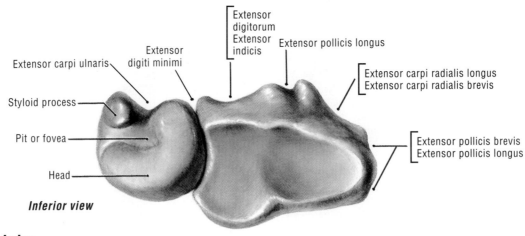

Extensor
digitorum
Extensor
indicis

Extensor pollicis longus

Extensor
digiti minimi

Extensor carpi ulnaris

Extensor carpi radialis longus
Extensor carpi radialis brevis

Styloid process

Pit or fovea

Extensor pollicis brevis
Extensor pollicis longus

Head

Inferior view

6.134
Distal ends of radius and ulna

Observe:
1. The four features of the distal end of the ulna, head, fovea, styloid process, and groove for the tendon of extensor carpi ulnaris;

2. The grooves for the tendons at the posterior aspect of the wrist; Figure 6.105 shows these tendons in their synovial sheaths.

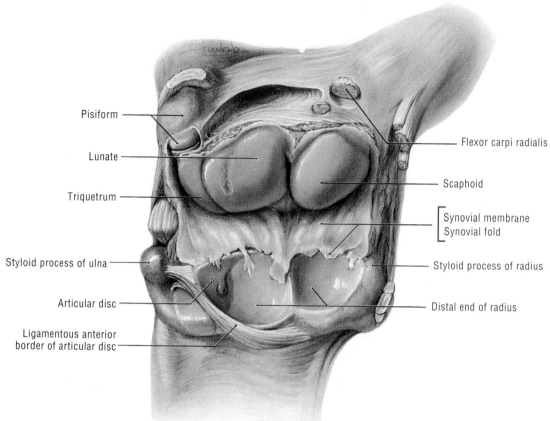

Pisiform

Lunate

Triquetrum

Styloid process of ulna

Articular disc

Ligamentous anterior
border of articular disc

Flexor carpi radialis

Scaphoid

Synovial membrane
Synovial fold

Styloid process of radius

Distal end of radius

6.135
Surfaces of the radiocarpal or wrist joint, opened anteriorly

Observe:

1. The nearly equal proximal articular surfaces of the scaphoid and lunate;

2. The lunate articulating with the radius and the articular disc; only during adduction of the wrist does the triquetrum come into articulation with the disc;

3. The perforation in the disc and the associated roughened surface of the lunate; this is a common occurrence;

4. The pisiform joint communicating with the radiocarpal joint.

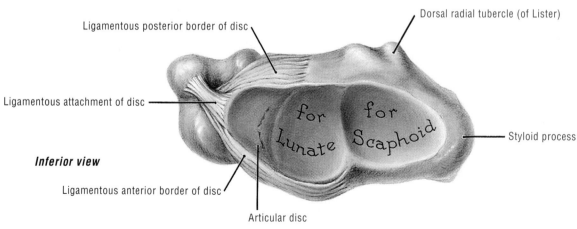

Ligamentous posterior border of disc

Dorsal radial tubercle (of Lister)

Ligamentous attachment of disc

Inferior view

Ligamentous anterior border of disc

Articular disc

for Lunate   for Scaphoid

Styloid process

6.136
Articular disc of the distal radioulnar joint

This disc is the bond of union between the distal ends of the radius and ulna; it is fibrocartilaginous, smooth, and stiff at the triangular area compressed between the head of the ulna and the lunate, but it is ligamentous and pliable elsewhere; the cartilaginous part is commonly fissured, as here, but the ligamentous parts are not.

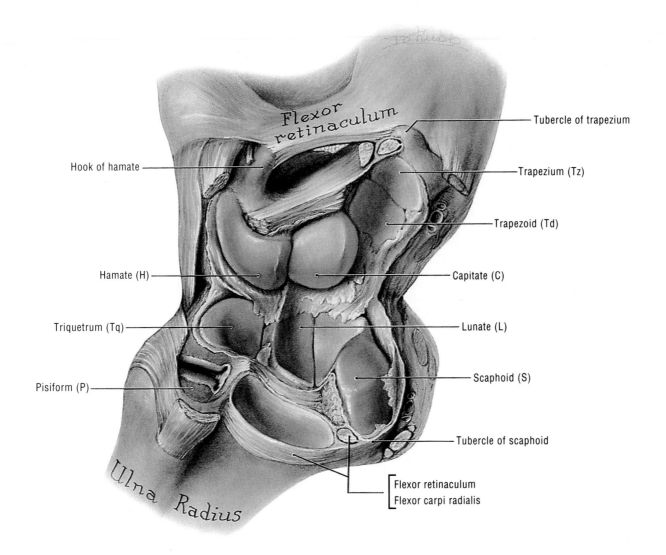

6.137
Surfaces of the midcarpal (transverse carpal) joint, opened anteriorly

The letters in parentheses refer to Figure 6.138. Observe:
1. The flexor retinaculum has been divided;

2. The sinuous surfaces of the opposed bones; the trapezium and trapezoid together presenting a concave, oval surface to the scaphoid; the capitate and hamate together presenting a convex surface to the scaphoid, lunate, and triquetrum, which is slightly broken by the linear facet on the apex of the hamate for its counterpart on the lunate;

3. Synovial folds projecting into the joint;

4. The relative weakness of the proximal part of the flexor retinaculum, which stretches from the movable pisiform to the scaphoid, and the strength of the distal part, which stretches from the hook of the hamate to the tubercle of the trapezium.

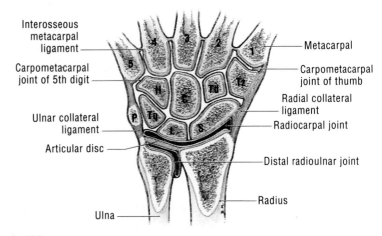

6.138
Coronal section of wrist and hand

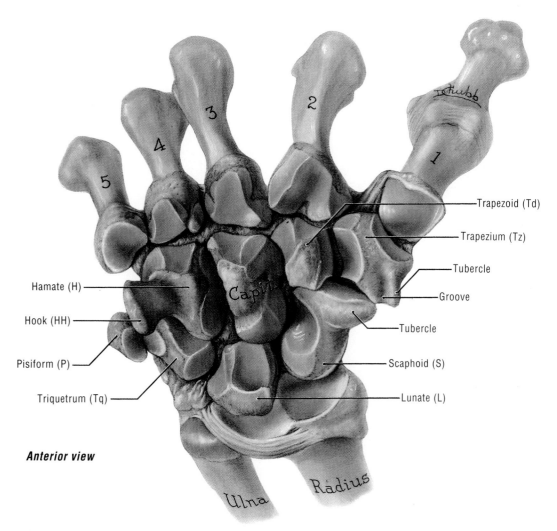

Hamate (H)

Hook (HH)

Pisiform (P)

Triquetrum (Tq)

Trapezoid (Td)

Trapezium (Tz)

Tubercle

Groove

Tubercle

Scaphoid (S)

Lunate (L)

Anterior view

6.139
Carpal bones and the bases of the metacarpals

The dorsal ligaments remain as a binding allowing study of the articular facets.

Observe:

1. The radius supporting two proximal carpals (scaphoid and lunate muscles); these, in turn, supporting three distal carpals (trapezium, trapezoid, and capitate) and articulating with the apex of the hamate; the four distal carpals supporting the five metacarpals; the triquetrum is unsupported;

2. The marginal projections (pisiform, hook of hamate, tubercle of scaphoid, and tubercle of trapezium) to which the flexor retinaculum attaches;

3. The triquetrum having an isolated facet for the pisiform muscle;

4. The capitate articulating with three metacarpals (2nd, 3rd, and 4th);

5. The 2nd metacarpal articulating with three carpals (trapezium, trapezoid, and capitate);

6. The 2nd and 3rd carpometacarpal joints are practically immobile; the 1st, saddle-shaped; the 4th and 5th, hinge-shaped.

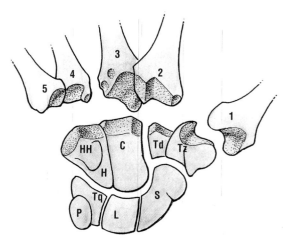

6.140
Diagram of the articular surfaces of the carpometacarpal joints

C - Capitate.

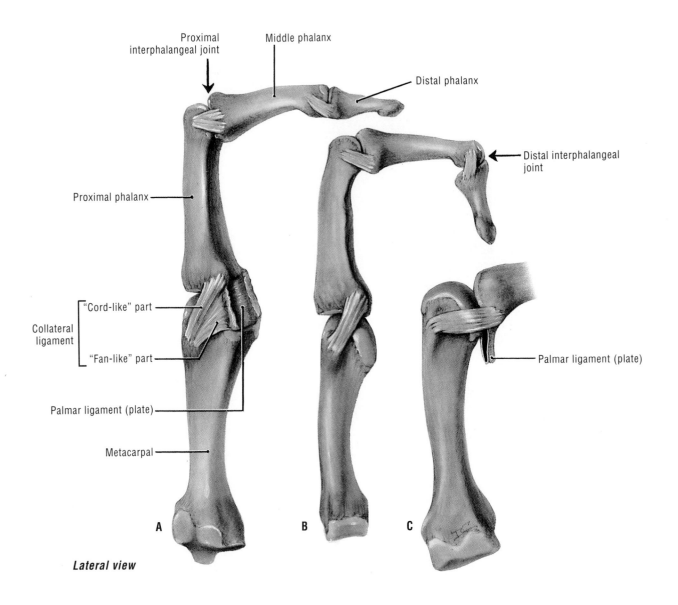

Proximal interphalangeal joint

Middle phalanx

Distal phalanx

Distal interphalangeal joint

Proximal phalanx

"Cord-like" part

Collateral ligament

"Fan-like" part

Palmar ligament (plate)

Palmar ligament (plate)

Metacarpal

A   B   C

Lateral view

6.141
Metacarpophalangeal and interphalangeal joints

Observe:

1. A fibrocartilaginous plate, the palmar ligament, hanging from the base of the proximal phalanx; fixed to the head of the metacarpal by the weaker, fan-like part of the collateral ligament; and moving like a visor across the metacarpal head; the deep transverse metacarpal ligaments that unite the plates, and the insertions of the palmar aponeurosis into them (Fig. 6.99);

2. The extremely strong, cord-like parts of the collateral ligaments of this joint, being eccentrically attached to the metacarpal

heads; they are slack during extension and taut during flexion; hence the fingers cannot be spread (abducted) unless the hand is open;

3. The interphalangeal joints have corresponding ligaments but the distal ends of the proximal and middle phalanges, being flattened anteroposteriorly and having two small condyles, permit neither adduction nor abduction.

7   The Head

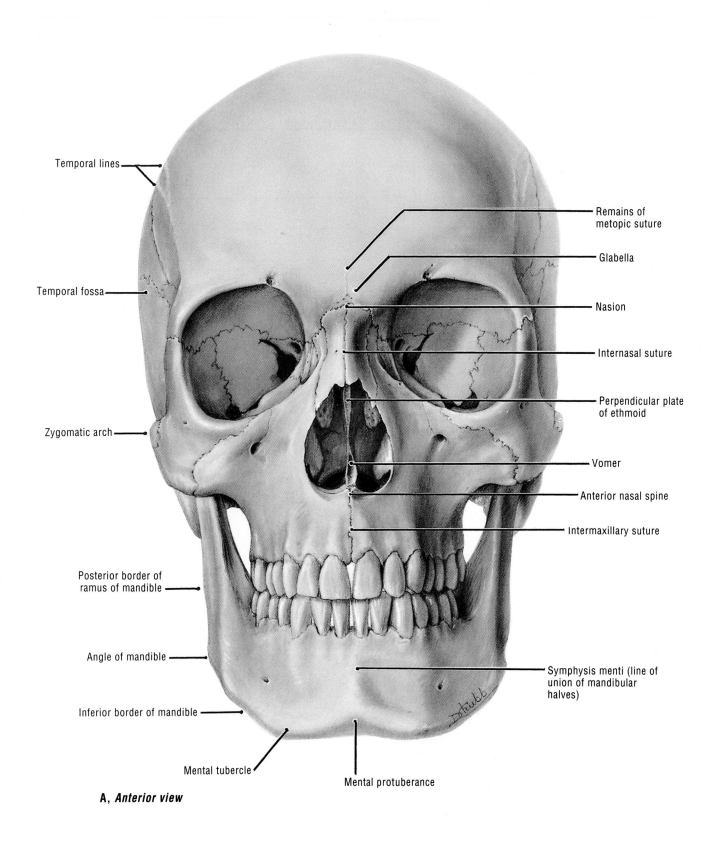

Temporal lines

Temporal fossa

Zygomatic arch

Posterior border of
ramus of mandible

Angle of mandible

Inferior border of mandible

Mental tubercle

Remains of
metopic suture

Glabella

Nasion

Internasal suture

Perpendicular plate
of ethmoid

Vomer

Anterior nasal spine

Intermaxillary suture

Symphysis menti (line of
union of mandibular
halves)

Mental protuberance

A, *Anterior view*

7.1
Skull

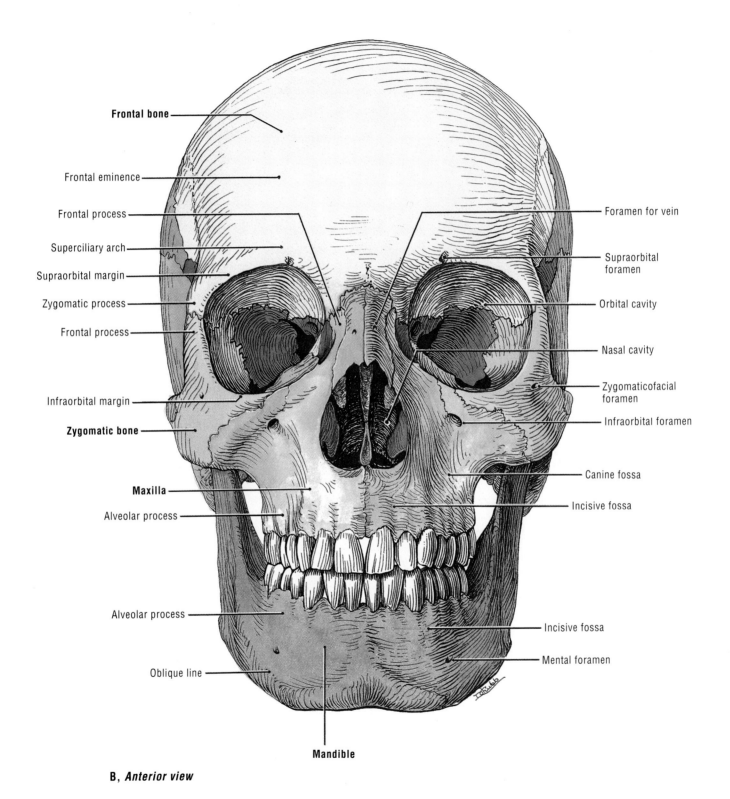

Frontal bone

Frontal eminence

Frontal process

Superciliary arch

Supraorbital margin

Zygomatic process

Frontal process

Infraorbital margin

Zygomatic bone

Maxilla

Alveolar process

Alveolar process

Oblique line

Foramen for vein

Supraorbital foramen

Orbital cavity

Nasal cavity

Zygomaticofacial foramen

Infraorbital foramen

Canine fossa

Incisive fossa

Incisive fossa

Mental foramen

Mandible

B, *Anterior view*

7.1
Skull *(continued)*

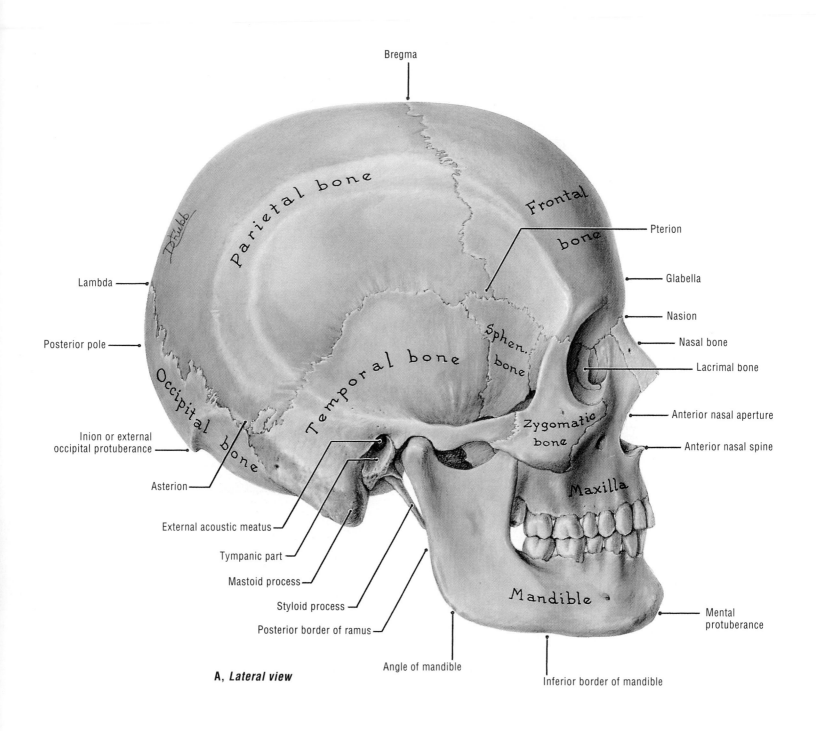

Bregma

Parietal bone

Frontal bone

Pterion

Lambda

Glabella

Nasion

Posterior pole

Nasal bone

Sphen. bone

Lacrimal bone

Temporal bone

Occipital bone

Zygomatic bone

Anterior nasal aperture

Inion or external occipital protuberance

Anterior nasal spine

Asterion

Maxilla

External acoustic meatus

Tympanic part

Mandible

Mastoid process

Styloid process

Posterior border of ramus

Mental protuberance

A, *Lateral view*

Angle of mandible

Inferior border of mandible

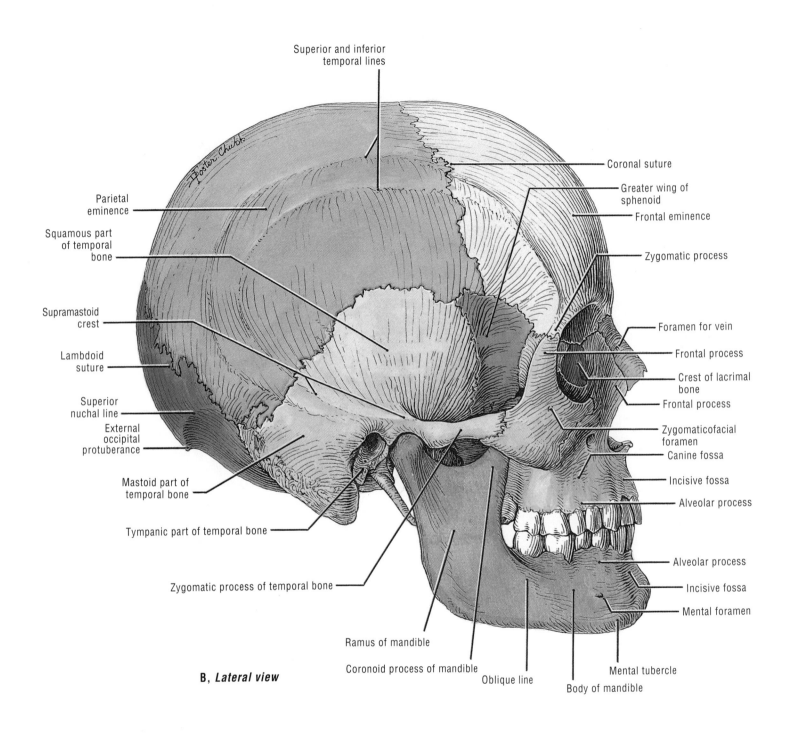

Superior and inferior
temporal lines

Parietal
eminence

Squamous part
of temporal
bone

Supramastoid
crest

Lambdoid
suture

Superior
nuchal line

External
occipital
protuberance

Mastoid part of
temporal bone

Tympanic part of temporal bone

Zygomatic process of temporal bone

Coronal suture

Greater wing of
sphenoid

Frontal eminence

Zygomatic process

Foramen for vein

Frontal process

Crest of lacrimal
bone

Frontal process

Zygomaticofacial
foramen

Canine fossa

Incisive fossa

Alveolar process

Alveolar process

Incisive fossa

Mental foramen

Ramus of mandible

Coronoid process of mandible

Oblique line

Mental tubercle

Body of mandible

B, *Lateral view*

**7.2
Skull *(continued)***

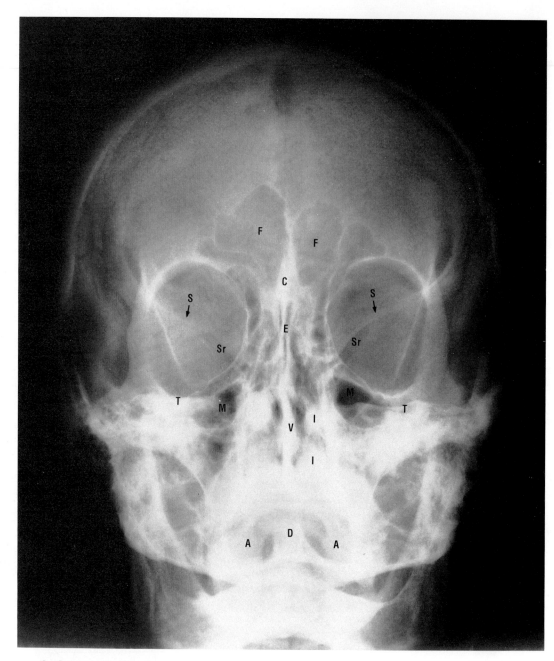

A, *Anteroposterior view*

7.3
Radiograph of the skull

Observe in **A**:

1. The superior orbital fissure *(Sr)*, the lesser wing of sphenoid *(S)*, and the superior surface of the petrous part of the temporal bone *(T)*;

2. The nasal septum is formed by the perpendicular plate of the ethmoid *(E)* and the vomer *(V)*; the inferior and middle conchae *(I)* of the lateral wall of the nose;

3. The crista galli *(C)*; the frontal sinus *(F)* and the maxillary sinus *(M)*;

4. Superimposed on the facial skeleton is the dens *(D)* and the lateral masses of the atlas *(A)*. (Courtesy of Dr. E. Becker, Associate Professor of Radiology, University of Toronto, Toronto, Ontario, Canada.)

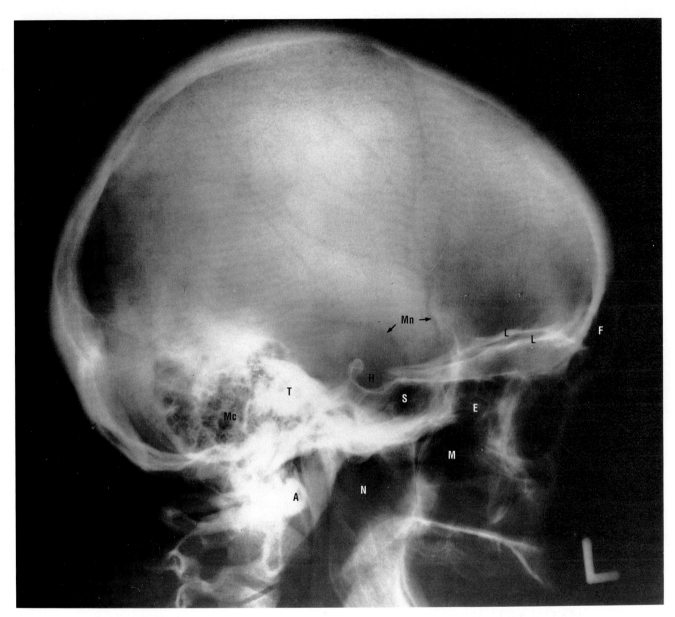

B, *Lateral view*

7.3
Radiograph of the skull *(continued)*

Observe in **B**:

1. The paranasal sinuses: frontal *(F)*, ethmoidal *(E)*, sphenoidal *(S)*, and maxillary *(M)*;

2. The hypophyseal fossa *(H)* for the pituitary gland;

3. The great density of the petrous part of the temporal bone *(T)* and the mastoid cells *(Mc)*;

4. The right and left orbital plates of the frontal bone are not superimposed and, thus, the floor of the anterior cranial fossa appears as two lines *(L)*;

5. The grooves for the branches of the middle meningeal vessels *(Mn)*;

6. The arch of the atlas *(A)* and the nasopharynx *(N)*. (Courtesy of Dr. E. Becker, Associate Professor of Radiology, University of Toronto, Toronto, Ontario, Canada.)

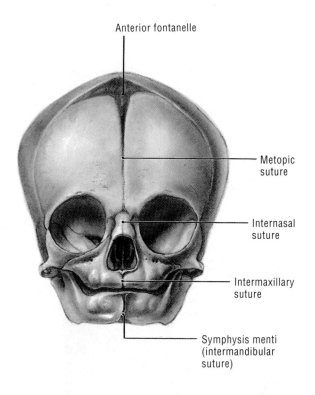

Anterior fontanelle

Metopic suture

Internasal suture

Intermaxillary suture

Symphysis menti (intermandibular suture)

A, Anterior view

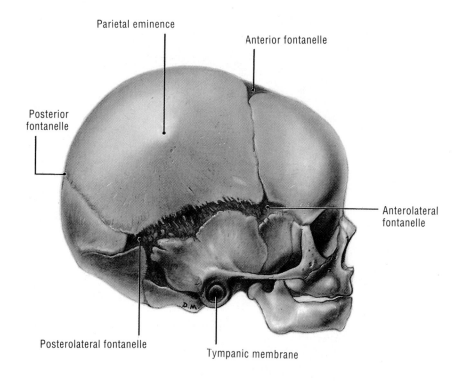

Parietal eminence

Anterior fontanelle

Posterior fontanelle

Anterolateral fontanelle

Posterolateral fontanelle

Tympanic membrane

B, Lateral view

7.4
Skull at birth

Observe:

1. The teeth have not erupted; the paranasal sinuses are rudimentary, the maxilla and the mandible are small, the angle of the mandible is obtuse and so the ramus and body of the mandible are nearly in line, and the inferior border of the mandible is on a level with the foramen magnum; the orbital cavities are large, but the nasal cavities are not deep; the face is small, forming 1/8 of the whole skull; whereas in the adult it forms 1/3;

2. The symphysis menti (intermandibular suture), which closes during the 2nd year, and the metopic suture, which closes during the 6th year, are still open;

3. The eminence of the parietal bone – like that of the frontal bone – is conical; ossification, which starts at the eminences and spreads in centrifugal waves, has not yet reached the four angles of the parietal bone; accordingly, these are still membranous and the membrane is blended with the pericranium externally and the dura mater internally to form the fontanelles; of the fontanelles, the anterior and largest closes during the 2nd year;

4. There being no mastoid process until the 2nd year, the stylomastoid foramen, which transmits the facial nerve, opens beneath the skin surface; the external acoustic meatus having no length, the tympanic membrane is close to the surface of the skull.

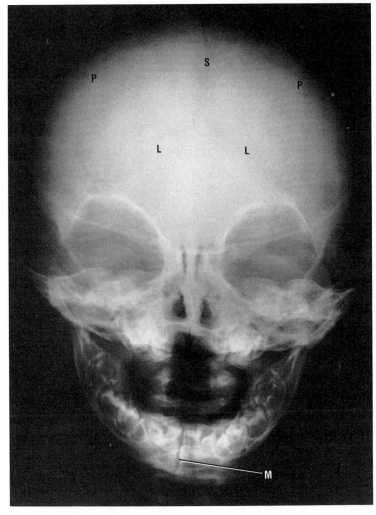

A, *Posteroanterior view*

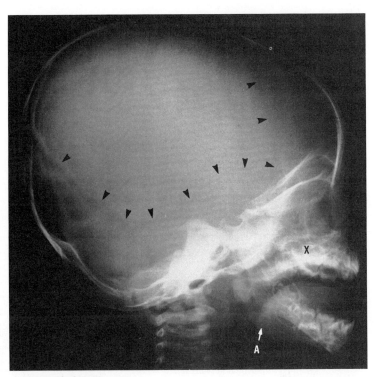

B, *Lateral view*

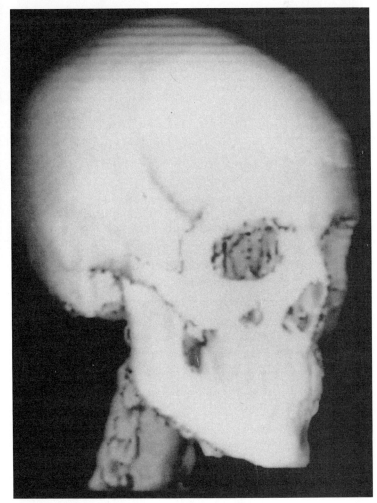

C, *Anterolateral view*

7.5
Radiographs of a child's skull

A and **B**. Radiographs of a 6 1/2-month-old child. *A* - Angle of mandible, *X* - Maxilla, *M* - Symphysis menti, *S* - Sagittal suture, *L* - Lambdoid suture, *P* - Parietal eminence, *arrowheads* - Membranous outline of the parietal bone. For explanation of labeled structures, see text of Figure 7.4.

C. Three-dimensional computer-generated image of a child's skull. (Courtesy of Dr. D. Armstrong, Associate Professor of Radiology, University of Toronto, Toronto, Ontario, Canada.)

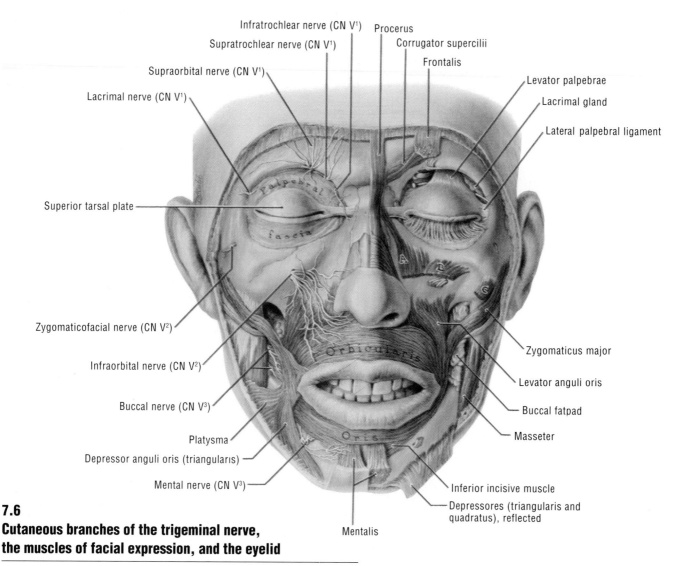

Infratrochlear nerve (CN V¹)   Procerus
Supratrochlear nerve (CN V¹)   Corrugator supercilii
Supraorbital nerve (CN V¹)   Frontalis
Lacrimal nerve (CN V¹)   Levator palpebrae
    Lacrimal gland
    Lateral palpebral ligament
Superior tarsal plate
Zygomaticofacial nerve (CN V²)   Zygomaticus major
Infraorbital nerve (CN V²)   Levator anguli oris
Buccal nerve (CN V³)   Buccal fatpad
    Masseter
Platysma
Depressor anguli oris (triangularis)   Inferior incisive muscle
Mental nerve (CN V³)   Depressores (triangularis and quadratus), reflected
    Mentalis

7.6
Cutaneous branches of the trigeminal nerve, the muscles of facial expression, and the eyelid

Observe:

1. The five cutaneous branches of the ophthalmic nerve (CN V¹); of these, the external nasal branch is shown but not labeled; the cornea is supplied by the nasociliary nerve;

2. The three cutaneous branches of the maxillary nerve (CN V²): the infraorbital branch, the zygomaticofacial, and the zygomaticotemporal branches (Fig. 7.64);

3. The three cutaneous branches of the mandibular nerve (CN V³): the mental, the buccal, and the auriculotemporal (Fig. 7.10) branches;

4. Three sectioned muscles: A, levator labii superioris alaeque nasi; B, levator labii superioris; C, zygomaticus minor;

5. The buccal pad of fat, filling the space between buccinator medially and the ramus of the jaw and masseter laterally;

6. The palpebral fascia (orbital septum), attached to the orbital margin, and medially passing posterior to the lacrimal sac to the crest of the lacrimal bone;

7. The medial palpebral ligament, crossing anterior to the lacrimal sac, and attaching the elliptical superior and the rod-like inferior tarsal plate to the frontal process of the maxilla.

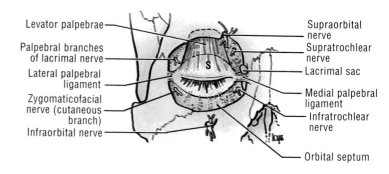

Levator palpebrae   Supraorbital nerve
Palpebral branches of lacrimal nerve   Supratrochlear nerve
Lateral palpebral ligament   Lacrimal sac
Zygomaticofacial nerve (cutaneous branch)   Medial palpebral ligament
    Infratrochlear nerve
Infraorbital nerve   Orbital septum

7.7
Skeleton and innervation of the eyelids

This diagram shows the superior (S) and inferior (I) tarsal plates and their attachments. Their ciliary margins are free; but peripherally the margins are attached to the orbital septum (palpebral fascia in the eyelid). The angles are anchored by medial and lateral palpebral ligaments. The fan-shaped aponeurosis of levator palpebrae superioris, is attached to the anterior surface and superior edge of the superior tarsal plate.

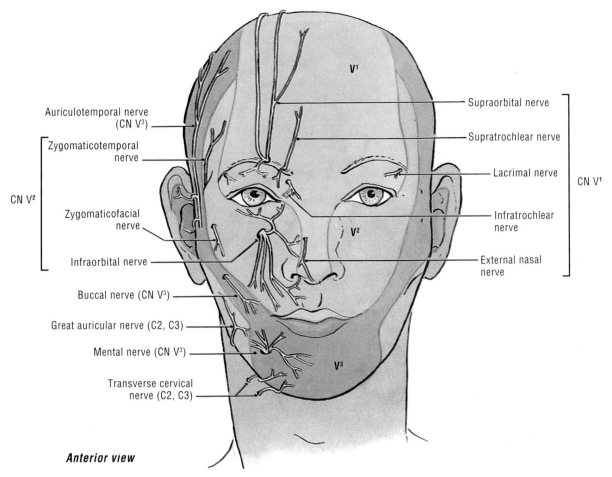

Auriculotemporal nerve
(CN V³)

Zygomaticotemporal
nerve

CN V²

Zygomaticofacial
nerve

Infraorbital nerve

Buccal nerve (CN V³)

Great auricular nerve (C2, C3)

Mental nerve (CN V³)

Transverse cervical
nerve (C2, C3)

V¹

Supraorbital nerve

Supratrochlear nerve

Lacrimal nerve

CN V¹

Infratrochlear
nerve

External nasal
nerve

V²

V³

Anterior view

7.8
Sensory nerves of face

The three divisions of the trigeminal nerve (CN V) correspond in their distribution, nearly but not absolutely, to the three embryological regions of the face. Thus, the ophthalmic nerve (CN V¹) supplies the frontonasal prominence; the maxillary nerve (CN V²), the maxillary prominence; and the mandibular nerve (CN V³), the mandibular prominence. They supply the whole thickness of the prominences – from skin to mucous surface – indeed, to the median plane (i.e., falx cerebri, nasal septum, and septum of tongue).

Cutaneous branches (supraorbital and auriculotemporal) have spread posteriorly in the scalp to meet the greater and lesser occipital nerves (Fig. 7.13**A**). The great auricular nerve has spread into the parotid region. The buccal nerve supplies the skin and mucous membrane of the cheek, reaching the angle of the mouth.

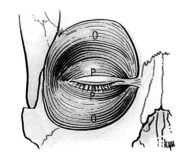

A

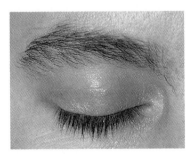

B

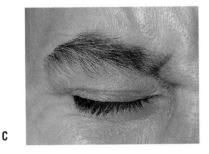

C

7.9
Orbicularis oculi

A. Diagram showing palpebral (P) and orbital (O) parts of the orbicularis oculi. **B.** Palpebral part gently closes the eyelids. **C.** Orbital part tightly closes the eyelids (see also Fig. 7.12). The lacrimal portion (not shown) passes posterior to the lacrimal sac to attach to the tarsal plates and lateral margin of the lacrimal sac and aids in the spread of lacrimal secretions by holding the eyelids close to the eyeballs.

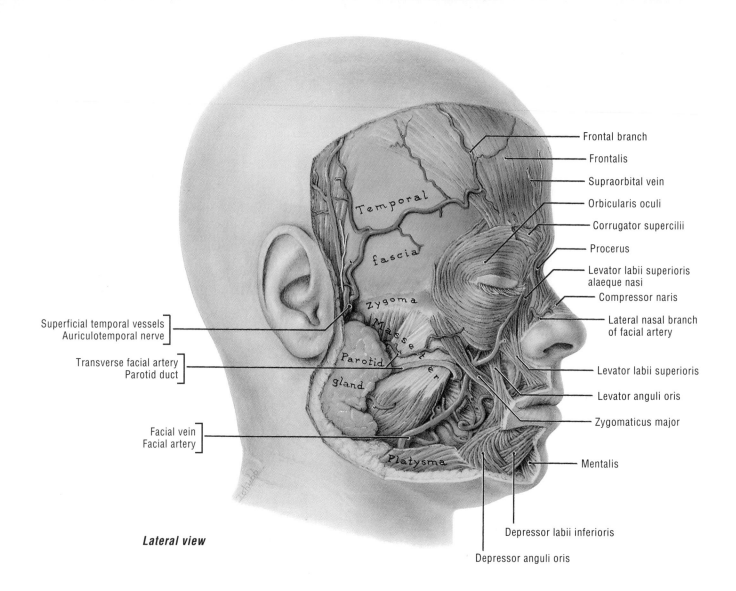

Frontal branch

Frontalis

Supraorbital vein

Orbicularis oculi

Corrugator supercilii

Procerus

Levator labii superioris alaeque nasi

Compressor naris

Lateral nasal branch of facial artery

Levator labii superioris

Levator anguli oris

Zygomaticus major

Mentalis

Depressor labii inferioris

Depressor anguli oris

Superficial temporal vessels
Auriculotemporal nerve

Transverse facial artery
Parotid duct

Facial vein
Facial artery

Temporal

fascia

Zygoma

Masseter

Parotid

gland

Platysma

Lateral view

7.10
Muscles of expression and arteries of face

Observe:

1. The "muscles of facial expression" are superficial sphincters and dilators of the orifices of the head; all are supplied by the facial nerve (CN VII);

2. The muscles of facial expression around the eye, ear, nose, and mouth and blending into the upper lip, lower lip, chin, and cheek;

3. The facial artery, usually sinuous but here tortuous, crossing the base of the mandible at the anterior border of the masseter muscle, passing within 1 cm of the angle of the mouth, and lying anterior to the facial vein, which takes a straight and more superficial course;

4. The auriculotemporal nerve, ascending with the superficial temporal vessels;

5. Masseter and temporalis (covered by temporal fascia) are muscles of mastication and are innervated by the trigeminal nerve.

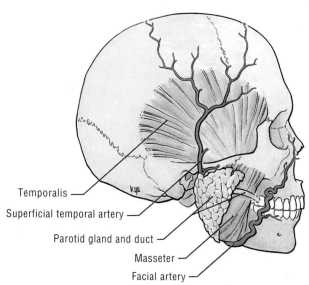

Temporalis

Superficial temporal artery

Parotid gland and duct

Masseter

Facial artery

7.11
Parotid gland and facial and superficial temporal arteries

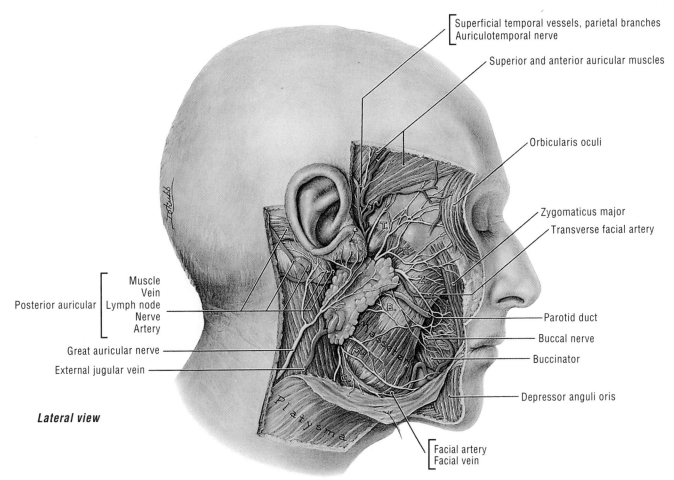

Superficial temporal vessels, parietal branches
Auriculotemporal nerve

Superior and anterior auricular muscles

Orbicularis oculi

Zygomaticus major

Transverse facial artery

Muscle
Vein
Posterior auricular | Lymph node
Nerve
Artery

Parotid duct

Buccal nerve

Great auricular nerve

Buccinator

External jugular vein

Depressor anguli oris

Lateral view

Facial artery
Facial vein

7.12
Face: terminal branches of the facial nerve

Observe:

1. The parotid gland, and the parotid duct crossing the masseter muscle a finger's breadth inferior to the zygomatic arch and turning medially to pierce buccinator;

2. The facial nerve, motor to the muscles of facial expression, is in jeopardy in surgery of the parotid gland; its branches radiate from under cover of the gland like digits from an outstretched hand, anastomosing with each other and with the branches of the trigeminal nerve, and entering the muscles on their deep surfaces except where the muscles are two layers thick, i.e., the deeper layer is then entered on its superficial surface, e.g., buccinator; the nerve is divided somewhat arbitrarily into temporal *(T)*, zygomatic *(Z)*, buccal *(B)*, mandibular *(M)*, and cervical *(C)* branches;

3. The cervical branch, running inferior to the angle of the mandible and, after supplying branches to the platysma, crossing the anterior border of the masseter, supplies the muscles of the lower lip and chin;

4. The buccal branch, which is motor to the buccinator, anastomosing with the buccal nerve (a branch of the trigeminal), which is sensory;

5. The greater auricular nerve (C2, C3), here lying just posterior to the external jugular vein, but commonly in contact with it;

6. The posterior auricular nerve, which is motor to auricularis posterior and occipitalis, joined by a twig from the great auricular nerve.

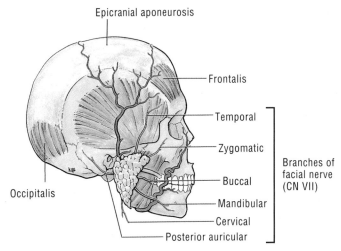

Epicranial aponeurosis

Frontalis

Temporal

Zygomatic

Branches of facial nerve (CN VII)

Buccal

Occipitalis

Mandibular

Cervical

Posterior auricular

7.13
Branches of the facial nerve and the epicranial aponeurosis

Arteries and nerves of the scalp

Observe:

1. The arteries, anastomosing freely; the supraorbital and supratrochlear are derived from the internal carotid artery via the ophthalmic artery; the three others are branches of the external carotid artery; hemorrhage from a scalp injury is often profuse, due to the vascularity of the scalp and the lack of constriction of the arterial vessels on injury;

2. The nerves, appearing in sequence: CN V[1], CN V[2], CN V[3], ventral rami of C2 and C3, and dorsal rami of C2 and C3 (C1 has no cutaneous branch).

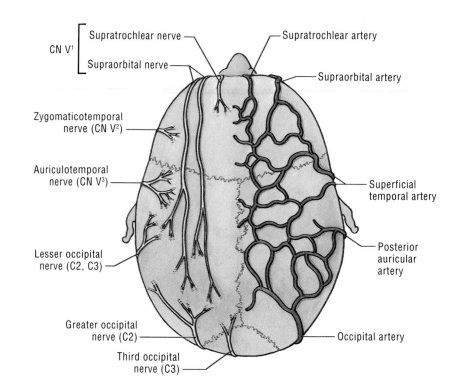

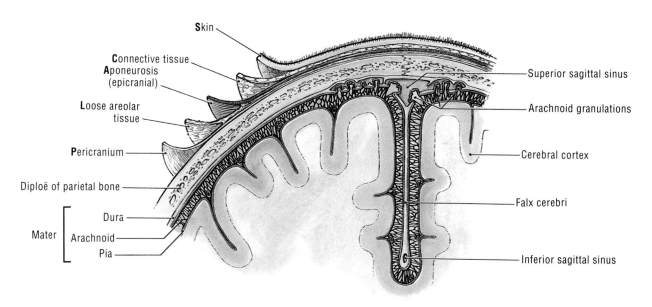

7.15

The scalp, skull, and meninges, coronal section

Observe:

1. *The layers of the scalp:* the skin is bound tightly to the epicranial aponeurosis, which is attached to the skull laterally and to the two fleshy muscles for which it serves as intermediate tendon (Fig. 7.13); occipitalis attaches to bone while frontalis attaches superficially to subcutaneous tissue; thus blood from a torn vessel may spread widely over the skull deep to the aponeurosis and leak out anteriorly, appearing as bruising in the area of the eyelids;

2. The outer tough dura mater (gray) encloses venous sinuses;

3. The arachnoid mater (purple) in contact with the dura and bridging over sulci on the cortical surface;

4. The pia mater (red), a delicate, intimate investment of the brain;

5. Between dura and arachnoid, a potential subdural space into which hemorrhage may occur;

6. Between arachnoid and pia, the subarachnoid space containing cerebrospinal fluid;

7. The arachnoid granulations, which are responsible for absorption of cerebrospinal fluid from the subarachnoid space into the venous system.

7.16
Diploic veins

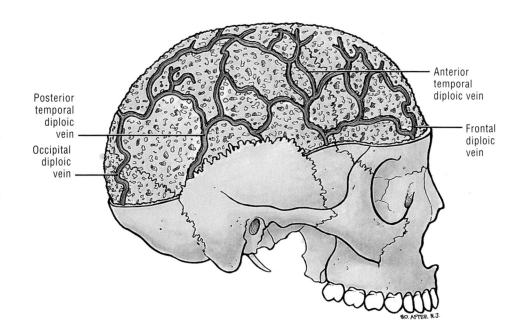

Observe:

1. The outer table of the skull has been filed away and the channels for the diploic veins thereby opened;

2. Of the four (paired) diploic veins, the frontal opens into the supraorbital vein at the supraorbital notch; the anterior temporal opens into the sphenoparietal sinus; the posterior temporal and the occipital both open into the transverse sinus – but they may open into surface veins;

3. There are no accompanying diploic arteries; the meningeal and pericranial arteries provide the arterial blood;

4. Connections with intracranial and extracranial venous channels allow infection to travel freely between scalp, skull, meninges, and brain.

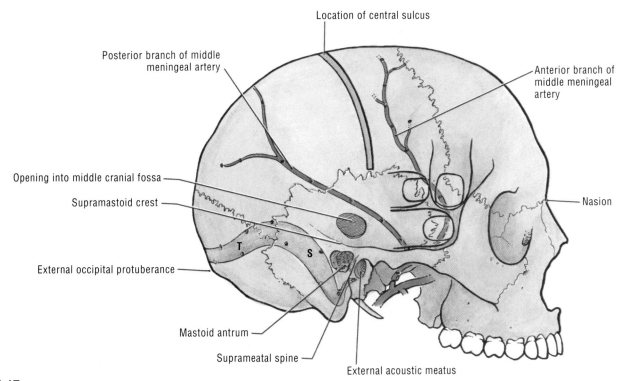

7.17
Surface anatomy of the cranium

The artery (red) and venous sinus (blue) were related to the outside of the skull by drilling holes along the grooves on the inside.

Observe:

1. The pterion, two fingers' breadth superior to the zygomatic arch and a thumb's breadth posterior to the frontal process of the zygomatic bone; the anterior branch of the middle meningeal artery crosses the pterion;

2. The supramastoid crest approximately at the level of the floor of the middle cranial fossa; hence, a hole drilled inferior to the crest and superior to the suprameatal spine enters the mastoid (tympanic) antrum; whereas one drilled superior to the crest enters the middle cranial fossa;

3. The transverse *(T)* and sigmoid *(S)* sinuses.

7.18
External surface of the dura mater: arachnoid granulations

Observe:

1. The calvaria (skull cap) is removed; in the median plane, the thick roof of the superior sagittal sinus is partly pinned aside and, laterally, the thin roofs of two lacunae laterales are reflected;

2. On the right, an angular flap of dura is turned anteriorly; the subdural space is thereby opened; and the convolutions of the cerebral cortex are visible through the cobweb-like arachnoid mater;

3. Each artery lying in a venous channel (middle meningeal veins), which enlarges superiorly into a lake, lacuna lateralis; a channel or channels, draining the lacuna lateralis into the superior sagittal sinus;

4. The arachnoid granulations, in the lacunae; they are responsible for absorption of cerebrospinal fluid.

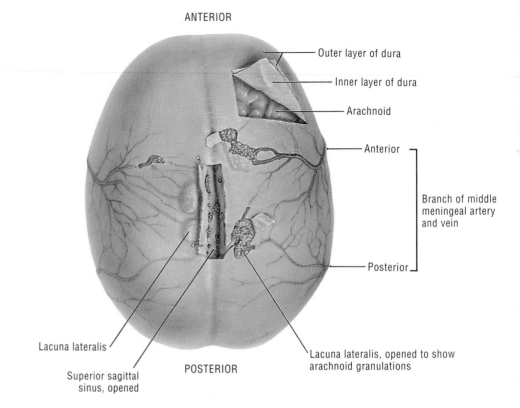

ANTERIOR

Outer layer of dura

Inner layer of dura

Arachnoid

Anterior

Branch of middle meningeal artery and vein

Posterior

Lacuna lateralis, opened to show arachnoid granulations

Lacuna lateralis

POSTERIOR

Superior sagittal sinus, opened

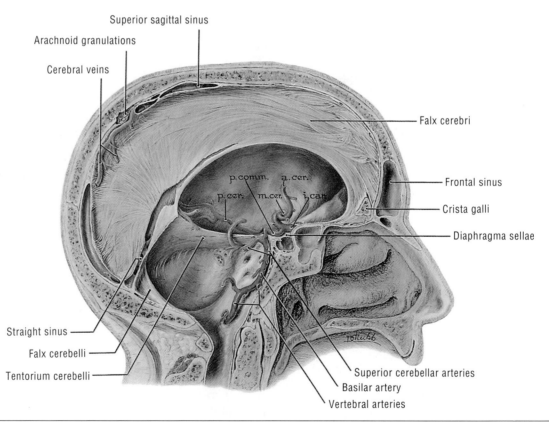

Superior sagittal sinus

Arachnoid granulations

Cerebral veins

Falx cerebri

p.comm. a.cer.

p.cer. m.cer. i.car.

Frontal sinus

Crista galli

Diaphragma sellae

Straight sinus

Falx cerebelli

Tentorium cerebelli

Superior cerebellar arteries

Basilar artery

Vertebral arteries

7.19
The dura mater

Observe:

1. Two sickle-shaped folds, the falx cerebri and the falx cerebelli, which lie vertically in the median plane; and two roof-like folds, the tentorium cerebelli and the diaphragma sellae, which lie horizontally;

2. The two paired arteries that supply the brain – the internal carotid and the vertebral arteries.

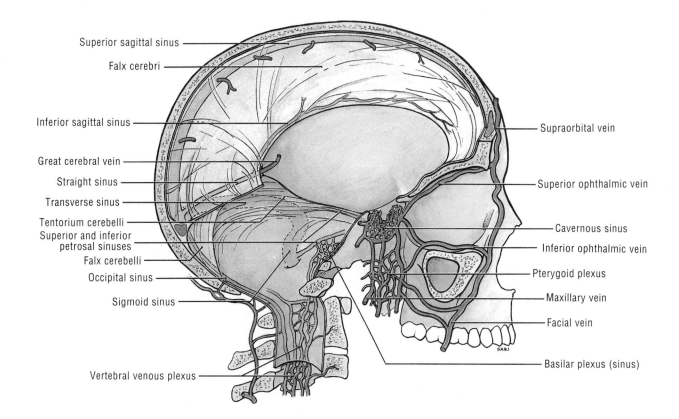

- Superior sagittal sinus
- Falx cerebri
- Inferior sagittal sinus
- Great cerebral vein
- Straight sinus
- Transverse sinus
- Tentorium cerebelli
- Superior and inferior petrosal sinuses
- Falx cerebelli
- Occipital sinus
- Sigmoid sinus
- Vertebral venous plexus
- Supraorbital vein
- Superior ophthalmic vein
- Cavernous sinus
- Inferior ophthalmic vein
- Pterygoid plexus
- Maxillary vein
- Facial vein
- Basilar plexus (sinus)

7.20
Venous sinuses of the dura mater

Observe:

1. The superior sagittal sinus at the superior border of the falx cerebri; the inferior sagittal sinus in its free border; the great cerebral vein joining the inferior sagittal sinus to form the straight sinus that runs obliquely in the junction between falx cerebri and tentorium cerebelli; the occipital sinus in the attached border of the falx cerebelli;

2. The superior sagittal sinus usually becomes: the right transverse sinus, right sigmoid sinus, right internal jugular vein; the straight sinus behaves similarly on the left side;

3. The cavernous sinus communicating with the veins of the face via the ophthalmic veins and the pterygoid plexus, and emptying via the superior and inferior petrosal sinuses;

4. The basilar sinus connecting the inferior petrosal sinuses of the opposite sides and, like the occipital sinus, communicating inferiorly with the vertebral venous plexus.

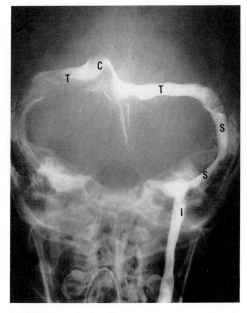

A, Anteroposterior view

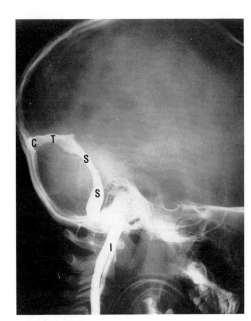

B, Lateral view

7.21
Venograms of sinuses

C - Confluence of sinuses, T - Transverse sinus, S - Sigmoid sinus, I - Internal jugular vein. (Courtesy of Dr. D. Armstrong, Associate Professor of Radiology, University of Toronto, Toronto, Ontario, Canada.)

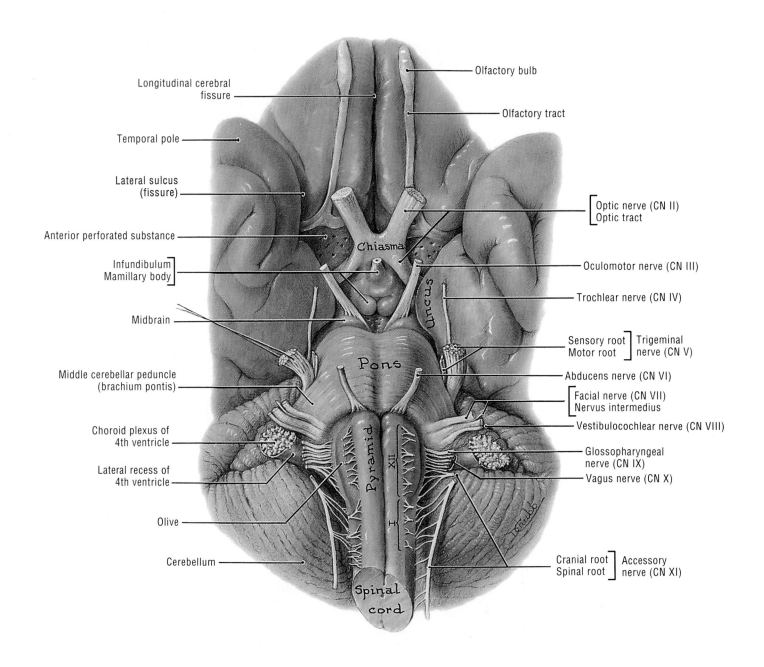

Longitudinal cerebral fissure

Temporal pole

Lateral sulcus (fissure)

Anterior perforated substance

Infundibulum
Mamillary body

Midbrain

Middle cerebellar peduncle (brachium pontis)

Choroid plexus of 4th ventricle

Lateral recess of 4th ventricle

Olive

Cerebellum

Olfactory bulb

Olfactory tract

Optic nerve (CN II)
Optic tract

Oculomotor nerve (CN III)

Trochlear nerve (CN IV)

Sensory root ⎤ Trigeminal
Motor root ⎦ nerve (CN V)

Abducens nerve (CN VI)

Facial nerve (CN VII)
Nervus intermedius

Vestibulocochlear nerve (CN VIII)

Glossopharyngeal nerve (CN IX)

Vagus nerve (CN X)

Cranial root ⎤ Accessory
Spinal root ⎦ nerve (CN XI)

Chiasma

Uncus

Pons

Pyramid

XII

XI

Spinal cord

7.22
Base of the brain: the superficial origins of the cranial nerves

Observe:

1. The olfactory bulb, in which the olfactory nerves (CN I) (not shown) end;

2. The superficial origin of the trochlear nerve (CN IV) is shown in Figure 7.33;

3. The fila of the hypoglossal nerve (CN XII), arising between the pyramid and the olive, and in line with the ventral rootlets of the 1st cervical nerve.

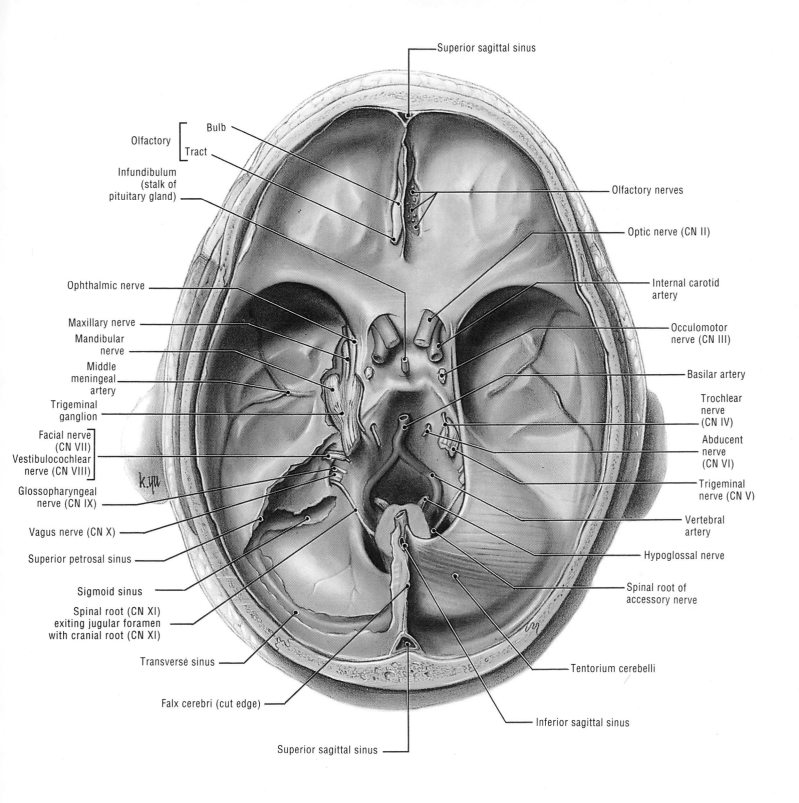

Superior sagittal sinus

Olfactory { Bulb / Tract

Infundibulum (stalk of pituitary gland)

Olfactory nerves

Optic nerve (CN II)

Ophthalmic nerve

Internal carotid artery

Maxillary nerve

Mandibular nerve

Occulomotor nerve (CN III)

Middle meningeal artery

Basilar artery

Trigeminal ganglion

Trochlear nerve (CN IV)

Facial nerve (CN VII)
Vestibulocochlear nerve (CN VIII)

Abducent nerve (CN VI)

Glossopharyngeal nerve (CN IX)

Trigeminal nerve (CN V)

Vagus nerve (CN X)

Vertebral artery

Superior petrosal sinus

Hypoglossal nerve

Sigmoid sinus

Spinal root of accessory nerve

Spinal root (CN XI) exiting jugular foramen with cranial root (CN XI)

Transverse sinus

Tentorium cerebelli

Falx cerebri (cut edge)

Inferior sagittal sinus

Superior sagittal sinus

7.23

Interior of the base of the skull: the cranial nerves, dura mater and blood vessels

Observe:

1. On the left side the dura mater is cut away to expose the trigeminal nerve and its three branches and the sigmoid sinus; the tentorium cerebelli is removed to reveal the transverse and superior petrosal sinuses;

2. The frontal lobes are located in the anterior cranial fossa, the

temporal lobes in the middle cranial fossa, the brain stem and cerebellum in the posterior cranial fossa;

3. The location of the twelve cranial nerves, the internal carotid, vertebral, basilar, and middle meningeal arteries.

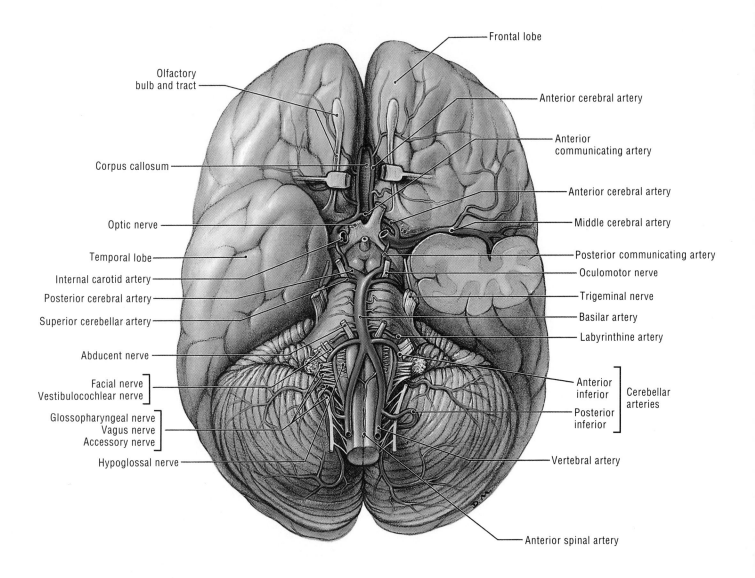

Frontal lobe

Olfactory bulb and tract

Anterior cerebral artery

Anterior communicating artery

Corpus callosum

Anterior cerebral artery

Optic nerve

Middle cerebral artery

Temporal lobe

Posterior communicating artery

Internal carotid artery

Oculomotor nerve

Posterior cerebral artery

Trigeminal nerve

Superior cerebellar artery

Basilar artery

Labyrinthine artery

Abducent nerve

Facial nerve
Vestibulocochlear nerve

Anterior inferior

Cerebellar arteries

Glossopharyngeal nerve
Vagus nerve
Accessory nerve

Posterior inferior

Hypoglossal nerve

Vertebral artery

Anterior spinal artery

7.24
Base of the brain: cerebral arterial circle (of Willis)

Three arterial stems ascend to supply the brain: right and left internal carotids and the basilar artery, which results from the union of the two vertebral arteries. Observe that these three stems form an arterial circle (the circle of Willis) at the base of the brain through the linkages provided by the anterior communicating artery and the two posterior communicating arteries. The cerebellum is mainly supplied by branches from the vertebral and basilar arteries.

The left temporal pole is removed to enable visualization of the middle cerebral artery in the lateral fissure. The frontal lobes are separated to expose the anterior cerebral arteries and the corpus callosum.

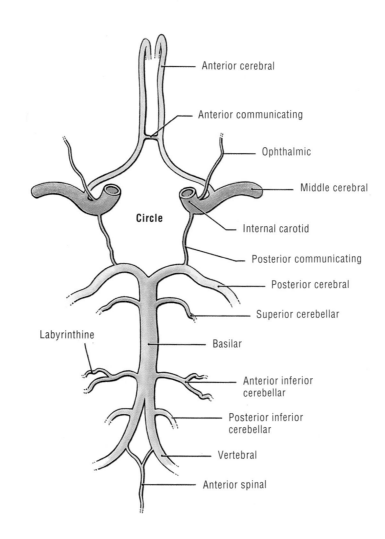

Anterior cerebral

Anterior communicating

Ophthalmic

Middle cerebral

Circle

Internal carotid

Posterior communicating

Posterior cerebral

Superior cerebellar

Labyrinthine

Basilar

Anterior inferior cerebellar

Posterior inferior cerebellar

Vertebral

Anterior spinal

7.25
Cerebral arterial circle (of Willis)

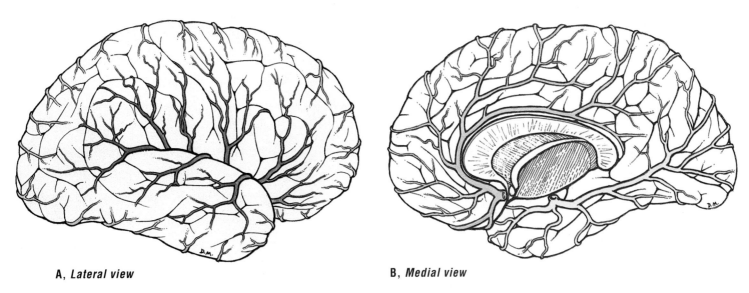

A, *Lateral view*

B, *Medial view*

7.26
Blood supply of cerebral hemispheres

Blood supply to the cerebral hemispheres is shared by the anterior and middle cerebral arteries from the internal carotids and the posterior cerebral arteries from the basilar.

In these schematic diagrams, the general areas of supply are shown for the three cerebral arteries: anterior (green), middle (purple), and posterior (yellow).

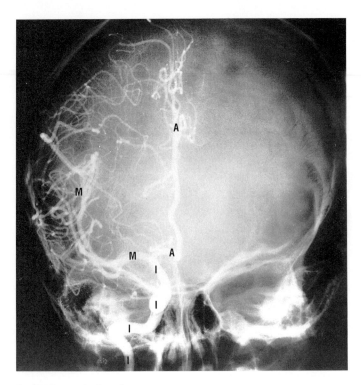

A, *Posteroanterior view*

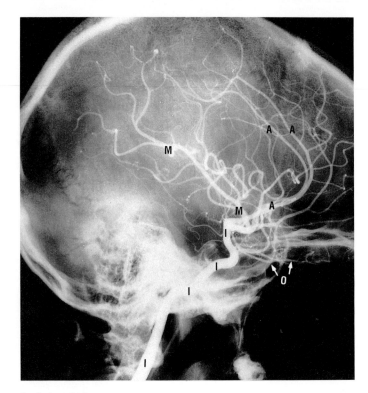

B, *Lateral view*

7.27
Carotid arteriograms

Observe:

1. The four letter *I*'s indicate the parts of the internal carotid artery: cervical, before entering the skull; petrous, within the temporal bone; cavernous, within that venous sinus; and cerebral, within the cranial subarachnoid space;

2. The anterior cerebral artery and its branches *(A)*; the middle cerebral artery and its branches *(M)*; the ophthalmic artery *(O)*. (Courtesy of Dr. D. Armstrong, Associate Professor of Radiology, University of Toronto, Toronto, Ontario, Canada.)

7.28
Vertebral arteriogram

Observe:

1. The curve made by the vertebral artery to lie in contact with the posterior arch of the atlas prior to its passage through the dura mater *(1)*;

2. The vertebral artery entering the skull through the foramen magnum *(2)* (within the subarachnoid space);

3. Posterior inferior cerebellar artery *(3)*;

4. Anterior inferior cerebellar artery *(4)*;

5. The basilar artery *(5)* formed by the union of right and left vertebral arteries;

6. Superior cerebellar artery *(6)*;

7. Posterior cerebral artery *(7)* with branches going to occipital and temporal lobes;

8. Posterior communicating arteries *(8)*.

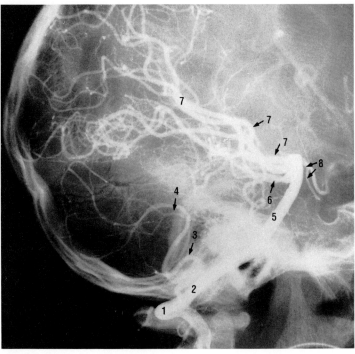

Lateral view

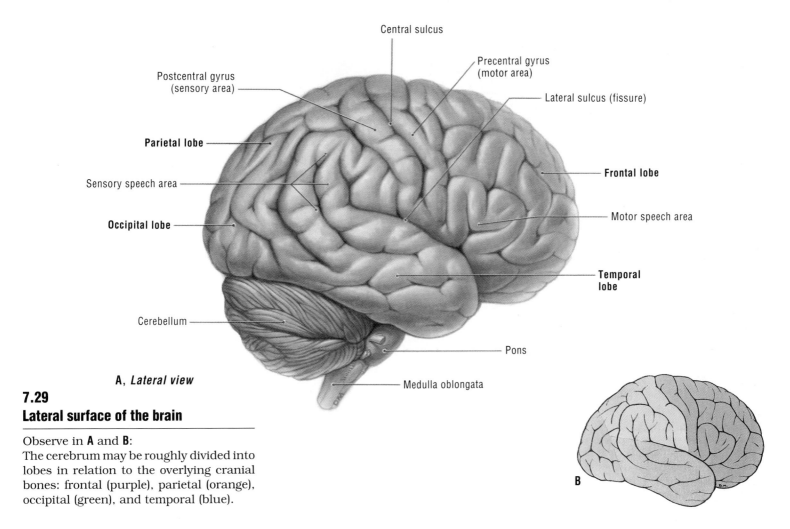

Central sulcus

Precentral gyrus (motor area)

Postcentral gyrus (sensory area)

Lateral sulcus (fissure)

Parietal lobe

Frontal lobe

Sensory speech area

Motor speech area

Occipital lobe

Temporal lobe

Cerebellum

Pons

A, *Lateral view*

Medulla oblongata

B

7.29
Lateral surface of the brain

Observe in **A** and **B**:
The cerebrum may be roughly divided into lobes in relation to the overlying cranial bones: frontal (purple), parietal (orange), occipital (green), and temporal (blue).

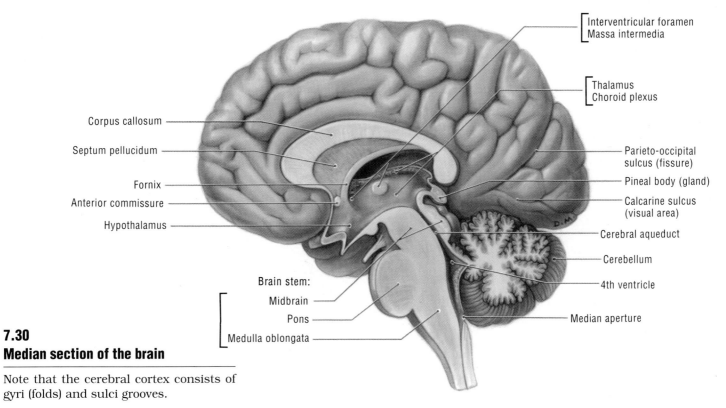

Interventricular foramen
Massa intermedia

Thalamus
Choroid plexus

Corpus callosum

Septum pellucidum

Parieto-occipital sulcus (fissure)

Fornix

Pineal body (gland)

Anterior commissure

Calcarine sulcus (visual area)

Hypothalamus

Cerebral aqueduct

Cerebellum

Brain stem:

4th ventricle

Midbrain

Pons

Median aperture

7.30
Median section of the brain

Medulla oblongata

Note that the cerebral cortex consists of gyri (folds) and sulci grooves.

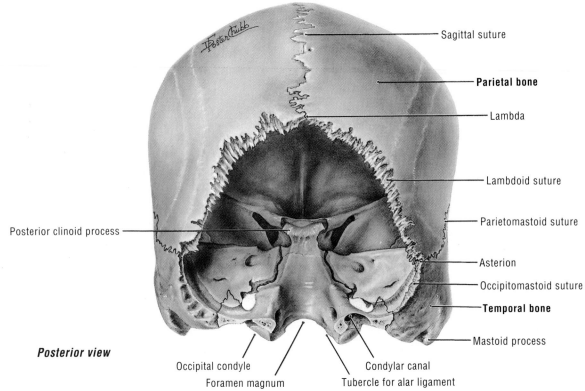

Sagittal suture

Parietal bone

Lambda

Lambdoid suture

Parietomastoid suture

Asterion

Occipitomastoid suture

Temporal bone

Mastoid process

Posterior clinoid process

Posterior view

Occipital condyle

Foramen magnum

Condylar canal

Tubercle for alar ligament

7.31

Posterior cranial fossa

Part of the occipital bone has been removed. Observe:
1. The dorsum sellae is the squarish plate of bone rising from the body of the sphenoid; at its superior angles are the posterior clinoid processes;

2. The clivus is the sloping surface between the dorsum sellae and the foramen magnum; it is formed by the basilar part of the occipital bone (basiocciput) with some assistance from the body of the sphenoid;

3. The grooves for the sigmoid sinus and the inferior petrosal sinus both lead inferiorly to the jugular foramen.

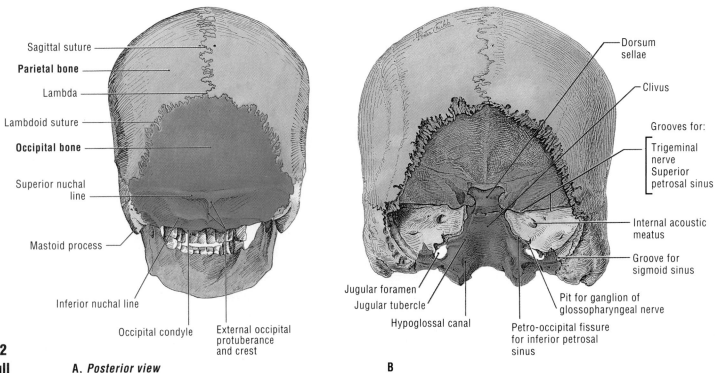

Sagittal suture

Parietal bone

Lambda

Lambdoid suture

Occipital bone

Superior nuchal line

Mastoid process

Inferior nuchal line

Occipital condyle

External occipital protuberance and crest

Dorsum sellae

Clivus

Grooves for:

Trigeminal nerve
Superior petrosal sinus

Internal acoustic meatus

Groove for sigmoid sinus

Pit for ganglion of glossopharyngeal nerve

Jugular foramen

Jugular tubercle

Hypoglossal canal

Petro-occipital fissure for inferior petrosal sinus

7.32

Skull

A, *Posterior view*

B

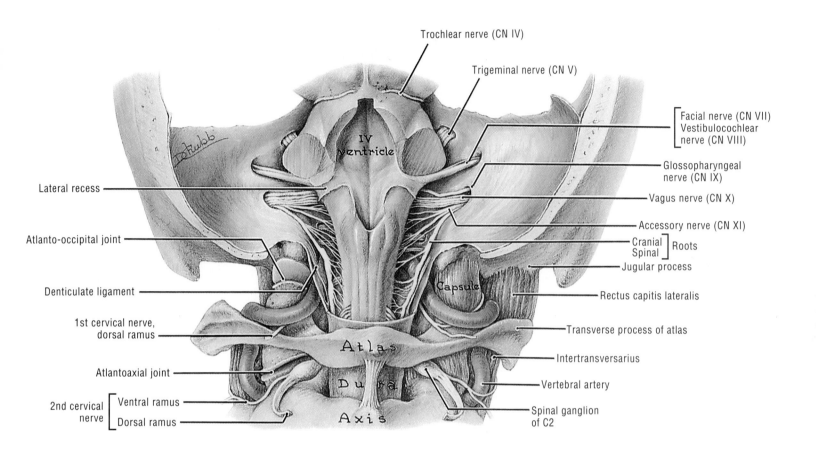

Trochlear nerve (CN IV)

Trigeminal nerve (CN V)

Facial nerve (CN VII)
Vestibulocochlear
nerve (CN VIII)

Glossopharyngeal
nerve (CN IX)

Vagus nerve (CN X)

Accessory nerve (CN XI)

Cranial ⎤
Spinal ⎦ Roots

Jugular process

Rectus capitis lateralis

Transverse process of atlas

Intertransversarius

Vertebral artery

Spinal ganglion
of C2

IV ventricle

Capsule

Atlas

Dura

Axis

Lateral recess

Atlanto-occipital joint

Denticulate ligament

1st cervical nerve,
dorsal ramus

Atlantoaxial joint

2nd cervical nerve ⎡ Ventral ramus
                    ⎣ Dorsal ramus

7.33
Cranial nerves, exposed posteriorly

Observe:

1. The trochlear nerves (CN IV), arising from the dorsal aspect of midbrain just inferior to the inferior colliculi; the trigeminal nerves (CN V), ascending to enter the mouths of the trigeminal caves; the facial (CN VII) and vestibulocochlear (CN VIII) nerves coursing superiorly to the internal acoustic meatus; the glosso-pharyngeal nerves (CN IX) piercing the dura mater separately and passing with the vagus (CN X) and accessory (CN XI) nerves through the jugular foramina; the fila of the accessory nerves of opposite sides, leaving the medulla and spinal cord asymmetrically;

2. The abducens nerves (CN VI) are not in view; the hypoglossal nerves (CN XII) are seen vaguely anterior to the spinal roots of nerves XI and just superior to the vertebral arteries;

3. The transverse process of the atlas, joined to the jugular

process of the occipital bone by rectus capitis lateralis muscle, which morphologically is an intertransverse muscle;

4. The vertebral arteries, raised from their beds on the posterior arch of the atlas;

5. The 1st cervical nerve, here having no sensory component; its dorsal ramus (suboccipital nerve) passing between the vertebral artery and the posterior arch of the atlas; its ventral ramus (not labeled), curving around the atlanto-occipital joint;

6. The 2nd cervical nerve, largely sensory, having a large spinal ganglion, a large dorsal ramus (or greater occipital nerve), and a smaller ventral ramus; the fila of its dorsal root are seen just superior to the cut edge of the dura and posterior to the spinal root of CN XI.

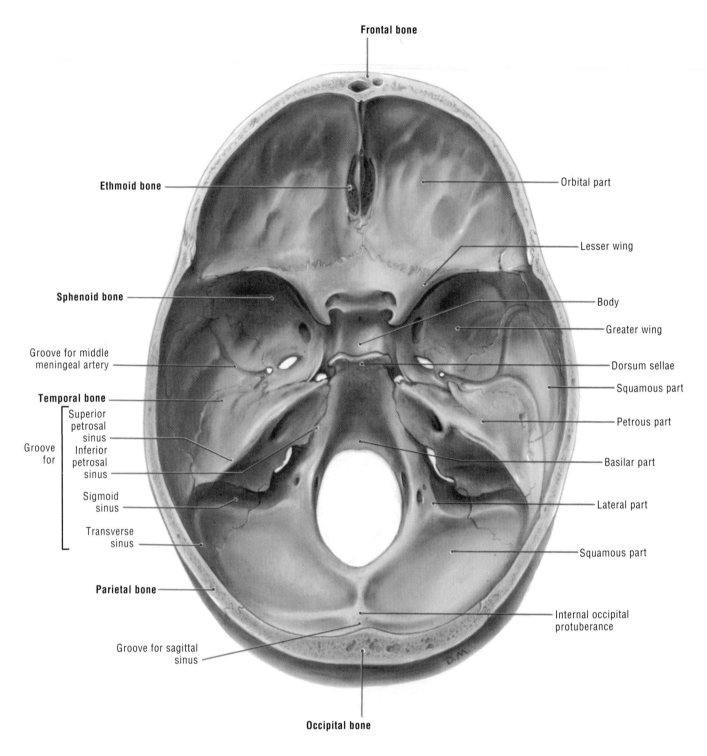

Frontal bone

Ethmoid bone

Sphenoid bone

Groove for middle
meningeal artery

Temporal bone

Superior
petrosal
sinus
Groove | Inferior
for | petrosal
sinus

Sigmoid
sinus

Transverse
sinus

Parietal bone

Groove for sagittal
sinus

Occipital bone

Orbital part

Lesser wing

Body

Greater wing

Dorsum sellae

Squamous part

Petrous part

Basilar part

Lateral part

Squamous part

Internal occipital
protuberance

7.34
Interior of the base of the skull

Observe:

1. The three bones contributing to the anterior cranial fossa: orbital plate of frontal, cribriform plate of ethmoid, and lesser wing of sphenoid;

2. The four developmental parts of the occipital bone: basilar, right and left lateral, and squamous;

3. Of the two paired clinoid processes for the attachment of the tentorium, the anterior on the lesser wing of the sphenoid is conical; the posterior, on the angle of the dorsum sellae, is beak-like.

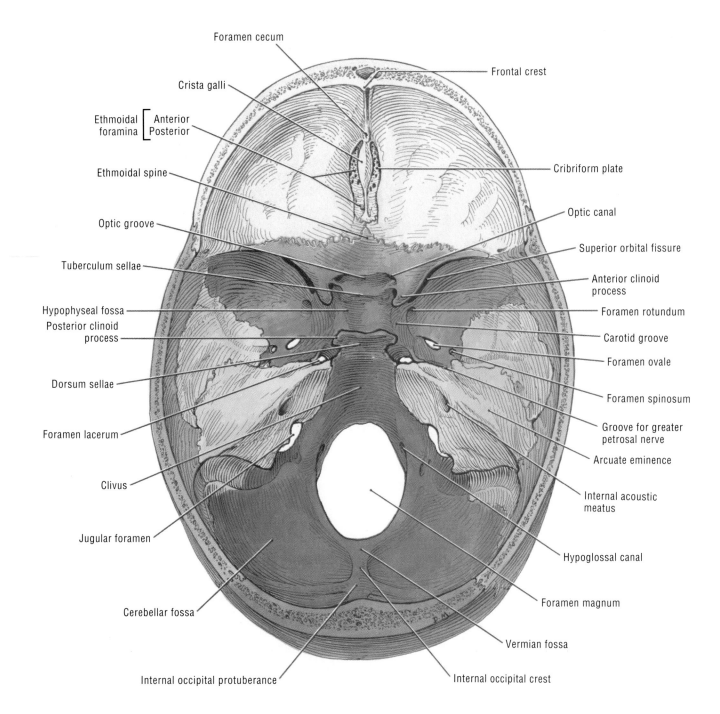

Foramen cecum

Crista galli

Ethmoidal foramina { Anterior / Posterior

Ethmoidal spine

Optic groove

Tuberculum sellae

Hypophyseal fossa

Posterior clinoid process

Dorsum sellae

Foramen lacerum

Clivus

Jugular foramen

Cerebellar fossa

Internal occipital protuberance

Frontal crest

Cribriform plate

Optic canal

Superior orbital fissure

Anterior clinoid process

Foramen rotundum

Carotid groove

Foramen ovale

Foramen spinosum

Groove for greater petrosal nerve

Arcuate eminence

Internal acoustic meatus

Hypoglossal canal

Foramen magnum

Vermian fossa

Internal occipital crest

7.35
Interior of the base of the skull

Observe the following features in the median plane:
1. In the anterior cranial fossa: frontal crest and crista galli for attachment of the falx cerebri; between them, the foramen cecum – not usually blind – which transmits a vein connecting the superior sagittal sinus with the veins of the frontal sinus and root of the nose;

2. In the middle cranial fossa: the optic groove leading from one optic canal to the other, but not lodging the optic chiasma; three features – tuberculum sellae, hypophyseal fossa, and dorsum sellae constitute the sella turcica or Turkish saddle;

3. In the posterior cranial fossa: clivus, foramen magnum, vermian fossa (for vermis of the cerebellum), internal occipital crest for attachment of the falx cerebelli, and the internal occipital protuberance from which grooves for the transverse sinuses curve laterally.

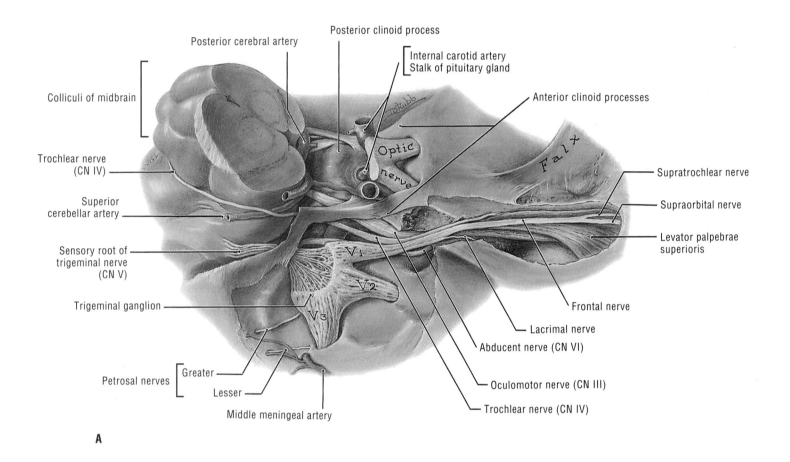

Posterior cerebral artery

Posterior clinoid process

Internal carotid artery
Stalk of pituitary gland

Colliculi of midbrain

Anterior clinoid processes

Optic nerve

Falx

Trochlear nerve
(CN IV)

Supratrochlear nerve

Superior
cerebellar artery

Supraorbital nerve

Levator palpebrae
superioris

Sensory root of
trigeminal nerve
(CN V)

V1

Trigeminal ganglion

V2

Frontal nerve

V3

Lacrimal nerve

Abducent nerve (CN VI)

Petrosal nerves [Greater

Oculomotor nerve (CN III)

Lesser

Trochlear nerve (CN IV)

Middle meningeal artery

A

7.36
Nerves of the middle cranial fossa

A. Superficial dissection. **B**. Orientation drawing. The tentorium cerebelli is cut away to reveal the courses of the trochlear and trigeminal nerves in the posterior cranial fossa. The dura is largely removed from the middle cranial fossa. The roof of the orbit is partly removed.

Observe:

1. The trigeminal (semilunar) ganglion and its three divisions;

2. The mandibular nerve (CN V³), dropping inferiorly through the foramen ovale into the infratemporal fossa;

3. The maxillary nerve (CN V²), passing anteriorly through the foramen rotundum into the pterygopalatine fossa;

4. The ophthalmic nerve (CN V¹), ascending slightly, closely applied to the trochlear nerve (CN IV), and dividing into frontal and lacrimal branches; these three (trochlear, frontal, lacrimal) nerves, running anteriorly through the superior orbital fissure and applied to the roof of the orbital cavity (removed).

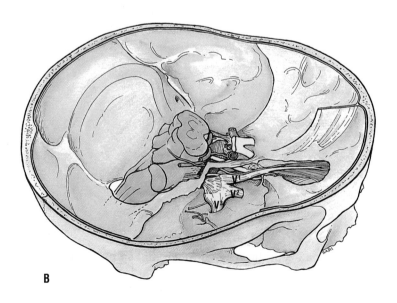

B

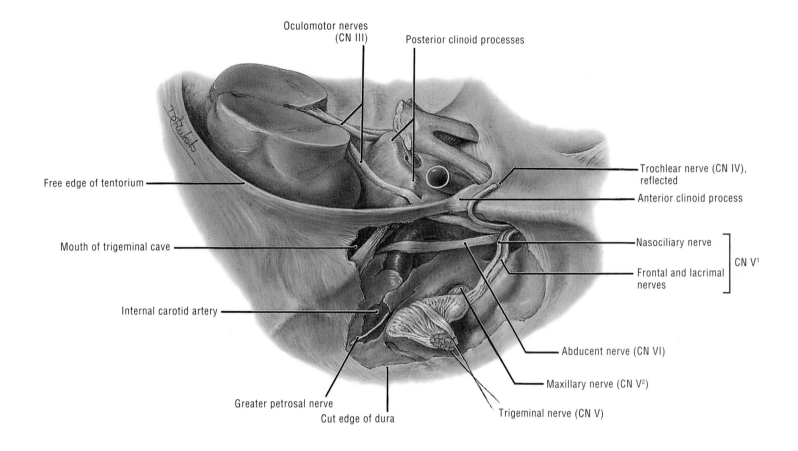

Oculomotor nerves (CN III)

Posterior clinoid processes

Free edge of tentorium

Mouth of trigeminal cave

Internal carotid artery

Greater petrosal nerve

Cut edge of dura

Trochlear nerve (CN IV), reflected

Anterior clinoid process

Nasociliary nerve

Frontal and lacrimal nerves

CN V¹

Abducent nerve (CN VI)

Maxillary nerve (CN V²)

Trigeminal nerve (CN V)

7.37
Nerves in the middle cranial fossa, deep dissection

The trigeminal nerve is divided, withdrawn from the mouth of the trigeminal cave, and turned anteriorly. The trochlear nerve also is reflected anteriorly.

Observe:

1. The bed of the trigeminal ganglion is partly formed by the greater petrosal nerve and the internal carotid artery, dura intervening;

2. The motor root of nerve CN V (the nerve to the muscles of mastication), crossing the ganglion diagonally, to join CN V³;

3. CN V¹, giving off the nasociliary nerve, and crowding with cranial nerves III, IV, and VI through the superior orbital fissure;

4. The anterior clinoid process, "pulled posteriorly" by the free edge of the tentorium cerebelli between the optic nerve and internal carotid artery medially, and the oculomotor nerve inferiorly;

5. The abducent nerve (CN VI), making a right-angled turn at the apex of the petrous bone and then, as it runs horizontally anteriorly, hugging the internal carotid artery, which flattens it;

6. The sinuous course of the internal carotid artery.

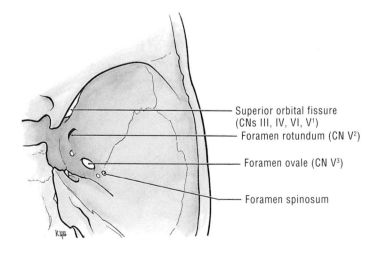

Superior orbital fissure (CNs III, IV, VI, V¹)

Foramen rotundum (CN V²)

Foramen ovale (CN V³)

Foramen spinosum

7.38
Crescent of foramina in the middle cranial fossa

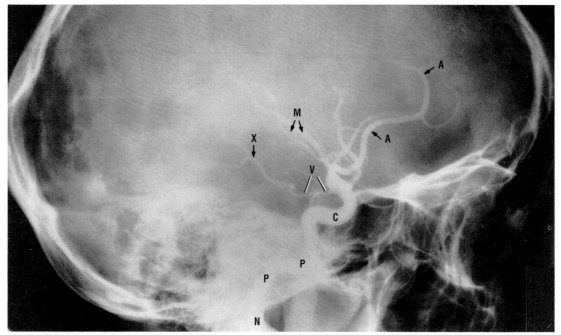

Lateral view

7.39
Arteriogram of carotid siphon

Compare the arteriogram to the diagram below. Note the course of the internal carotid artery in the neck *(N)*, in the petrous temporal bone *(P)*, in the cavernous sinus *(C)* and its terminal branches, the anterior *(A)* and middle *(M)* cerebral arteries.

Also note the posterior cerebral *(X)*, and posterior communicating *(V)* arteries. (Courtesy of Dr. D. Armstrong, Associate Professor of Radiology, University of Toronto, Toronto, Ontario, Canada.)

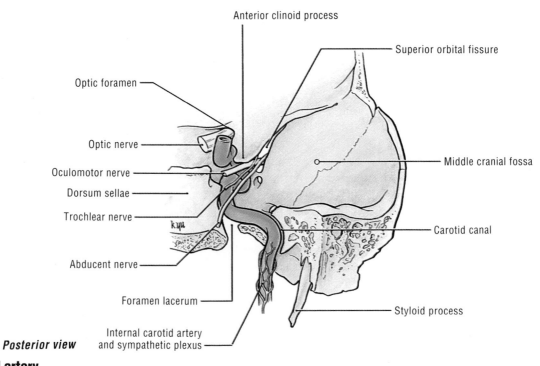

Anterior clinoid process

Superior orbital fissure

Optic foramen

Optic nerve

Oculomotor nerve

Middle cranial fossa

Dorsum sellae

Trochlear nerve

Abducent nerve

Carotid canal

Foramen lacerum

Styloid process

Internal carotid artery
and sympathetic plexus

7.40   *Posterior view*

Internal carotid artery

This is a coronal section through the carotid canal showing the internal carotid artery in the carotid canal and cavernous sinus. The artery takes an inverted L-shaped course from the inferior surface of the petrous bone to its apex. There, at the superior end of foramen lacerum, it enters the cranial cavity and takes an S-shaped course. Note its contacts.

7.41
Cavernous sinus, coronal section

Observe:

1. This venous sinus is situated bilaterally at the lateral aspect of the sphenoidal air sinus and of the hypophyseal fossa;

2. Cranial nerves III, IV, V^1, and V^2 are in a sheath in the lateral wall of the sinus;

3. The internal carotid artery surrounded by the internal carotid plexus (not drawn) and the abducent nerve (CN VI) run through the cavernous sinus and so are vulnerable in thrombosis of the sinus;

4. The internal carotid artery, having made an acute bend, is cut twice; this artery and the oculomotor nerve groove the anterior clinoid process;

5. The ophthalmic veins drain into the cavernous sinus.

B. Orientation drawing for Figures 7.41**A** and 7.42.

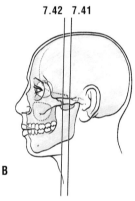

B

7.42
Apex of orbital cavity, coronal section

Observe:

1. The optic nerve within its pial, arachnoid, and dural sheaths and the subarachnoid space; the ophthalmic artery emerging from the optic canal;

2. Other nerves crowded together, tightly packed, passing through the medial end of the superior orbital fissure; they are: the superior and the inferior branch of the oculomotor nerve (CN III), the trochlear nerve (CN IV); the frontal, lacrimal, and nasociliary branches of the ophthalmic nerve (CN V^1); and the abducent nerve (CN VI);

3. The ophthalmic vein, about to open into the cavernous sinus, in turn to be drained by the superior and inferior petrosal sinuses (Fig. 7.20).

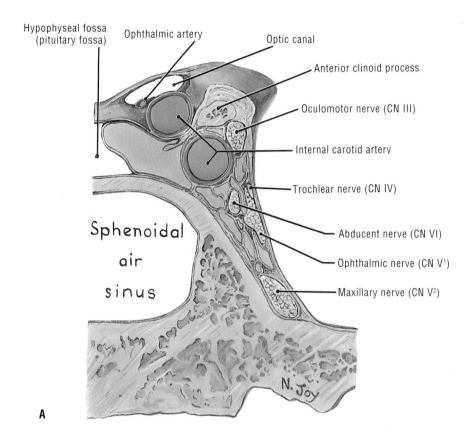

Hypophyseal fossa (pituitary fossa)
Ophthalmic artery
Optic canal
Anterior clinoid process
Oculomotor nerve (CN III)
Internal carotid artery
Trochlear nerve (CN IV)
Abducent nerve (CN VI)
Ophthalmic nerve (CN V^1)
Maxillary nerve (CN V^2)
Sphenoidal air sinus
N. Joy

A

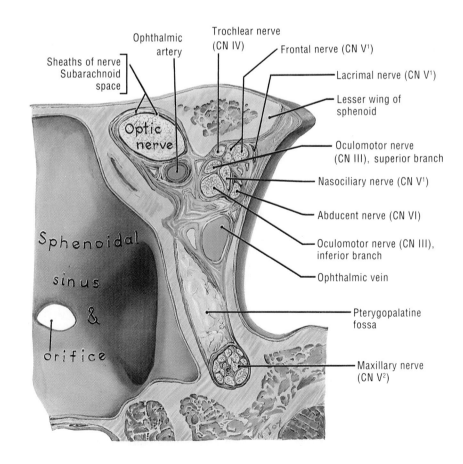

Ophthalmic artery
Trochlear nerve (CN IV)
Frontal nerve (CN V^1)
Sheaths of nerve Subarachnoid space
Lacrimal nerve (CN V^1)
Lesser wing of sphenoid
Optic nerve
Oculomotor nerve (CN III), superior branch
Nasociliary nerve (CN V^1)
Abducent nerve (CN VI)
Oculomotor nerve (CN III), inferior branch
Ophthalmic vein
Sphenoidal sinus & orifice
Pterygopalatine fossa
Maxillary nerve (CN V^2)

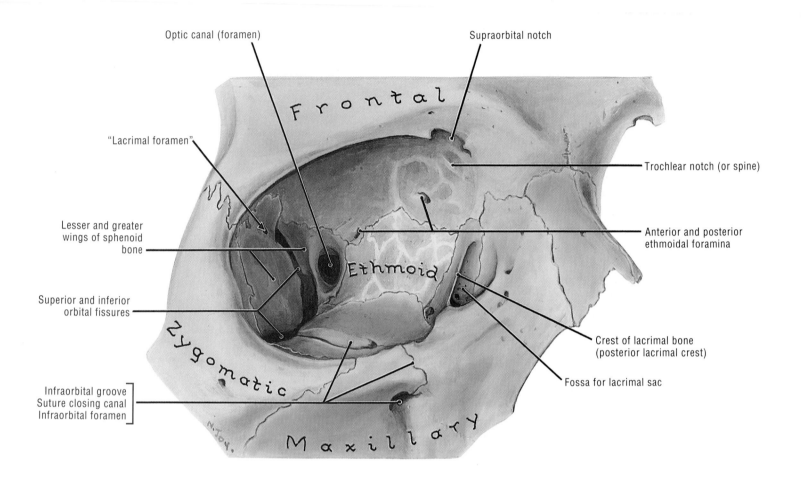

Optic canal (foramen)

Supraorbital notch

Frontal

"Lacrimal foramen"

Trochlear notch (or spine)

Lesser and greater
wings of sphenoid
bone

Ethmoid

Anterior and posterior
ethmoidal foramina

Superior and inferior
orbital fissures

Zygomatic

Crest of lacrimal bone
(posterior lacrimal crest)

N.Joy.

Fossa for lacrimal sac

Infraorbital groove
Suture closing canal
Infraorbital foramen

Maxillary

7.43
Orbital cavity

Observe:

1. The quadrangular orbital margin, at the base of the cavity, to which the frontal, maxillary, and zygomatic bones contribute;

2. The spiral form of the medial part of this margin; it is spiral since the supraorbital margin leads to the crest of the lacrimal bone (posterior lacrimal crest), whereas the infraorbital margin is continuous with the crest on the frontal process of the maxilla (anterior lacrimal crest);

3. The fossa for the lacrimal sac, between these two crests;

4. The optic canal, situated at the apex of the pear-shaped orbital cavity, and placed between the body of the sphenoid and the two roots of the lesser wing; a straight probe must pass along the lateral wall of the cavity, if it is to traverse the canal;

5. The superior wall or roof, formed by the orbital plate of the frontal bone;

6. The inferior wall or floor, formed by the orbital plate of the maxilla and slightly by the zygomatic bone, and crossed by the infraorbital groove, the anterior end of which is converted into the infraorbital canal that ends at the infraorbital foramen;

7. The stout lateral wall, formed by the frontal process of the zygomatic bone and by the greater wing of the sphenoid; the superior and inferior orbital fissures, together forming a V-shaped fissure, which limits the greater wing of the sphenoid;

8. The fragile medial wall, formed by the papery lacrimal bone and the papery orbital plate of the ethmoid bone; the anterior and posterior ethmoidal foramina, which developed in the suture between the frontal and ethmoidal bones, but are now, in this specimen, enveloped by the frontal bone;

9. The "lacrimal foramen," just beyond the superolateral end of the superior orbital fissure, for the anastomosis between the middle meningeal and lacrimal arteries; the zygomatic foramen on the orbital surface of the zygomatic bone is not in view.

7.44
Dissection of the orbital cavity

The eyelids, orbital septum, levator palpebrae superioris, and some fat are removed. Observe:

1. The ocular conjunctiva, loose and wrinkled over the sclera, but adherent to the cornea;

2. The aponeurotic insertions of the four recti, inserted 6 to 8 mm posterior to the sclerocorneal junction;

3. The tendon of the superior oblique muscle, playing in a cartilaginous pulley or trochlea, which is fixed by ligamentous fibers just posterior to the superomedial angle of the orbital margin;

4. The nerve to the inferior oblique muscle entering its posterior border;

5. The lacrimal gland, placed between the bony orbital wall laterally and the eyeball and lateral rectus muscle medially.

7.45
The eye

A. Surface features. Observe:

1. The tough white fibrous outer coat of the eyeball, the sclera;

2. The central transparent cornea, through which can be seen the pigmented iris with its aperture, the pupil;

3. Superior and inferior lids meet at angles, the medial and lateral canthi;

4. The inferior lid has been everted to show the reflection of conjunctiva from the anterior surface of the eyeball to the inner surface of the lid;

5. An *arrow* points to the inferior lacrimal punctum;

6. Near the medial angle, a vertical fold of conjunctiva, the plica semilunaris *(S)*;

7. In the medial angle, an unattractive mound of modified skin, the lacrimal caruncle *(C)*;

B. Lacrimal apparatus. Tears are secreted into the conjunctival sac by the lacrimal gland *(L)* located in the superolateral angle of the bony orbit; tears, after passing over the eyeball, drain into the lacrimal sac *(S)* through puncta in superior and inferior lids, leading to the lacrimal canaliculi *(C)*; the lacrimal sac drains into the nasolacrimal duct *(N)*, which empties into the inferior meatus *(I)* of the nose.

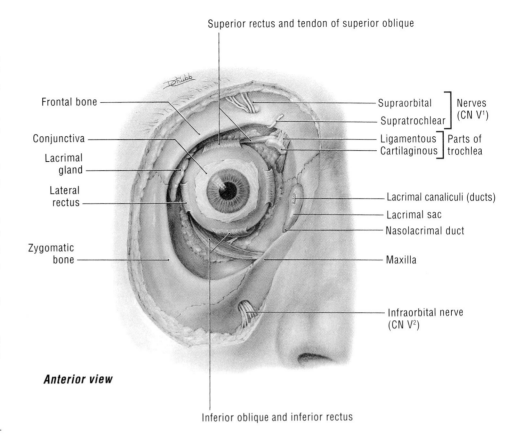

Superior rectus and tendon of superior oblique

Frontal bone

Conjunctiva

Lacrimal gland

Lateral rectus

Zygomatic bone

Supraorbital
Supratrochlear — Nerves (CN V¹)

Ligamentous
Cartilaginous — Parts of trochlea

Lacrimal canaliculi (ducts)

Lacrimal sac

Nasolacrimal duct

Maxilla

Infraorbital nerve (CN V²)

Anterior view

Inferior oblique and inferior rectus

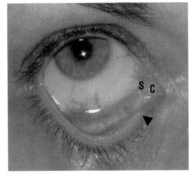

A

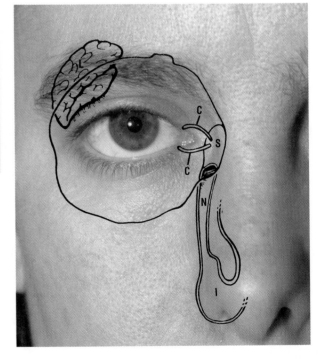

B

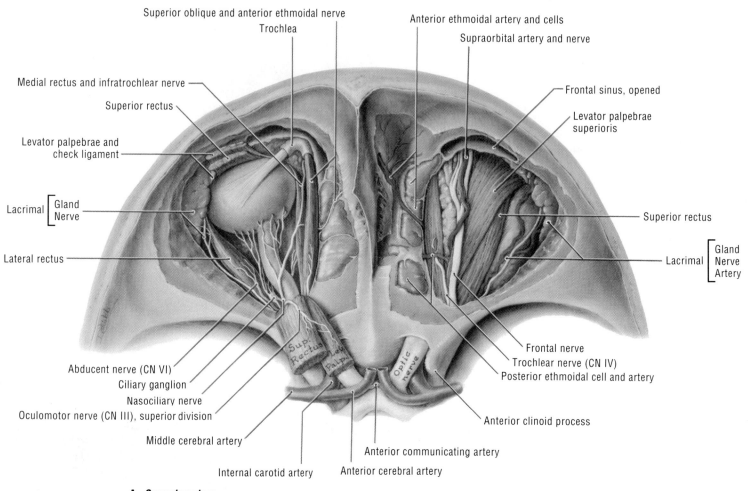

Superior oblique and anterior ethmoidal nerve
Trochlea
Medial rectus and infratrochlear nerve
Superior rectus
Levator palpebrae and check ligament
Lacrimal [Gland / Nerve]
Lateral rectus

Anterior ethmoidal artery and cells
Supraorbital artery and nerve
Frontal sinus, opened
Levator palpebrae superioris
Superior rectus
Lacrimal [Gland / Nerve / Artery]

Abducent nerve (CN VI)
Ciliary ganglion
Nasociliary nerve
Oculomotor nerve (CN III), superior division
Middle cerebral artery
Internal carotid artery
Anterior cerebral artery
Anterior communicating artery

Frontal nerve
Trochlear nerve (CN IV)
Posterior ethmoidal cell and artery
Anterior clinoid process

Sup. Rectus
Palp.
Optic nerve

A, *Superior view*

7.46
Orbital cavity

Observe on the right side of **A**:

1. The orbital plate of the frontal bone is removed.

2. Levator palpebrae superioris muscle, overlying the superior rectus muscle;

3. The three nerves applied to the roof of the orbital cavity– trochlear, frontal, lacrimal;

4. Four of the branches of the ophthalmic artery.

Observe on the left side of **A**:

1. The levator palpebrae and superior rectus muscles have been reflected;

2. The superior division of nerve III supplying the superior rectus and levator palpebrae muscles;

3. The entire course of the superior oblique muscle and the trochlear nerve (CN IV) supplying it;

4. The lateral rectus muscle and the abducent nerve (CN VI) supplying it;

5. The medial rectus muscle and a branch of the oculomotor nerve (CN III) supplying it;

6. The lacrimal nerve, running superior to the lateral rectus muscle to the lacrimal gland;

7. The ciliary ganglion, placed between the lateral rectus muscle and the optic nerve and giving off many short ciliary nerves;

8. The nasociliary nerve, giving off two long ciliary nerves that anastomose with each other and with the short ciliary nerves.

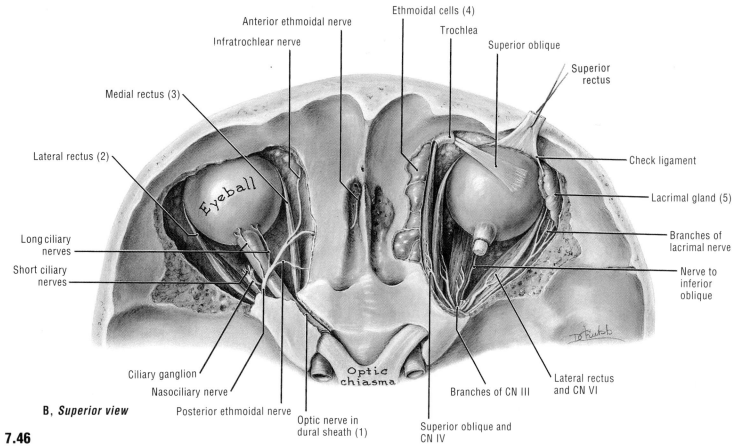

Medial rectus (3)

Lateral rectus (2)

Long ciliary nerves

Short ciliary nerves

Anterior ethmoidal nerve

Infratrochlear nerve

Ethmoidal cells (4)

Trochlea

Superior oblique

Superior rectus

Check ligament

Lacrimal gland (5)

Branches of lacrimal nerve

Nerve to inferior oblique

Ciliary ganglion

Nasociliary nerve

Posterior ethmoidal nerve

Optic nerve in dural sheath (1)

Optic chiasma

Superior oblique and CN IV

Branches of CN III

Lateral rectus and CN VI

B, *Superior view*

7.46
Orbital cavity *(continued)*

Observe on the right side of **B**:

1. The nerves to the six ocular muscles – four recti and two obliques – the trochlear to the superior oblique muscle, the abducent to the lateral rectus muscle, and the oculomotor to the remaining four and also to levator palpebrae superioris;

2. The four recti (superior, medial, inferior, lateral), supplied on their ocular surfaces; the two obliques (superior, inferior) near their borders; the superior rectus and inferior obliques are not in view.

Observe on the left side of **B**:

1. The eyeball, occupying the anterior half on the 5 cm long orbital cavity;

2. The ciliary ganglion, lying posteriorly between the lateral rectus muscle and the sheath of the optic nerve, receiving a twig (sensory and sympathetic) from the nasociliary nerve and a twig (motor to sphincter pupillae and ciliary muscle) from the nerve to the inferior oblique muscle, and giving off short ciliary nerves (cut short);

3. The nasociliary nerve, sending a twig to the ciliary ganglion, crossing the optic nerve, giving off two long ciliary nerves (sensory to the eyeball and cornea), and the posterior ethmoidal nerve (to the sphenoidal sinus and posterior ethmoidal cells), and dividing into the anterior ethmoidal and intratrochlear nerves.

C. Transverse MRI (magnetic resonance image). Numbers refer to structures in **B**. (Courtesy of Dr. W. Kucharczyk, Clinical Director of Tri-Hospital Resonance Centre, Toronto, Ontario, Canada.)

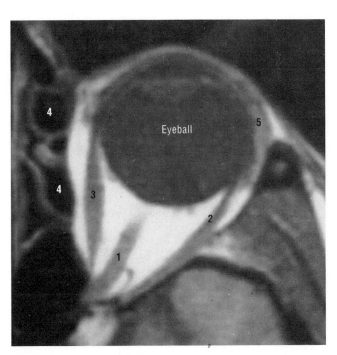

Eyeball

C

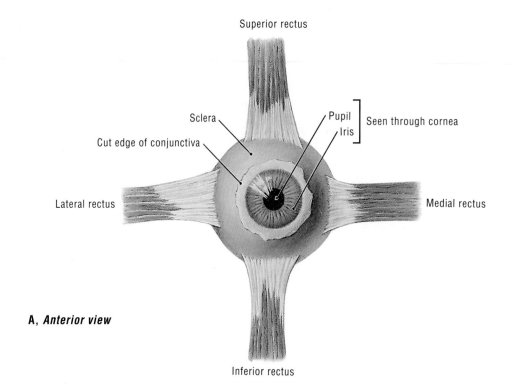

Superior rectus

Sclera ⌐ Pupil ⌐
                Iris ⌐ Seen through cornea

Cut edge of conjunctiva

Lateral rectus   Medial rectus

A, *Anterior view*

Inferior rectus

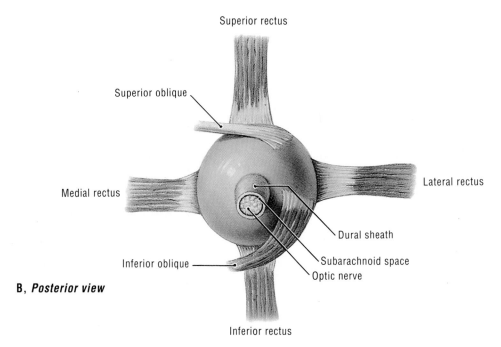

Superior rectus

Superior oblique

Medial rectus   Lateral rectus

                                Dural sheath

Inferior oblique   Subarachnoid space
                        Optic nerve

B, *Posterior view*

Inferior rectus

7.47
Eyeball and insertions

A. Insertions of the four recti. The four recti are spread out to show the insertions of their aponeuroses into the anterior half of the bulb or eyeball, 6 to 8 mm posterior to the sclerocorneal junction.

B. Insertions of the two obliques. The two obliques are inserted by aponeuroses into the posterolateral quadrant of the eyeball. When in situ, the inferior rectus passes superior to the inferior oblique muscle.

Superior rectus (CN III)　　　　Inferior oblique
　　　　　　　　　　　　　　　　(CN III)

Lateral rectus (CN VI)　　　　Medial rectus
　　　　　　　　　　　　　　　(CN III)

Inferior rectus　　　　　Superior
(CN III)　　　　　oblique (CN IV)

Superior rectus (CN III)

Lateral rectus (CN VI)

Inferior rectus (CN III)

7.48
Actions of the extrinsic ocular muscles

The *arrows* indicate the direction of movement of the cornea; this is a simple way to test the functioning of the extraocular muscles clinically, but in order to understand these actions, movement of the eyeball must be considered around three axes (vertical, horizontal, anteroposterior).

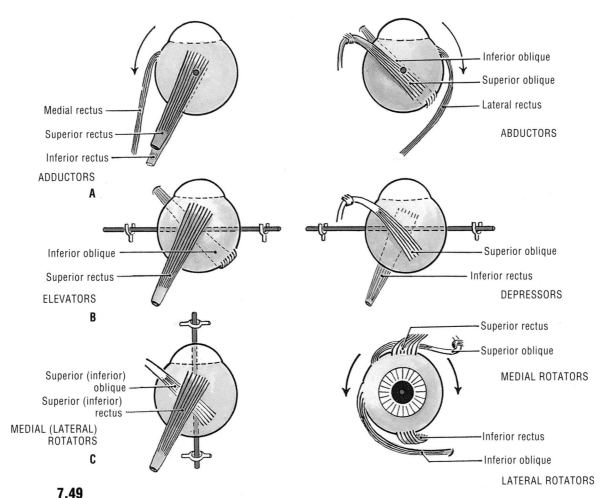

Medial rectus
Superior rectus
Inferior rectus
ADDUCTORS
A

Inferior oblique
Superior oblique
Lateral rectus
ABDUCTORS

Inferior oblique
Superior rectus
ELEVATORS
B

Superior oblique
Inferior rectus
DEPRESSORS

Superior (inferior) oblique
Superior (inferior) rectus
MEDIAL (LATERAL) ROTATORS
C

Superior rectus
Superior oblique
MEDIAL ROTATORS

Inferior rectus
Inferior oblique
LATERAL ROTATORS

7.49
Movement of the eyeball around the vertical, horizontal, and anteroposterior axes

A. Vertical axis. **B.** Horizontal axis. **C.** Anteroposterior axis. In each instance, it is the right eyeball that is represented. Of the six ocular muscles, the medial rectus and the lateral rectus move the eyeball on one axis only; each of the four other muscles moves it on all three axes. The two obliques also protract (protrude) the eyeball, whereas the four recti retract it.

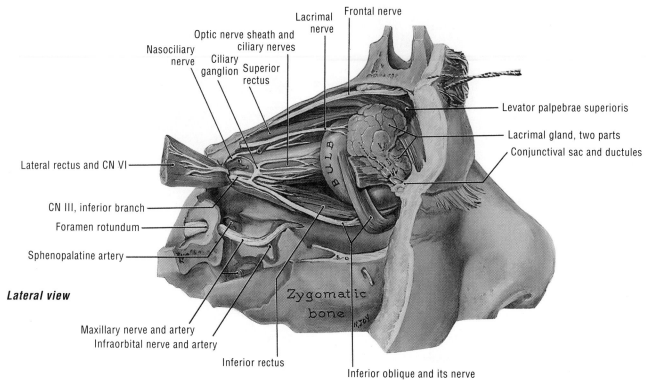

7.50
Dissection of orbit

Lateral view

Labels (clockwise): Optic nerve sheath and ciliary nerves — Lacrimal nerve — Frontal nerve — Levator palpebrae superioris — Lacrimal gland, two parts — Conjunctival sac and ductules — Nasociliary nerve — Ciliary ganglion — Superior rectus — BULB — Lateral rectus and CN VI — CN III, inferior branch — Foramen rotundum — Sphenopalatine artery — Zygomatic bone — Maxillary nerve and artery — Infraorbital nerve and artery — Inferior rectus — Inferior oblique and its nerve

Note in particular the ciliary ganglion that receives sensory fibers from the nasociliary branches of V^1, sympathetic fibers from the internal carotid plexus traveling around the ophthalmic artery, and parasympathetic fibers (which synapse in the ganglion) from the inferior branch of the oculomotor nerve. Eight to ten short ciliary nerves go to the eyeball.

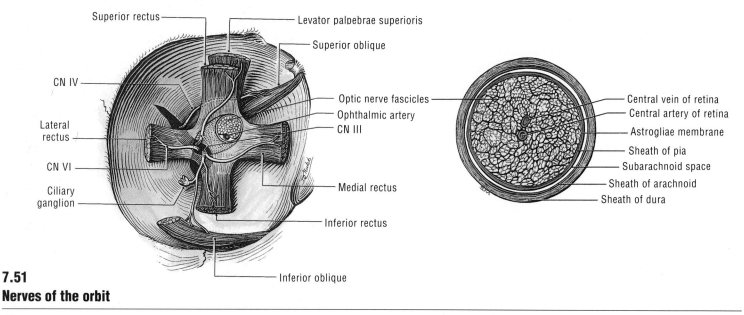

7.51
Nerves of the orbit

Labels (left figure): Superior rectus — Levator palpebrae superioris — Superior oblique — CN IV — Optic nerve fascicles — Ophthalmic artery — CN III — Lateral rectus — CN VI — Ciliary ganglion — Medial rectus — Inferior rectus — Inferior oblique

Labels (right figure): Central vein of retina — Central artery of retina — Astrogliae membrane — Sheath of pia — Subarachnoid space — Sheath of arachnoid — Sheath of dura

Observe:

1. The optic nerve within its pial, arachnoid, and dural sheaths;

2. The four recti arising from a fibrous cuff, called the anulus tendineus, that encircles: the dural sheath of the optic nerve, CN VI, and the superior and inferior branches of CN III; the nasociliary nerve (not shown) also passes through this cuff, but CN IV clings to the bony roof of the cavity;

3. Cranial nerves IV and VI supplying one muscle each, and CN III supplying the remaining five orbital muscles: two via its superior branch, three via its inferior branch;

4. The oculomotor (CN III) through the ciliary ganglion supplies parasympathetic fibers to the ciliary muscle and sphincter iridis.

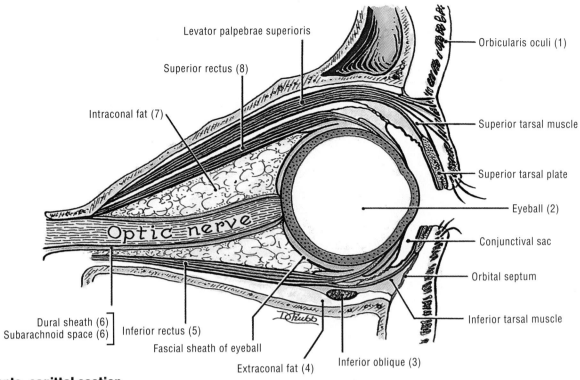

7.52
Orbital contents, sagittal section

The numbers in parentheses refer to Figure 7.54.

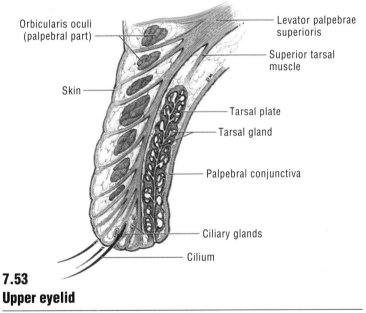

7.53
Upper eyelid

This diagram of a sagittal section through the upper eyelid is redrawn from Whitnall SE. In *Anatomy of the Human Orbit*, London: Oxford Medical Publications, 1921. The lid has a superficial ciliary part and a deeper tarsal part. The ciliary part is covered with skin, contains the fibers of the palpebral part of orbicularis oculi, and bears the eyelashes or cilia. The tarsal part is lined with conjunctiva, has a fibrous tissue plate (the tarsal plate) forming its skeleton, and embedded in the tarsal plate are modified sebaceous glands that open on the margin of the eyelid.

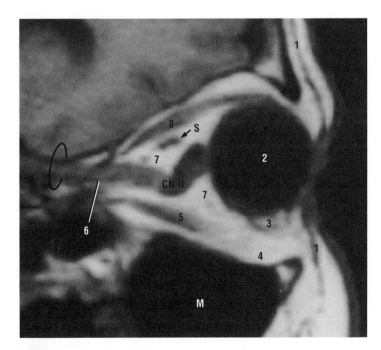

7.54
Sagittal MRI (magnetic resonance image) through the optic nerve

S - Superior ophthalmic vein, *M* - Maxillary sinus, *circled* - Optic foramen. (Courtesy of Dr. W. Kucharczyk, Clinical Director of Tri-Hospital Resonance Centre, Toronto, Ontario, Canada.)

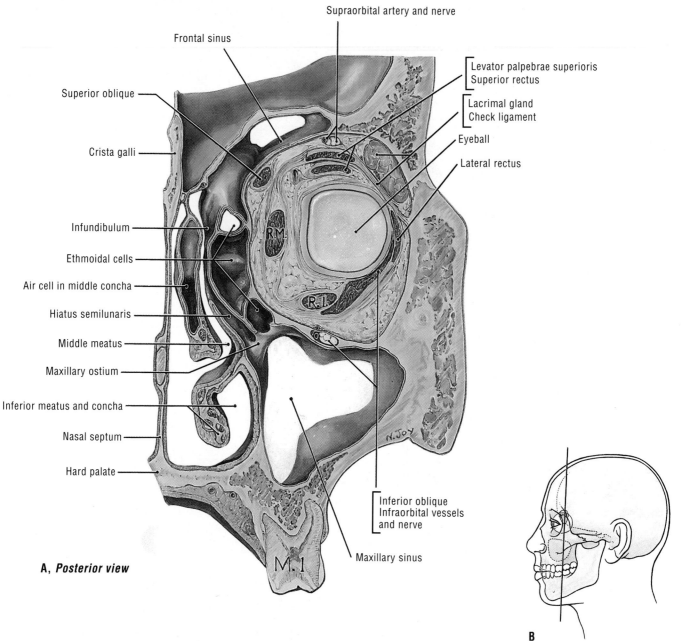

Supraorbital artery and nerve

Frontal sinus

Superior oblique

Crista galli

Infundibulum

Ethmoidal cells

Air cell in middle concha

Hiatus semilunaris

Middle meatus

Maxillary ostium

Inferior meatus and concha

Nasal septum

Hard palate

Levator palpebrae superioris
Superior rectus

Lacrimal gland
Check ligament

Eyeball

Lateral rectus

R.M.

R.I.

N.JOY

M.I

Inferior oblique
Infraorbital vessels
and nerve

Maxillary sinus

A, *Posterior view*

B

7.55
Coronal section of the right side of the head

Observe:

1. The eyeball within the somewhat circular orbital cavity; the stout, thick lateral bony wall; the thin, papery roof, medial wall, and floor surrounded with paranasal sinuses – frontal, ethmoidal, and maxillary;

2. The four recti and two obliques arranged around the bulb, the inferior oblique inserted by a tendon; levator palpebrae superioris superior to the superior rectus muscle, and the check ligament passing from it;

3. The lacrimal gland lying between the check ligament and the frontal bone;

4. The four recti and the fascia uniting them forming a circle around the bulb; the medial rectus (R.M.) and the inferior rectus (R.I.);

5. The nasal septum (semidiagrammatic); the middle concha, here, contains an air cell; the entrance to the frontal sinus through the infundibulum, which is at the most inferior point of the sinus;

6. The entrance to the maxillary sinus through the hiatus semilunaris, which is at the level of the roof of the sinus; the most inferior point of the sinus, here as commonly, is inferior to the level of the floor of the nasal cavity; the nasal wall of the sinus is very thin in the inferior meatus.

B. Orientation drawing of **A**.

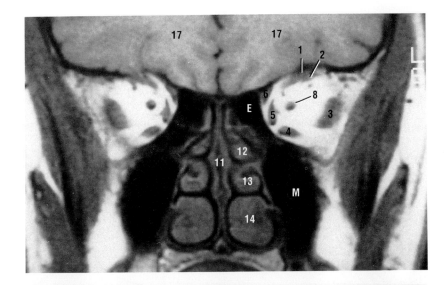

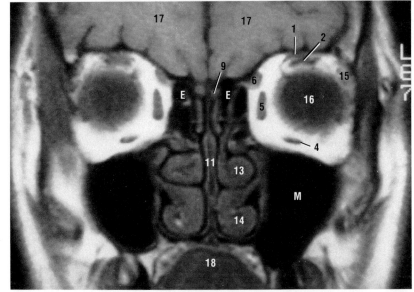

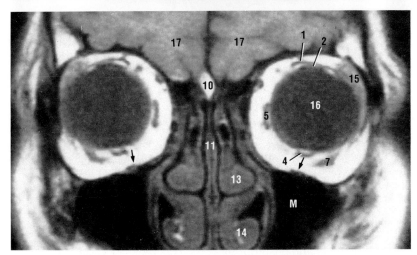

1	Levator palpabrae superioris
2	Superior rectus
3	Lateral rectus
4	Inferior rectus
5	Medial rectus
6	Superior oblique
7	Inferior oblique
8	Optic nerve
9	Olfactory bulb
10	Crista galli
11	Nasal septum
12	Superior concha
13	Middle concha
14	Inferior concha
15	Lacrimal gland
16	Eyeball
17	Frontal lobe
18	Tongue
M	Maxillary sinus
E	Ethmoidal sinus
arrowhead	Infra-orbital vessels and nerve

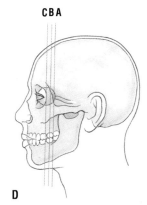

7.56
Coronal MRIs (magnetic resonance images) through the orbit

(Courtesy of Dr. W. Kucharczyk, Clinical Director of Tri-Hospital Resonance Centre, Toronto, Ontario, Canada.)

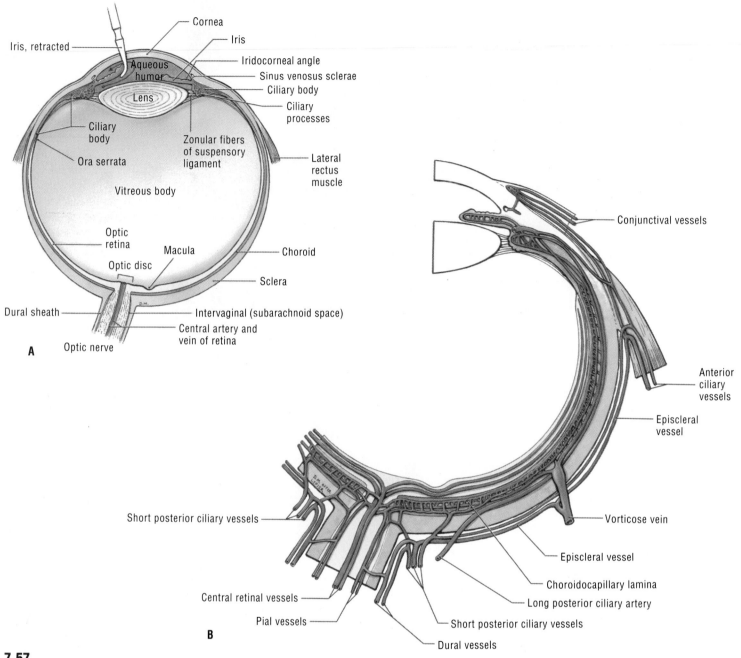

A

Iris, retracted

Cornea

Iris

Iridocorneal angle

Aqueous humor

Sinus venosus sclerae

Lens

Ciliary body

Ciliary processes

Ciliary body

Zonular fibers of suspensory ligament

Ora serrata

Lateral rectus muscle

Vitreous body

Optic retina

Macula

Choroid

Optic disc

Sclera

Dural sheath

Intervaginal (subarachnoid space)

Central artery and vein of retina

Optic nerve

B

Conjunctival vessels

Anterior ciliary vessels

Episcleral vessel

Short posterior ciliary vessels

Vorticose vein

Episcleral vessel

Choroidocapillary lamina

Long posterior ciliary artery

Central retinal vessels

Short posterior ciliary vessels

Pial vessels

Dural vessels

7.57
Right eyeball, horizontal section

Observe:

1. The eyeball or bulbus oculi has three coats (see **A**); external or fibrous coat: sclera and cornea; middle or vascular coat: choroid, ciliary body, and iris; internal or retinal coat: (a) outer layer of pigmented cells; (b) inner layer of cells that are optic (visual) posterior to the ora serrata, thin and mostly pigmented anterior to it; these extend to the pupillary margin (see **A**);

2. The four refractive media are: (a) the cornea; and posterior to it (b) the aqueous humor, which fills two chambers – an anterior in front of the iris and a posterior behind the iris; (c) the lens; and (d) the vitreous body, a jelly-like substance within a capsule, the vitreous (hyaloid) membrane, and occupying the vitreous chamber;

3. The central artery of the retina, a branch of the ophthalmic artery (Fig. 7.59), is an end artery; of the eight or so posterior ciliary arteries, six supply the choroid, which, in turn, nourishes the outer nonvascular layer of the retina, whereas two long posterior ciliary arteries, one on each side of the eyeball, run between sclera and choroid to anastomose with anterior ciliary arteries, which are derived from muscular branches (see **B**);

4. The vorticose veins (see **B**) (four to five in number) drain into the posterior ciliary and ophthalmic veins (Fig. 7.60).

7.58
Right ocular fundus

A photograph of the retina as seen through an ophthalmoscope.

Observe:

1. The oval optic disc with retinal vessels radiating from its center; composed of nerve fibers, the disc is the "blind spot";

2. Retinal veins are wider than the arteries;

3. The central retinal artery (a branch of the ophthalmic artery) enters the optic nerve posterior to the eyeball and divides into superior and inferior branches; each then divides into a medial (nasal) and lateral (temporal) branch;

4. The round dark area lateral to the disc is the macula; branches of vessels extend into this area but fail to reach its center, a depressed spot – the fovea centralis – which is the area of most acute vision; the fovea centralis is avascular and is nourished by the choroidal circulation. (Courtesy of Dr. J.R. Buncic, Associate Professor of Ophthalmology, University of Toronto, Toronto, Ontario, Canada.)

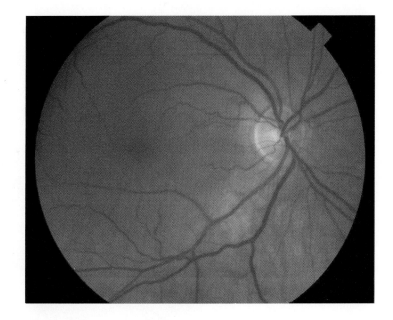

7.59
Ophthalmic artery

Observe:

1. This branch of the internal carotid artery enters the orbit via the optic canal within the dural sheath of the optic nerve; it supplies the contents of the orbit;

2. Of its branches, the central artery of the retina is an end artery;

3. Six branches pass beyond the orbit: (a) supratrochlear and (b) supraorbital arteries to the forehead, (c) dorsal nasal to the face, (d) lacrimal to the eyelid and, via its zygomatic branches, to the cheek and the temporal region, and (e and f) anterior and posterior ethmoidal arteries to the nasal cavity; these six arteries, which extend beyond the orbit, anastomose freely with branches of the external carotid artery;

4. The lacrimal artery commonly anastomoses with the middle meningeal artery, via the foramen lacrimale.

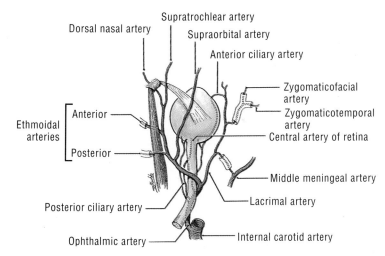

7.60
Ophthalmic veins

Observe:

1. The superior and inferior ophthalmic veins empty into the cavernous sinus posteriorly and communicate with the facial and supraorbital veins anteriorly;

2. The superior ophthalmic vein travels with the ophthalmic artery and its branches;

3. The inferior ophthalmic vein running in the floor of the orbit and entering the cavernous sinus; it may join the superior ophthalmic vein prior to entering the sinus.

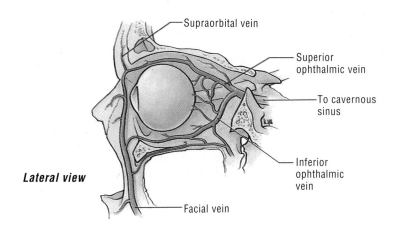

Lateral view

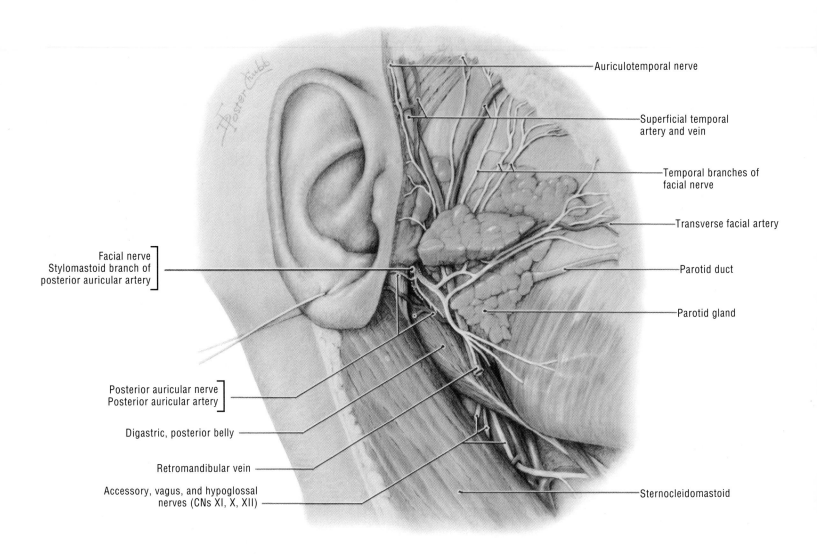

Auriculotemporal nerve

Superficial temporal artery and vein

Temporal branches of facial nerve

Transverse facial artery

Parotid duct

Parotid gland

Sternocleidomastoid

Facial nerve
Stylomastoid branch of posterior auricular artery

Posterior auricular nerve
Posterior auricular artery

Digastric, posterior belly

Retromandibular vein

Accessory, vagus, and hypoglossal nerves (CNs XI, X, XII)

7.61
Parotid region

See Figure 7.12 for a more superficial dissection.

Observe:

1. The stem of the facial nerve descending from the stylomastoid foramen for about 1 cm before curving anteriorly to penetrate the deeper part of the parotid gland;

2. The nerve to the posterior belly of the digastric muscle arising from the stem of the facial nerve;

3. The posterior auricular artery giving off a branch, the stylomastoid artery, which accompanies the facial nerve through the stylomastoid foramen into the facial canal;

4. The relatively superficial position of the landmark in the superior part of the neck, posterior belly of the digastric muscle; only three structures cross superficial to it: the cervical branch of

the facial nerve, branches of the retromandibular vein, and the branches of the great auricular nerve shown in Figure 7.12; all other crossing structures cross deep to it;

5. Preauricular lymph nodes;

6. Auricular and temporal branches of the auriculotemporal nerve;

7. Enlargement of the parotid and other salivary glands occurs in certain metabolic and endocrine diseases as well as in nutritional deficiency including anorexia nervosa; the resulting facial swelling is often not reversible (see Walsh BT, Croft CB, Katz JL. *Anorexia nervosa and salivary gland enlargement*. Int J Psychiatr Med 1981; 11:255-261).

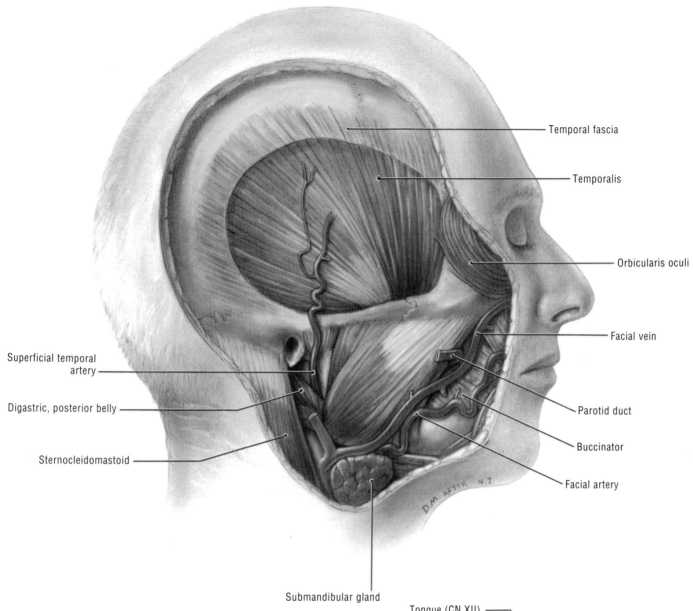

Temporal fascia

Temporalis

Orbicularis oculi

Facial vein

Superficial temporal artery

Parotid duct

Digastric, posterior belly

Buccinator

Sternocleidomastoid

Facial artery

Submandibular gland

7.62
Great muscles on the side of the skull

Observe:

1. The temporalis and masseter muscles; both are supplied by the trigeminal nerve and both close the jaw; temporalis arises, in part, from the overlying fascia;

2. Orbicularis oculi and buccinator, both supplied by the facial nerve; one closes the eye; the other prevents food from collecting between cheeks and teeth (Fig. 7.63);

3. Sternocleidomastoid, which is the chief flexor of the head and neck, forming the posterior boundary of the parotid region; and the digastric muscle, which limits this region inferiorly;

4. The submandibular gland, with the facial artery passing deep to it and the facial vein passing superficial.

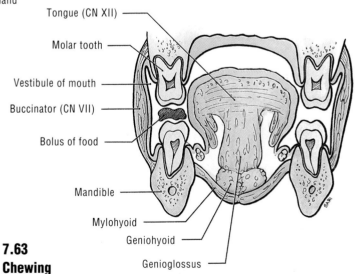

Tongue (CN XII)

Molar tooth

Vestibule of mouth

Buccinator (CN VII)

Bolus of food

Mandible

Mylohyoid

Geniohyoid

Genioglossus

7.63
Chewing

The tongue and the buccinator retain food between the molar teeth during the act of chewing.

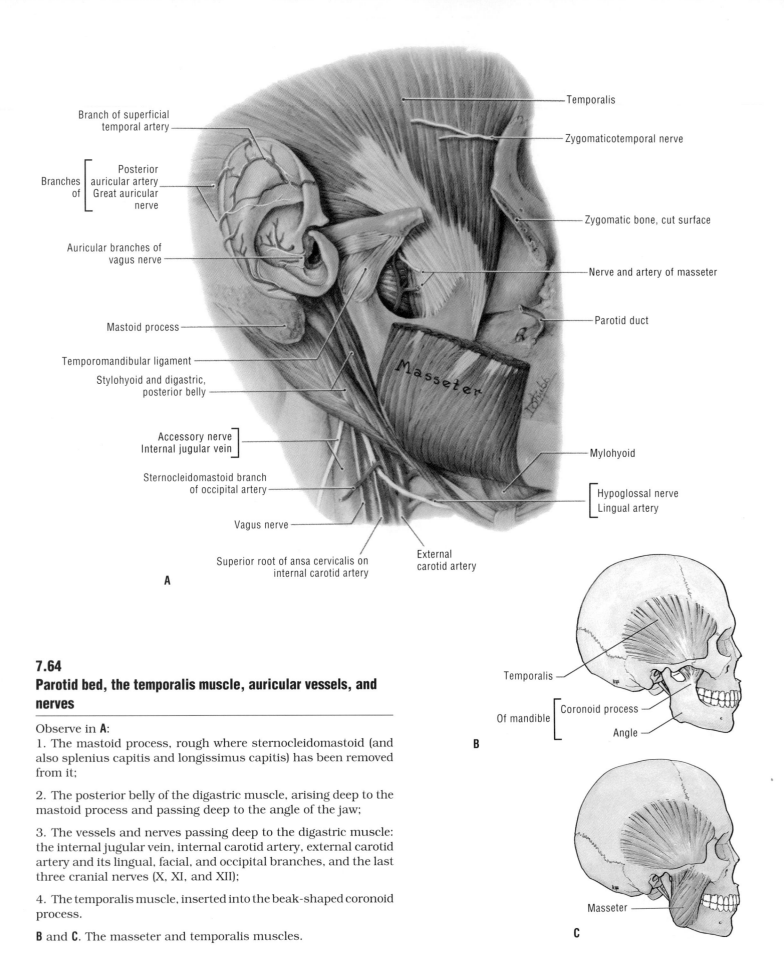

Branch of superficial temporal artery

Branches of { Posterior auricular artery / Great auricular nerve }

Auricular branches of vagus nerve

Mastoid process

Temporomandibular ligament

Stylohyoid and digastric, posterior belly

Accessory nerve / Internal jugular vein

Sternocleidomastoid branch of occipital artery

Vagus nerve

Superior root of ansa cervicalis on internal carotid artery

Temporalis

Zygomaticotemporal nerve

Zygomatic bone, cut surface

Nerve and artery of masseter

Parotid duct

Masseter

Mylohyoid

Hypoglossal nerve / Lingual artery

External carotid artery

A

7.64

Parotid bed, the temporalis muscle, auricular vessels, and nerves

Observe in **A**:

1. The mastoid process, rough where sternocleidomastoid (and also splenius capitis and longissimus capitis) has been removed from it;

2. The posterior belly of the digastric muscle, arising deep to the mastoid process and passing deep to the angle of the jaw;

3. The vessels and nerves passing deep to the digastric muscle: the internal jugular vein, internal carotid artery, external carotid artery and its lingual, facial, and occipital branches, and the last three cranial nerves (X, XI, and XII);

4. The temporalis muscle, inserted into the beak-shaped coronoid process.

B and **C**. The masseter and temporalis muscles.

Temporalis

Of mandible { Coronoid process / Angle }

B

Masseter

C

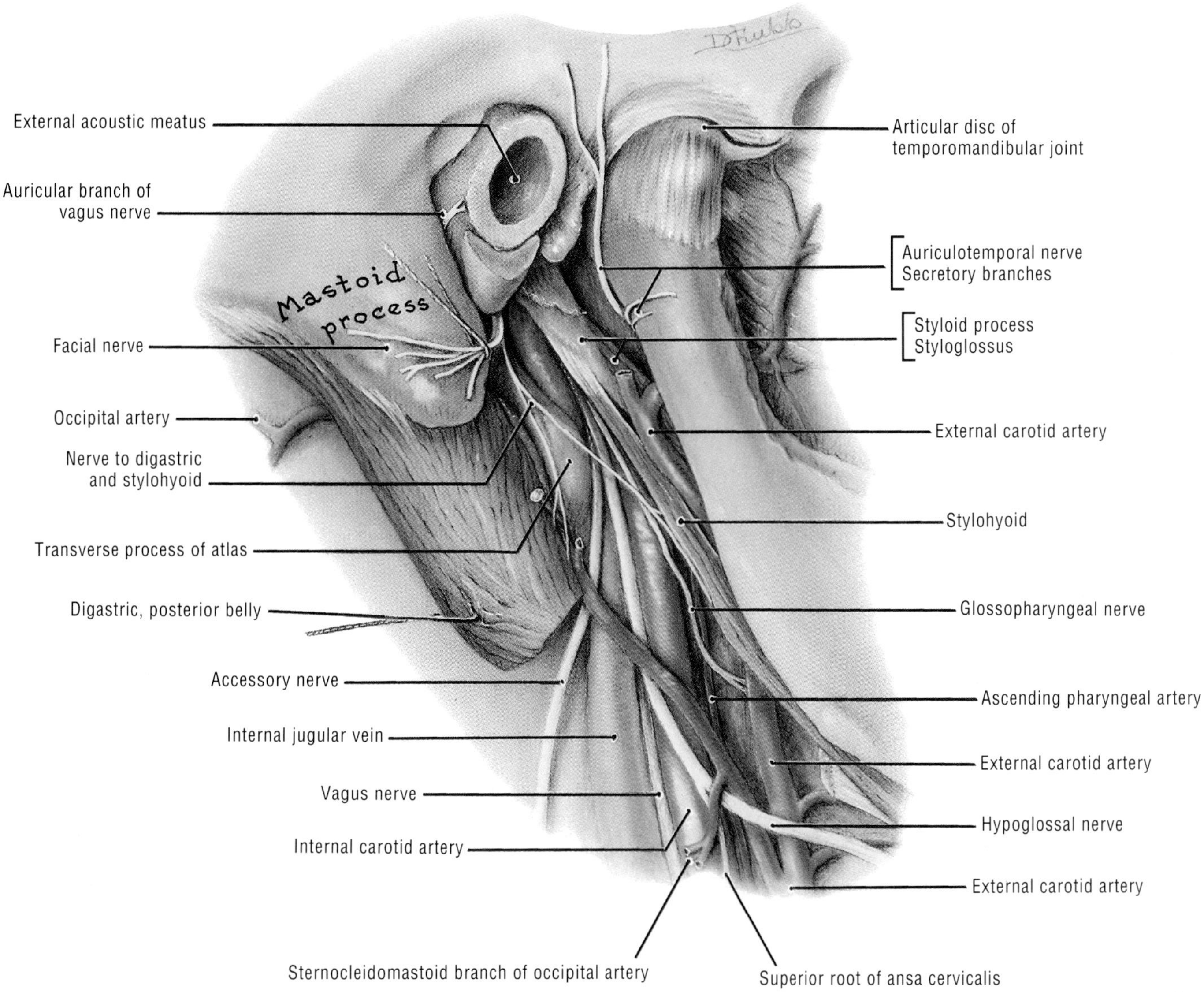
External acoustic meatus
Auricular branch of vagus nerve
Mastoid process
Facial nerve
Occipital artery
Nerve to digastric and stylohyoid
Transverse process of atlas
Digastric, posterior belly
Accessory nerve
Internal jugular vein
Vagus nerve
Internal carotid artery
Sternocleidomastoid branch of occipital artery
Superior root of ansa cervicalis
Articular disc of temporomandibular joint
Auriculotemporal nerve
Secretory branches
Styloid process
Styloglossus
External carotid artery
Stylohyoid
Glossopharyngeal nerve
Ascending pharyngeal artery
External carotid artery
Hypoglossal nerve
External carotid artery

7.65
Structures deep to the parotid bed

The facial nerve, the posterior belly of the digastric muscle, and the nerve to this belly are retracted, whereas the external carotid artery, stylohyoid, and the nerve to stylohyoid remain in situ.

Observe:

1. The tip of the transverse process of the atlas, about midway between the tip of the mastoid process and the angle of the mandible;

2. The internal jugular vein, the internal carotid artery, and the last four cranial nerves crossing anterior to the transverse process and deep to the styloid process;

3. The internal and external carotids separated from each other by the styloid process;

4. The two nerves that pass anteriorly to the tongue: (a) glossopharyngeal (CN IX) being superior to the level of the angle of the mandible and passing between the two carotid arteries, and (b) hypoglossal (CN XII) being inferior to the angle of the mandible and passing superficial to both carotids, and indeed, to all the arteries it meets, except the occipital artery and its sternocleidomastoid branch;

5. The thickness of the skin lining the cartilage of the external acoustic meatus, and the stems of the two nerves – auricular branch of the vagus and auriculotemporal – that supply the meatus and the external surface of the tympanic membrane.

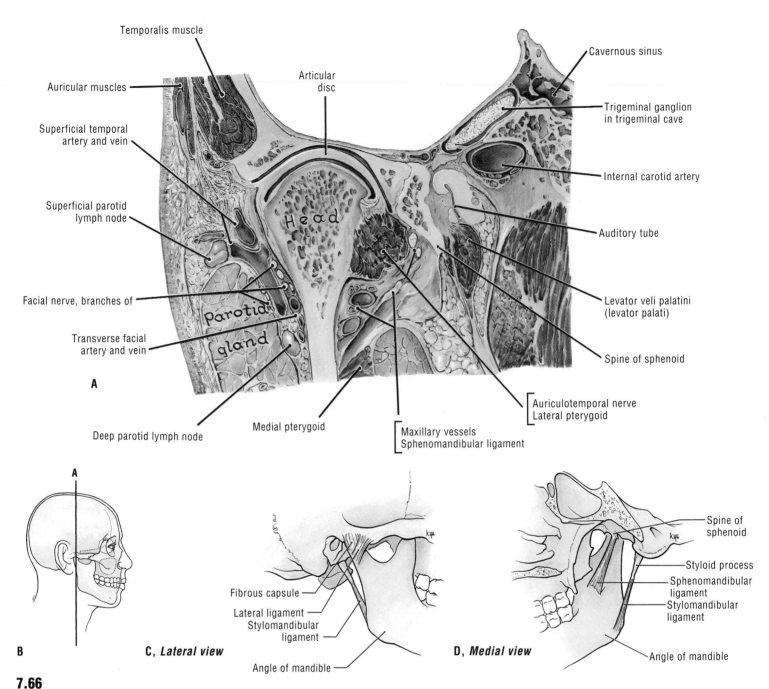

Temporalis muscle

Articular disc

Cavernous sinus

Auricular muscles

Trigeminal ganglion in trigeminal cave

Superficial temporal artery and vein

Internal carotid artery

Superficial parotid lymph node

Head

Auditory tube

Facial nerve, branches of

Parotid gland

Transverse facial artery and vein

Levator veli palatini (levator palati)

A

Spine of sphenoid

Deep parotid lymph node

Medial pterygoid

Maxillary vessels
Sphenomandibular ligament

Auriculotemporal nerve
Lateral pterygoid

A

B

C, *Lateral view*

Fibrous capsule

Lateral ligament
Stylomandibular ligament

Angle of mandible

D, *Medial view*

Spine of sphenoid

Styloid process

Sphenomandibular ligament

Stylomandibular ligament

Angle of mandible

7.66
Temporomandibular joint

A. Coronal section. **B.** Orientation drawing. **C** and **D.** Temporomandibular joint and the stylomandibular and sphenomandibular ligaments.

Observe:
1. The articular disc attached to the neck of the mandible medially and laterally, partly in conjunction with the lateral pterygoid;

2. The roof of the mandibular fossa, which separates head and disc from the middle cranial fossa, is thin centrally but thick elsewhere;

3. The spine of the sphenoid at the medial end of the fossa, and the two roots of the auriculotemporal nerve crossing lateral to it;

4. The auditory tube with closed slit-like lumen, and the levator veli palatini (levator palati) lying inferior to it;

5. The trigeminal ganglion in its trigeminal cave, the mouth of which opens inferior to the tentorium (cerebelli); and separated from the internal carotid artery by membrane (bone being deficient) and, therefore, subjected to the pulsations of that artery;

6. The maxillary vessels crossing the neck of the mandible on its medial side;

7. The "aponeurotic" tendon of temporalis, buried in the muscle for it receives fleshy fibers from the temporal fossa on one side and from the temporal fascia on the other.

7.67
Temporomandibular joint

A sagittal section is shown. Note the articular disc dividing the articular cavity into a superior and an inferior compartment, and the lateral pterygoid inserted, in part, into the anterior aspect of the disc. For the articular part of the mandibular fossa and articular tubercle, see Figure 7.73.

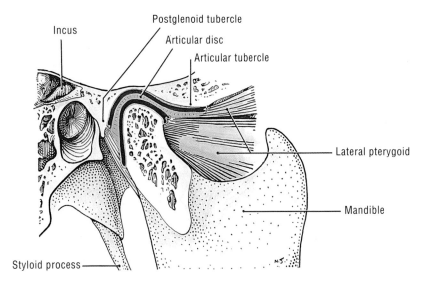

Incus — Postglenoid tubercle — Articular disc — Articular tubercle — Lateral pterygoid — Mandible — Styloid process

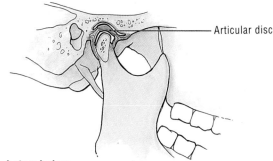

Articular disc

A, Lateral view

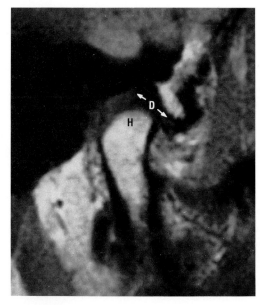

B, Sagittal view

7.68
Temporomandibular joint, mouth closed, sagittal section

Note the position of the articular disc (D) in relation to the head of the mandible (H) and mandibular fossa of the temporal bone (F). (MRI scans courtesy of Dr. W. Kucharczyk, Clinical Director of Tri-Hospital Resonance Centre, Toronto, Ontario, Canada.)

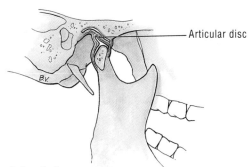

Articular disc

A, Lateral view

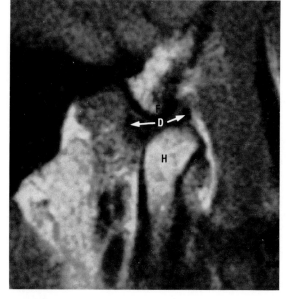

B, Sagittal view

7.69
Temporomandibular joint, mouth open, sagittal section

Letter labels refer to structures in Figure 7.68.

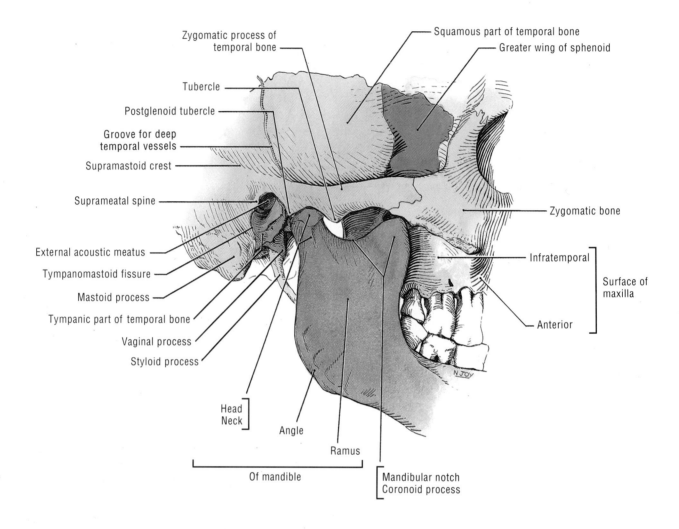

Zygomatic process of temporal bone

Squamous part of temporal bone

Greater wing of sphenoid

Tubercle

Postglenoid tubercle

Groove for deep temporal vessels

Supramastoid crest

Suprameatal spine

Zygomatic bone

External acoustic meatus

Tympanomastoid fissure

Mastoid process

Tympanic part of temporal bone

Vaginal process

Styloid process

Infratemporal

Surface of maxilla

Anterior

Head
Neck

Angle

Ramus

Of mandible

Mandibular notch
Coronoid process

7.70
Infratemporal fossa, lateral wall

Observe:

1. The lateral wall of the infratemporal fossa is the ramus of the mandible;

2. The zygomatic process of the squamous part of the temporal bone plus the zygomatic bone constitute the zygomatic arch;

3. The zygomatic process lies at the boundary line between the temporal fossa superiorly and the infratemporal fossa inferiorly;

4. Inferior to the tubercle of the zygomatic process and anterior to the neck of the mandible, there is a clear passage across the base of the skull through which a pencil can be passed.

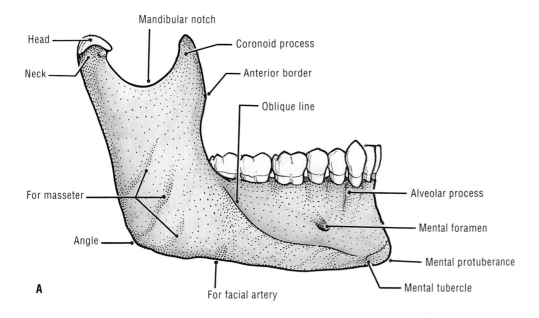

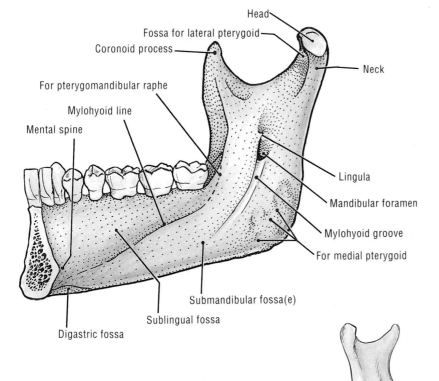

7.71
Mandible

A. External surface. Observe: The coronoid process and the mental tubercle imperfectly connected by (a) the anterior border of the ramus, and (b) the oblique line that crosses the body diagonally.

B. Internal surface. Observe: The coronoid process and the symphysis menti imperfectly connected by the site of attachment of the pterygomandibular raphe, and the mylohyoid line, which crosses the body of the mandible diagonally to end between the mental spine and digastric fossa.

7.72
Mental foramen in edentulous jaws

The position of the mental foramen in edentulous jaws varies with the extent of the absorption of the alveolar process. Pressure of a dental prosthesis on a vulnerable mental nerve in an edentulous jaw may produce pain.

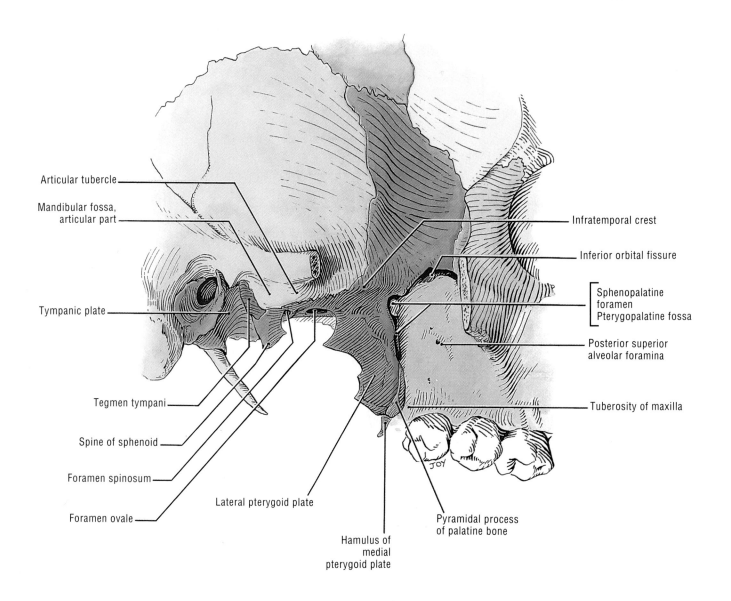

Articular tubercle

Mandibular fossa,
articular part

Tympanic plate

Tegmen tympani

Spine of sphenoid

Foramen spinosum

Foramen ovale

Lateral pterygoid plate

Hamulus of
medial
pterygoid plate

Infratemporal crest

Inferior orbital fissure

Sphenopalatine
foramen
Pterygopalatine fossa

Posterior superior
alveolar foramina

Tuberosity of maxilla

Pyramidal process
of palatine bone

7.73
Infratemporal fossa: roof and medial and lateral walls

Observe:

1. The medial wall of the fossa is formed by the lateral pterygoid plate;

2. The posterior free border of this plate, when followed superiorly, leads to the foramen ovale in the roof of the fossa; posterior to the foramen ovale, at the root of the spine of the sphenoid is the foramen spinosum; the roof is separated from the temporal fossa by the infratemporal crest;

3. Inferiorly, the anterior border of the lateral plate is separated from the maxilla by the pyramidal process of the palatine bone, which is insinuated as a buffer between the two; superiorly, the border is free and forms the posterior limit of the pterygomaxillary fissure, which is the entrance to the pterygopalatine fossa on the medial wall of which can be seen the sphenopalatine foramen, which leads to the nasal cavity;

4. The rounded anterior wall of the fossa is the infratemporal surface of the maxilla, which is of eggshell thickness, is limited superiorly by the inferior orbital fissure, and is pierced by two (or more) posterior superior alveolar foramina for the vessels and nerves of the same name.

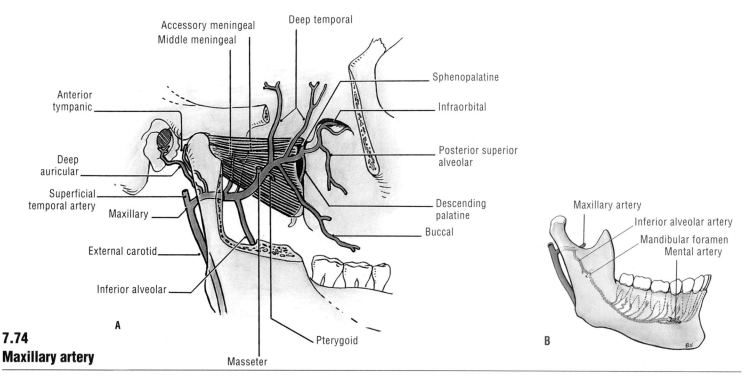

A

- Accessory meningeal
- Middle meningeal
- Deep temporal
- Anterior tympanic
- Sphenopalatine
- Infraorbital
- Deep auricular
- Posterior superior alveolar
- Superficial temporal artery
- Maxillary
- Descending palatine
- External carotid
- Buccal
- Inferior alveolar
- Pterygoid
- Masseter

B

- Maxillary artery
- Inferior alveolar artery
- Mandibular foramen
- Mental artery

7.74
Maxillary artery

Observe:

1. The maxillary artery, arising at the neck of the mandible and divided into three parts by lateral pterygoid; it may pass medial or lateral to the lateral pterygoid;

2. The branches of the first part pass through foramina or canals: deep auricular to external acoustic meatus, anterior tympanic to the tympanum, middle and accessory meningeal to the cranial cavity, and inferior alveolar to the mandible and teeth;

3. The branches of the second part supply muscles, by masseteric, deep temporal, pterygoid, and buccal branches;

4. The branches of the third part arise just before and within the pterygopalatine fossa: posterior superior alveolar, infraorbital, descending palatine and sphenopalatine arteries.

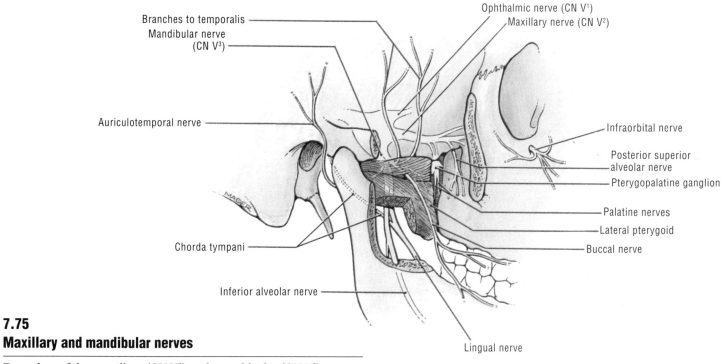

- Branches to temporalis
- Mandibular nerve (CN V^3)
- Ophthalmic nerve (CN V^1)
- Maxillary nerve (CN V^2)
- Auriculotemporal nerve
- Infraorbital nerve
- Posterior superior alveolar nerve
- Pterygopalatine ganglion
- Palatine nerves
- Lateral pterygoid
- Chorda tympani
- Buccal nerve
- Inferior alveolar nerve
- Lingual nerve

7.75
Maxillary and mandibular nerves

Branches of the maxillary (CN V^2) and mandibular (CN V^3) nerves accompany branches from the three parts of the maxillary artery.

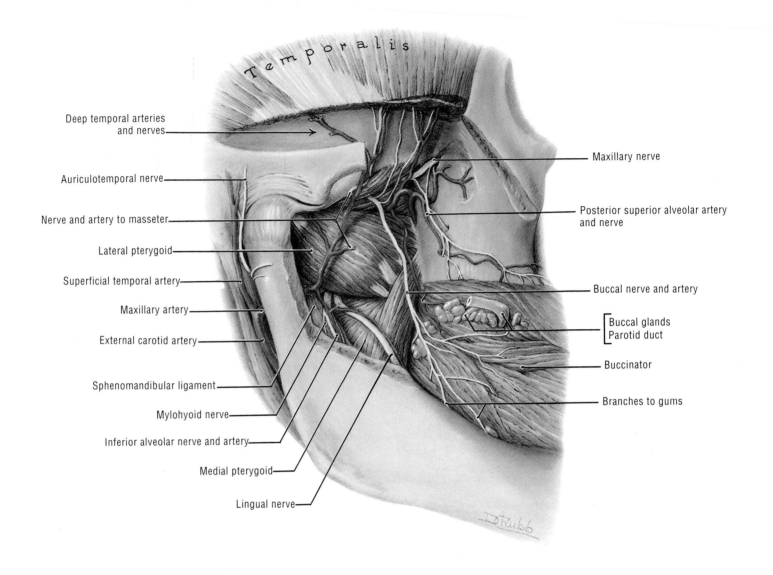

Deep temporal arteries and nerves

Auriculotemporal nerve

Nerve and artery to masseter

Lateral pterygoid

Superficial temporal artery

Maxillary artery

External carotid artery

Sphenomandibular ligament

Mylohyoid nerve

Inferior alveolar nerve and artery

Medial pterygoid

Lingual nerve

Temporalis

Maxillary nerve

Posterior superior alveolar artery and nerve

Buccal nerve and artery

Buccal glands
Parotid duct

Buccinator

Branches to gums

7.76
Infratemporal region, superficial dissection

Observe:

1. Three muscles: lateral pterygoid, medial pterygoid, and buccinator;

2. The maxillary (CN V^2) becoming the infraorbital nerve and passing through the inferior orbital fissure after giving off the posterior superior alveolar nerve;

3. Branches of the mandibular (CN V^3), both sensory and motor;

4. The maxillary artery, the larger of two terminal branches of the external carotid, divided into three parts by its relationship to the lateral pterygoid muscle; the first part sends branches accompanying branches of CN V^3, the second part supplies blood to the muscles of the region, and the third part sends branches accompanying branches of CN V^2;

5. Buccinator is pierced by the parotid duct, the ducts of buccal (molar) glands, and branches (sensory) of the buccal nerve;

6. The lateral pterygoid muscle arising by two heads, from the roof and medial wall of the infratemporal fossa; it inserts into the articular disc of the temporomandibular joint and into the anterior aspect of the neck of the mandible; the more superior head is active during jaw closing while the inferior head is active during jaw opening and protrusion (see Grant PG. *Lateral pterygoid: two muscles? Am J Anat* 1973; 138:1-10).

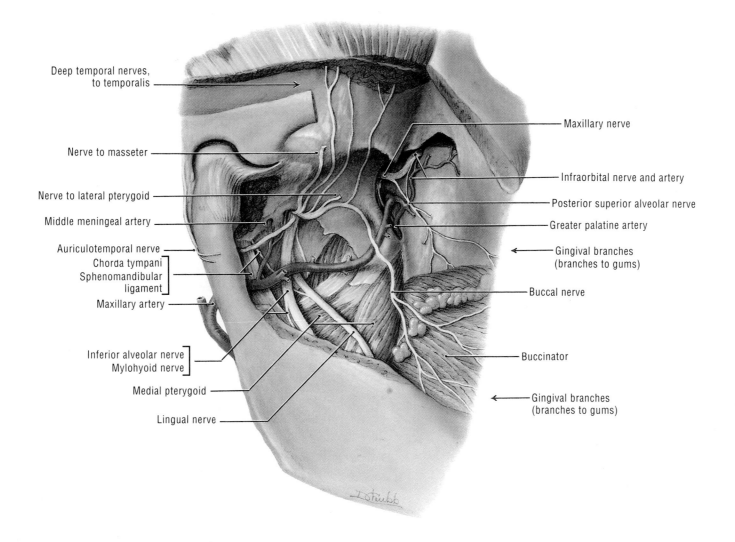

Deep temporal nerves, to temporalis

Nerve to masseter

Nerve to lateral pterygoid

Middle meningeal artery

Auriculotemporal nerve

Chorda tympani
Sphenomandibular ligament

Maxillary artery

Inferior alveolar nerve
Mylohyoid nerve

Medial pterygoid

Lingual nerve

Maxillary nerve

Infraorbital nerve and artery

Posterior superior alveolar nerve

Greater palatine artery

Gingival branches (branches to gums)

Buccal nerve

Buccinator

Gingival branches (branches to gums)

7.77
Infratemporal region, deeper dissection

The lateral pterygoid muscle and most branches of the maxillary artery have been removed.

Observe:

1. The medial pterygoid muscle arising from the medial surface of the lateral pterygoid plate and having a small superficial head that arises from the pyramidal process of the palatine bone (Fig. 7.73);

2. The sphenomandibular ligament, which, as a fascial band, descends from near the spine of the sphenoid to the lingula of the mandible;

3. The maxillary artery and the auriculotemporal nerve passing between the ligament and the neck of the mandible;

4. The mandibular (CN V³) entering the infratemporal fossa through the roof, via the foramen ovale, which also transmits the accessory meningeal artery (not labeled);

5. The middle meningeal artery and vein passing through the roof via the foramen spinosum;

6. The inferior alveolar and lingual nerves descending on the medial pterygoid muscle; the former giving off the mylohyoid nerve (to the mylohyoid muscle and anterior belly of the digastric muscle); the latter receiving the chorda tympani (which carries secretory sympathetic fibers and fibers of taste);

7. The nerves to four muscles of mastication: masseter, temporalis, and lateral pterygoid, which are labeled, and the nerve to medial pterygoid muscle, which is not labeled; note that the buccal branch of the mandibular nerve is sensory; the buccal branch of the facial nerve is the motor supply to the buccinator muscle;

8. The maxillary (CN V²) becoming the infraorbital nerve that enters the infraorbital groove at the inferior orbital fissure.

Observe in **A**:

1. The cut surface of the mylohyoid muscle becoming progressively thinner as traced anteriorly;

2. The sublingual salivary gland, almond-shaped, almost touching its fellow of the opposite side posterior to the symphysis menti and in contact with the deep part of the submandibular gland posteriorly;

3. The dozen or more fine ducts passing from the superior border of the sublingual gland to open on the sublingual fold;

4. Several individual or detached lobules of the sublingual gland, each having a fine duct, posterior to the main mass of the gland, and labial glands in the lip (unlabeled);

5. The mylohyoid nerve and artery (cut short) and the lingual nerve and artery clamped between the medial pterygoid muscle and the ramus of the mandible;

6. The lingual nerve lying between the sublingual gland and the deep or oral part of the submandibular gland;

7. The submandibular ganglion is suspended from the lingual nerve, and various branches leave it.

B. Tongue excised. Observe:

1. Undisturbed: the geniohyoid muscle inferiorly, the middle constrictor posteriorly, and the cut edge of the mucous membrane superiorly;

2. Three divided muscles: genioglossus anteriorly, hyoglossus inferiorly, and styloglossus posteriorly;

3. The lingual nerve appearing between the medial pterygoid muscle and the ramus of the mandible and making three-quarters of a spiral around the submandibular duct; the hypoglossal nerve separated from the lingual artery by the hyoglossus muscle;

4. The deep or oral part of the submandibular gland in the angle between the lingual nerve and the submandibular duct, which separates it from the sublingual gland; the orifice of the duct is seen at the anterior end of the sublingual fold;

5. The submandibular duct adhering to the medial side of the sublingual gland, and here receiving, as it sometimes does, a large accessory duct from the inferior part of the sublingual gland.

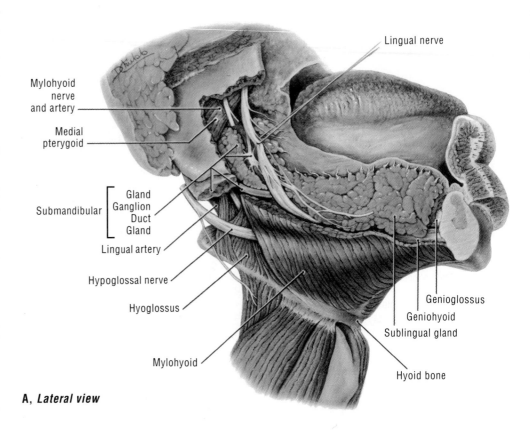

A, *Lateral view*

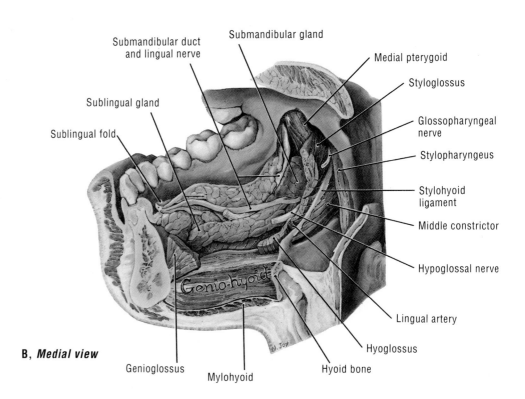

B, *Medial view*

7.79

Muscles and vessels of the mandible and base of the skull

Observe:

1. The mylohyoid muscle with a thick, free, posterior border thinning anteriorly where inferior to the origins of the genial muscles, it may be deficient, as here, with a resulting thin, free, anterior border;

2. The medial pterygoid muscle taking much the same direction on the medial side of the ramus of the mandible as the masseter muscle takes on the lateral;

3. The tensor veli palatini muscle, here sending some fibers to the hamulus;

4. The lingual nerve joined superior to the medial pterygoid muscle by the chorda tympani and appearing in the mouth at the anterior border of that muscle;

5. The otic ganglion lying medial to the mandibular (CN V³), and between the foramen ovale superiorly and the medial pterygoid muscle inferiorly; the tensor veli palatini muscle usually covers the ganglion; the otic ganglion receives sensory fibers from the auriculotemporal branch of CN V³, sympathetic fibers from the plexus on the middle meningeal artery, and contains the synapse of parasympathetic fibers from the lesser superficial petrosal branch of CN IX; it connects with CN VII and allows the motor fibers to the tensors to pass through it.

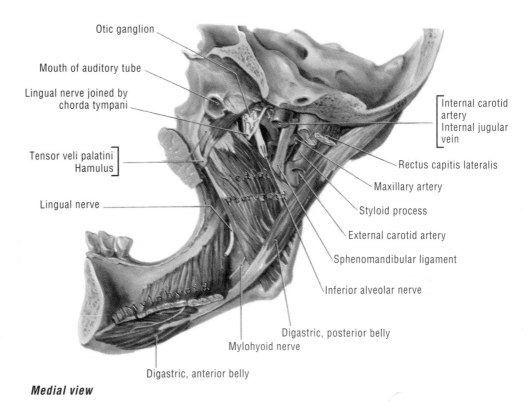

Otic ganglion
Mouth of auditory tube
Lingual nerve joined by chorda tympani
Tensor veli palatini
Hamulus
Lingual nerve
Internal carotid artery
Internal jugular vein
Rectus capitis lateralis
Maxillary artery
Styloid process
External carotid artery
Sphenomandibular ligament
Inferior alveolar nerve
Digastric, posterior belly
Mylohyoid nerve
Digastric, anterior belly

Medial view

7.80

Muscles of the floor of the mouth

Observe:

1. The geniohyoid muscles, paired, triangular, and occupying a horizontal plane, with apex at the mental spine, base at the body of the hyoid bone, medial border in contact with its fellow, and lateral border in contact with the mylohyoid muscle;

2. The mylohyoid muscle arising from the mylohyoid line of the mandible; having a thick, free, posterior border; thinning as it is traced anteriorly; and ending in a delicate, free, anterior border as it nears the origin of the genial muscles.

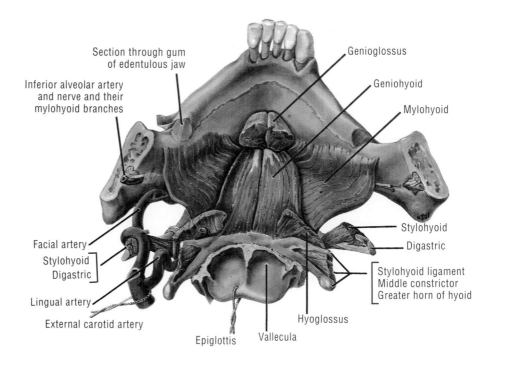

Section through gum of edentulous jaw
Inferior alveolar artery and nerve and their mylohyoid branches
Genioglossus
Geniohyoid
Mylohyoid
Facial artery
Stylohyoid
Digastric
Lingual artery
External carotid artery
Epiglottis
Vallecula
Hyoglossus
Stylohyoid
Digastric
Stylohyoid ligament
Middle constrictor
Greater horn of hyoid

7.81
Tongue and floor of the mouth, median section

Observe:

1. The tongue is composed mainly of muscles: extrinsic (which alter the position of the tongue) and intrinsic (which alter its shape); in this illustration, extrinsic muscles are represented by the genioglossus muscle and intrinsic by the superior longitudinal muscle;

2. The foramen cecum, which is the patent upper end of the primitive thyroglossal duct, and the limbs of the V-shaped sulcus terminalis, which diverge from the foramen, lie slightly posterior to the vallate papillae, and demarcate the developmentally different, posterior one-third of the tongue from the anterior two-thirds;

3. The anterior lingual gland, covered with a layer of muscle; the several ducts of this mixed mucoserous gland open inferior to the tongue, but are not in view;

4. Lingual follicles of lymphoid tissues constituting the lingual tonsil;

5. In Figure 7.83: the vallate papillae, variable in number, and four other shapes of papillae.

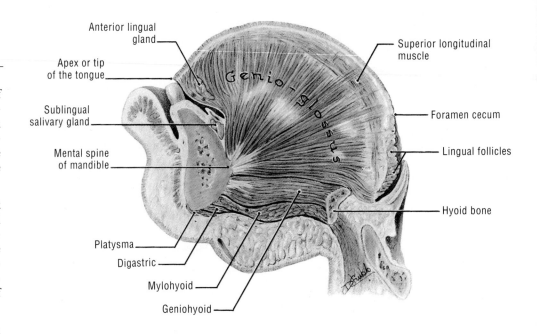

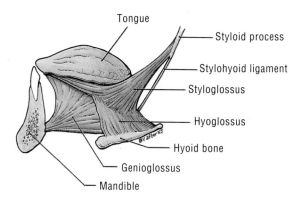

7.82
Extrinsic muscles of the tongue

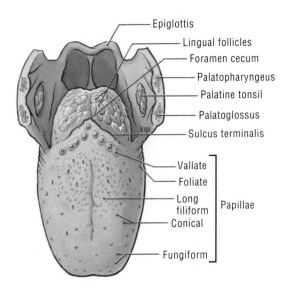

7.83
Dorsum of the tongue

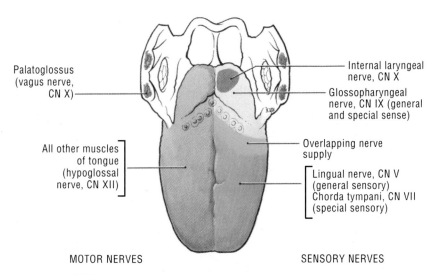

MOTOR NERVES   SENSORY NERVES

7.84
Nerve supply to the tongue

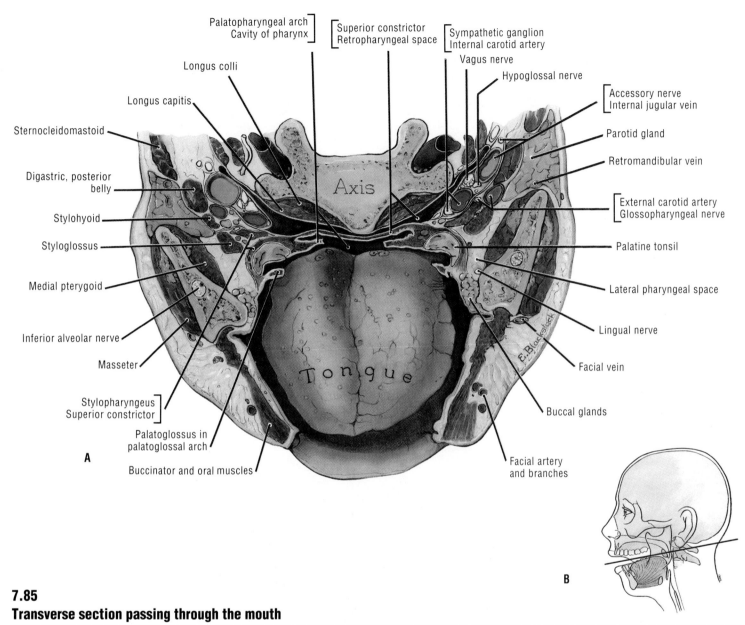

Palatopharyngeal arch
Cavity of pharynx

Superior constrictor
Retropharyngeal space

Sympathetic ganglion
Internal carotid artery

Vagus nerve

Hypoglossal nerve

Longus colli

Longus capitis

Sternocleidomastoid

Accessory nerve
Internal jugular vein

Parotid gland

Retromandibular vein

Digastric, posterior
belly

Axis

External carotid artery
Glossopharyngeal nerve

Stylohyoid

Styloglossus

Palatine tonsil

Medial pterygoid

Lateral pharyngeal space

Inferior alveolar nerve

Lingual nerve

Masseter

Facial vein

Tongue

Stylopharyngeus
Superior constrictor

Buccal glands

Palatoglossus in
palatoglossal arch

A

Facial artery
and branches

Buccinator and oral muscles

B

7.85
Transverse section passing through the mouth

Observe in **A**:

1. The parotid gland filling its wedge-shaped bed; the digastric and stylohyoid muscles intervening between the parotid gland and the great vessels and nerves of the neck;

2. The masseter muscle inserted into the lateral surface of the ramus of the mandible and the medial pterygoid muscle inserted into the medial surface;

3. The lingual nerve in contact with the ramus of the mandible;

4. Anterior to the ribbon-like palatoglossus muscle and its arch is the mouth; posterior to it is the pharynx;

5. The pharynx is flattened anteroposteriorly, and the palatine tonsil is in its wall;

6. The tonsil bed formed by superior constrictor and

palatopharyngeus muscles, an areolar space intervening, and limited anteriorly and posteriorly by the palatine arches;

7. The retropharyngeal space, here opened up, which allows the pharnyx to contract and relax during swallowing; it is closed laterally at the carotid sheath and is limited posteriorly by the prevertebral fascia;

8. The three styloid muscles: stylohyoid, styloglossus, and stylopharyngeus; all three muscles arise from the styloid process; their names reveal their insertions; each is supplied by a different cranial nerve: stylohyoid, CN VII; stylopharyngeus, CN IX; and styloglossus, CN XII.

B. Orientation drawing of **A**.

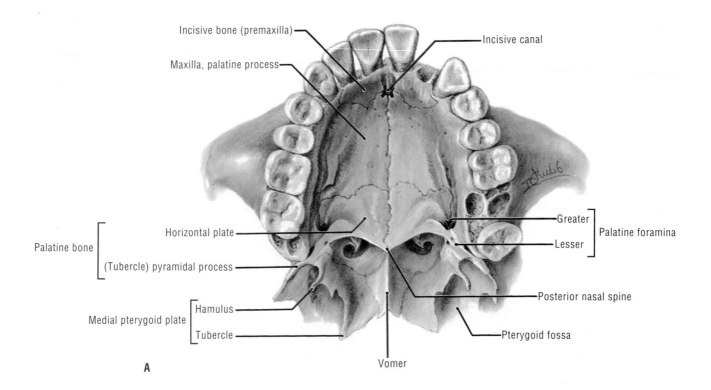

Incisive bone (premaxilla)
Incisive canal
Maxilla, palatine process
Horizontal plate
Greater
Lesser
Palatine foramina
Palatine bone
(Tubercle) pyramidal process
Posterior nasal spine
Medial pterygoid plate
Hamulus
Tubercle
Pterygoid fossa
Vomer

A

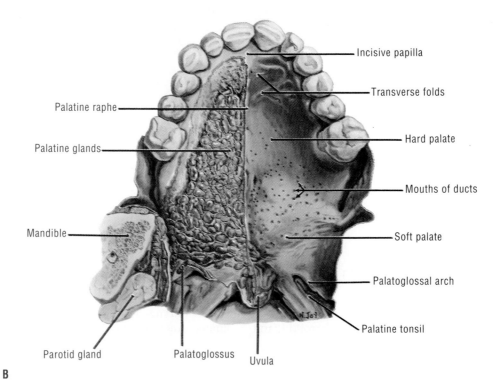

Incisive papilla
Transverse folds
Palatine raphe
Hard palate
Palatine glands
Mouths of ducts
Mandible
Soft palate
Palatoglossal arch
Palatine tonsil
Parotid gland
Palatoglossus
Uvula

B

7.86
The palate

A. Bones of the hard palate. B. Mucous membrane and glands of the palate. Observe in B:

1. The orifices of the ducts of the palatine glands, which give the mucous membrane an orange-skin appearance;

2. The palatine glands forming a very thick layer in the soft palate, a thin one in the hard palate, and absent in the region of the incisive bone and anterior part of the median raphe;

3. Posteriorly, the palate ending medially in the uvula, and on each side in the palatopharyngeal arch; the palatoglossus muscle and the palatoglossal arch extending to the undersurface of the soft palate.

7.87
Nerves and vessels of the palate

Observe:

1. The palate having bony, aponeurotic, and muscular parts;

2. The tensor veli palatini muscle hooking around the hamulus to join the palatine aponeurosis;

3. A crest on the bony palate, having a branch of the greater palatine nerve on each side and the artery on the lateral side;

4. The lateral branch of the nerve expended mainly on the gums, the medial branch on the hard palate, the nasopalatine nerve in the incisive region, and the lesser palatine nerves in the soft palate;

5. Four palatine arteries, two on the hard palate and two on the soft: greater palatine, terminal branch of sphenopalatine artery (posterior nasal septal), lesser palatine, and ascending palatine.

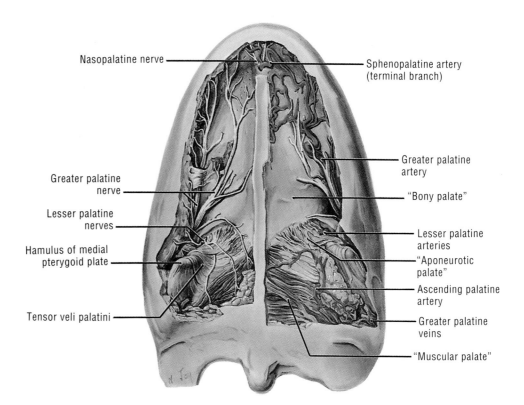

Nasopalatine nerve

Greater palatine nerve

Lesser palatine nerves

Hamulus of medial pterygoid plate

Tensor veli palatini

Sphenopalatine artery (terminal branch)

Greater palatine artery

"Bony palate"

Lesser palatine arteries

"Aponeurotic palate"

Ascending palatine artery

Greater palatine veins

"Muscular palate"

7.88
Palatine nerves and vessels, lateral wall of nasal cavity

Observe:

1. The mucous membrane, containing a layer of mucous glands, has been separated by blunt dissection; the layer of glands is thin on the bony palate where it is part of a mucoperiosteum; it is thickest on the aponeurotic part; and it is less thick on the muscular part;

2. The posterior ends (1 cm) of the middle and inferior conchae are cut through; these and the mucoperiosteum are peeled off the side wall of the nose as far as the posterior border of the medial pterygoid plate; the papery perpendicular plate of the palatine bone is broken through and the palatine nerves and arteries are thereby exposed.

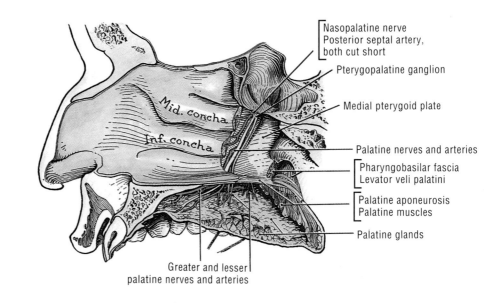

Mid. concha

Inf. concha

Nasopalatine nerve Posterior septal artery, both cut short

Pterygopalatine ganglion

Medial pterygoid plate

Palatine nerves and arteries

Pharyngobasilar fascia Levator veli palatini

Palatine aponeurosis Palatine muscles

Palatine glands

Greater and lesser palatine nerves and arteries

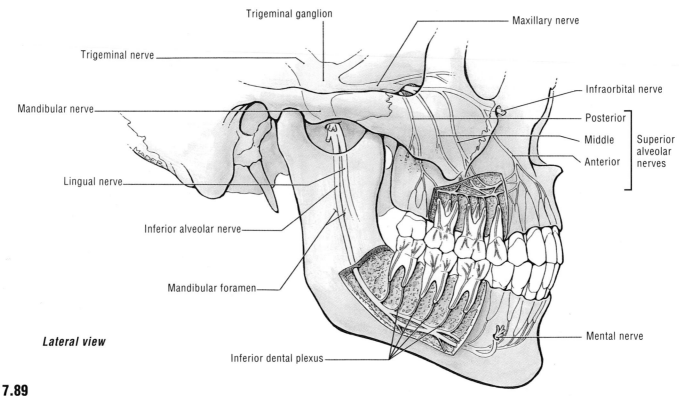

Lateral view

7.89
Innervation of the teeth

Observe:

1. The upper teeth innervated by the superior alveolar nerves from the maxillary nerve; the posterior and middle alveolar nerves arising from the maxillary nerve and the anterior from the infraorbital nerve.

2. The lower teeth innervated by the inferior alveolar branch of the mandibular nerve; the nerve entering the mandibular foramen on the medial surface of the ramus of the mandible.

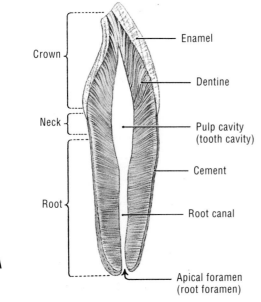

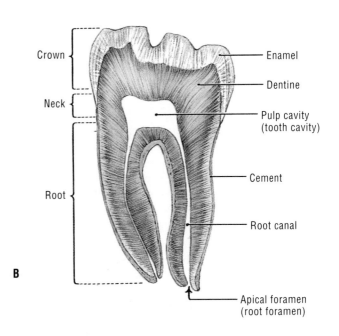

7.90
Longitudinal section of tooth

A. Incisor tooth. **B**. Molar tooth.

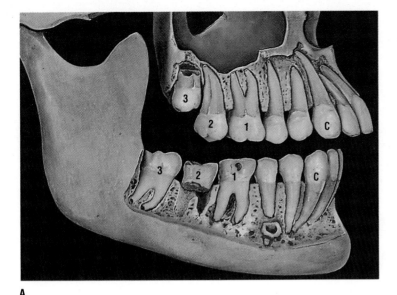

A

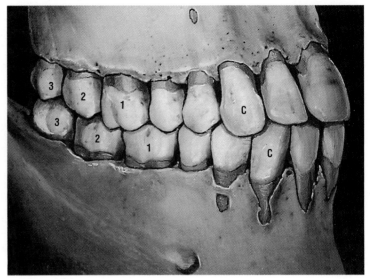

B

7.91
Permanent teeth

A. Roots exposed. Observe:

1. The upper canine ("eye tooth") has the longest root; this is the longest tooth;

2. The roots of the upper premolars, in this specimen, are at some distance from the maxillary sinus or antrum, but the roots of the three molars almost penetrate into the sinus;

3. The root of the 2nd lower premolar, very long in this specimen, does not usually extend below the level of the mental foramen;

4. The roots of the 2nd lower molar have been removed, thereby revealing the cribriform nature of the wall of a socket;

5. The upper and lower 3rd molars are not yet fully developed; the lower is more advanced than the upper – the root foramina of the lower are still large, whereas the roots of the upper have not yet formed.

B. Observe:

1. The maxillary (upper) and mandibular (lower) teeth in centric occlusion;

2. The lower central incisor is the smallest of the incisors, and the 3rd upper molar is the smallest of the molars; except for these two teeth – the first in the lower row and the last in the upper – all teeth, when in occlusion, bite on two opposing teeth;

3. The upper dental arch overlaps the lower dental arch;

4. The lower incisors bite against the lingual surface of the upper incisors; as a variant, there may be variable overjet (**A**).

7.92
Pantomographic radiograph of the mandible and maxilla

I - Inscisors, *C* - Canine, *PM* - Premolars, *M1, M2, M3* - Molars. Left lower M3 is not present. (Courtesy of M.J. Pharoah, Associate Professor of Dental Radiology, Faculty of Dentistry, University of Toronto, Toronto, Ontario, Canada.)

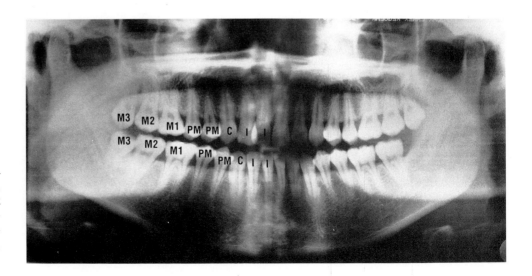

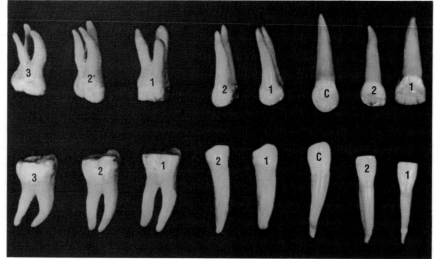

Buccal view

7.93
Roots of permanent teeth

Observe:

1. Mandibular (lower) teeth: the incisor, canine, and premolar (bicuspid) teeth each have one root, whereas the molars have two roots, a mesial (anterior) and a distal (posterior); the mesial roots generally have two root canals; the roots are flattened mesiodistally (i.e., from central incisor posterior to the 3rd molar); the sockets for the lower incisor teeth are near the labial surface of the mandible, those for the lower molars are near the lingual surface;

2. Maxillary (upper) teeth: the incisor and canine teeth each have

one root; the premolars each have either one or two roots, the 1st premolar usually having two, a lingual and a labial, and the 2nd usually having one – although sometimes, as here, both premolars have two roots; each of the three molars has three roots, one being lingual and two being labial (buccal); the roots are flattened mesiodistally, except the root of the central incisor and the lingual root of each of the three molars, which are circular on transverse section.

7.94
Permanent teeth and their sockets

Observe:

1. There are 32 permanent teeth, of which eight are on each side of each dental arch – two incisors, one canine, two premolars, and three molars;

2. Maxillary (upper) incisor teeth are larger than lower or mandibular incisor teeth; the upper central incisors are the largest of the incisors and the lower central are the smallest; in each dental arch, the 1st molar tooth is usually the largest molar and the 3rd molar is the smallest, although the 3rd lower molar may be very large, as here;

3. Crowns: an incisor tooth has a cutting edge; a canine tooth (cuspid) has one cusp on its crown; a premolar tooth (bicuspid) has two (or three) cusps; and a molar tooth has from three to five cusps; the crowns of the upper molars are either square or rhomboidal; the 1st usually has four cusps; the 2nd either four or three, and the 3rd has three; the crowns of the lower molars are oblong; the 1st usually has five cusps, the 2nd has four, and the 3rd has from three to five; the crowns, here, are somewhat worn.

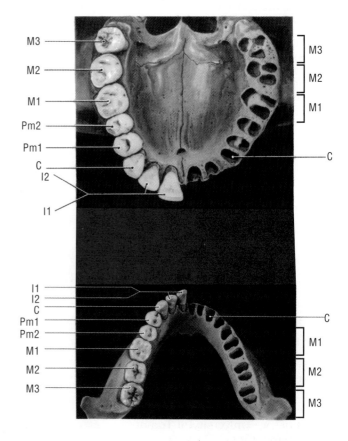

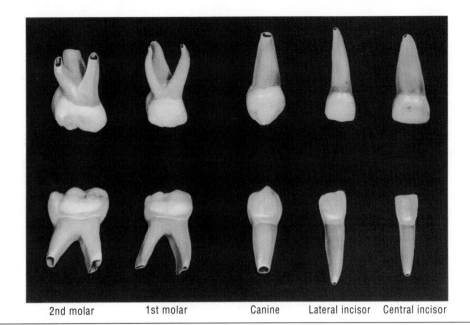

7.95
Primary teeth

2nd molar   1st molar   Canine   Lateral incisor   Central incisor

Observe:

1. There are 20 primary or deciduous teeth, five being in each half of the mandible and five in each maxilla; they are named: central incisor, lateral incisor, canine, 1st molar, and 2nd molar;

2. Of these 20 primary teeth, the first to erupt through the gums are the lower central incisors, about the 6th month, and the last to erupt are the 2nd upper molars, about the end of the 2nd year;

the three roots of the upper or maxillary molars and the two roots of the lower or mandibular molars are spread to grasp the developing permanent premolars;

3. Primary teeth differ from permanent teeth in being smaller and whiter ("milk teeth"); the molars have more bulbous crowns and more divergent roots.

7.96
Primary dentition, age under 2 years

Observe:

1. The canines have not fully erupted, the 2nd molars have just started to erupt – the sequence of eruption being incisors, 1st molars, canines, 2nd molars;

2. The 2nd molars have much larger crowns than the 1st molars;

3. The socket for the three-pronged root of the 1st upper molar is seen;

4. The foramina, seen on the lingual side of the primary incisors, lead to the alveoli for the permanent incisors;

5. Permanent teeth are colored orange; the crowns of the unerupted 1st and 2nd permanent molars are partly visible.

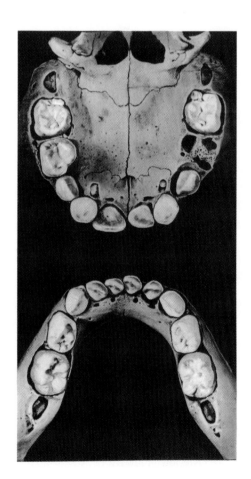

A

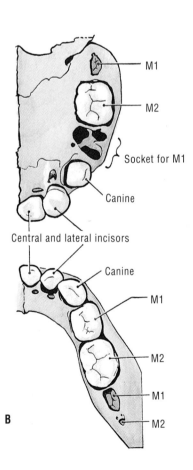

B

M1

M2

Socket for M1

Canine

Central and lateral incisors

Canine

M1

M2

M1

M2

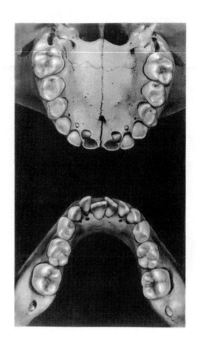

A

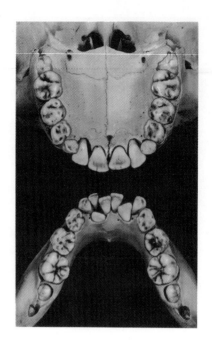

B

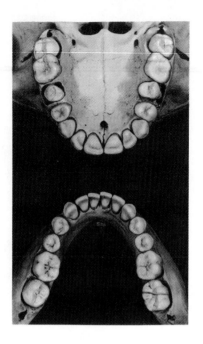

C

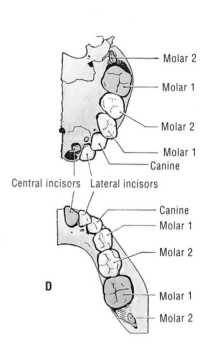

Molar 2
Molar 1
Molar 2
Molar 1
Canine
Central incisors   Lateral incisors

Canine
Molar 1
Molar 2
Molar 1
Molar 2

D

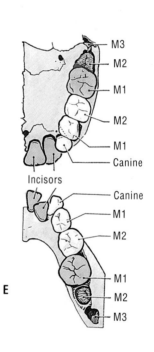

M3
M2
M1
M2
M1
Canine

Incisors

Canine
M1
M2
M1
M2
M3

E

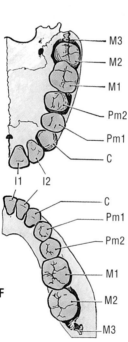

M3
M2
M1
Pm2
Pm1
C

I1   I2

C
Pm1
Pm2
M1
M2
M3

F

7.97
Progress in the eruption of permanent teeth

A. Aged 6 to 7 years. **B.** Aged 8 years. **C.** Aged 12 years. **D.** Schematic drawing of **A**. **E.** Schematic drawing of **B**. **F.** Schematic drawing of **C**.

Between the 6th and 12th years, the primary teeth are shed and are succeeded by permanent teeth (orange).

A and **D**. The 1st molars (6-year molars) have fully erupted; the primary central incisors have been shed; the lower central incisors have nearly fully erupted and the upper central incisors are moving downward into the empty sockets.

B and **E**. All the permanent incisors have erupted, the upper and lower central and the upper lateral fully and the lower lateral

partially; note that the alveolus has not yet closed around the upper lateral incisors; here, the root of the left lower lateral primary incisor has not been resorbed, so the tooth has not been shed.

C and **F**. The 20 primary teeth have been replaced by 20 permanent teeth, and the 1st molars and the 2nd molars (12-year molars) have erupted; but the canines, 2nd premolars, and 2nd molars – especially those in the upper jaw – have not erupted fully nor have their bony sockets closed around them; by the age of 12 years, 28 permanent teeth are in evidence; the last four teeth, the 3rd molars, may erupt any time after this, or never.

7.98
Dentition of a child, aged 6 to 7 years

Alveolar bone has been ground away from the specimen shown in Figure 7.63, aged 6 to 7 years. The permanent incisors and canines develop and erupt on the lingual side of the primary incisors and canines, the lateral incisors being the most posterior. Indeed, the upper lateral incisors extend into the bony palate. The premolar teeth develop between the spread roots of the primary molars. The permanent molars have no predecessor; they erupt posterior to the deciduous teeth in the dental arch.

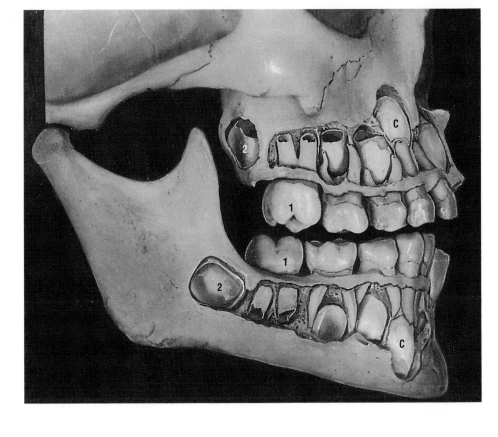

Lateral view

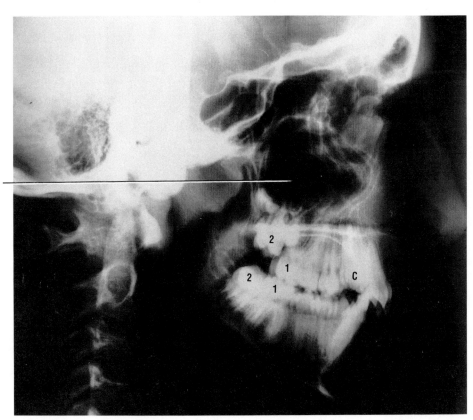

Maxillary sinus —

Lateral view

7.99
Radiograph of the skull

(Courtesy of Dr. M.J. Pharoah, Associate Professor of Dental Radiology, Faculty of Dentistry, University of Toronto, Toronto, Ontario, Canada.)

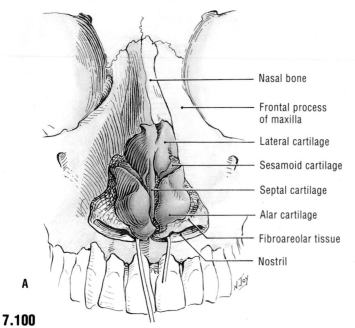

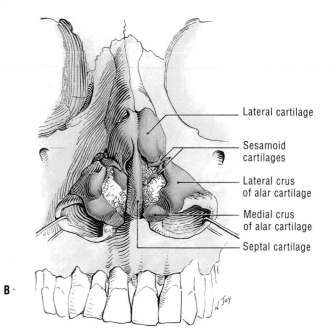

Nasal bone

Frontal process
of maxilla

Lateral cartilage

Sesamoid cartilage

Septal cartilage

Alar cartilage

Fibroareolar tissue

Nostril

A

Lateral cartilage

Sesamoid
cartilages

Lateral crus
of alar cartilage

Medial crus
of alar cartilage

Septal cartilage

B

7.100
Cartilages of the nose

Observe:

1. In **A**, the alar cartilages have been pulled down to expose the sesamoid cartilages; in **B**, the alar cartilages are separated by dissection and retracted laterally;

2. The lateral nasal cartilages, fixed by suture to the nasal bones and continuous with the septal cartilage;

3. The alar nasal cartilages, free, movable, and U-shaped;

4. The medial crus of the right and of the left U, when in apposition, forming part of the septum of the nose;

5. The distal part of the ala of the nose, formed of fibroareolar tissue; the nasal cartilages are hyaline cartilage; the cartilage of the auricle is elastic cartilage.

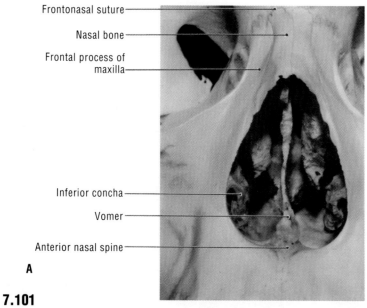

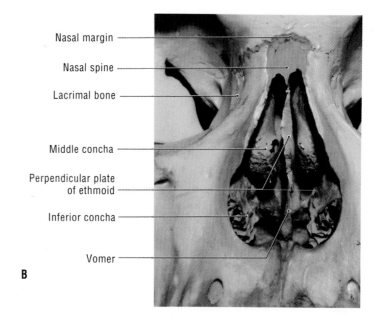

Frontonasal suture

Nasal bone

Frontal process of
maxilla

Inferior concha

Vomer

Anterior nasal spine

A

Nasal margin

Nasal spine

Lacrimal bone

Middle concha

Perpendicular plate
of ethmoid

Inferior concha

Vomer

B

7.101
Bones of the nose

Observe:

A. The margin of the anterior nasal aperture, is sharp and is formed by the maxillae and the nasal bones.

B. On removing the nasal bones, the areas on the frontal processes

of the maxillae and on the frontal bone that articulate with the nasal bones are seen; so is the nasal septum.

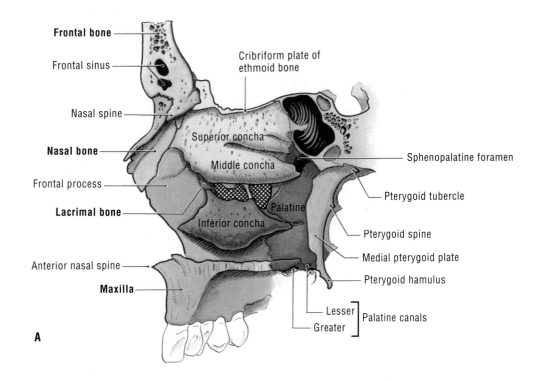

Frontal bone

Frontal sinus

Nasal spine

Nasal bone

Frontal process

Lacrimal bone

Anterior nasal spine

Maxilla

Cribriform plate of ethmoid bone

Superior concha

Middle concha

Palatine

Inferior concha

Sphenopalatine foramen

Pterygoid tubercle

Pterygoid spine

Medial pterygoid plate

Pterygoid hamulus

Lesser ⎤
Greater ⎦ Palatine canals

A

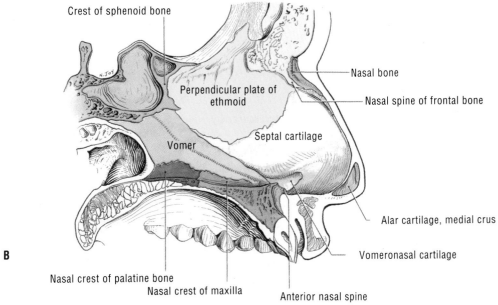

Crest of sphenoid bone

Perpendicular plate of ethmoid

Septal cartilage

Vomer

Nasal bone

Nasal spine of frontal bone

Alar cartilage, medial crus

Vomeronasal cartilage

B

Nasal crest of palatine bone

Nasal crest of maxilla

Anterior nasal spine

7.102
Lateral wall and the septum of the nose

A. Lateral wall of the nose. **B.** Septum of the nose. Observe:
1. Like the palate, the septum of the nose has a hard part and a soft or mobile part; the skeleton of the hard septum consists of three parts – perpendicular plate of ethmoid, septal cartilage, vomer – and, around the circumference of these, the adjacent bones (frontal, nasal, maxillary, palatine, and sphenoid) make minor contributions;

2. The mobile septum composed of: the medial limbs (crura) of the U-shaped alar cartilages, and the skin and soft tissues between

the tip of the nose and the anterior nasal spine; posterior to the vomer, an extension of the mucoperiosteum of the septum forms a second, although unimportant, mobile septum;

3. The superior and middle conchae are parts of the ethmoid bone, whereas the inferior concha is a bone of itself;

4. The fragile, perpendicular plate of the palatine bone has a notch at its superior border, which, when in articulation with the body of the sphenoid bone, forms the sphenopalatine foramen.

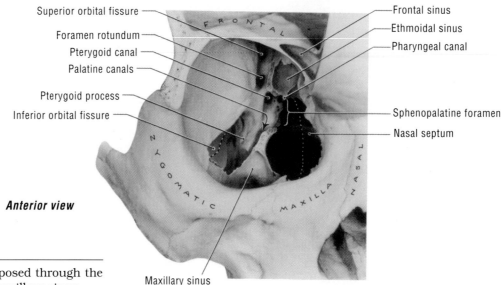

Superior orbital fissure
Foramen rotundum
Pterygoid canal
Palatine canals
Pterygoid process
Inferior orbital fissure

Frontal sinus
Ethmoidal sinus
Pharyngeal canal

Sphenopalatine foramen
Nasal septum

Anterior view

Maxillary sinus

7.103
Pterygopalatine fossa

The fossa has been exposed through the floor of the orbit and maxillary sinus.

7.104
Maxillary artery, 3rd part

Observe:

1. The stem of this artery is divided into three parts by the lateral pterygoid (Fig. 7.74**A**); the branches of 3rd part arise just before and within the pterygopalatine fossa: infraorbital, posterior superior alveolar, descending palatine, artery of pterygoid canal, pharyngeal, and sphenopalatine arteries; the descending palatine artery divides into the greater and lesser palatine arteries (Fig. 7.88); the sphenopalatine artery divides into the posterior nasal and posterior lateral nasal arteries (Fig. 7.106);

2. The 3rd part of the artery, often very tortuous, lies anterior to the maxillary nerve and its branches.

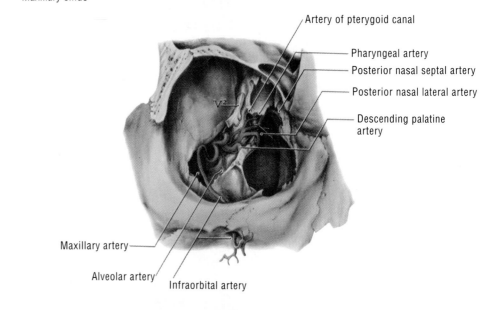

Artery of pterygoid canal
Pharyngeal artery
Posterior nasal septal artery
Posterior nasal lateral artery
Descending palatine artery

Maxillary artery
Alveolar artery
Infraorbital artery

7.105
Maxillary nerve

Observe:

1. Lateral and medial branches of the nerve are separated by the maxillary sinus; for medial branches, see Figure 7.107;

2. The greater petrosal nerve, via the nerve of pterygoid canal, brings parasympathetic fibers to the pterygopalatine ganglion, there to be relayed and distributed, with branches of CN V², as secretomotor fibers.

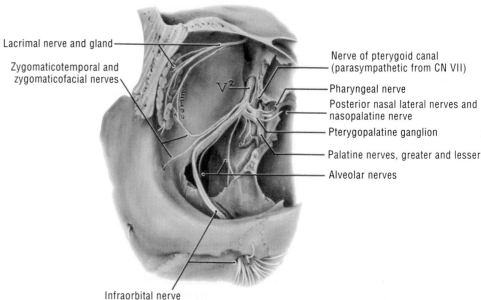

Lacrimal nerve and gland
Zygomaticotemporal and zygomaticofacial nerves

Nerve of pterygoid canal (parasympathetic from CN VII)
Pharyngeal nerve
Posterior nasal lateral nerves and nasopalatine nerve
Pterygopalatine ganglion
Palatine nerves, greater and lesser
Alveolar nerves

Infraorbital nerve

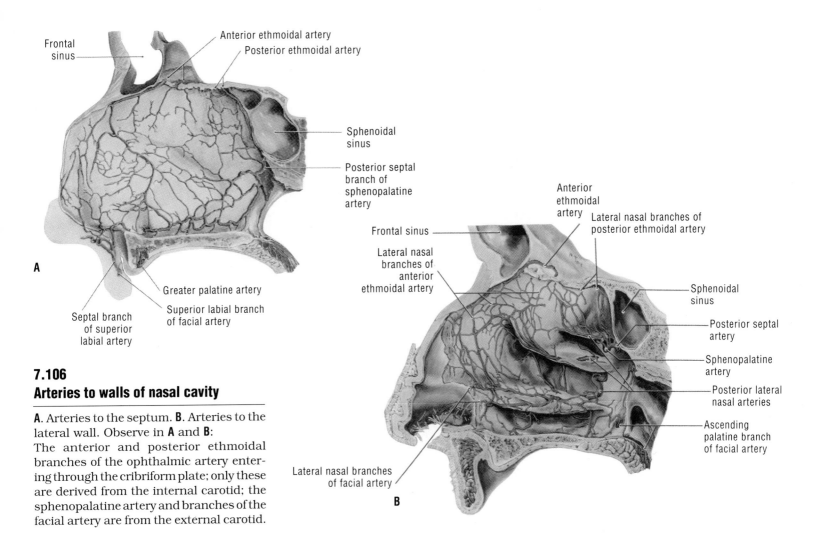

Frontal sinus — Anterior ethmoidal artery / Posterior ethmoidal artery

Sphenoidal sinus

Posterior septal branch of sphenopalatine artery

A

Greater palatine artery

Septal branch of superior labial artery

Superior labial branch of facial artery

Frontal sinus

Lateral nasal branches of anterior ethmoidal artery

Anterior ethmoidal artery

Lateral nasal branches of posterior ethmoidal artery

Sphenoidal sinus

Posterior septal artery

Sphenopalatine artery

Posterior lateral nasal arteries

Ascending palatine branch of facial artery

Lateral nasal branches of facial artery

B

7.106
Arteries to walls of nasal cavity

A. Arteries to the septum. **B**. Arteries to the lateral wall. Observe in **A** and **B**:
The anterior and posterior ethmoidal branches of the ophthalmic artery entering through the cribriform plate; only these are derived from the internal carotid; the sphenopalatine artery and branches of the facial artery are from the external carotid.

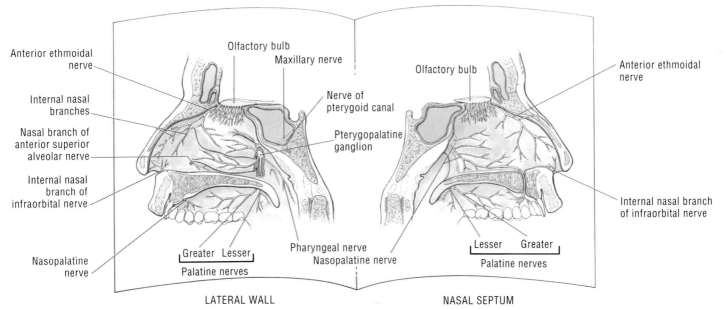

Anterior ethmoidal nerve

Olfactory bulb

Maxillary nerve

Internal nasal branches

Nasal branch of anterior superior alveolar nerve

Internal nasal branch of infraorbital nerve

Nasopalatine nerve

Nerve of pterygoid canal

Pterygopalatine ganglion

Olfactory bulb

Anterior ethmoidal nerve

Internal nasal branch of infraorbital nerve

Greater Lesser
Palatine nerves

Pharyngeal nerve
Nasopalatine nerve

Lesser Greater
Palatine nerves

LATERAL WALL

NASAL SEPTUM

7.107
Innervation of the walls of the nasal cavity

The pterygopalatine ganglion sends the nasopalatine nerve through the sphenopalatine foramen, the greater and lesser palatine nerves through canals of the same name, and the pharyngeal nerve through the pharyngeal canal.

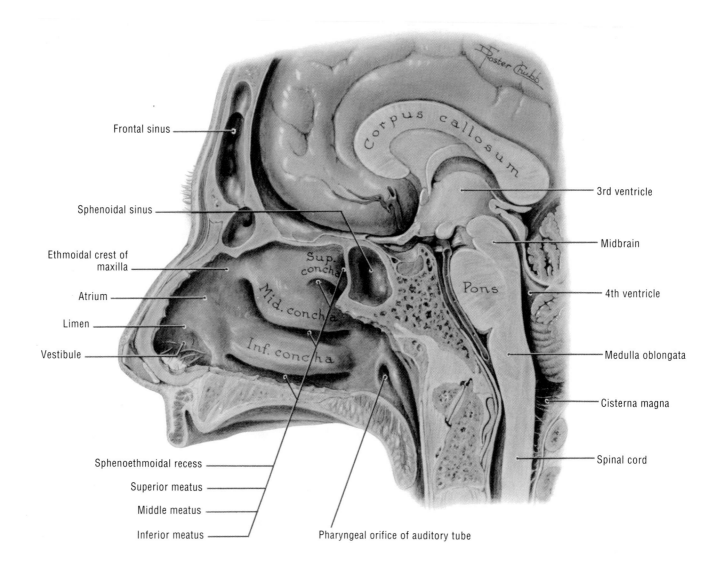

Frontal sinus

Sphenoidal sinus

Ethmoidal crest of maxilla

Atrium

Limen

Vestibule

Corpus callosum

3rd ventricle

Midbrain

Pons

4th ventricle

Sup. concha

Mid. concha

Inf. concha

Medulla oblongata

Cisterna magna

Spinal cord

Sphenoethmoidal recess

Superior meatus

Middle meatus

Inferior meatus

Pharyngeal orifice of auditory tube

7.108
Lateral wall of nasal cavity

Observe:

1. The vestibule, superior to the nostril and anterior to the inferior meatus; the hairs growing from its skin-lined surface, spreading in all directions;

2. The atrium, superior to the vestibule and anterior to the middle meatus;

3. The inferior and middle conchae, curving inferiorly and medially from the lateral wall, dividing it into three nearly equal parts, and covering the inferior and middle meatuses, respectively;

4. The superior concha, small and anterior to the sphenoidal sinus; the middle concha, with an angled inferior border, ending inferior to the sphenoidal sinus; the inferior concha, with a slightly curved inferior border, ending inferior to the middle

concha, about 1 cm anterior to the orifice of the auditory tube, i.e., about the width of the medial pterygoid plate;

5. The floor of the nose, inclined slightly inferiorly and posteriorly, at the level of the atlas;

6. The roof composed of: an anterior sloping part, corresponding to the bridge of the nose; an intermediate horizontal part, formed by the delicate cribriform plate; a perpendicular part anterior to the sphenoidal sinus, and a curved part, inferior to the sinus, which is confluent with the roof of the nasopharynx;

7. The pons and the 4th ventricle of the brain at the level of the sphenoidal sinus.

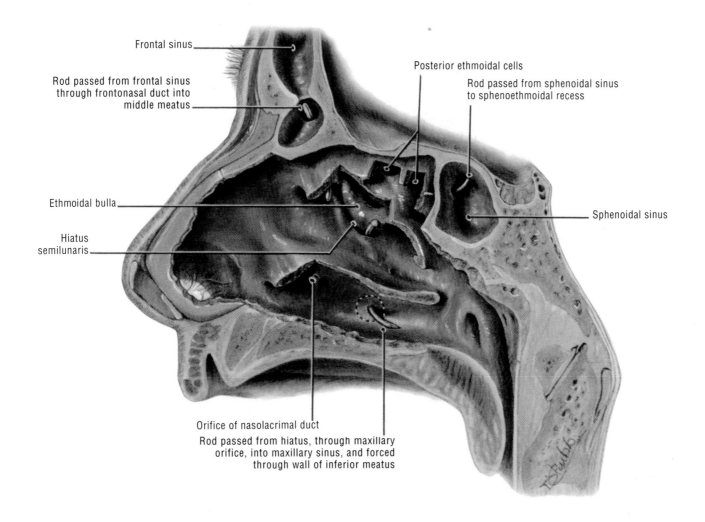

Frontal sinus

Rod passed from frontal sinus
through frontonasal duct into
middle meatus

Ethmoidal bulla

Hiatus
semilunaris

Posterior ethmoidal cells

Rod passed from sphenoidal sinus
to sphenoethmoidal recess

Sphenoidal sinus

Orifice of nasolacrimal duct

Rod passed from hiatus, through maxillary
orifice, into maxillary sinus, and forced
through wall of inferior meatus

7.109
Dissection of the lateral wall of nasal cavity

Parts of the superior, middle, and inferior conchae are cut away.

Observe:

1. The sphenoidal sinus in the body of the sphenoid bone; its orifice, superior to the middle of its anterior wall, opens into the sphenoethmoidal recess;

2. The orifices of posterior ethmoidal cells open into the superior meatus;

3. A cell, in this specimen, opening onto the superior surface of the ethmoidal bulla;

4. The attachment of the inferior concha, steep in its anterior one-third, but gently sloping in its posterior two-thirds; the orifice of the nasolacrimal duct, a short (variable) distance inferior to the angle of union of the anterior one-third and posterior two-thirds;

5. The sharp probe forced through the thinnest portion of the medial wall of the maxillary sinus, well superior to the level of the floor of the nasal cavity.

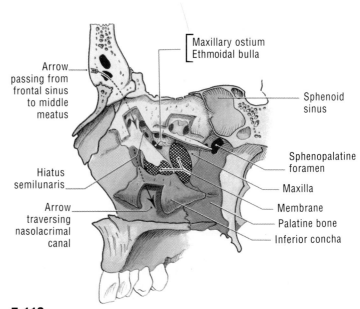

Arrow
passing from
frontal sinus
to middle
meatus

Maxillary ostium
Ethmoidal bulla

Sphenoid
sinus

Sphenopalatine
foramen

Maxilla

Membrane

Palatine bone

Inferior concha

Hiatus
semilunaris

Arrow
traversing
nasolacrimal
canal

7.110
Diagram of the bones of lateral wall of nasal cavity following dissection

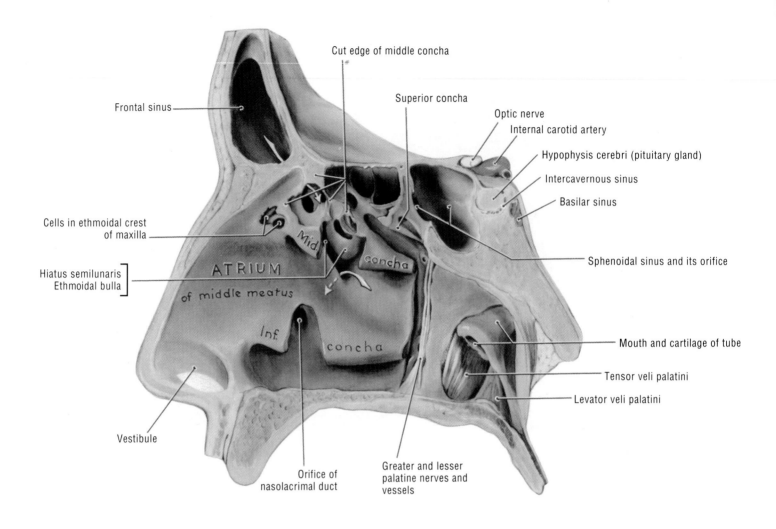

Cut edge of middle concha

Frontal sinus

Superior concha

Optic nerve

Internal carotid artery

Hypophysis cerebri (pituitary gland)

Intercavernous sinus

Basilar sinus

Cells in ethmoidal crest of maxilla

Hiatus semilunaris
Ethmoidal bulla

Sphenoidal sinus and its orifice

ATRIUM
of middle meatus

Mouth and cartilage of tube

Tensor veli palatini

Levator veli palatini

Vestibule

Orifice of
nasolacrimal duct

Greater and lesser
palatine nerves and
vessels

7.111
Paranasal air sinuses and hypophysis cerebri

Observe:

1. The frontal sinus with its outlet at its most inferior point, leading into the middle meatus medial to the hiatus semilunaris; the hiatus ends blindly anteriorly as an anterior ethmoidal cell, and posteriorly as the maxillary orifice, indicated by an *arrow*;

2. The sphenoidal sinus of average size, and with a very large orifice.

7.112
Accessory maxillary orifices

Observe:

1. In addition to the primary or normal ostium (not in view), there are four secondary or acquired ostia resulting from the breaking down of the membrane shown in cross-hatching in Figure 7.110;

2. The septum between the right and left sphenoidal sinus, here occupies the median plane – it is usually deflected to one side or the other.

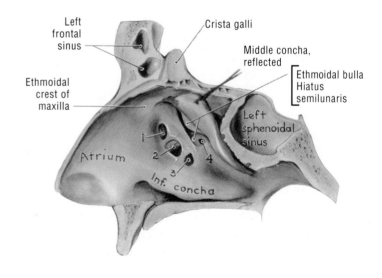

Left
frontal
sinus

Crista galli

Middle concha,
reflected

Ethmoidal bulla
Hiatus
semilunaris

Ethmoidal
crest of
maxilla

Left
sphenoidal
sinus

Atrium

Inf. concha

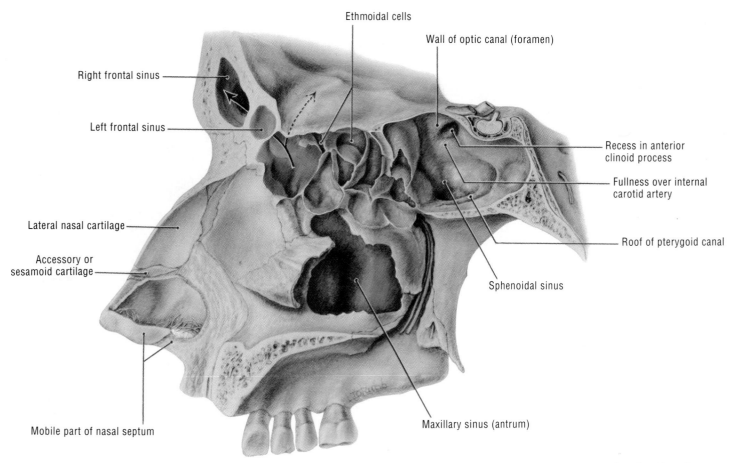

Ethmoidal cells

Wall of optic canal (foramen)

Right frontal sinus

Left frontal sinus

Recess in anterior clinoid process

Fullness over internal carotid artery

Lateral nasal cartilage

Accessory or sesamoid cartilage

Roof of pterygoid canal

Sphenoidal sinus

Mobile part of nasal septum

Maxillary sinus (antrum)

7.113
Paranasal sinuses, opened

Observe:

1. The ethmoidal cells (blue), collectively called a sinus, like a honeycomb, has the thin orbital plate of the frontal bone for a roof;

2. An anterior ethmoidal cell (pink) invading the diploe of the squama of the frontal bone to become a frontal sinus; it is ethmoidal in origin, but frontal in location; an offshoot *(broken arrow)* invades the orbital plate of the frontal bone;

3. The sphenoidal sinus (yellow) in this specimen is very extensive – extending (a) posteriorly inferior to the hypophysis cerebri to the dorsum sellae, (b) laterally, inferior to the optic nerve, into the anterior clinoid process, and (c) inferiorly to the pterygoid process, but leaving the pterygoid canal rising as a ridge on the floor of the sinus;

4. The maxillary sinus (purple) is pyramidal in shape; its base (largely nibbled away) contributes to the lateral wall of the nasal cavity, its apex is in the zygomatic process.

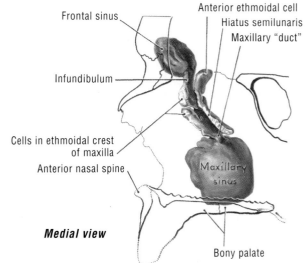

Frontal sinus

Anterior ethmoidal cell

Hiatus semilunaris

Maxillary "duct"

Infundibulum

Cells in ethmoidal crest of maxilla

Anterior nasal spine

Maxillary sinus

Medial view

Bony palate

7.114
Cast, frontal and maxillary sinuses

Observe:

1. The frontal sinus lies superior to the orbital cavity and has its opening at its most inferior point, whereas the maxillary sinus lies inferior to the orbital cavity and has its opening on a level with its most superior point;

2. Had this frontal sinus failed to develop, the anterior ethmoidal cell (shown) would have taken its place in default.

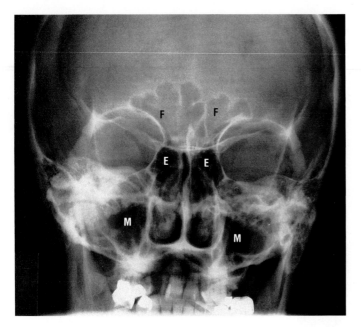

A, *Posteroanterior view*

B, *Lateral view*

7.115
Radiographs of paranasal sinuses

F - Frontal sinus, *E* - Ethmoidal sinus, *S* - Sphenoidal sinus, *M* - Maxillary sinus, *P* - Pharynx. (Courtesy of Dr. E. Becker, Associate Professor of Radiology, University of Toronto, Toronto, Ontario, Canada.)

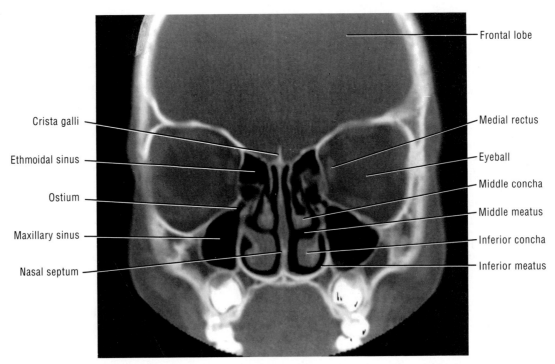

Frontal lobe

Crista galli

Medial rectus

Ethmoidal sinus

Eyeball

Ostium

Middle concha

Middle meatus

Maxillary sinus

Inferior concha

Nasal septum

Inferior meatus

7.116
Coronal CT (computed tomographic) scan

(Courtesy of Dr. D. Armstrong, Associate Professor of Radiology, University of Toronto, Toronto, Ontario, Canada.)

7.117

Medial wall of orbital cavity and lateral view of the maxillary sinus

Observe:

1. The site of the hiatus semilunaris between the bulla of the ethmoid bone superiorly and the uncinate process inferiorly;

2. The pterygopalatine fossa between pterygoid process, maxilla, palatine bone, and sphenoid bone; the foramen rotundum opens into the fossa from the middle cranial fossa and the sphenopalatine foramen opens into the nasal cavity.

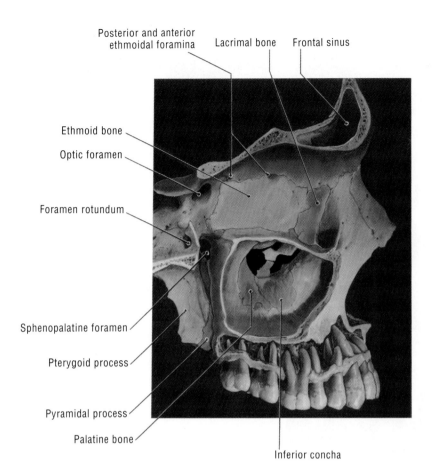

Posterior and anterior ethmoidal foramina — Lacrimal bone — Frontal sinus

Ethmoid bone

Optic foramen

Foramen rotundum

Sphenopalatine foramen

Pterygoid process

Pyramidal process

Palatine bone

Inferior concha

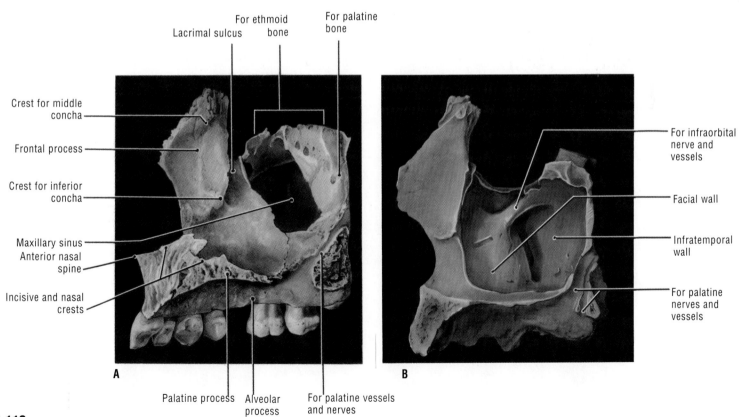

Lacrimal sulcus — For ethmoid bone — For palatine bone

Crest for middle concha

Frontal process

Crest for inferior concha

Maxillary sinus
Anterior nasal spine

Incisive and nasal crests

For infraorbital nerve and vessels

Facial wall

Infratemporal wall

For palatine nerves and vessels

A

B

Palatine process — Alveolar process — For palatine vessels and nerves

7.118

Medial aspect of maxilla and maxillary sinus

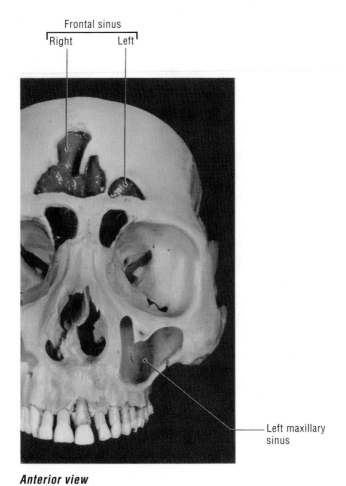

Frontal sinus
Right   Left

Left maxillary
sinus

Anterior view

7.119
Frontal and maxillary sinuses

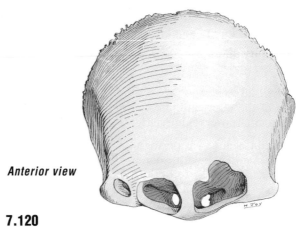

Anterior view

7.120
Frontal sinuses

The orifices of the sinuses are at the most inferior points of the sinuses.

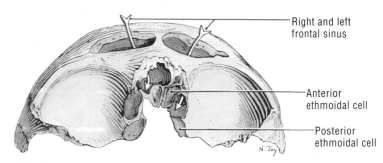

Right and left
frontal sinus

Anterior
ethmoidal cell

Posterior
ethmoidal cell

Inferior view

7.121
Frontal and ethmoidal sinuses

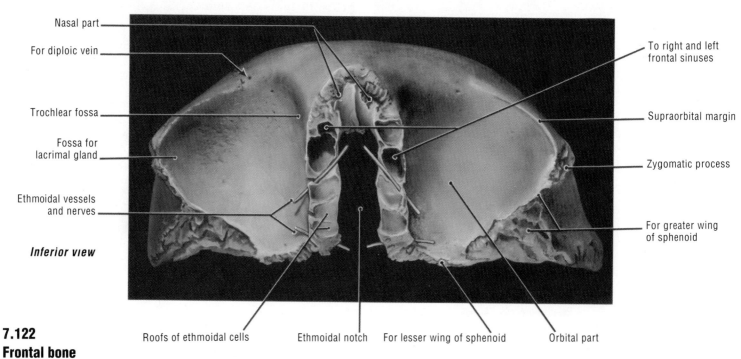

Nasal part

For diploic vein

Trochlear fossa

Fossa for
lacrimal gland

Ethmoidal vessels
and nerves

To right and left
frontal sinuses

Supraorbital margin

Zygomatic process

For greater wing
of sphenoid

Inferior view

Roofs of ethmoidal cells   Ethmoidal notch   For lesser wing of sphenoid   Orbital part

7.122
Frontal bone

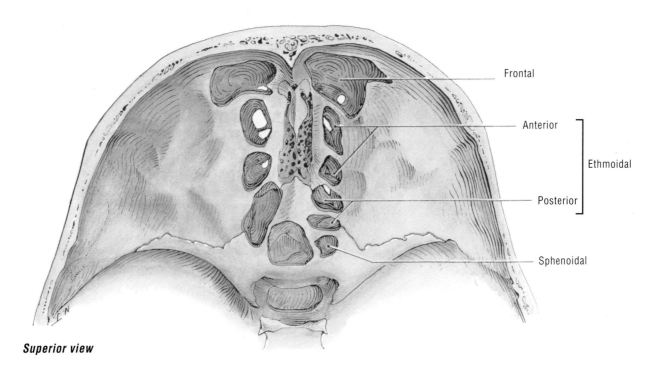

Superior view

7.123
Sinuses surrounding the cribriform plate

Frontal

Anterior ⎤
⎥ Ethmoidal
Posterior ⎦

Sphenoidal

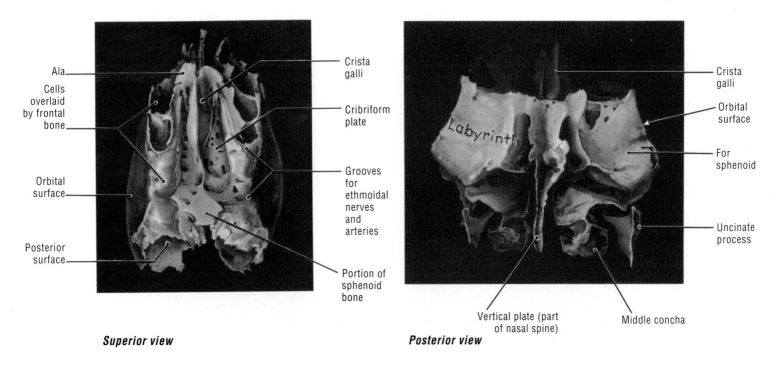

Ala

Cells
overlaid
by frontal
bone

Orbital
surface

Posterior
surface

Crista
galli

Cribriform
plate

Grooves
for
ethmoidal
nerves
and
arteries

Portion of
sphenoid
bone

Superior view

7.124
Ethmoid bone, crista galli and cribriform plate

Labyrinth

Crista
galli

Orbital
surface

For
sphenoid

Uncinate
process

Vertical plate (part
of nasal spine)

Middle concha

Posterior view

7.125
Ethmoid bone, concha and labyrinth

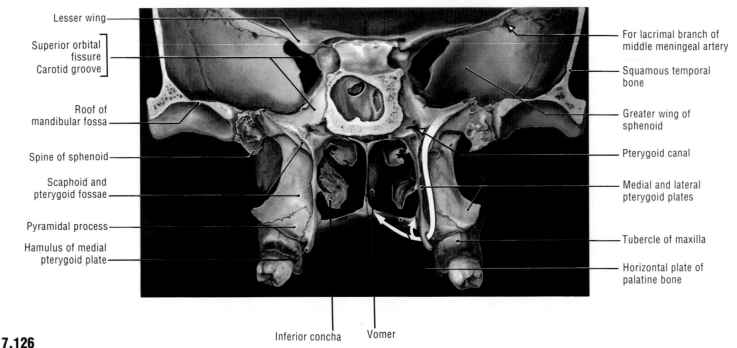

7.126
Coronal section of the skull

Observe:

1. The two posterior nasal apertures separated by the vomer, and each bounded inferiorly by the horizontal plate of the palatine bone, laterally by the medial pterygoid plate, and superiorly by the ala of the vomer and the vaginal process of the medial pterygoid plate (not labeled);

2. The pterygoid fossa, bounded medially by the medial pterygoid plate, which extends superiorly to the pterygoid canal and ends inferior to the level of the palate, as the hamulus; the tensor veli palatini *(arrow)*; the sphenoidal sinus (yellow).

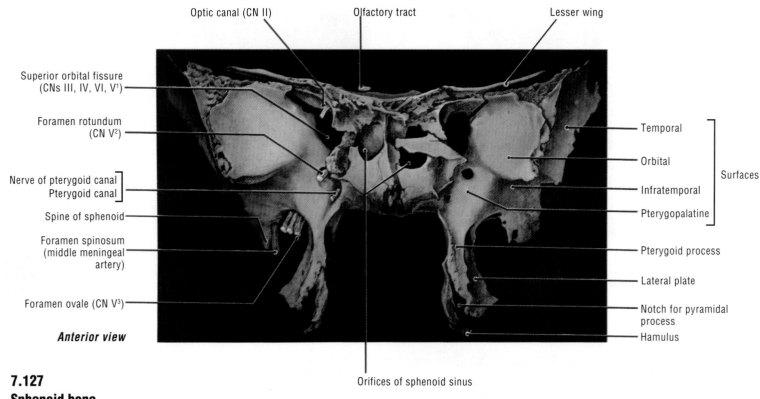

Anterior view

7.127
Sphenoid bone

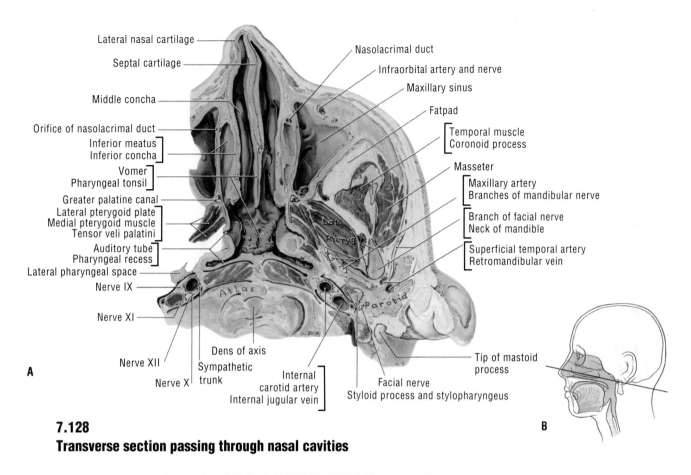

7.128

Transverse section passing through nasal cavities

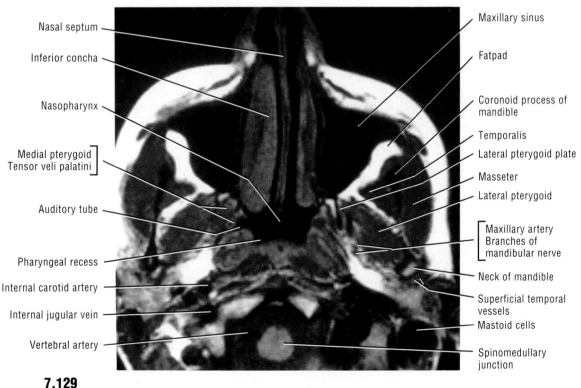

7.129

Transverse MRI (magnetic resonance image) through the nose

(Courtesy of Dr. W. Kucharczyk, Clinical Director of Tri-Hospital Resonance Centre, Toronto, Ontario, Canada.)

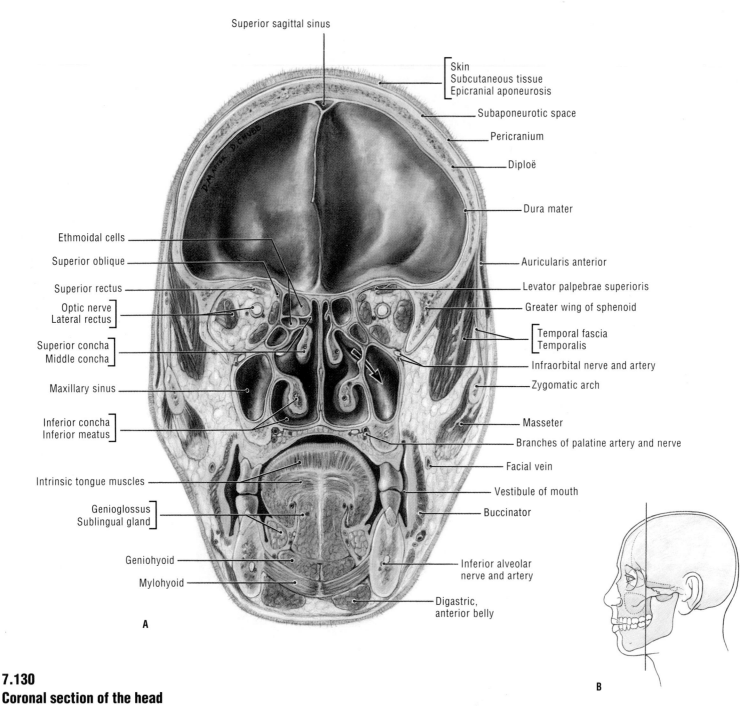

Superior sagittal sinus

Skin
Subcutaneous tissue
Epicranial aponeurosis

Subaponeurotic space

Pericranium

Diploë

Dura mater

Ethmoidal cells

Auricularis anterior

Superior oblique

Levator palpebrae superioris

Superior rectus

Greater wing of sphenoid

Optic nerve
Lateral rectus

Temporal fascia
Temporalis

Superior concha
Middle concha

Infraorbital nerve and artery

Maxillary sinus

Zygomatic arch

Inferior concha
Inferior meatus

Masseter

Branches of palatine artery and nerve

Intrinsic tongue muscles

Facial vein

Vestibule of mouth

Genioglossus
Sublingual gland

Buccinator

Geniohyoid

Inferior alveolar
nerve and artery

Mylohyoid

Digastric,
anterior belly

A

B

7.130
Coronal section of the head

Observe:

1. The central position of the ethmoid bone whose horizontal component forms the central part of the anterior cranial fossa superiorly and the roof of the nasal cavity inferiorly; the suspended ethmoidal cells give attachment to the superior and middle concha and form part of the medial wall of the orbit; the perpendicular plate of the ethmoid forms part of the nasal septum;

2. The thin orbital plate of the frontal bone forms a roof over the orbit and a floor for the anterior cranial fossa;

3. The palate forms the floor of the nasal cavity and the roof of the oral cavity;

4. The maxillary sinus forms the inferior part of the lateral wall of the nose; the middle concha shelters the hiatus semilunaris into which the maxillary ostium opens *(arrow)*;

5. In chewing, the tongue pushes food between the molar teeth into the vestibule and the buccinator muscle pushes it back again;

6. The mylohyoid muscle, slung like a hammock between right and left halves of the mandible, supports the structures of the oral cavity.

B. Orientation drawing of **A**.

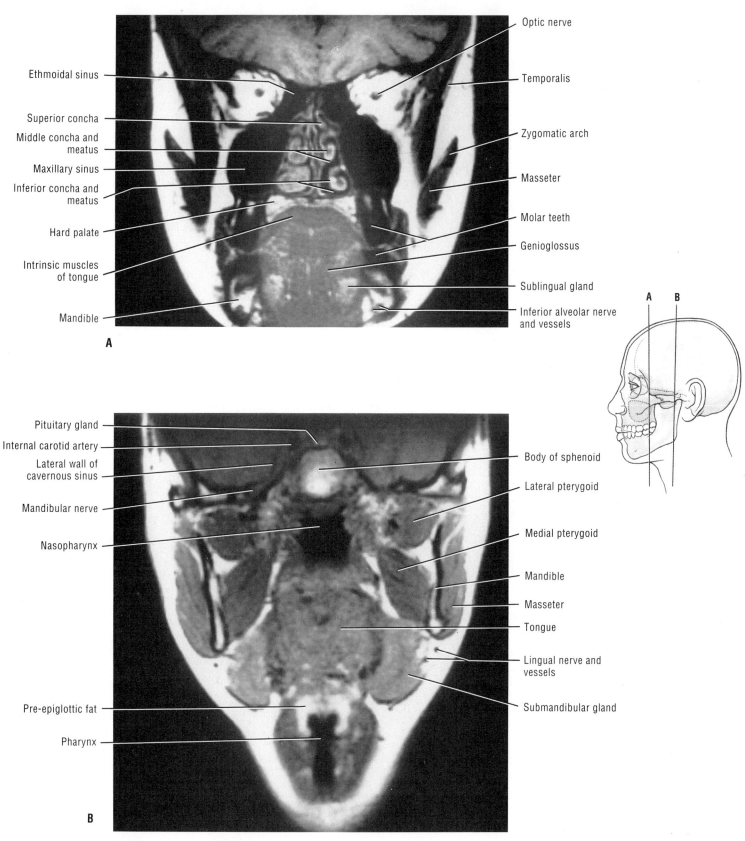

Ethmoidal sinus

Superior concha

Middle concha and meatus

Maxillary sinus

Inferior concha and meatus

Hard palate

Intrinsic muscles of tongue

Mandible

A

Optic nerve

Temporalis

Zygomatic arch

Masseter

Molar teeth

Genioglossus

Sublingual gland

Inferior alveolar nerve and vessels

Pituitary gland

Internal carotid artery

Lateral wall of cavernous sinus

Mandibular nerve

Nasopharynx

Pre-epiglottic fat

Pharynx

B

Body of sphenoid

Lateral pterygoid

Medial pterygoid

Mandible

Masseter

Tongue

Lingual nerve and vessels

Submandibular gland

7.131
Coronal MRIs (magnetic resonance images) of the head

(Courtesy of Dr. W. Kucharczyk, Clinical Director of Tri-Hospital Resonance Centre, Toronto, Ontario, Canada.)

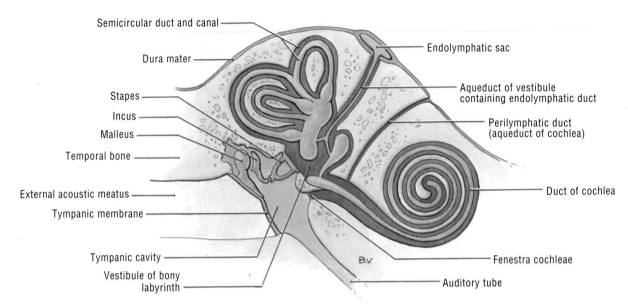

Semicircular duct and canal

Dura mater

Stapes

Incus

Malleus

Temporal bone

External acoustic meatus

Tympanic membrane

Tympanic cavity

Vestibule of bony labyrinth

Endolymphatic sac

Aqueduct of vestibule containing endolymphatic duct

Perilymphatic duct (aqueduct of cochlea)

Duct of cochlea

Fenestra cochleae

Auditory tube

7.132
General scheme of the ear

The ear is divisible into three parts – external, middle, internal. The *external ear* is comprised of the auricle and the external acoustic (auditory) meatus.

The *middle ear* (tympanum) lies between the tympanic membrane and the internal ear. Three ossicles, the malleus, incus, and stapes, stretch from the lateral to the medial wall of the tympanum. Of these, the malleus is attached to the tympanic membrane. The stapes is attached by an anular ligament to the fenestra vestibuli (oval window); and the incus connects these two ossicles. The auditory tube opens into the anterior wall of the tympanic cavity.

The *internal ear* is comprised of a closed system of membranous tubes and bulbs, called the membranous labyrinth, which is filled with fluid, called endolymph, and bathed in surrounding fluid called perilymph (purple).

When the tympanic membrane vibrates, the malleus vibrates with it and transmits the vibrations via the incus to the stapes. The stapes, being attached to the margins of the fenestra vestibuli by an anular ligament, transmits the vibrations to the perilymph within the vestibule. A secondary tympanic membrane that closes the fenestra cochleae (round window) receiving the vibrations transmitted to the incompressible perilymph is, itself, made to vibrate in turn.

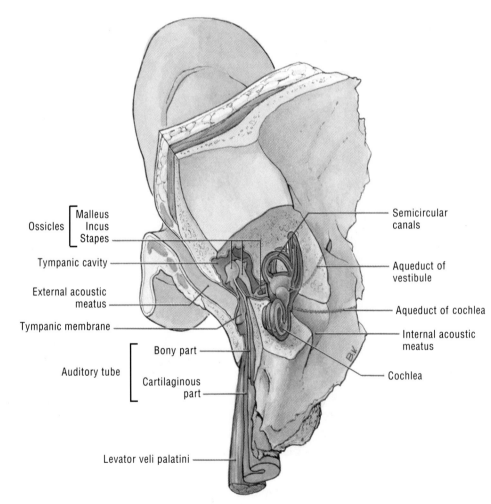

Ossicles
- Malleus
- Incus
- Stapes

Tympanic cavity

External acoustic meatus

Tympanic membrane

Auditory tube
- Bony part
- Cartilaginous part

Levator veli palatini

Semicircular canals

Aqueduct of vestibule

Aqueduct of cochlea

Internal acoustic meatus

Cochlea

7.133
The ear in situ

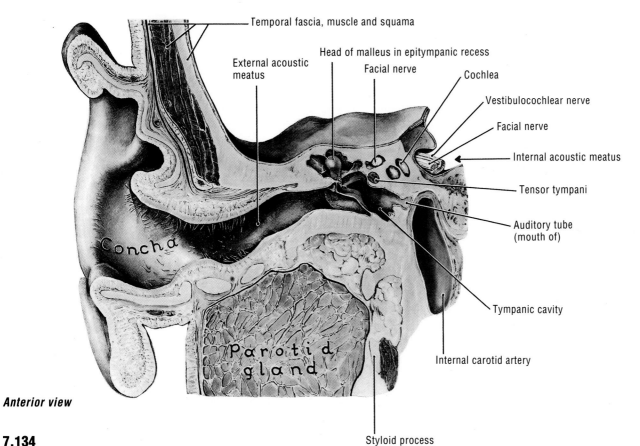

Temporal fascia, muscle and squama

Head of malleus in epitympanic recess

External acoustic meatus

Facial nerve

Cochlea

Vestibulocochlear nerve

Facial nerve

Internal acoustic meatus

Tensor tympani

Auditory tube (mouth of)

Tympanic cavity

Internal carotid artery

Styloid process

Concha

Parotid gland

Anterior view

7.134
Coronal section of the ear

Observe:

1. The external acoustic (auditory) meatus, which from tragus to eardrum is 3 cm long, half of its length being cartilaginous and half bony; it is narrowest near the drum due to the rise on the floor, hence the "well" where fluid might collect at the medial end of the meatus; it is innervated by the auriculotemporal branch of the mandibular nerve (CN V³) and the auricular branches of the vagus nerve (CN X), if the wall of the external acoustic meatus is irritated, reflex coughing or vomiting may occur; similarly, a toothache (CN V³ distribution) may refer pain to the ear;

2. The cartilaginous part of the external acoustic meatus, lined with thick skin and having hairs and the mouths of many glands; the bony part is lined with a thin epithelium that adheres to the periosteum and also forms the outermost layer of the tympanic membrane;

3. The obliquity of the tympanic membrane that meets the roof of the meatus at an obtuse angle and the floor at an acute one;

4. The middle ear or tympanic cavity, extending superior to the drum as the epitympanic recess, and the recess extending laterally superior to the bony meatus;

5. The tympanic cavity widest superiorly, narrow inferiorly, and narrowest at the level of the umbo where the membrane is indrawn and faces the promontory of the cochlea;

6. The thin shell of bone covering the facial nerve; the grooved anterior crus of the stapes and the anterior half of its base closing the fenestra vestibuli; the long axis of the stapes inclined superomedially.

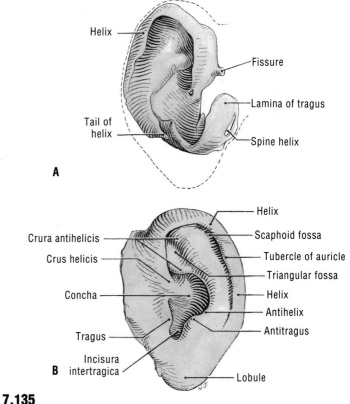

Helix

Fissure

Lamina of tragus

Tail of helix

Spine helix

A

Helix

Crura antihelicis

Scaphoid fossa

Crus helicis

Tubercle of auricle

Triangular fossa

Concha

Helix

Antihelix

Tragus

Antitragus

Incisura intertragica

B

Lobule

7.135
The auricle

A. Cartilage (gray) of the right auricle. **B.** Left auricle.

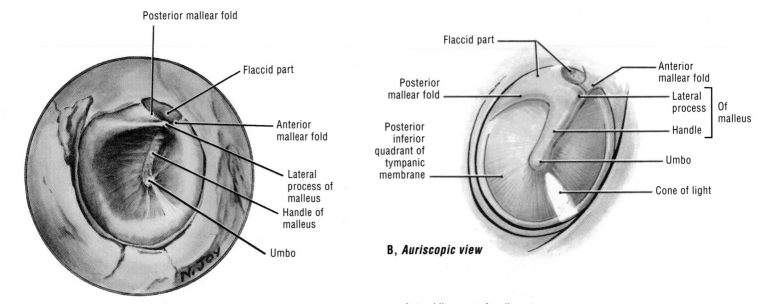

Posterior mallear fold

Flaccid part

Anterior mallear fold

Lateral process of malleus

Handle of malleus

Umbo

A, *Lateral view*

Flaccid part

Posterior mallear fold

Posterior inferior quadrant of tympanic membrane

Anterior mallear fold

Lateral process
Handle

Of malleus

Umbo

Cone of light

B, *Auriscopic view*

7.136
Tympanic membrane *(above)*

Observe:

1. The tympanic membrane, oval rather than round, and shaped like a funnel with rolled rim and a depressed part, called the umbo, at the tip of the handle of the malleus which is situated anteroinferior to the center of the membrane;

2. Superior to the lateral process of the malleus the membrane is thin and is called the flaccid part (pars flaccida); the flaccid part lacks the radial and circular fibers present in the remainder of the membrane (tense part or pars tensa); the junction between the two parts, flaccid and tense, is marked by an anterior and a posterior line, both of which run from the lateral process of the malleus to the free ends of the horseshoe-shaped tympanic ring;

3. The flaccid part (pars flaccida) forms the lateral wall of the superior recess of the tympanic cavity;

4. The lateral surface of the tympanic membrane is innervated by the auricular branch of the auriculotemporal nerve (CN V³) and the auricular branch of the vagus nerve (CN X); medially, it is innervated by tympanic branches of the CN IX;

5. In otitis media, to drain the middle ear, the tympanic membrane is incised in the posteroinferior quadrant.

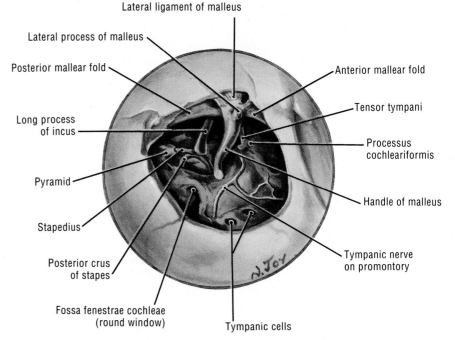

Lateral ligament of malleus

Lateral process of malleus

Posterior mallear fold

Long process of incus

Pyramid

Stapedius

Posterior crus of stapes

Fossa fenestrae cochleae (round window)

Anterior mallear fold

Tensor tympani

Processus cochleariformis

Handle of malleus

Tympanic nerve on promontory

Tympanic cells

Inferolateral view

7.137
Tympanic cavity after removal of the tympanic membrane

Observe:

1. The direction of the handle of the malleus and of the long process of the incus that lies posterior to it; the posterior and anterior mallear folds of mucous membrane in which the chorda tympani passes between the two bones;

2. The fullness of the promontory with grooves for the tympanic nerve (a branch of the glossopharyngeal nerve) and its connections;

3. The end of a fossa, at the deep end of which is the fenestra cochleae or round window, closed by the secondary tympanic membrane (not in view);

4. The lateral ligament of the malleus and the neck of the malleus forming the medial wall of the superior recess of the tympanic membrane.

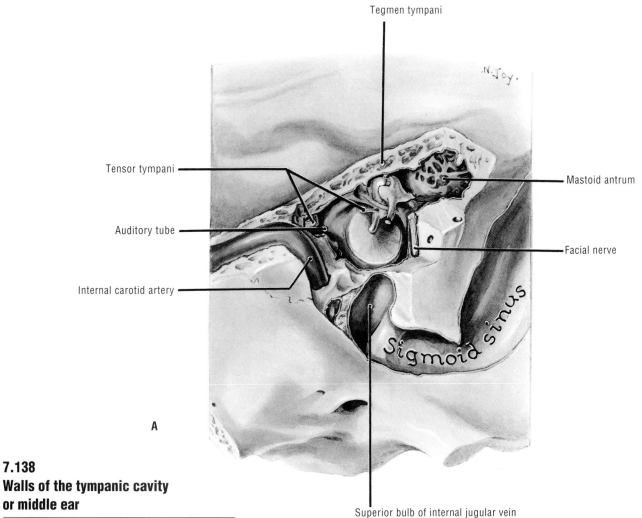

Tegmen tympani

Tensor tympani

Auditory tube

Internal carotid artery

Mastoid antrum

Facial nerve

Sigmoid sinus

A

Superior bulb of internal jugular vein

7.138
Walls of the tympanic cavity or middle ear

A. The specimen was dissected with a drill from the medial aspect. **B.** Schematic drawing of the middle ear. The anterior wall of the middle ear is removed.

Observe:

1. The tegmen tympani forming the roof of the tympanic cavity and mastoid antrum, here fairly thick but commonly papery in thinness;

2. The internal carotid artery as the main feature of the anterior wall; the internal jugular vein the main feature of the floor; and the facial nerve the main feature of the posterior wall;

3. The superolateral part of the anterior wall leading to the auditory tube and tensor tympani; the superolateral part of the posterior wall leading to the mastoid antrum;

4. The tympanic membrane forming much of the lateral wall; superior to it is the epitympanic recess in which are housed the larger parts of the malleus and incus.

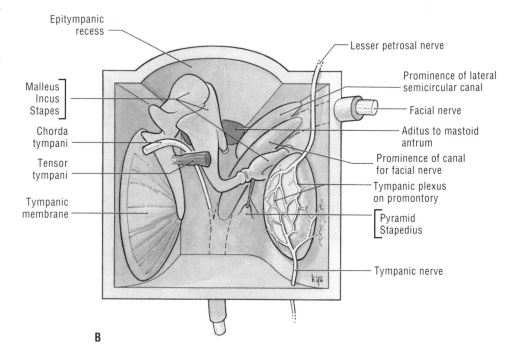

Epitympanic recess

Lesser petrosal nerve

Prominence of lateral semicircular canal

Malleus
Incus
Stapes

Facial nerve

Aditus to mastoid antrum

Chorda tympani

Prominence of canal for facial nerve

Tensor tympani

Tympanic plexus on promontory

Tympanic membrane

Pyramid
Stapedius

Tympanic nerve

B

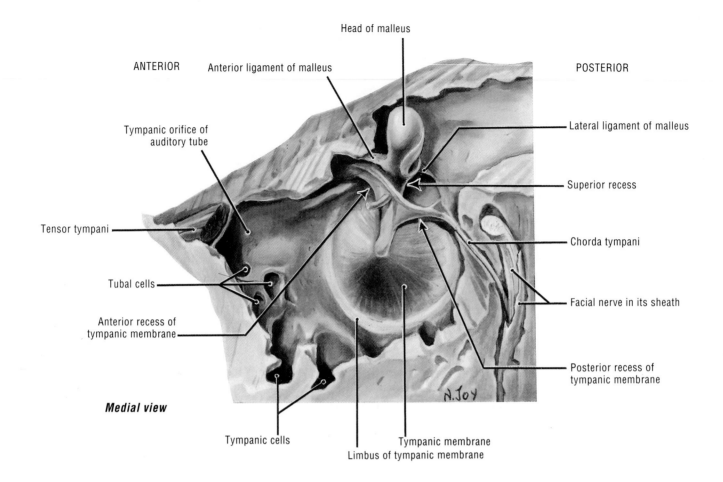

Head of malleus

ANTERIOR   Anterior ligament of malleus   POSTERIOR

Tympanic orifice of
auditory tube

Lateral ligament of malleus

Superior recess

Tensor tympani

Chorda tympani

Tubal cells

Anterior recess of
tympanic membrane

Facial nerve in its sheath

Posterior recess of
tympanic membrane

Medial view

Tympanic cells

Tympanic membrane

Limbus of tympanic membrane

7.139
Lateral wall of the tympanic cavity

Observe:

1. The oval tympanic membrane, with a greater vertical than horizontal diameter (9 mm x 8 mm);

2. The handle of the malleus incorporated in the membrane, its end being at the umbo;

3. The anterior process of the malleus anchored anteriorly by the anterior ligament;

4. The facial nerve within its tough periosteal tube; the chorda tympani leaving the facial nerve, and (a) lying within two crescentic folds of mucous membrane, (b) crossing the neck of the malleus superior to the tendon of tensor, and (c) following the anterior process and anterior ligament;

5. The three recesses of the tympanic membrane: anterior, posterior, and superior;

6. The fibrocartilaginous margin or limbus of the membrane, which fastens it to the sulcus in the tympanic bone.

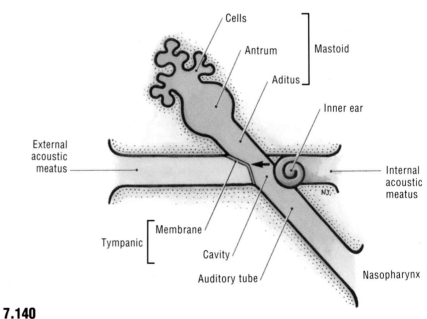

Cells

Antrum

Mastoid

Aditus

Inner ear

External
acoustic
meatus

Internal
acoustic
meatus

Membrane

Tympanic

Cavity

Auditory tube

Nasopharynx

7.140
Scheme of meatus and airway

This illustrates that the line of the external and internal meatus intersects at the tympanic cavity with the line of the airway from mastoid cells to nasopharynx. The *arrow* indicates the lateral wall of the tympanic cavity as viewed from its medial side as in Figure 7.139.

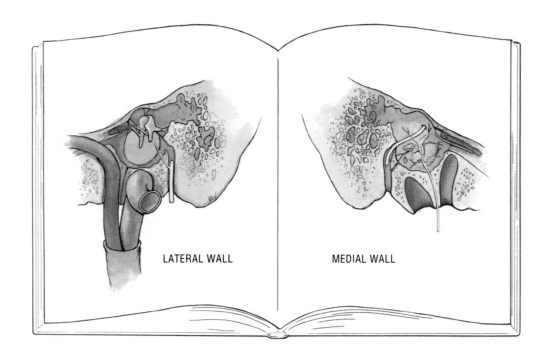

7.141
Tympanic cavity

LATERAL WALL

MEDIAL WALL

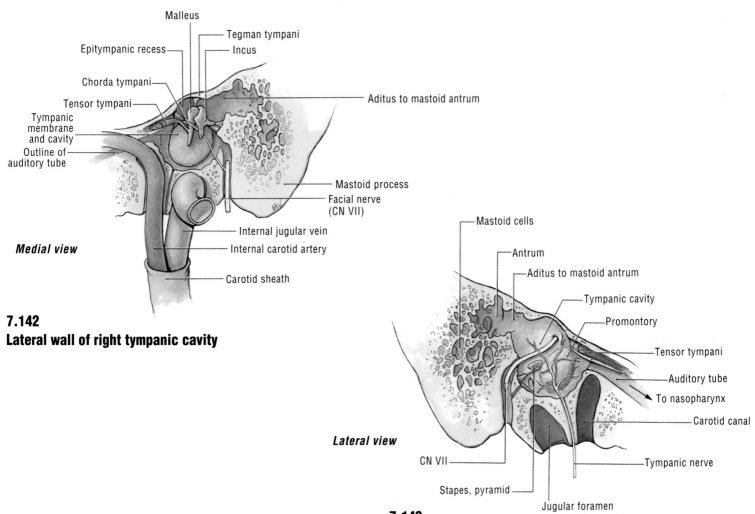

Malleus

Tegman tympani

Epitympanic recess

Incus

Chorda tympani

Tensor tympani

Aditus to mastoid antrum

Tympanic membrane and cavity

Outline of auditory tube

Mastoid process

Facial nerve (CN VII)

Internal jugular vein

Internal carotid artery

Medial view

Carotid sheath

7.142
Lateral wall of right tympanic cavity

Mastoid cells

Antrum

Aditus to mastoid antrum

Tympanic cavity

Promontory

Tensor tympani

Auditory tube

To nasopharynx

Carotid canal

Lateral view

CN VII

Tympanic nerve

Stapes, pyramid

Jugular foramen

7.143
Medial wall of right tympanic cavity

M - Malleus, *I* - Incus, *S* - Stapes, *EA* - External acoustic meatus, *T* - Tympanic membrane, *TC* - Tympanic cavity, *ER* - Epitympanic recess, *AT* - Auditory tube.

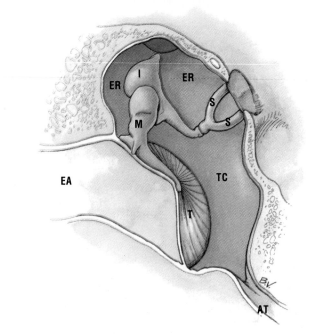

MALLEUS

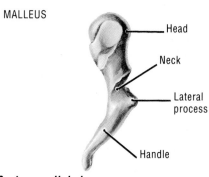

Head

Neck

Lateral process

Handle

A, *Posteromedial view*

MALLEUS

INCUS

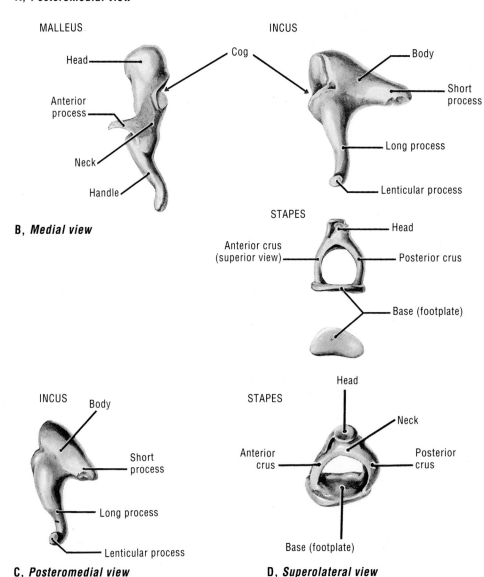

Head

Cog

Body

Anterior process

Short process

Neck

Long process

Handle

Lenticular process

B, *Medial view*

STAPES

Head

Anterior crus (superior view)

Posterior crus

Base (footplate)

INCUS

Body

Head

STAPES

Short process

Neck

Long process

Anterior crus

Posterior crus

Lenticular process

Base (footplate)

C, *Posteromedial view*

D, *Superolateral view*

7.145
Ossicles of the middle ear

A. Malleus. **B.** Malleus, incus, stapes. **C.** Incus. **D.** Stapes.

Observe:
1. The head of the malleus and the body and short process of the incus lie in the epitympanic recess;

2. The saddle-shaped articular surface of the head of the malleus and the reciprocally saddle-shaped articular surface of the body of the incus form the incudomallear synovial joint;

3. The anterior process of the malleus and the short process of the incus are in line and are moored anteriorly and posteriorly by ligaments;

4. The handle of the malleus, from lateral process to tip, is embedded in the tympanic membrane;

5. The end of the long process of the incus has a convex articular facet for articulation with the head of the stapes, at the incudostapedial synovial joint;

6. The hole in the stapes in the embryo transmits an artery, the stapedial artery; it is now closed by a membrane; the superior border of the footplate is convex and is deeper anteriorly than posteriorly; the two crura are grooved; the anterior crus is the more slender and straighter and it is fixed to a small area on the plate; the posterior crus is attached to the whole depth of the plate.

7.146
Auditory tube exposed from the lateral aspect

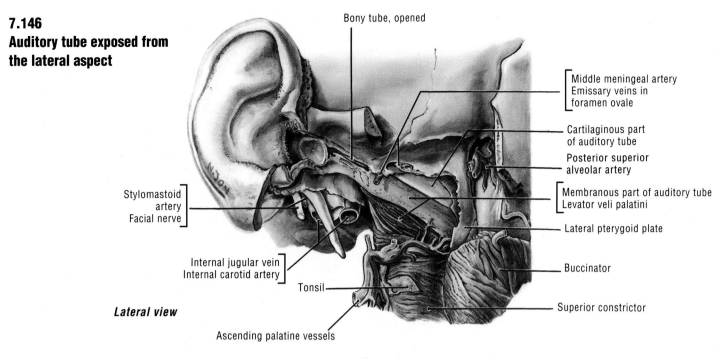

Bony tube, opened

Middle meningeal artery
Emissary veins in foramen ovale

Cartilaginous part of auditory tube

Posterior superior alveolar artery

Membranous part of auditory tube
Levator veli palatini

Lateral pterygoid plate

Buccinator

Superior constrictor

Stylomastoid artery
Facial nerve

Internal jugular vein
Internal carotid artery

Tonsil

Lateral view

Ascending palatine vessels

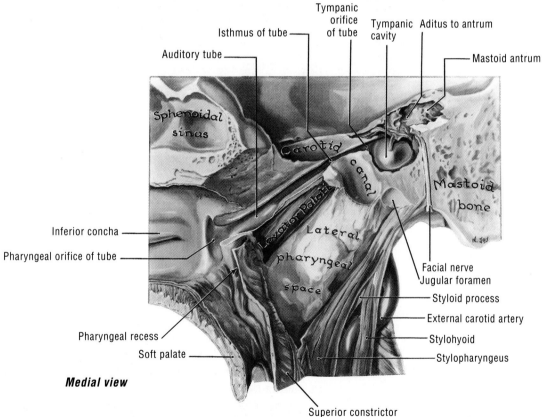

Tympanic orifice of tube

Tympanic cavity

Aditus to antrum

Isthmus of tube

Auditory tube

Mastoid antrum

Sphenoidal sinus

Carotid canal

Mastoid bone

Levator Palati

Lateral pharyngeal space

Inferior concha

Pharyngeal orifice of tube

Facial nerve
Jugular foramen

Styloid process

External carotid artery

Stylohyoid

Stylopharyngeus

Pharyngeal recess

Soft palate

Medial view

Superior constrictor

7.147
Auditory tube exposed from the pharyngeal (medial) aspect

Observe:

1. The general direction of the tube – superiorly, posteriorly, and laterally from the nasopharynx to tympanic cavity;

2. The funnel-shaped pharyngeal orifice of the tube, situated 1 cm posterior to the inferior concha of the nose;

3. The cartilaginous part of the tube, 2.5 cm long, resting throughout its length on levator veli palatini;

4. The bony part of the tube passing lateral to the carotid canal, about 1 cm long, narrow at the isthmus where it joins the cartilaginous part, wider at its tympanic orifice.

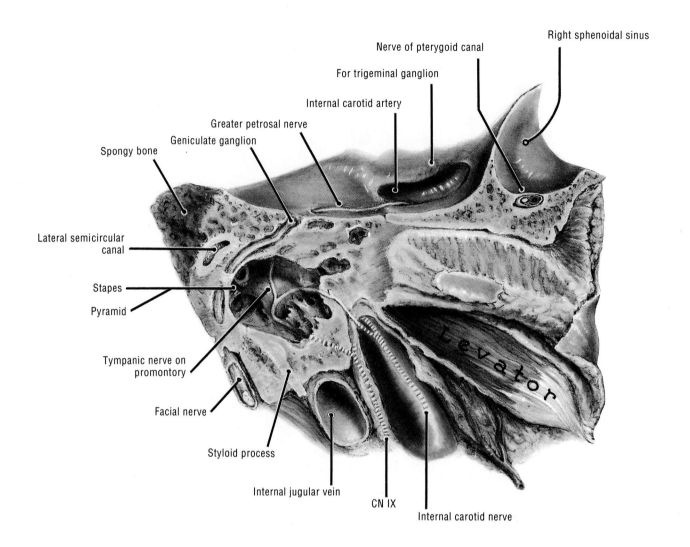

Right sphenoidal sinus

Nerve of pterygoid canal

For trigeminal ganglion

Internal carotid artery

Greater petrosal nerve

Geniculate ganglion

Spongy bone

Lateral semicircular canal

Stapes

Pyramid

Tympanic nerve on promontory

Facial nerve

Styloid process

Internal jugular vein

CN IX

Internal carotid nerve

Levator

7.148
The right auditory tube and tympanic cavity, split longitudinally – medial part

The cut surfaces of this longitudinally split specimen are shown on these two facing pages. (The procedure used was modified after Laurenson RD. *A rapid method of dissecting the middle ear. Anat Rec 1965; 151:503.*)

The squamous and mastoid parts of the temporal bone are sawn across coronally from suprameatal spine, through the mastoid antrum, into the posterior cranial fossa. The posterior part of the bone is then discarded.

The thin roof (tegmen) of the mastoid antrum and the aditus to the antrum are nibbled away until the incus comes into view. The incus is now picked from its articulation with malleus laterally and stapes medially.

A probe, passed from the pharynx up the auditory tube, until arrested at the isthmus, will serve as a directional guide.

Identify the internal carotid artery medially, beneath the trigeminal ganglion at the foramen lacerum, and the middle meningeal artery laterally, at the foramen spinosum.

A saw cut from the gap left by the incus to the space between the two arteries (carotid and meningeal) will pass between the greater and lesser petrosal nerves, being parallel, and continue into the tube.

The incus having been removed, the only structure that crosses the path of the saw is the tensor tympani tendon, which passes from the medial to lateral wall. In this specimen, a shaving of the medial wall (containing the fleshy tensor in its semicanal and the processus cochleariformis) was included with the lateral part, leaving the tendon intact.

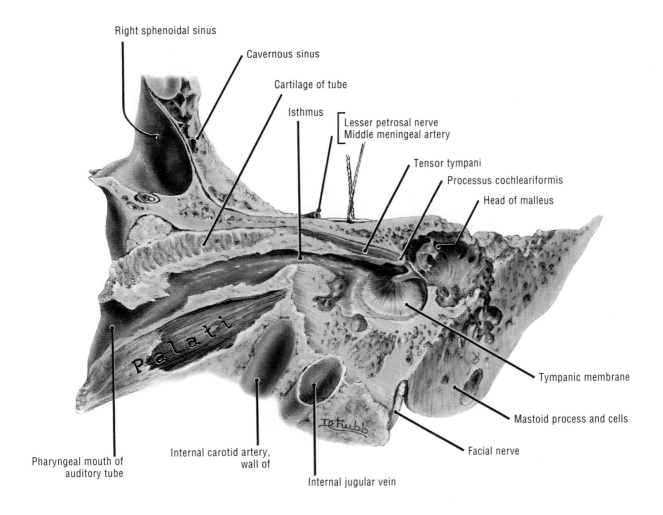

Right sphenoidal sinus

Cavernous sinus

Cartilage of tube

Isthmus

Lesser petrosal nerve
Middle meningeal artery

Tensor tympani

Processus cochleariformis

Head of malleus

Tympanic membrane

Mastoid process and cells

Facial nerve

Internal jugular vein

Internal carotid artery,
wall of

Pharyngeal mouth of
auditory tube

7.149
The right auditory tube and tympanic cavity, split longitudinally – lateral part

The lateral wall of the cavity is dominated by the tympanic membrane, handle of malleus, and chorda tympani nerve.

The medial wall has a broad bulging, the promontory, which overlies the first turn of the cochlea. On it, the tympanic nerve and caroticotympanic branches of the internal carotid plexus form the tympanic plexus, which supplies the region and gives off the lesser petrosal nerve.

Structures, divided and seen on both medial (Fig. 7.148) and lateral (this figure) parts include:

a) Levator veli palatini, supporting the auditory tube;
b) Auditory tube, cartilaginous superiorly and medially; membranous inferiorly and laterally;
c) Right sphenoidal sinus, with the pterygoid canal inferior to it;
d) Internal carotid artery;
e) Internal jugular vein;
f) Facial nerve;
g) A petrosal nerve, either greater or lesser.

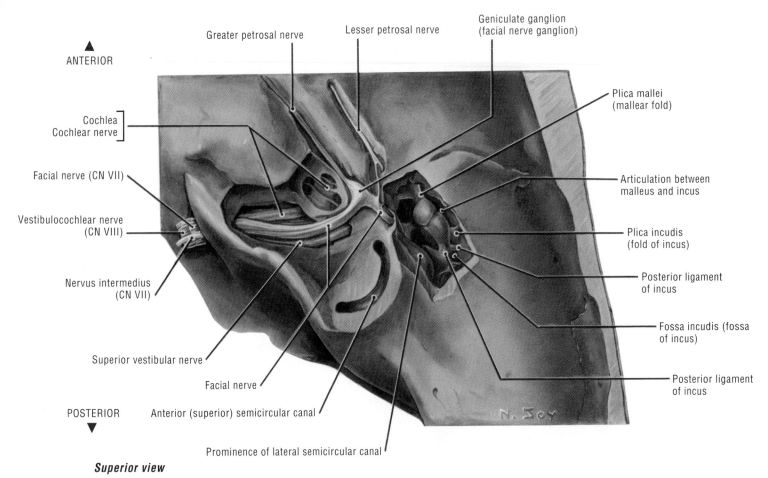

ANTERIOR ▲

Greater petrosal nerve

Lesser petrosal nerve

Geniculate ganglion (facial nerve ganglion)

Cochlea
Cochlear nerve

Plica mallei (mallear fold)

Facial nerve (CN VII)

Articulation between malleus and incus

Vestibulocochlear nerve (CN VIII)

Plica incudis (fold of incus)

Nervus intermedius (CN VII)

Posterior ligament of incus

Fossa incudis (fossa of incus)

Superior vestibular nerve

Posterior ligament of incus

Facial nerve

POSTERIOR ▼

Anterior (superior) semicircular canal

Prominence of lateral semicircular canal

Superior view

7.150
Geniculate ganglion

Observe:

1. The facial nerve, the nervus intermedius, and the vestibulocochlear nerve, entering and traversing the internal acoustic meatus; the facial nerve, joined by the nervus intermedius, running posterior to the cochlea and, therefore, across the roof of the vestibule to the geniculate ganglion and at the ganglion making a right angle bend, called the genu, and then curving posteroinferiorly within the bony facial canal, whose papery lateral wall separates it from the tympanic cavity;

2. The petrosal branch of the middle meningeal artery, which enters the canal at the hiatus, running with the nerve;

3. The geniculate ganglion, which is the cell station of fibers of general sensation and of taste; through the ganglion run fibers of the greater (superficial) petrosal nerve on their way to the pterygopalatine ganglion; from the facial nerve, beyond the ganglion, a communicating branch goes to the lesser (superficial) petrosal nerve on its way to the otic ganglion.

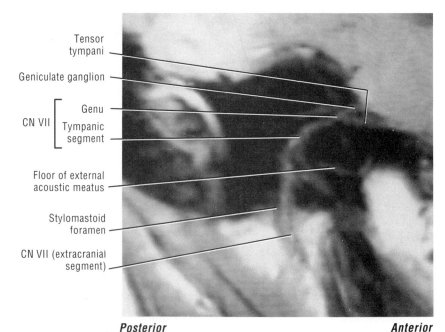

Tensor tympani

Geniculate ganglion

CN VII — Genu
Tympanic segment

Floor of external acoustic meatus

Stylomastoid foramen

CN VII (extracranial segment)

Posterior   *Anterior*

7.151
Oblique sagittal MRI (magnetic resonance image) showing the facial nerve and geniculate ganglion

Compare this figure to Figures 7.147 and 7.150. (Courtesy of Dr. W. Kucharczyk, Clinical Director of Tri-Hospital Resonance Centre, Toronto, Ontario, Canada.)

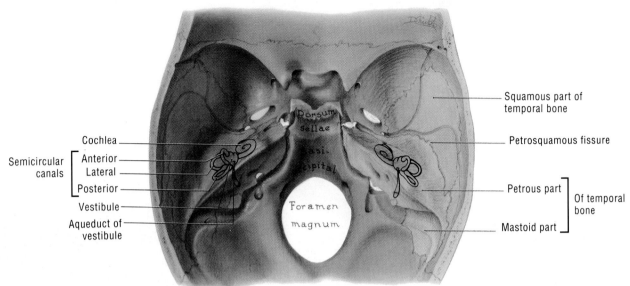

Cochlea

Semicircular canals
- Anterior
- Lateral
- Posterior

Vestibule

Aqueduct of vestibule

Dorsum sellae

Basi-occipital

Foramen magnum

Squamous part of temporal bone

Petrosquamous fissure

Petrous part
Mastoid part
} Of temporal bone

7.152

The temporal bone and osseous labyrinth, superior view of the interior of the base of the skull

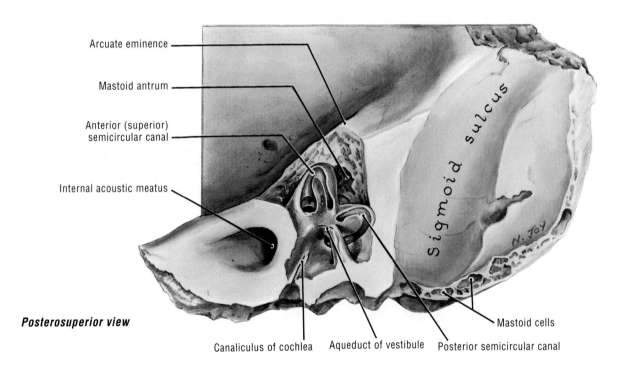

Arcuate eminence

Mastoid antrum

Anterior (superior) semicircular canal

Internal acoustic meatus

Sigmoid sulcus

N. Joy

Posterosuperior view

Canaliculus of cochlea   Aqueduct of vestibule   Posterior semicircular canal

Mastoid cells

7.153

Semicircular canals and the aqueducts

Observe:

1. The anterior semicircular canal, set vertically below the arcuate eminence, and making a right angle with the posterior surface of the petrous bone;

2. The posterior semicircular canal, nearly parallel to the posterior surface of the bone, close to that surface, and only 5 mm from the sigmoid sulcus;

3. The aqueduct of the vestibule, which contains the ductus endolymphaticus and opens medial to the posterior semicircular canal;

4. The canaliculus of the cochlea, which contains the perilymphatic duct (aqueduct of cochlea) and opens at the apex of the depression for the ganglion of nerve IX.

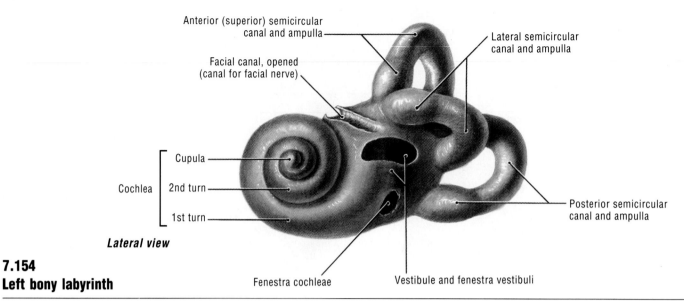

Anterior (superior) semicircular
canal and ampulla

Facial canal, opened
(canal for facial nerve)

Lateral semicircular
canal and ampulla

Cupula

Cochlea — 2nd turn

1st turn

Posterior semicircular
canal and ampulla

Lateral view

7.154
Left bony labyrinth

Fenestra cochleae

Vestibule and fenestra vestibuli

Observe:

1. The three parts of the bony internal ear or bony labyrinth: cochlea, anteriorly; vestibule in the middle; semicircular canals, posteriorly;

2. The 2 1/2 turns or coils of the cochlea; the first or basal coil, which lies deep to the medial wall of the tympanic cavity, communicating with the tympanic cavity through the fenestra cochleae (round window); in life, this fenestra is closed by the secondary tympanic membrane;

3. The vestibule, crossed superiorly by the facial canal and

communicating with the tympanic cavity through the fenestra vestibuli (oval window); in life, this window is closed by the base or footpiece of the stapes;

4. The three semicircular canals – anterior, posterior, and lateral; the anterior and posterior canals set vertically at a right angle to each other; the lateral canal set horizontally and at a right angle to the two others; each canal, forming about two-thirds of a circle, and each having an ampulla at one end; the lateral canal is the shortest; the posterior canal is the longest.

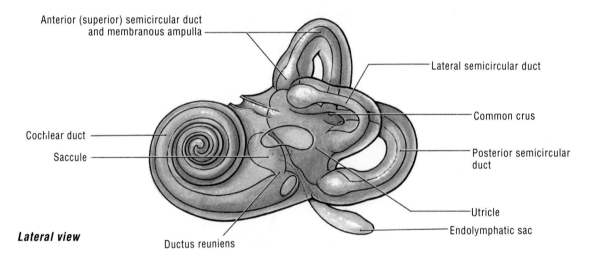

Anterior (superior) semicircular duct
and membranous ampulla

Lateral semicircular duct

Common crus

Cochlear duct

Saccule

Posterior semicircular
duct

Utricle

Endolymphatic sac

Lateral view

Ductus reuniens

7.155

Left membranous labyrinth, superimposed on the bony labyrinth

Observe:

1. The membranous labyrinth or membranous internal ear is contained within the bony labyrinth or bony internal ear; it is a closed system of ducts and chambers, filled with endolymph and surrounded with, or bathed in, perilymph;

2. It has three parts – the duct of the cochlea, within the cochlea; the saccule and the utricle, within the vestibule; and the three semicircular ducts, within the three semicircular canals;

3. One end of the duct of the cochlea is closed; the other end communicates with the saccule through the ductus reuniens;

4. The saccule, in turn, communicates with the utricle through the utriculosaccular duct (not labeled); from this duct springs the endolymphatic duct, which occupies the aqueduct of the vestibule and ends in the endolymphatic sac; the three semicircular ducts have five openings into the utricle.

Grant's Atlas of Anatomy

7.156
Posterior cranial fossa

Observe:

1. That at birth the subarcuate fossa was large and extended laterally, under the arc of the anterior semicircular canal;

2. That the aqueduct of the vestibule opened under the arc of the posterior semicircular canal; this aqueduct transmits the endolymphatic duct;

3. That the perilymphatic duct (within the canaliculus of the cochlea) opens at the base of the pyramidal pit for the glossopharyngeal ganglion; this capillary aqueduct is said to allow the perilymph of the internal ear to mix with the cerebrospinal fluid in the posterior cranial fossa, but there is also evidence that it ends as a closed sac.

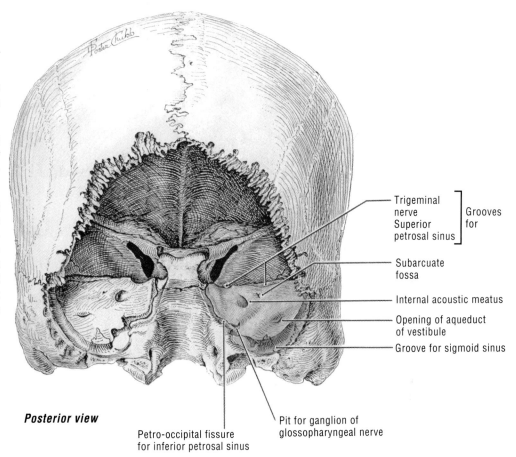

Trigeminal nerve
Superior petrosal sinus } Grooves for

Subarcuate fossa

Internal acoustic meatus

Opening of aqueduct of vestibule

Groove for sigmoid sinus

Posterior view

Petro-occipital fissure for inferior petrosal sinus

Pit for ganglion of glossopharyngeal nerve

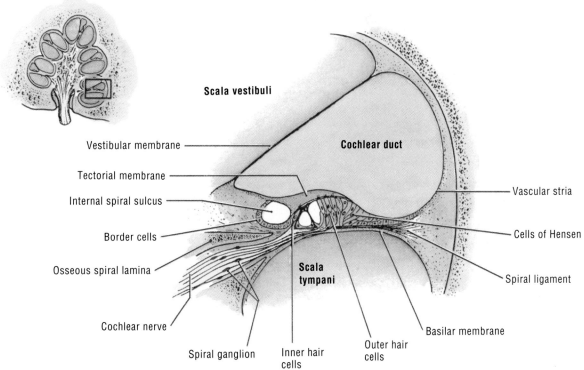

Scala vestibuli

Vestibular membrane

Tectorial membrane

Internal spiral sulcus

Border cells

Osseous spiral lamina

Cochlear nerve

Cochlear duct

Vascular stria

Cells of Hensen

Spiral ligament

Scala tympani

Basilar membrane

Spiral ganglion

Inner hair cells

Outer hair cells

7.157
Diagram of radial section through the cochlea

Note the cochlear duct, the basilar membrane, the spiral organ (of Corti), and the tectorial membrane; in the upper left is a small drawing of an axial section of the cochlea; the large drawing shows details of the area enclosed in the rectangle.

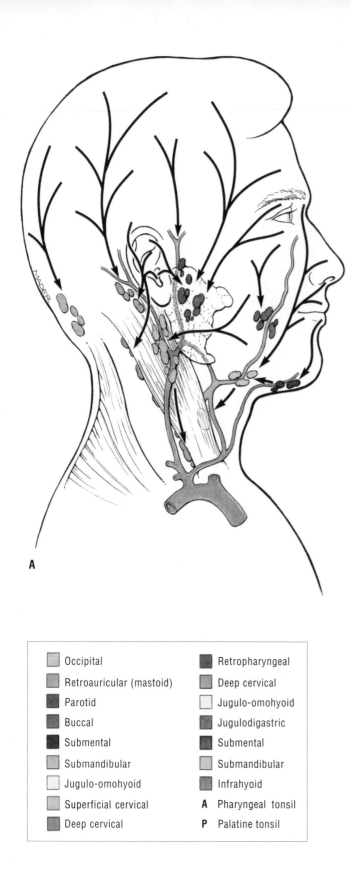

A

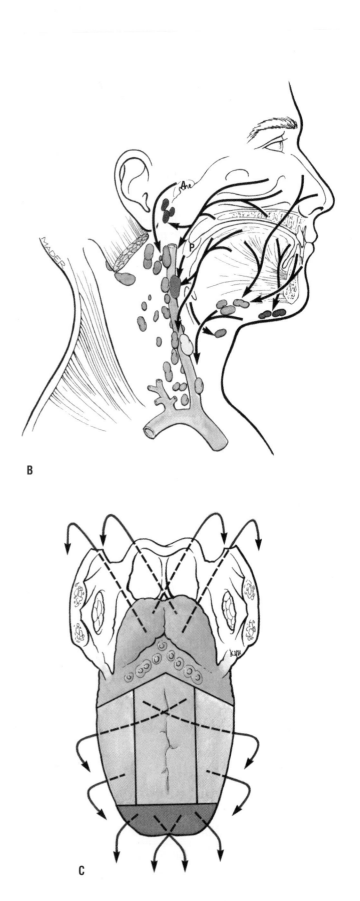

B

▢ Occipital	▢ Retropharyngeal
▢ Retroauricular (mastoid)	▢ Deep cervical
▢ Parotid	▢ Jugulo-omohyoid
▢ Buccal	▢ Jugulodigastric
▢ Submental	▢ Submental
▢ Submandibular	▢ Submandibular
▢ Jugulo-omohyoid	▢ Infrahyoid
▢ Superficial cervical	**A** Pharyngeal tonsil
▢ Deep cervical	**P** Palatine tonsil

7.158
Drainage of the head and neck

A. Superficial. **B**. Deep. **C**. Tongue.

C

8   The Neck

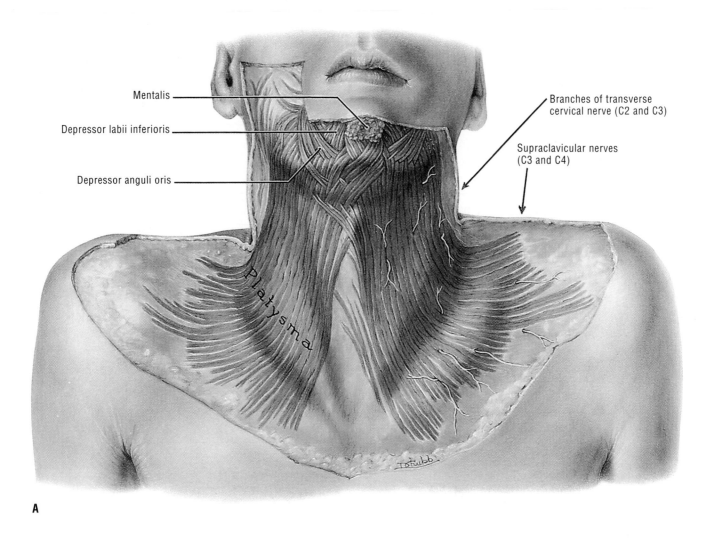

Mentalis

Depressor labii inferioris

Depressor anguli oris

Branches of transverse
cervical nerve (C2 and C3)

Supraclavicular nerves
(C3 and C4)

Platysma

A

8.1
Platysma muscle

Observe the dissection (**A**) and the surface anatomy photo (**B**):
1. The platysma muscle, spreading subcutaneously like a sheet, pierced by cutaneous nerves, crossing the whole length of the inferior border of the mandible superiorly, crossing the whole length of the clavicle inferiorly, and extending inferiorly to the level of the 1st or 2nd rib and to the acromion;

2. The anterior borders of the two platysma muscles, decussating posterior to the chin in the submental region and inferior to that free and diverging, and so leaving the median part of the neck uncovered;

3. Its posterior border, free, covering the anteroinferior part of the posterior triangle, and continuing superiorly across the inferior border of the mandible to the angle of the mouth.

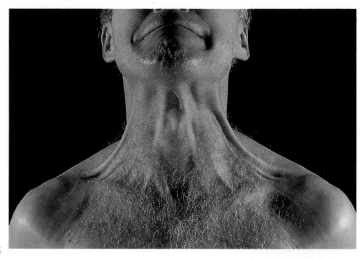

B

8.2
Triangles of the neck

The obliquely set sternocleidomastoid muscle divides the lateral aspect of the neck into an anterior and a posterior triangle.

The anterior triangle is subdivided into three small triangles: submandibular (blue), carotid (orange), and muscular (green).

The posterior triangle is divisible into a supraclavicular (purple) and an occipital (pink) triangle. Note the area superior to the accessory nerve (CN XI) contains little of importance, but the area inferior to CN XI contains numerous structures of great importance.

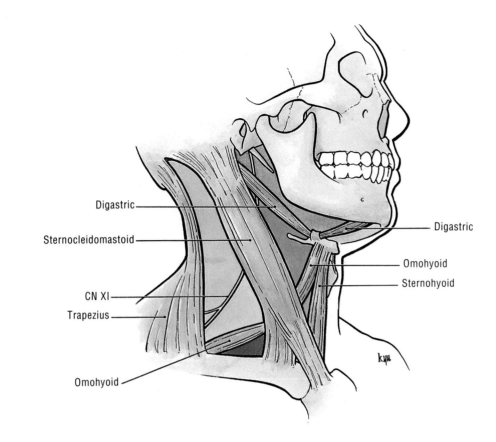

8.3
Bony landmarks of the neck

Observe:

1. The external occipital protuberance and the mastoid process (and the superior nuchal line uniting them) are created by the downward pull of the trapezius and sternocleidomastoid muscles;

2. The transverse process of the atlas, being the most prominent of the cervical transverse processes, is felt with the fingertip by pressing superiorly between the angle of the mandible and the mastoid process;

3. The body of the hyoid bone lies at the angle between the floor of the mouth and the anterior aspect of the neck; the greater horn of one side of the hyoid bone is palpable only when the greater horn of the opposite side is steadied;

4. The arch of the cricoid cartilage projects beyond the rings of the trachea and is thereby readily identified in life; it is the guide to the level of C6;

5. The coracoid process, located 2.5 cm inferior to the clavicle, under the edge of the deltoid muscle, is palpable by pressing laterally with the finger in the deltopectoral triangle.

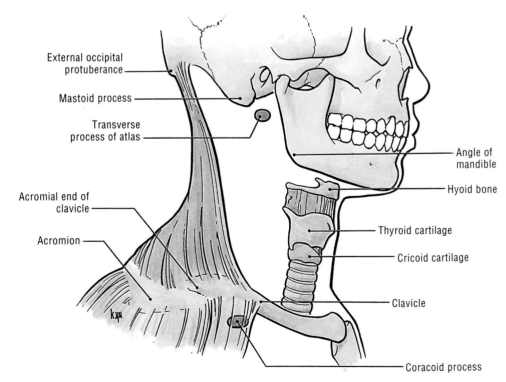

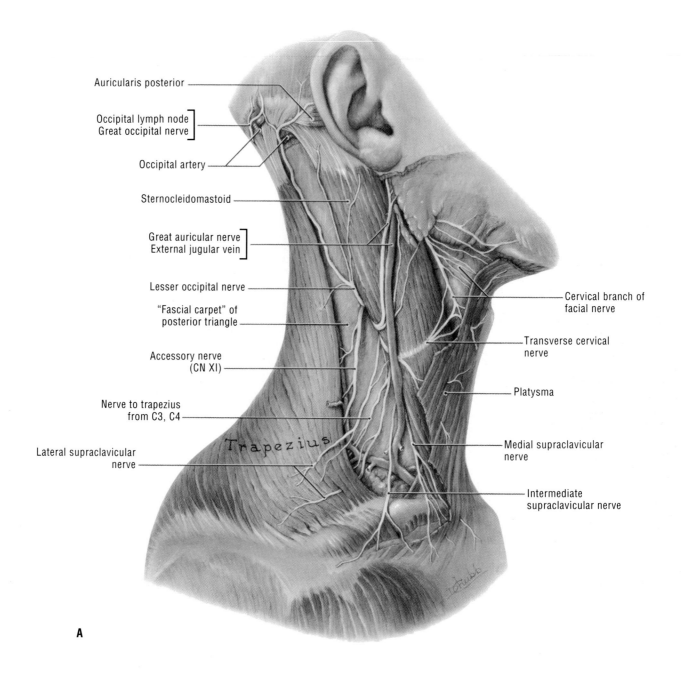

Auricularis posterior

Occipital lymph node
Great occipital nerve

Occipital artery

Sternocleidomastoid

Great auricular nerve
External jugular vein

Lesser occipital nerve

"Fascial carpet" of
posterior triangle

Accessory nerve
(CN XI)

Nerve to trapezius
from C3, C4

Lateral supraclavicular
nerve

Cervical branch of
facial nerve

Transverse cervical
nerve

Platysma

Medial supraclavicular
nerve

Intermediate
supraclavicular nerve

Trapezius

A

8.4
Posterior triangle of the neck

A. Superficial structures. Observe:

1. The three sides of the triangle: the trapezius muscle, the sternocleidomastoid muscle, and the middle third of the clavicle; the apex is where the aponeuroses of the two muscles blend just inferior to the superior nuchal line;

2. The platysma muscle (partly cut away), covering the inferior part of the triangle;

3. The external jugular vein, descending vertically from posterior to the angle of the mandible, across the sternocleidomastoid muscle to its posterior border where, an inch superior to the clavicle, it pierces the investing deep fascia;

4. The "fascial carpet" that covers the muscular floor;

5. The accessory nerve (CN XI) – the only motor nerve superficial to the "fascial carpet" – descending within the deep fascia, and disappearing about 2 fingers' breadth superior to the clavicle;

6. The cutaneous nerves (C2, C3, C4), radiating from the posterior border of the sternocleidomastoid muscle, inferior to the accessory nerve.

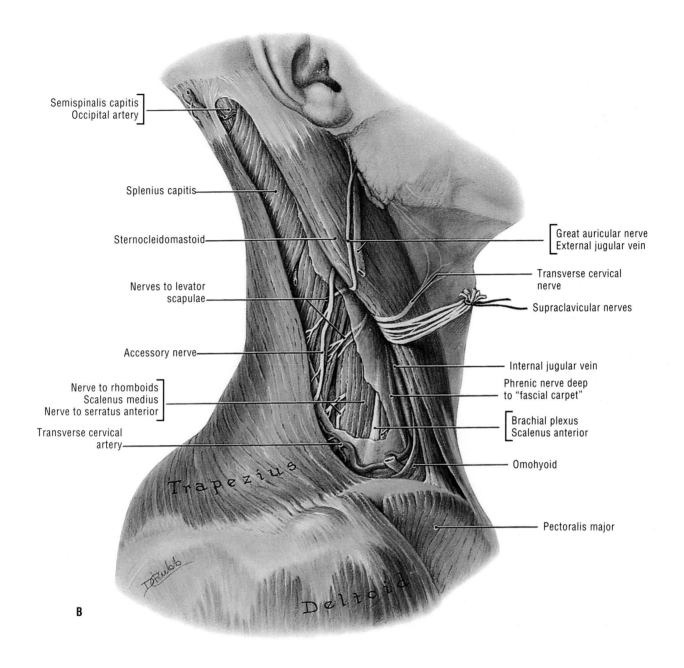

Semispinalis capitis
Occipital artery

Splenius capitis

Sternocleidomastoid

Nerves to levator
scapulae

Accessory nerve

Nerve to rhomboids
Scalenus medius
Nerve to serratus anterior

Transverse cervical
artery

Trapezius

Deltoid

Great auricular nerve
External jugular vein

Transverse cervical
nerve

Supraclavicular nerves

Internal jugular vein

Phrenic nerve deep
to "fascial carpet"

Brachial plexus
Scalenus anterior

Omohyoid

Pectoralis major

B

8.4
Posterior triangle of the neck *(continued)*

B. Motor nerves deep to fascial carpet. Observe:

1. The muscles forming the floor of the superior part of the triangle (semispinalis capitis, splenius capitis, levator scapulae muscles); the muscles forming the inferior part of the floor are shown in **D**;

2. The accessory nerve (i.e., the nerve to the sternocleidomastoid and the trapezius muscles), lying along the levator scapulae muscle but separated by the "fascial carpet";

3. Three motor nerves to upper limb muscles, lying (a) in the plane between the fascial carpet and the muscular floor, and (b) between the accessory nerve superiorly and the brachial plexus inferiorly; they are: nerves to the levator scapulae (C3, C4), to the rhomboids (C5), and to the serratus anterior (C5, C6; the branch from C7 lies protected posterior to the plexus);

4. Two structures of surgical importance, situated just beyond the geometrical confines of the triangle: (a) the phrenic nerve to the diaphragm (C3, C4, C5), placed between the carpet and the floor; (b) the internal jugular vein, superficial to the carpet.

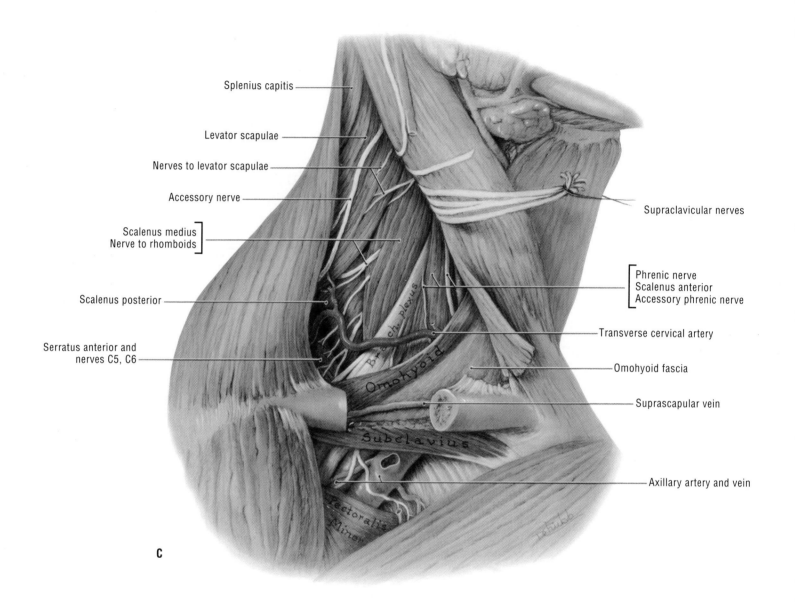

Splenius capitis

Levator scapulae

Nerves to levator scapulae

Accessory nerve

Scalenus medius
Nerve to rhomboids

Scalenus posterior

Serratus anterior and
nerves C5, C6

Supraclavicular nerves

Phrenic nerve
Scalenus anterior
Accessory phrenic nerve

Transverse cervical artery

Omohyoid fascia

Suprascapular vein

Axillary artery and vein

Br.ch. plexus

Omohyoid

Subclavius

Pectoralis Minor

C

8.4
Posterior triangle of the neck *(continued)*

C. Omohyoid and its fascia. The clavicular head of the pectoralis major muscle and part of the clavicle have been excised. Observe:
1. The posterior belly of the omohyoid muscle, held down by a sheet of "omohyoid" fascia to the fascia ensheathing the subclavius muscle; and the resulting pocket between this fascia posteriorly and the investing deep fascia and the sternocleidomastoid muscle anteriorly;

2. The brachial plexus, appearing between the scalenus anterior and the scalenus medius muscles and here, as commonly, giving off an accessory phrenic nerve from C5;

3. The posterior border of the scalenus anterior muscle, nearly parallel to the posterior border of the sternocleidomastoid muscle, and slightly posterior to it; hence one is a guide to the other.

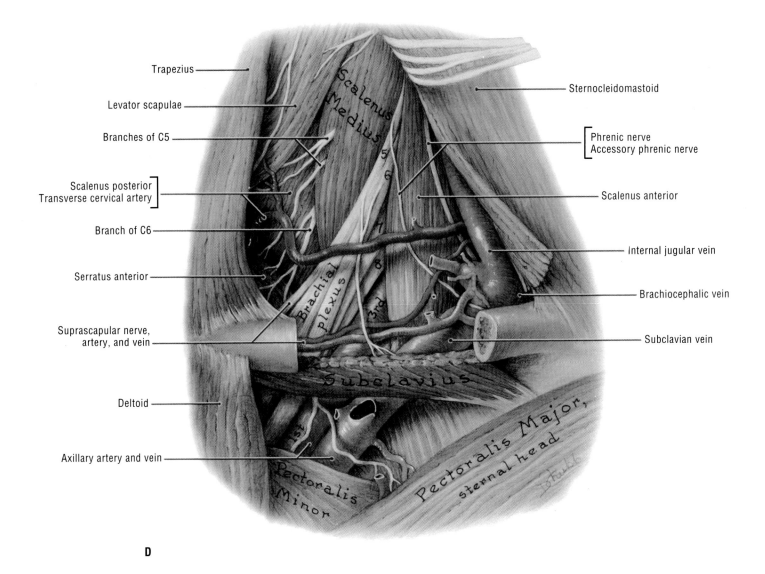

Trapezius

Levator scapulae

Branches of C5

Scalenus posterior
Transverse cervical artery

Branch of C6

Serratus anterior

Suprascapular nerve,
artery, and vein

Deltoid

Axillary artery and vein

Sternocleidomastoid

Phrenic nerve
Accessory phrenic nerve

Scalenus anterior

Internal jugular vein

Brachiocephalic vein

Subclavian vein

D

8.4
Posterior triangle of the neck *(continued)*

D. Brachial plexus and subclavian vessels. Observe:
1. The third part of the subclavian artery and the first part of the axillary artery are labeled;

2. The muscles forming the floor of the inferior part of the triangle (scaleni posterior, medius, and anterior, and serratus anterior muscles);

3. The brachial plexus and subclavian artery, appearing between the scalenus medius and scalenus anterior muscles; the most inferior root of the plexus (T1) is concealed by the third part of the artery;

4. The subclavian vein, separated from the second part of the subclavian artery by the scalenus anterior muscle;

5. Subclavius, unimportant as a muscle, but valuable as a buffer between a fractured clavicle and the subclavian vessels; by voluntarily forcing the upper limb posteroinferiorly, the clavicle and subclavius compress the subclavian vessels against the 1st rib and so arrest the pulse.

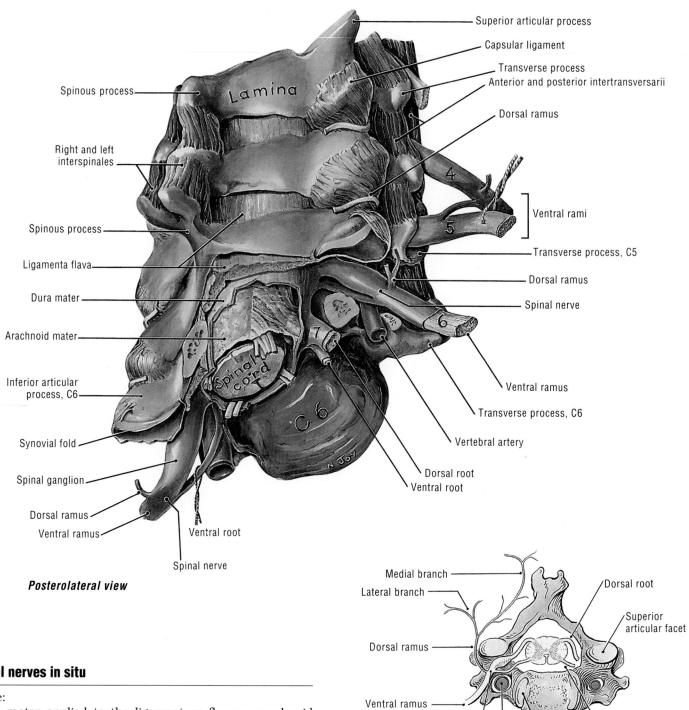

Spinous process — Lamina

Right and left interspinales

Spinous process

Ligamenta flava

Dura mater

Arachnoid mater

Inferior articular process, C6

Synovial fold

Spinal ganglion

Dorsal ramus

Ventral ramus

Ventral root

Spinal nerve

Superior articular process

Capsular ligament

Transverse process
Anterior and posterior intertransversarii

Dorsal ramus

Ventral rami

Transverse process, C5

Dorsal ramus

Spinal nerve

Ventral ramus

Transverse process, C6

Vertebral artery

Dorsal root
Ventral root

Spinal cord

C6

N Joy

Posterolateral view

Medial branch

Lateral branch

Dorsal ramus

Ventral ramus

Spinal nerve

Dorsal root

Superior articular facet

Ventral root

Articular surface of uncovertebral joint

Superior view   Vertebral artery

8.5
Cervical nerves in situ

Observe:

1. Dura mater applied to the ligamentum flavum; arachnoid mater applied to dura and separated from pia mater, by cerebrospinal fluid, which has escaped;

2. A dorsal root and its swelling, the dorsal root (spinal) ganglion; the ventral and dorsal roots, each in a separate dural sheath, uniting beyond the ganglion to form a mixed spinal nerve; the spinal nerve, about 1 cm long, dividing into a small dorsal and a large ventral ramus;

3. The roots and the spinal nerve crossing posterior to the vertebral artery; the dorsal ramus curving dorsally, applied to the root of a superior articular process; the ventral ramus resting on the transverse process, which is grooved to support it.

8.6
The formation of the spinal nerve

This diagram reminds us of the vulnerability of vertebral artery, spinal cord, and nerve roots to arthritic expansion from articular processes and the vertebral body, especially the lateral edge of the superior surface of the body: the uncovertebral joint (joint of Luschka).

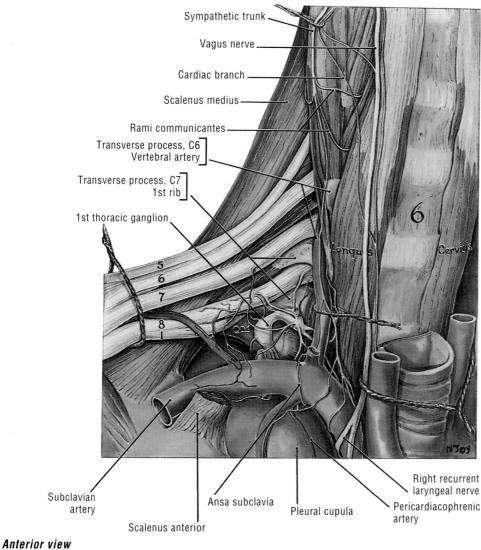

Anterior view labels:
Sympathetic trunk
Vagus nerve
Cardiac branch
Scalenus medius
Rami communicantes
Transverse process, C6
Vertebral artery
Transverse process, C7
1st rib
1st thoracic ganglion

Subclavian artery
Scalenus anterior
Ansa subclavia
Pleural cupula
Right recurrent laryngeal nerve
Pericardiacophrenic artery

Anterior view

8.7
Stellate ganglion and sympathetic trunk

The pleura has been depressed and the vertebral artery retracted.

Observe:

1. The inferior trunk of the branchial plexus (C8 and T1) raised from the groove it occupies on the 1st rib posterior to the subclavian artery; the dorsal scapular artery (not labeled) passing through the plexus;

2. The sympathetic trunk (retracted laterally) sending a communicating branch to the vagus, and gray rami communicantes (postganglionic fibers) to the roots of the cervical nerves, and cardiac branches;

3. The vertebral artery, retracted medially in order to uncover the stellate ganglion (the combined inferior cervical and 1st thoracic ganglia);

4. Fine branches passing from the stellate ganglion to nerves C7, C8, and T1, and to adjacent arteries.

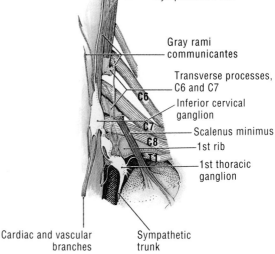

Sympathetic trunk
Gray rami communicantes
Transverse processes, C6 and C7
Inferior cervical ganglion
Scalenus minimus
1st rib
1st thoracic ganglion
Cardiac and vascular branches
Sympathetic trunk

8.8
Brachial plexus and sympathetic trunk

This illustration is a tracing of a photograph of the left side of the specimen in Figure 8.7, revealing a very different pattern; here, the inferior cervical ganglion occupies its more usual position between the transverse process of C7 and the 1st rib, ganglion T1 being on and inferior to the 1st rib.

8.9
Superficial veins

Outside the skull, superficial temporal and maxillary veins form the retromandibular vein whose posterior division unites with the posterior auricular to form the external jugular vein. The facial vein receives the anterior division of the retromandibular vein before emptying into the internal jugular vein.

A - Splenius muscle, *B* - Levator scapulae muscle, *C* - Scalenus medius and scalenus posterior muscles.

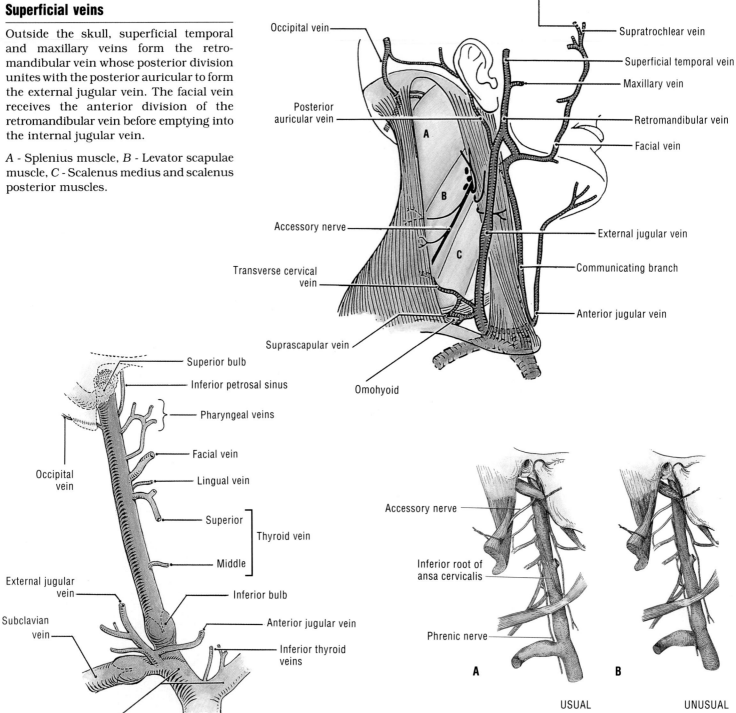

8.10
Internal jugular vein and its tributaries

Note the dilation or bulb at each end of the internal jugular vein. The superior jugular bulb is separated from the floor of the middle ear by a delicate bony plate. The inferior jugular bulb, like the corresponding bulb at the end of the subclavian vein, contains a bicuspid valve that permits the flow of blood toward the heart. There are no valves in the brachiocephalic veins or in the superior vena cava.

8.11
Variable relationships of the accessory, descending cervical, and phrenic nerves to the great veins

The accessory nerve crossed anterior to the internal jugular vein in 70% of 188 instances, and it crossed posterior to it in 30%.

The phrenic nerve (C3, C4, and C5) passes posterior to the site of union of the subclavian, internal jugular, and brachiocephalic veins but, occasionally, the branch from C5 or, less commonly, the entire phrenic nerve, passes anterior to the subclavian vein.

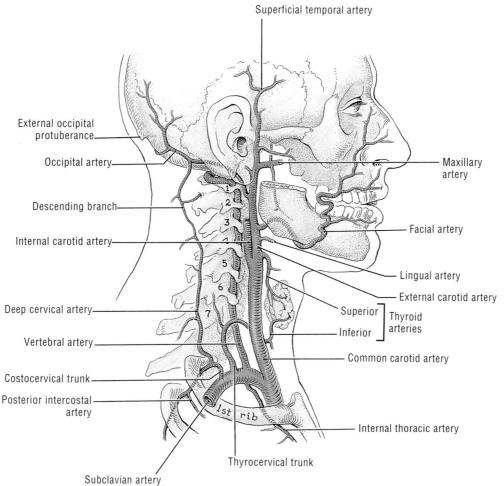

Superficial temporal artery

External occipital
protuberance

Occipital artery

Descending branch

Internal carotid artery

Deep cervical artery

Vertebral artery

Costocervical trunk

Posterior intercostal
artery

Subclavian artery

Maxillary
artery

Facial artery

Lingual artery

External carotid artery

Superior ⎤ Thyroid
Inferior ⎦ arteries

Common carotid artery

Internal thoracic artery

Thyrocervical trunk

1st rib

8.12

The four chief arterial connections between the arch of the aorta and the head

Blood supply to the head comes from the common carotid and subclavian arteries. The vertebral artery, a branch of the subclavian artery, enters the foramen magnum and contributes to the cerebral arterial circle (of Willis). The common carotid artery terminates as the internal and external carotids. In general, the internal carotid supplies structures inside the head and the external carotid supplies the exterior. However, the ophthalmic artery (from the internal carotid) sends supraorbital and supratrochlear arteries to the forehead. Note that the deep cervical artery (from the costocervical trunk) anastomoses with the descending branch of the occipital artery and with branches of the vertebral artery.

8.13

Oblique carotid arteriogram

B - Brachiocephalic artery, *S* - Subclavian artery, *V* - Vertebral artery, *I* - Internal thoracic artery, *C* - Thyrocervical trunk, *CC* - Common carotid artery, *IC* - Internal carotid artery, *EC* - External carotid artery, *T* - Superior thyroid artery, *F* - Facial artery, *L* - Lingual artery, *A* - Ascending pharyngeal artery. (Courtesy of Dr. D. Armstrong, Associate Professor of Radiology, University of Toronto, Toronto, Ontario, Canada.)

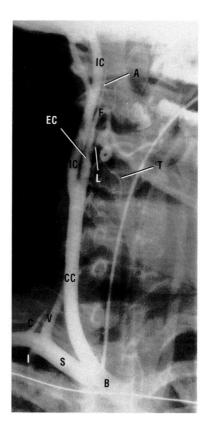

8 : T h e N e c k

559

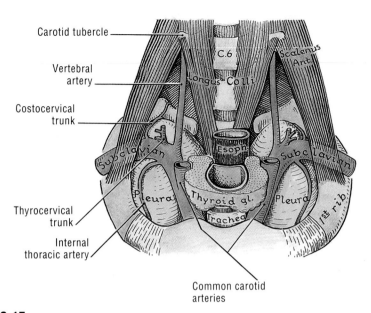

Carotid tubercle — C.6 — Scalenus Ant.

Vertebral artery — Longus Colli

Costocervical trunk — Subclavian

Esoph.

Subclavian

Thyrocervical trunk — Pleura — Thyroid gl. — Pleura — 1st rib

Internal thoracic artery — Trachea

Common carotid arteries

8.15
The vertebral artery

In 6.4% of 1000 half heads, the vertebral artery enters not the foramen of the 6th cervical transverse process but another – the 5th in 4.5%, the 7th in 1.2%, and the 4th in 0.7% (see Adachi B. Anteria vertebralis. In *Das Arteriensystem der Japaner*, vol. 1, p. 138. Kyoto, Japan; 1928).

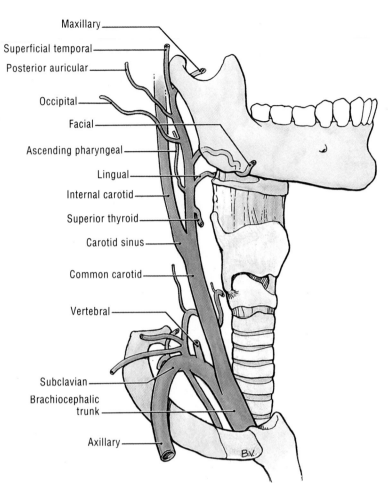

Maxillary
Superficial temporal
Posterior auricular
Occipital
Facial
Ascending pharyngeal
Lingual
Internal carotid
Superior thyroid
Carotid sinus
Common carotid
Vertebral
Subclavian
Brachiocephalic trunk
Axillary

B.V.

8.14
Subclavian and carotid arteries

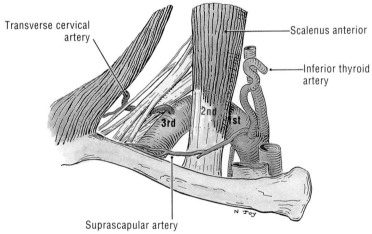

Transverse cervical artery — Scalenus anterior

Inferior thyroid artery

3rd — 2nd — 1st

Suprascapular artery

N Joy

8.17
Branches of the third part of the subclavian artery

Almost as a rule, some branch springs from the third part of this artery, or else from its short second part, and passes laterally through the brachial plexus; the dorsal scapular artery does this in about 50% of cases; the transverse cervical artery in about 20%, and the suprascapular artery in about 10% (see Huelke DF. *A study of the transverse cervical and dorsal scapular arteries.* Anat Rec 1958;132:233).

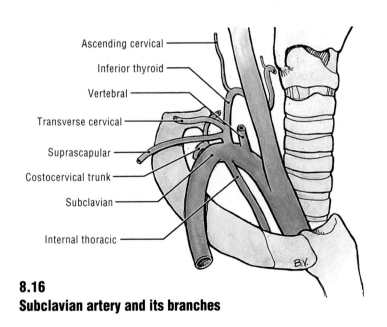

Ascending cervical
Inferior thyroid
Vertebral
Transverse cervical
Suprascapular
Costocervical trunk
Subclavian
Internal thoracic

B.V.

8.16
Subclavian artery and its branches

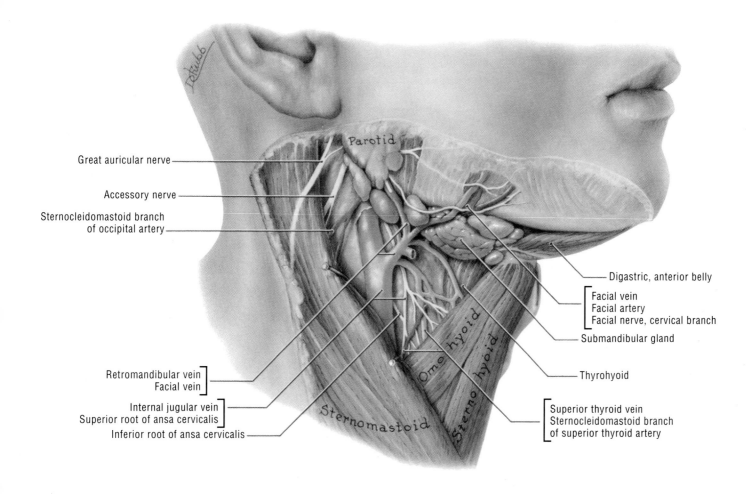

Great auricular nerve

Accessory nerve

Sternocleidomastoid branch
of occipital artery

Parotid

Digastric, anterior belly

Facial vein
Facial artery
Facial nerve, cervical branch

Submandibular gland

Thyrohyoid

Retromandibular vein
Facial vein

Internal jugular vein
Superior root of ansa cervicalis
Inferior root of ansa cervicalis

Superior thyroid vein
Sternocleidomastoid branch
of superior thyroid artery

8.18
Anterior triangle of the neck –
superficial dissection

Observe:

1. The accessory nerve entering the deep
surface of the sternocleidomastoid muscle
about 5 cm inferior to the tip of the mastoid process, and joined along its inferior
border by the sternocleidomastoid branch
of the occipital artery;

2. The internal jugular vein joined anteriorly by several veins, notably the common
facial vein, about the level of the hyoid
bone;

3. The sternocleidomastoid branch of the
superior thyroid artery descending near
the superior border of the omohyoid
muscle;

4. The submandibular gland and lymph
nodes; the retromandibular and facial veins
running superficial to the gland.

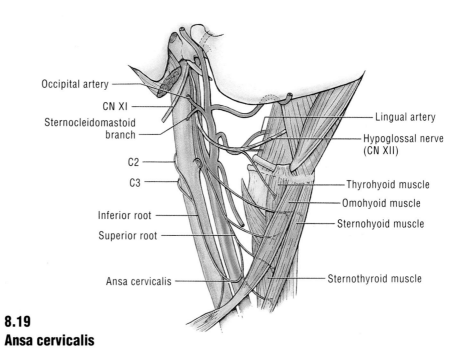

Occipital artery

CN XI

Sternocleidomastoid
branch

C2

C3

Inferior root

Superior root

Ansa cervicalis

Lingual artery

Hypoglossal nerve
(CN XII)

Thyrohyoid muscle

Omohyoid muscle

Sternohyoid muscle

Sternothyroid muscle

8.19
Ansa cervicalis

8.20

Diagram of structures related to the posterior belly of the digastric

Observe:

1. The superficial and key position of the posterior belly of the digastric muscle that runs from the mastoid process to the hyoid bone;

2. All vessels and nerves cross deep to this belly except for: (a) cervical branches of the facial nerve, (b) facial branches of the great auricular nerve, and (c) the external jugular vein and its connections (Fig. 8.8).

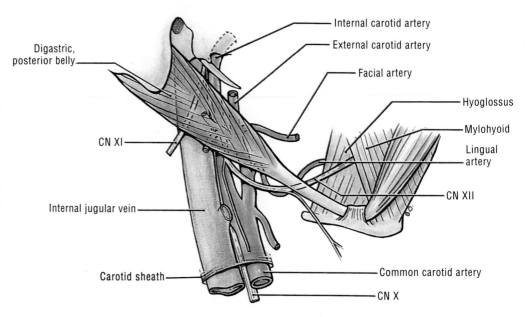

8.21

Diagram of structures related to the hyoid bone

The tip of the greater horn is the reference point for many structures – muscles, nerves, and arteries.

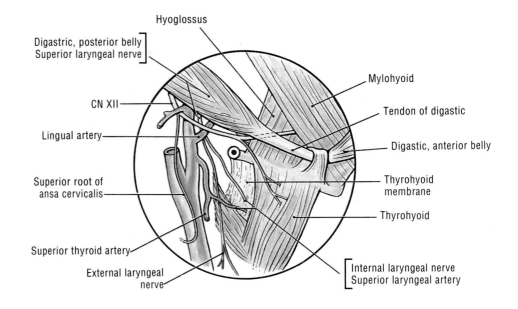

8.22

Origin of the lingual artery

Variation in origin was studied in 211 specimens. In 80%, the superior thyroid, lingual, and facial arteries arose separately as in **A**; in 20%, the lingual and facial arteries arose from a common stem inferiorly (**B**) or high on the external carotid artery (**C**); in one specimen, the superior thyroid and lingual arteries arose from a common stem.

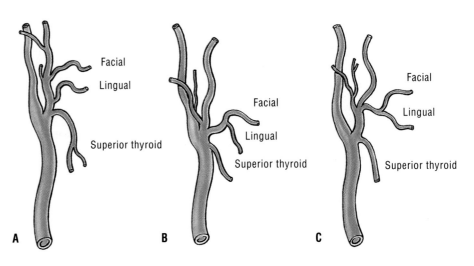

562

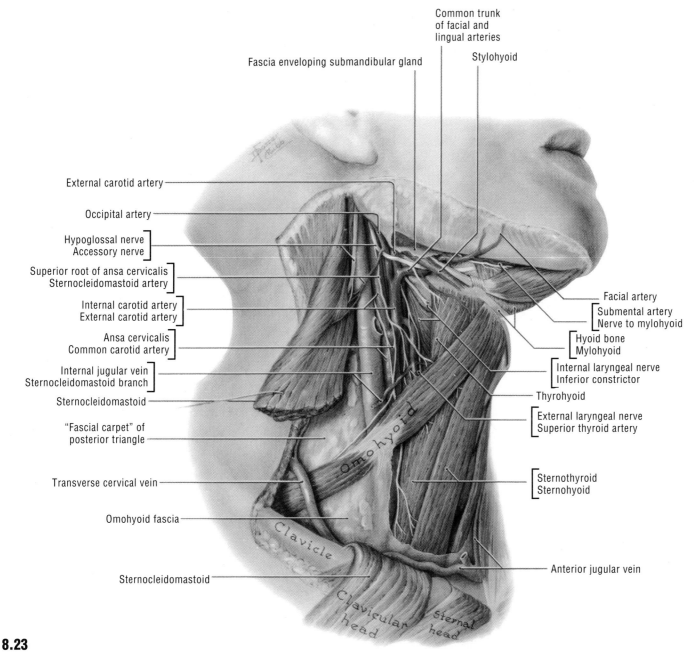

Common trunk
of facial and
lingual arteries

Fascia enveloping submandibular gland

Stylohyoid

External carotid artery

Occipital artery

Hypoglossal nerve
Accessory nerve

Superior root of ansa cervicalis
Sternocleidomastoid artery

Internal carotid artery
External carotid artery

Ansa cervicalis
Common carotid artery

Internal jugular vein
Sternocleidomastoid branch

Sternocleidomastoid

"Fascial carpet" of
posterior triangle

Transverse cervical vein

Omohyoid fascia

Sternocleidomastoid

Facial artery

Submental artery
Nerve to mylohyoid

Hyoid bone
Mylohyoid

Internal laryngeal nerve
Inferior constrictor

Thyrohyoid

External laryngeal nerve
Superior thyroid artery

Sternothyroid
Sternohyoid

Anterior jugular vein

Omohyoid

Clavicle

Clavicular head

Sternal head

8.23
Anterior triangle of the neck, deeper dissection

Observe:

1. The intermediate tendon of the digastric muscle held down to the hyoid bone by a fascial sling; the intermediate tendon of the omohyoid muscle similarly held down to the clavicle;

2. The facial and lingual arteries, here arising by a common stem and passing deep to the stylohyoid and digastric muscles;

3. The thyrohyoid and inferior constrictor muscles forming the floor or medial wall of the carotid triangle;

4. The hypoglossal nerve passing deep to the digastric muscle twice, crossing the internal and external carotid arteries, and giving off two branches: the superior root of the ansa cervicalis and the nerve to the thyrohyoid muscle;

5. The internal and external laryngeal nerves appearing deep to the external carotid artery.

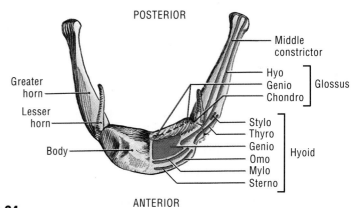

POSTERIOR

Middle
constrictor

Greater
horn

Lesser
horn

Body

Hyo
Genio
Chondro

Glossus

Stylo
Thyro
Genio
Omo
Mylo
Sterno

Hyoid

ANTERIOR

8.24
Hyoid bone

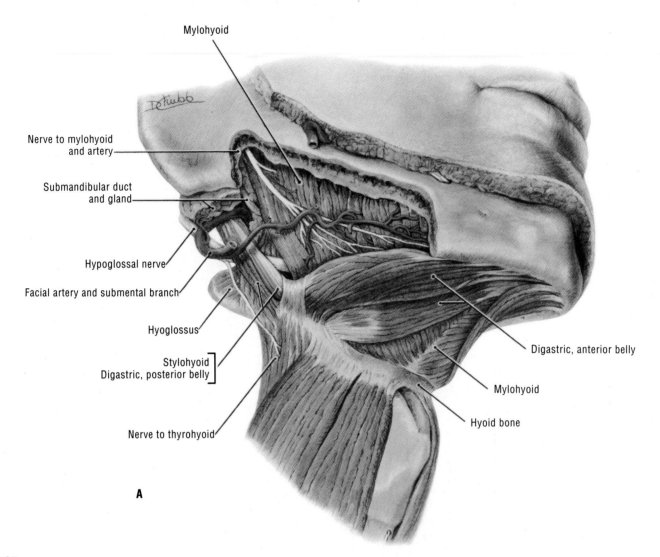

Mylohyoid

Nerve to mylohyoid and artery

Submandibular duct and gland

Hypoglossal nerve

Facial artery and submental branch

Hyoglossus

Stylohyoid
Digastric, posterior belly

Nerve to thyrohyoid

Digastric, anterior belly

Mylohyoid

Hyoid bone

A

8.25
Suprahyoid region–I

Observe in **A**:

1. The stylohyoid and the posterior belly of the digastric muscles forming the posterior side of the submandibular triangle; the facial artery arching superficial to these; the anterior belly of the digastric muscle forming the anterior side; here this belly has an extra origin from the hyoid bone;

2. The mylohyoid muscle forming the medial wall of the triangle and having a free, thick posterior border;

3. The nerve to mylohyoid, which supplies the mylohyoid muscle and anterior belly of the digastric muscle, accompanied by the mylohyoid branch of the inferior alveolar artery posteriorly and by the submental branch of the facial artery anteriorly;

4. The hypoglossal nerve, the submandibular gland, and the submandibular duct passing anteriorly deep to the posterior border of mylohyoid muscle.

B. Diagram of the suprahyoid muscles. Note that the muscles are in four layers: digastric *(D)*, mylohyoid *(M)*, hyoglossus *(H)*, and middle constrictor *(MC)*.

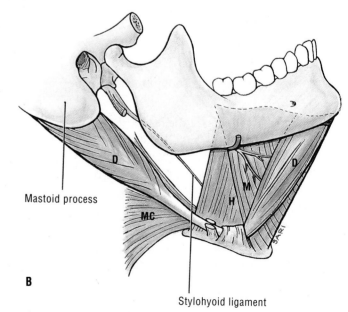

Mastoid process

B

Stylohyoid ligament

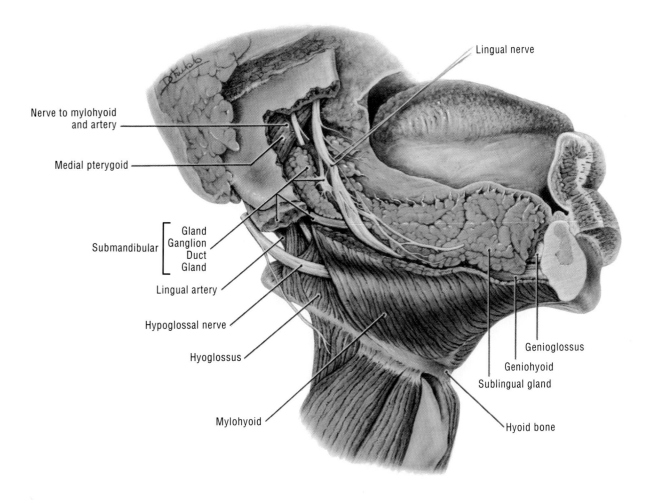

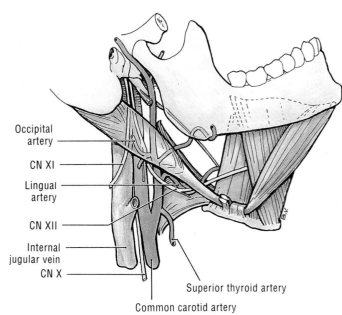

8.26
Suprahyoid region–II

Observe:

1. The cut surface of the mylohyoid muscle becoming progressively thinner as traced anteriorly;

2. The sublingual salivary gland, almond-shaped, almost touching its fellow of the opposite side posterior to the symphysis menti and in contact with the deep part of the submandibular gland posteriorly;

3. The dozen or more fine ducts passing from the superior border of the sublingual gland to open on the sublingual fold;

4. Several individual or detached lobules of the sublingual gland, each having a fine duct, posterior to the main mass of the gland, and labial glands in the lip (unlabeled);

5. The nerve to the mylohyoid and artery (cut short) and the lingual nerve clamped between the medial pterygoid muscle and the ramus of the mandible;

6. The lingual nerve lying between the sublingual gland and the deep or oral part of the submandibular gland; the submandibular ganglion is suspended from this nerve.

8.27
Diagram of the relationships of nerves and vessels to the suprahyoid muscles

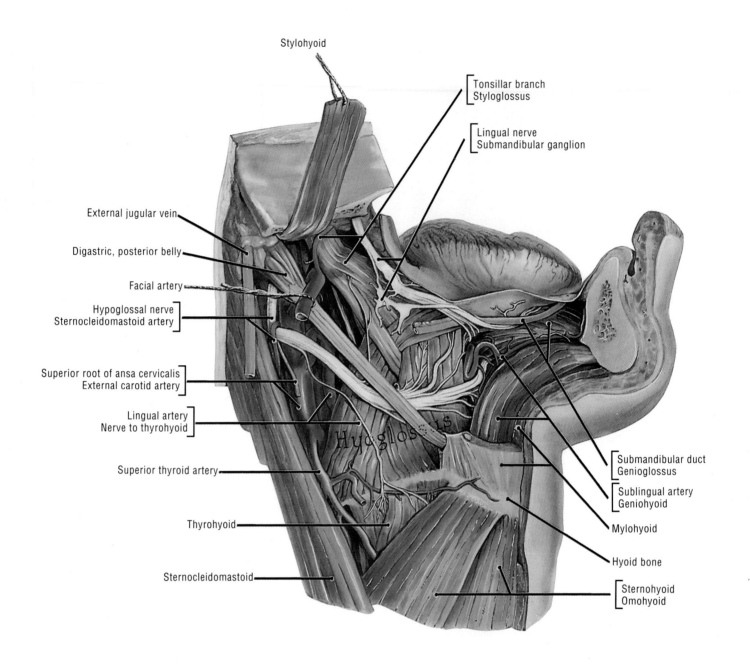

Stylohyoid

Tonsillar branch
Styloglossus

Lingual nerve
Submandibular ganglion

External jugular vein

Digastric, posterior belly

Facial artery

Hypoglossal nerve
Sternocleidomastoid artery

Superior root of ansa cervicalis
External carotid artery

Lingual artery
Nerve to thyrohyoid

Hyoglossus

Superior thyroid artery

Submandibular duct
Genioglossus

Sublingual artery
Geniohyoid

Mylohyoid

Thyrohyoid

Hyoid bone

Sternocleidomastoid

Sternohyoid
Omohyoid

8.28
Suprahyoid region–III

Observe:

1. The stylohyoid muscle is reflected superiorly; the posterior belly of the digastric muscle left in situ, as a landmark;

2. The hyoglossus muscle ascending from the greater horn and body of the hyoid bone to the side of the tongue; the styloglossus muscle, posterosuperiorly, crossed by the tonsillar branch of the facial artery and interdigitating with bundles of the hyoglossus muscle; and the genioglossus muscle, anteriorly, fanning out into the tongue; these are three extrinsic muscles of the tongue, all supplied by the hypoglossal nerve;

3. The hypoglossal nerve, crossed twice by the digastric muscle, crossing twice the lingual artery, and supplying all the muscles of

the tongue, both extrinsic and intrinsic, palatoglossus muscle excepted; the branches of the hypoglossal nerve before the second crossing of the digastric muscle, leaving its inferior border; hence, the wise dissector works along the superior border;

4. The submandibular duct running anteriorly, across the hyoglossus and genioglossus muscles, to its orifice;

5. The lingual nerve in contact with the mandible posteriorly, making a partial spiral around the submandibular duct, and ending in the tongue; the submandibular ganglion suspended from the nerve, and twigs leaving the nerve to supply the mucous membrane.

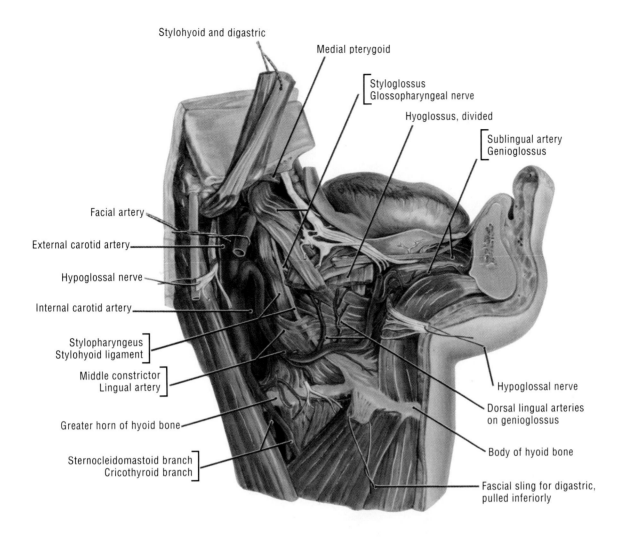

Stylohyoid and digastric

Medial pterygoid

Styloglossus
Glossopharyngeal nerve

Hyoglossus, divided

Sublingual artery
Genioglossus

Facial artery

External carotid artery

Hypoglossal nerve

Internal carotid artery

Stylopharyngeus
Stylohyoid ligament

Middle constrictor
Lingual artery

Greater horn of hyoid bone

Sternocleidomastoid branch
Cricothyroid branch

Hypoglossal nerve

Dorsal lingual arteries
on genioglossus

Body of hyoid bone

Fascial sling for digastric,
pulled inferiorly

8.29
Suprahyoid region–IV

The stylohyoid and posterior belly of the digastric muscles are reflected superiorly, the hypoglossal nerve is divided, and the hyoglossus muscle is mostly removed.

Observe:

1. The lingual artery, crossed twice by the hypoglossal nerve; then passing deep to the hyoglossus muscle, parallel to greater horn of hyoid bone, and lying on the middle constrictor muscle, stylohyoid ligament, and the genioglossus muscle; finally ascending at the anterior border of the hyoglossus muscle, which partly overlaps it, and turning into the tongue as the deep lingual arteries (see Fig. 8.30);

2. The branches of the lingual artery: (a) muscular, (b) dorsal lingual, that reach the tonsil bed, and (c) the sublingual, which supplies the sublingual gland and the anterior part of the floor of the mouth;

3. The stylopharyngeus muscle, appearing deep to the styloglossus muscle and disappearing deep to the middle constrictor muscle; the glossopharyngeal nerve, not making the usual spiral descent lateral to the stylopharyngeus muscle but descending medial to it.

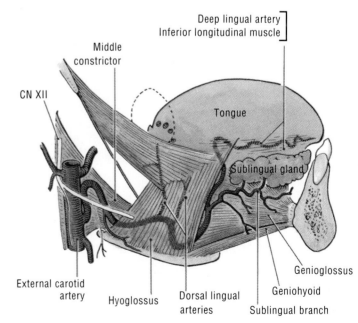

Deep lingual artery
Inferior longitudinal muscle

Middle constrictor

CN XII

Tongue

Sublingual gland

External carotid artery

Hyoglossus

Dorsal lingual arteries

Genioglossus

Geniohyoid

Sublingual branch

8.30
Diagram of the course of the lingual artery

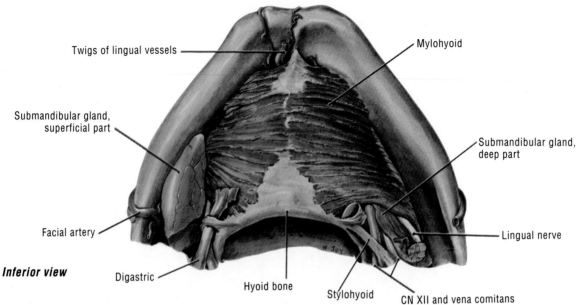

Twigs of lingual vessels

Mylohyoid

Submandibular gland, superficial part

Submandibular gland, deep part

Facial artery

Lingual nerve

Inferior view

Digastric

Hyoid bone

Stylohyoid

CN XII and vena comitans

8.31
The mylohyoid muscles of the floor of the mouth

The anterior bellies of the digastric muscles have been removed. Observe:

1. The right and left mylohyoid muscles, which together form the "oral diaphragm," arising from the mylohyoid line of the mandible, and inserted into an indefinite median raphe and into the hyoid bone;

2. The submandibular gland turning round the posterior border of the mylohyoid muscle;

3. The hypoglossal nerve and its companion vein passing deep to the same posterior border; the lingual nerve applied to the mandible.

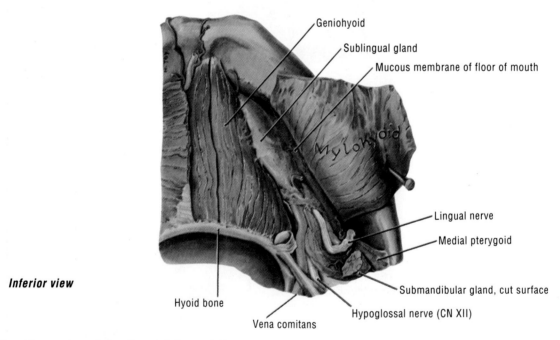

Geniohyoid

Sublingual gland

Mucous membrane of floor of mouth

Mylohyoid

Lingual nerve

Medial pterygoid

Inferior view

Submandibular gland, cut surface

Hyoid bone

Hypoglossal nerve (CN XII)

Vena comitans

8.32
The geniohyoid muscles of the floor of the mouth

The left mylohyoid muscle and part of the right are reflected. Observe:

1. The geniohyoid muscle, extending from the mental spine of the mandible to the body of the hyoid bone;

2. The hypoglossal nerve, deep part of the submandibular gland, and lingual nerve;

3. The areolar cover of the sublingual gland, and lateral to it the mucous membrane of the mouth with twigs of the sublingual artery.

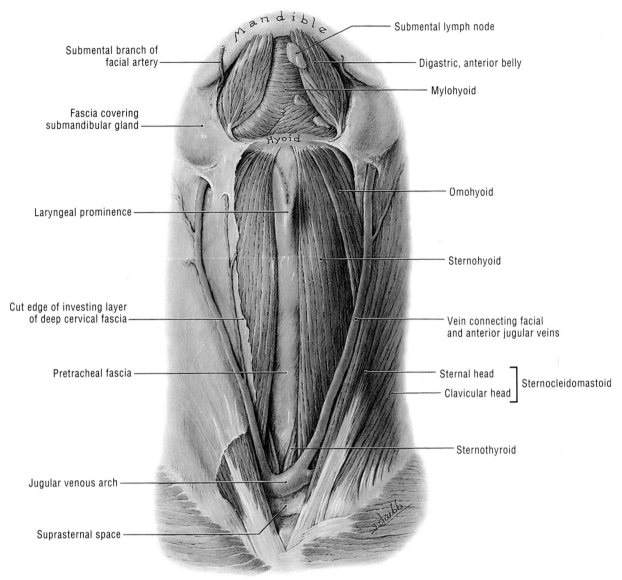

Submental branch of
facial artery

Fascia covering
submandibular gland

Laryngeal prominence

Cut edge of investing layer
of deep cervical fascia

Pretracheal fascia

Jugular venous arch

Suprasternal space

Mandible

Submental lymph node

Digastric, anterior belly

Mylohyoid

Hyoid

Omohyoid

Sternohyoid

Vein connecting facial
and anterior jugular veins

Sternal head
Clavicular head — Sternocleidomastoid

Sternothyroid

8.33
Anterior neck – superficial dissection

Observe:

1. This region extends from the mandible superiorly to the sternum inferiorly and is divided by the hyoid bone into a suprahyoid and an infrahyoid part;

2. The suprahyoid part or submental triangle (floor of the mouth) having the anterior bellies of the digastric muscles for its sides, the hyoid bone for its base, the mylohyoid muscles for its floor, and some submental lymph nodes for contents;

3. The infrahyoid part, shaped like an elongated diamond, and bounded on each side by the sternohyoid muscle superiorly and the sternothyroid muscle inferiorly;

4. The suprasternal (fascial) space, containing a cross-connecting vein called the jugular venous arch; in this specimen, the anterior jugular veins were absent, as such, in the median part of the neck, but were present superior to the clavicles.

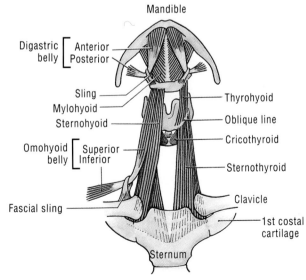

Mandible

Digastric { Anterior
belly { Posterior

Sling
Mylohyoid
Sternohyoid

Omohyoid { Superior
belly { Inferior

Fascial sling

Thyrohyoid

Oblique line

Cricothyroid

Sternothyroid

Clavicle

1st costal
cartilage

Sternum

8.34
Diagram of the infrahyoid (strap) muscles

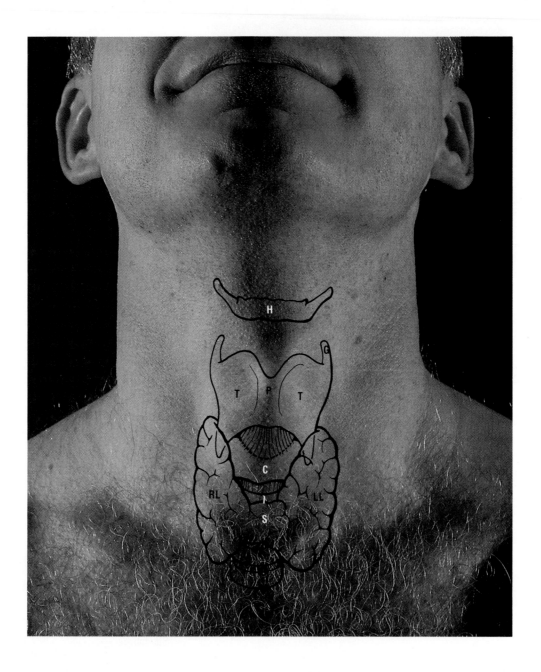

8.35
Anterior neck, location of larynx, trachea, hyoid bone, and thyroid gland

Observe:

1. The hyoid bone (H) lies at the angle between the floor of the mouth and the anterior aspect of the neck; the greater horn of one side of the hyoid bone is palpable only when the greater horn of the opposite side is steadied;

2. The laminae of the thyroid cartilage (T) projecting anteriorly above the point of union to form the laryngeal prominence (P); the palpable superior horn (G);

3. The arch of the cricoid cartilage (C) projects further anteriorly than the rings of the trachea and is thereby readily identified in life; it is the guide to the level of C6;

4. The first tracheal ring (I);

5. The thyroid gland consisting of right (RL) and left (LL) lobes and a connecting isthmus (S).

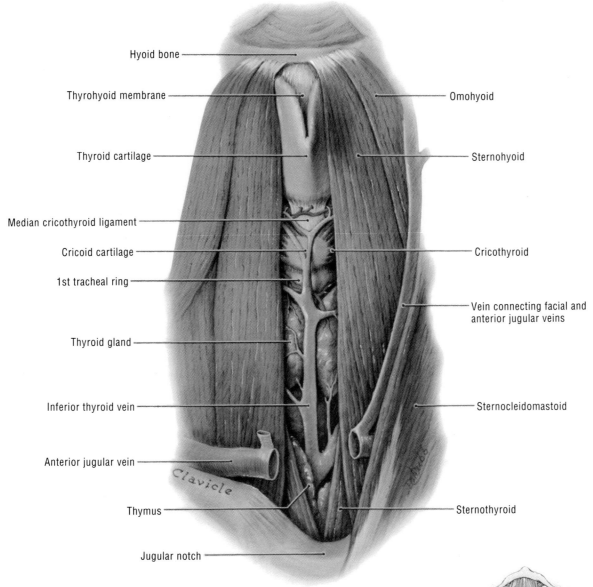

Hyoid bone

Thyrohyoid membrane

Omohyoid

Thyroid cartilage

Sternohyoid

Median cricothyroid ligament

Cricoid cartilage

Cricothyroid

1st tracheal ring

Vein connecting facial and anterior jugular veins

Thyroid gland

Inferior thyroid vein

Sternocleidomastoid

Anterior jugular vein

Clavicle

Thymus

Sternothyroid

Jugular notch

8.36
Anterior neck

Superficial infrahyoid (strap) muscles.

Observe:

1. The structures in the median plane labeled on the left side of the picture;

2. The unlabeled anastomoses between the cricothyroid arteries, between the superior thyroid arteries, and between the anterior jugular veins (excised);

3. The enlarged thymus projecting superiorly from the thorax;

4. The two superficial depressors of the larynx ("strap muscles"): omohyoid (superior belly) and sternohyoid.

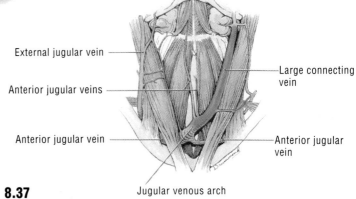

External jugular vein

Large connecting vein

Anterior jugular veins

Anterior jugular vein

Anterior jugular vein

Jugular venous arch

8.37
Large connecting vein

A small vein that lies along the anterior border of the sternocleidomastoid muscle and connects the facial vein to the anterior jugular vein may attain great size. It may, indeed, be greater than even the internal jugular vein and it is, at times, mistaken for it.

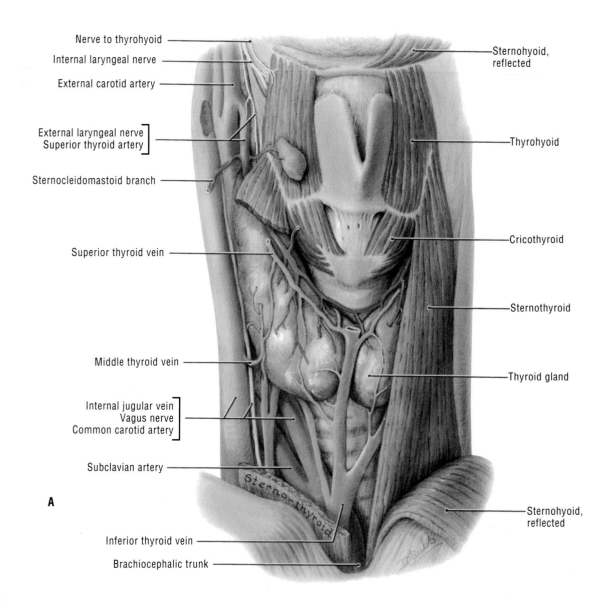

Nerve to thyrohyoid

Internal laryngeal nerve

External carotid artery

External laryngeal nerve
Superior thyroid artery

Sternocleidomastoid branch

Superior thyroid vein

Middle thyroid vein

Internal jugular vein
Vagus nerve
Common carotid artery

Subclavian artery

A

Inferior thyroid vein

Brachiocephalic trunk

Sternohyoid, reflected

Thyrohyoid

Cricothyroid

Sternothyroid

Thyroid gland

Sternohyoid, reflected

8.38
Thyroid gland

A. Anterior neck. On the left side, the sternohyoid and omohyoid muscles are reflected exposing the deeply lying sternothyroid and the thyrohyoid muscles; on the right side, the sternothyroid muscle is largely excised.

Observe:

1. The two lobes of the thyroid gland, united across the median plane by an isthmus;

2. The surface network of veins on the gland, drained by the superior, middle, and inferior thyroid veins;

3. The right lobe of the gland, overlying the common carotid artery; the superior thyroid artery and external laryngeal nerve;

4. An accessory thyroid gland, or detached lobule, is occasionally present.

B. Relations of the thyroid gland and the deep strap muscles.

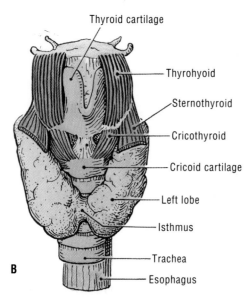

Thyroid cartilage

Thyrohyoid

Sternothyroid

Cricothyroid

Cricoid cartilage

Left lobe

Isthmus

Trachea

B

Esophagus

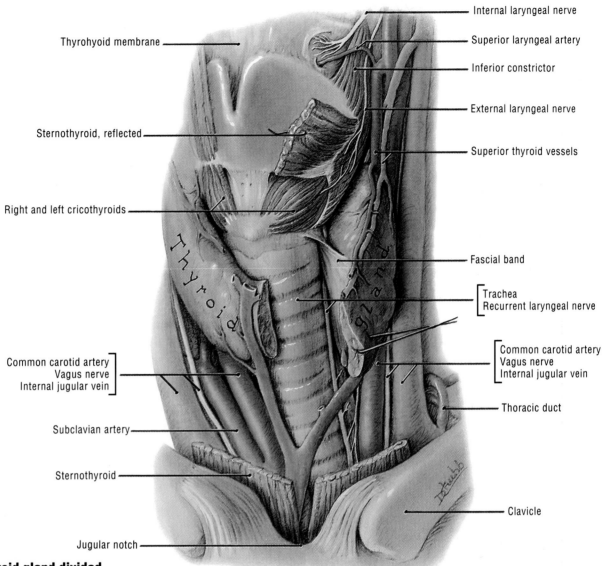

Thyrohyoid membrane

Sternothyroid, reflected

Right and left cricothyroids

Common carotid artery
Vagus nerve
Internal jugular vein

Subclavian artery

Sternothyroid

Jugular notch

Internal laryngeal nerve

Superior laryngeal artery

Inferior constrictor

External laryngeal nerve

Superior thyroid vessels

Fascial band

Trachea
Recurrent laryngeal nerve

Common carotid artery
Vagus nerve
Internal jugular vein

Thoracic duct

Clavicle

8.39
Anterior neck – thyroid gland divided

The isthmus of the thyroid gland is divided and the left lobe is retracted. Observe:

1. The retaining fascial band, attaching the capsule of the thyroid gland to the crico-tracheal ligament and cricoid cartilage;

2. The left recurrent laryngeal nerve, on the lateral aspect of the trachea, just ante-rior to the angle between the trachea and esophagus, and posterior to the retaining band;

3. The internal laryngeal nerve, running along the superior border of the inferior constrictor muscle, and piercing the thyrohyoid membrane as several branches;

4. The external laryngeal nerve, applied to the inferior constrictor, running along the anterior border of the superior thyroid artery, passing deep to the insertion of the sternothyroid muscle, and giving twigs to the inferior constrictor muscle and piercing it before ending in the cricothyroid muscle.

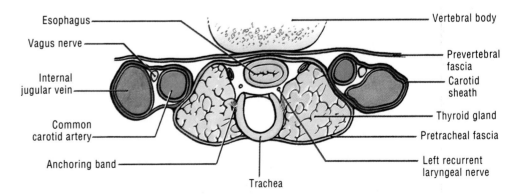

Esophagus

Vagus nerve

Internal
jugular vein

Common
carotid artery

Anchoring band

Trachea

Vertebral body

Prevertebral
fascia

Carotid
sheath

Thyroid gland

Pretracheal fascia

Left recurrent
laryngeal nerve

8.40
Relations of the thyroid gland

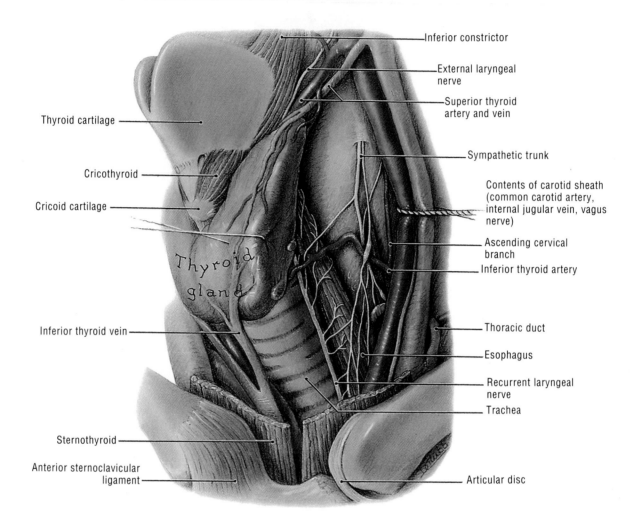

Thyroid cartilage

Cricothyroid

Cricoid cartilage

Thyroid gland

Inferior thyroid vein

Sternothyroid

Anterior sternoclavicular ligament

Inferior constrictor

External laryngeal nerve

Superior thyroid artery and vein

Sympathetic trunk

Contents of carotid sheath (common carotid artery, internal jugular vein, vagus nerve)

Ascending cervical branch

Inferior thyroid artery

Thoracic duct

Esophagus

Recurrent laryngeal nerve

Trachea

Articular disc

8.41
Root of the neck, left side

Observe:

1. The three structures contained in the carotid sheath (internal jugular vein, common carotid artery, and vagus nerve), retracted;

2. The esophagus, bulging to the left of the trachea; it does not bulge to the right;

3. The left recurrent laryngeal nerve, ascending on the lateral aspect of the trachea just anterior to the angle between the trachea and esophagus, giving twigs to the esophagus and trachea (not in view), and receiving twigs from the sympathetic trunk;

4. The thoracic duct, passing from the lateral aspect of the esophagus to its termination and, in so doing, arching immediately posterior to the three structures contained in the carotid sheath;

5. The middle cervical (sympathetic) ganglion, here in two parts: one anterior to the inferior thyroid artery; the other, just superior to the thoracic duct, is called the vertebral ganglion.

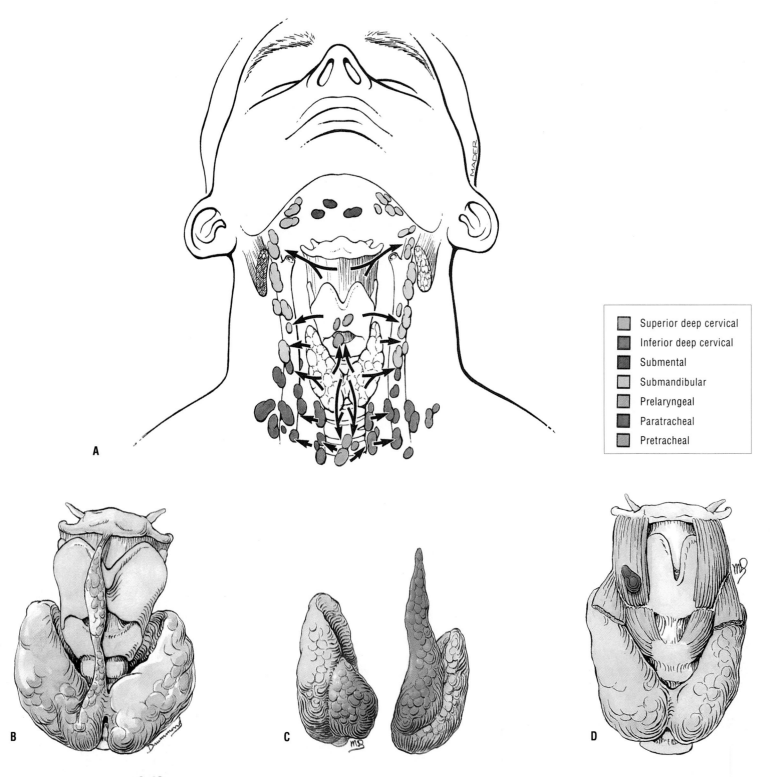

A

■	Superior deep cervical
■	Inferior deep cervical
■	Submental
□	Submandibular
■	Prelaryngeal
■	Paratracheal
■	Pretracheal

8.42
Thyroid gland

A. Lymphatic drainage of the thyroid gland, larynx, and trachea. **B**, **C**, **D**. Variations: **B**. Accessory thyroid tissue. This may occur along the course of the thyroglossal duct. **C**. Pyramidal lobe – absence of isthmus. About 50% of glands have a pyramidal lobe that extends from near the isthmus to, or toward, the hyoid bone; the isthmus is occasionally absent, the gland being then in two parts. **D**. An accessory thyroid gland that may occur between the suprahyoid region and the arch of the aorta.

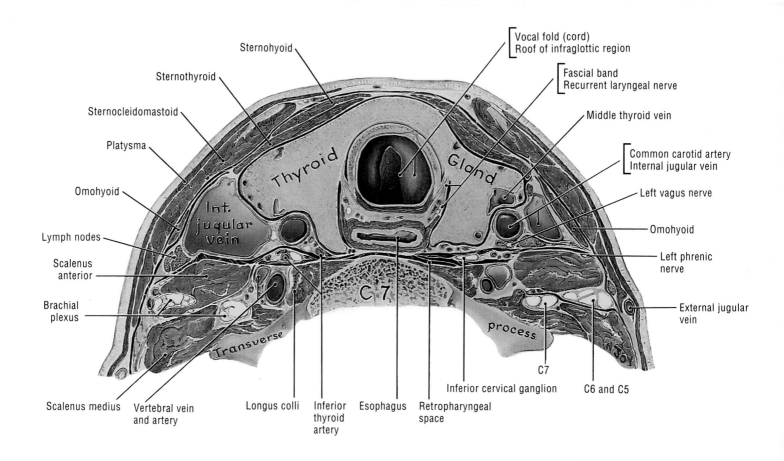

Sternohyoid

Sternothyroid

Sternocleidomastoid

Platysma

Omohyoid

Lymph nodes

Scalenus anterior

Brachial plexus

Scalenus medius

Vertebral vein and artery

Longus colli

Inferior thyroid artery

Esophagus

Retropharyngeal space

Inferior cervical ganglion

C7

C6 and C5

External jugular vein

Left phrenic nerve

Omohyoid

Left vagus nerve

Common carotid artery
Internal jugular vein

Middle thyroid vein

Fascial band
Recurrent laryngeal nerve

Vocal fold (cord)
Roof of infraglottic region

Thyroid

Gland

Int. jugular vein

C 7

Transverse

process

8.43
Transverse section of neck through the thyroid gland

Observe:

1. The thyroid gland, within its sheath, asymmetrically enlarged and overflowing the carotid sheath and its contents (common carotid artery, internal jugular vein, and vagus nerve) on one side and thrusting it laterally on the other;

2. The internal jugular veins, of unequal size as sometimes happens, and usually unequal vertebral arteries;

3. The retropharyngeal space of loose areolar tissue, extending far laterally posterior to the carotid sheath; the approach to the space is from the posterior border to the sternocleidomastoid muscle;

4. The scalenus anterior muscle deep to the posterior border of the sternocleidomastoid muscle;

5. The vertebral artery and vein between the longus colli and the scalenus anterior muscles;

6. The brachial plexus passing inferolaterally between the scalenus anterior and the scalenus medius muscles;

7. The inferior thyroid artery (sectioned twice) and the middle cervical ganglion on a plane between the carotid sheath and the vertebral artery;

8. The fascial band that retains the thyroid gland and, posterior to it, the recurrent laryngeal nerve and the inferior laryngeal artery;

9. The vocal folds and the conus elasticus (cricovocal membranes), covered with mucous membrane; hence, air expelled forcibly from the lung would blow the vocal folds apart;

10. Note that the rich blood supply of the thyroid gland is from the superior thyroid artery, a branch of the external carotid, which enters it superficially, and the inferior thyroid artery, a branch of the thyrocervical trunk of the subclavian artery, which enters the deep surface of the gland.

8.44
Fascia of the neck, transverse section

Observe:

1. Pretracheal fascia (orange): a thin sheath surrounding the thyroid gland, esophagus, and trachea;

2. Carotid sheath (purple): surrounding the carotid artery, vagus nerve, and (loosely) the internal jugular vein;

3. Prevertebral fascia (blue): sheathes the muscles associated with the vertebrae; as components of the brachial plexus emerge in their gutter between the scalenus anterior and medius muscles, they carry an investment of this fascia forming the axillary sheath;

4. Investing fascia (red): surrounds the neck.

1 - Esophagus, *2* - Trachea, *3* - Thyroid gland, *4* - Trapezius, *5* - Sternocleidomastoid, *6* - Sternohyoid, *7* - Omohyoid, *8* - Sternothyroid, *9* - Common carotid artery, *10* - Internal jugular vein, *11* - Vagus nerve.

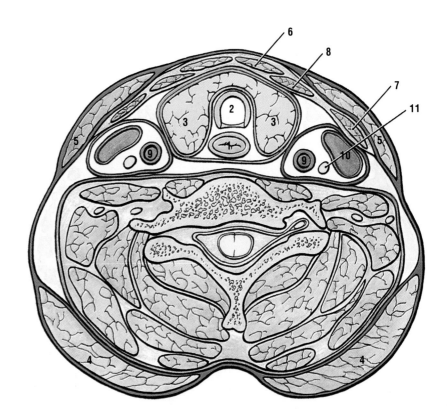

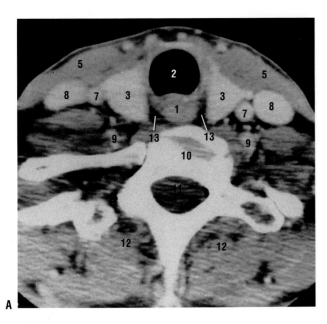

8.45
Transverse scans of the neck through the thyroid gland

A. CT (computed tomographic) scan through the lobes of the thyroid gland. (Courtesy of Dr. M. Keller, Assistant Professor of Radiology, University of Toronto, Toronto, Ontario, Canada.)

B. MRI (magnetic resonance image) through the isthmus of the thyroid gland. (Courtesy of Dr. W. Kucharczyk, Clinical Director of Tri-Hospital Resonance Centre, Toronto, Ontario, Canada.)

1 - Esophagus, *2* - Trachea, *3* - Lobes of thyroid gland, *4* - Thyroid isthmus, *5* - Sternocleidomastoid, *6* - Strap muscles, *7* - Common carotid artery, *8* - Internal jugular vein, *9* - Vertebral artery, *10* - Vertebral body, *11* - Spinal cord in cerebrospinal fluid, *12* - Deep muscles of back, *13* - Retropharyngeal space.

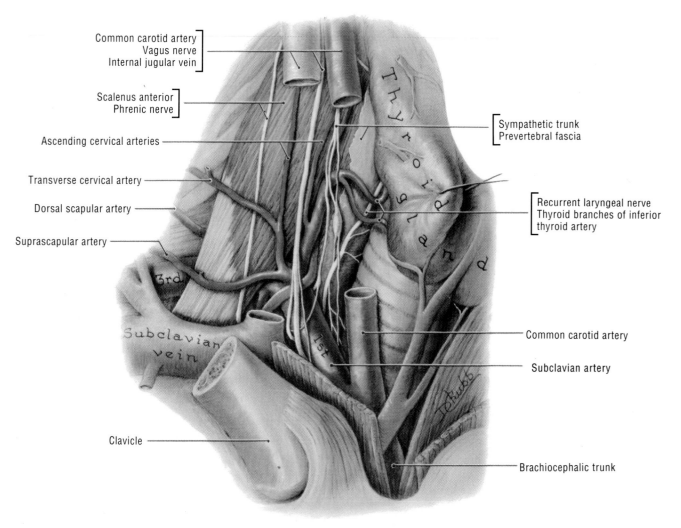

Common carotid artery
Vagus nerve
Internal jugular vein

Scalenus anterior
Phrenic nerve

Ascending cervical arteries

Transverse cervical artery

Dorsal scapular artery

Suprascapular artery

Clavicle

Sympathetic trunk
Prevertebral fascia

Recurrent laryngeal nerve
Thyroid branches of inferior
thyroid artery

Common carotid artery

Subclavian artery

Brachiocephalic trunk

8.46
Root of the neck, right side

The clavicle is removed, sections are taken from the common carotid artery and internal jugular vein, and the right lobe of the thyroid gland is retracted.

Observe:

1. The brachiocephalic trunk dividing posterior to the sternoclavicular joint into the right common carotid and right subclavian arteries;

2. The scalenus anterior muscle, dividing the subclavian artery into three parts and separating the second part from the subclavian vein; this vein, lying anteroinferior to the artery joins the internal jugular vein at the medial border of the scalenus anterior muscle to form the brachiocephalic vein;

3. Running vertically on the obliquely placed scalenus anterior muscle: (a) the common carotid artery, internal jugular vein, and vagus nerve (inside the carotid sheath); (b) the sympathetic trunk posterior to the common carotid artery (outside the sheath); (c) the ascending cervical artery (here represented by two vessels); and (d) most lateral of all, the phrenic nerve;

4. The vagus nerve, crossing the first part of the subclavian artery, and giving off an (inferior) cardiac branch and the right recurrent laryngeal nerve; the latter recurring inferior to the artery, crossing posterior to the common carotid artery on its way to the lateral aspect of the trachea, and giving twigs to the trachea and esophagus, and receiving twigs from the sympathetic trunk;

5. The middle cervical (sympathetic) ganglion is not labeled;

6. The thyrocervical trunk (not labeled), dividing into the inferior thyroid artery, which takes an S-shaped course, and the transverse cervical and suprascapular arteries, which cross the scalenus anterior muscle;

7. The dorsal scapular branch of the transverse cervical artery, springing from the second or third part of the subclavian artery; the vertebral vein (not labeled) crossing the first part of the artery.

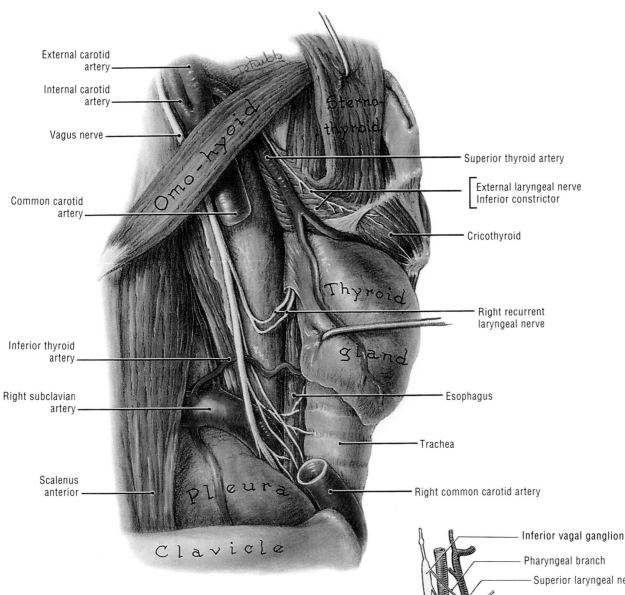

External carotid
artery

Internal carotid
artery

Vagus nerve

Common carotid
artery

Inferior thyroid
artery

Right subclavian
artery

Scalenus
anterior

Omo-hyoid

Sterno-
thyroid

Superior thyroid artery

External laryngeal nerve
Inferior constrictor

Cricothyroid

Thyroid

Right recurrent
laryngeal nerve

gland

Esophagus

Trachea

Right common carotid artery

Pleura

Clavicle

8.47
Anomalous right recurrent laryngeal nerve and subclavian artery

Occasionally, the right subclavian artery springs directly from the aortic arch, as its fourth branch, and passes posterior to the trachea and esophagus. For embryological reasons, the right recurrent nerve, having no artery around which to recur, takes an almost direct course to the larynx. As would be expected, many of its esophageal and tracheal branches then spring directly from the parent vagus nerve. The inferior thyroid artery here springs directly from the subclavian artery; the vertebral and internal thoracic arteries are not labeled.

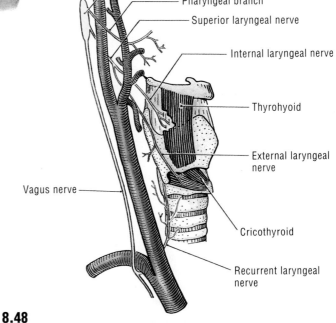

Inferior vagal ganglion

Pharyngeal branch

Superior laryngeal nerve

Internal laryngeal nerve

Thyrohyoid

External laryngeal
nerve

Vagus nerve

Cricothyroid

Recurrent laryngeal
nerve

8.48
Laryngeal branches of right vagus nerve

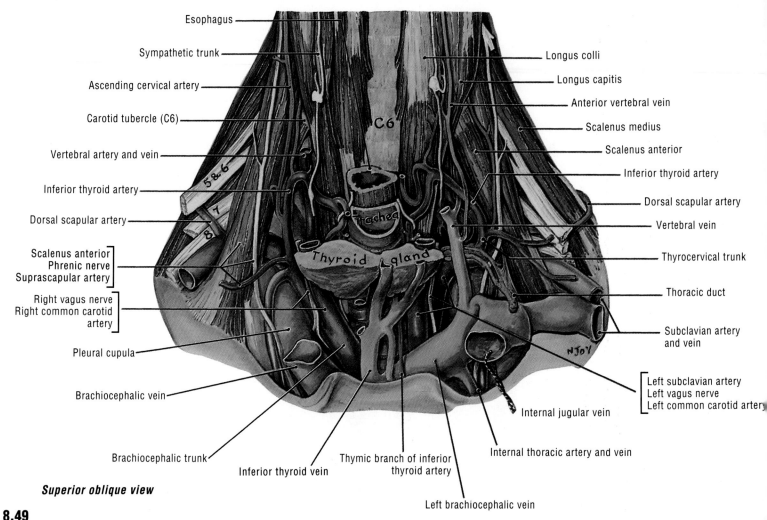

Esophagus

Sympathetic trunk

Ascending cervical artery

Carotid tubercle (C6)

Vertebral artery and vein

Inferior thyroid artery

Dorsal scapular artery

Scalenus anterior
Phrenic nerve
Suprascapular artery

Right vagus nerve
Right common carotid
artery

Pleural cupula

Brachiocephalic vein

Longus colli

Longus capitis

Anterior vertebral vein

Scalenus medius

Scalenus anterior

Inferior thyroid artery

Dorsal scapular artery

Vertebral vein

Thyrocervical trunk

Thoracic duct

Subclavian artery
and vein

Left subclavian artery
Left vagus nerve
Left common carotid artery

Internal jugular vein

Brachiocephalic trunk

Inferior thyroid vein

Thymic branch of inferior
thyroid artery

Internal thoracic artery and vein

Left brachiocephalic vein

Superior oblique view

8.49
Root of the neck

Observe:

1. *Laterally:* the pleural cupola, rising superior to the sternal end of the 1st rib; the subclavian artery, which arches over the pleura, divided into three unequal parts by the scalenus anterior muscle; the third part of the artery and the brachial plexus appearing between the scalenus anterior and scalenus medius muscles;

2. The phrenic nerve, descending almost vertically and crossing the scalenus anterior muscle obliquely, then lying on the pleura and crossing anterior to the internal thoracic artery before meeting the right brachiocephalic vein;

3. *In the median plane:* the esophagus applied to the vertebral column, the trachea applied to the esophagus, the thyroid gland applied to the trachea;

4. *Lateral to these median structures:* the carotid sheath surrounding the artery, vein, and nerve; the vagus nerves descending on the lateral side of the common carotid artery; the inferior thyroid artery arching medially to reach the thyroid gland as two branches, a superior and inferior; the recurrent laryngeal nerve bears a varying relationship to these arteries;

5. The thoracic duct pulled inferiorly by the reflected internal jugular vein.

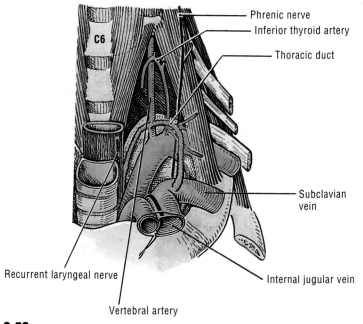

Phrenic nerve

Inferior thyroid artery

Thoracic duct

Subclavian
vein

Internal jugular vein

Recurrent laryngeal nerve

Vertebral artery

8.50
Termination of the thoracic duct

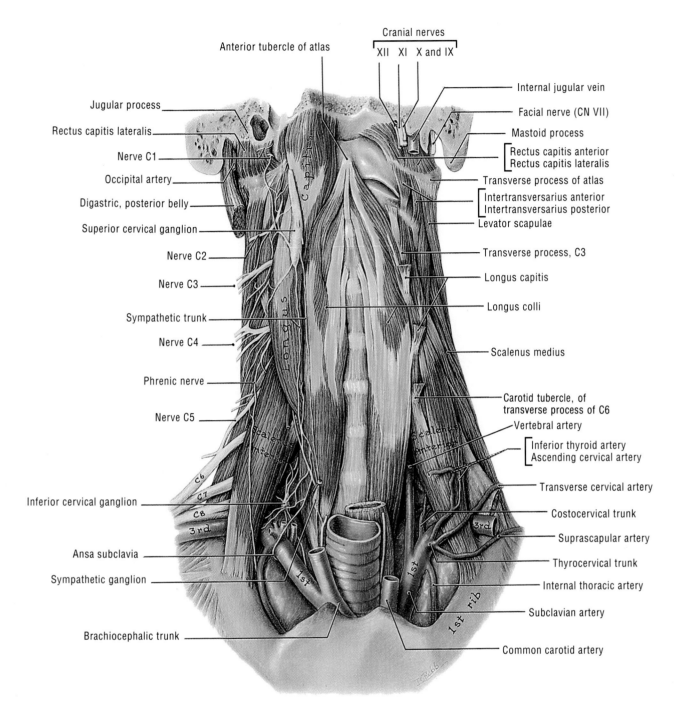

Cranial nerves
XII XI X and IX

Anterior tubercle of atlas

Jugular process

Rectus capitis lateralis

Nerve C1

Occipital artery

Digastric, posterior belly

Superior cervical ganglion

Nerve C2

Nerve C3

Sympathetic trunk

Nerve C4

Phrenic nerve

Nerve C5

Inferior cervical ganglion

Ansa subclavia

Sympathetic ganglion

Brachiocephalic trunk

Internal jugular vein

Facial nerve (CN VII)

Mastoid process

Rectus capitis anterior
Rectus capitis lateralis

Transverse process of atlas

Intertransversarius anterior
Intertransversarius posterior

Levator scapulae

Transverse process, C3

Longus capitis

Longus colli

Scalenus medius

Carotid tubercle, of
transverse process of C6

Vertebral artery

Inferior thyroid artery
Ascending cervical artery

Transverse cervical artery

Costocervical trunk

Suprascapular artery

Thyrocervical trunk

Internal thoracic artery

Subclavian artery

Common carotid artery

8.51
Prevertebral region: root of the neck

On the left side of the body, the longus capitis muscle is removed.

Observe:

1. The prevertebral and deep lateral muscles of the neck; of these muscles, three – the scalenus anterior, longus capitis, and longus colli muscles – are attached to the anterior tubercles of the transverse processes of vertebrae C3, C4, C5, and C6;

2. The transverse process of the atlas joined to the transverse process of the axis by intertransverse muscles and joined simi-

larly to the occipital bone by the rectus capitis lateralis muscle; the internal jugular vein crosses these structures;

3. The cervical plexus arising from ventral rami, C1, C2, C3, and C4; the brachial plexus from C5, C6, C7, C8, and T1;

4. The sympathetic trunk and ganglia and its gray rami communicantes;

5. The subclavian artery and its branches.

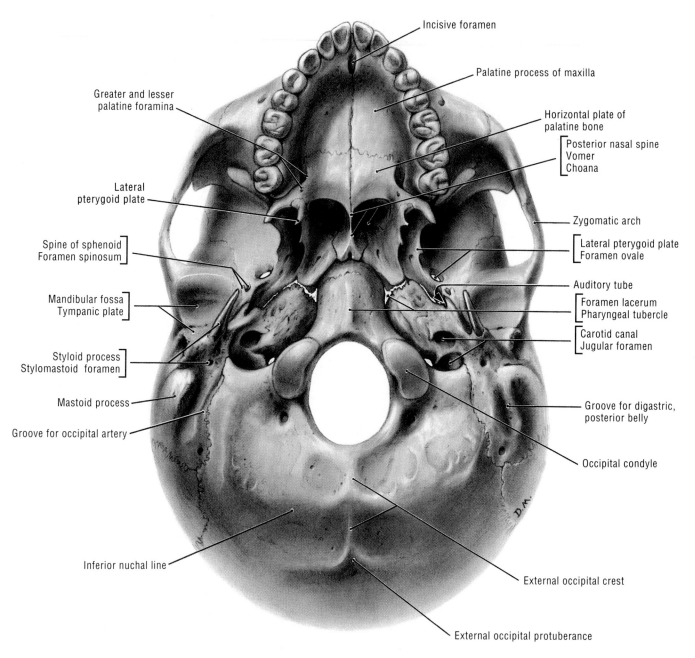

Incisive foramen

Palatine process of maxilla

Greater and lesser
palatine foramina

Horizontal plate of
palatine bone

Posterior nasal spine
Vomer
Choana

Lateral
pterygoid plate

Zygomatic arch

Lateral pterygoid plate
Foramen ovale

Spine of sphenoid
Foramen spinosum

Auditory tube

Foramen lacerum
Pharyngeal tubercle

Mandibular fossa
Tympanic plate

Carotid canal
Jugular foramen

Styloid process
Stylomastoid foramen

Mastoid process

Groove for digastric,
posterior belly

Groove for occipital artery

Occipital condyle

Inferior nuchal line

External occipital crest

External occipital protuberance

8.52
Exterior of the base of the skull–I

Observe:

1. The foramen ovale at the root of the lateral pterygoid plate;

2. The foramen lacerum at the root of the medial pterygoid plate;

3. The synchondrosis between the basioccipital and the body of the sphenoid;

4. A very small foramen not clearly seen, between the carotid canal and the jugular foramen, which transmits the tympanic branch of the glossopharyngeal nerve (CN IX);

5. The spine of the sphenoid for attachment of the sphenomandibular ligament, the hamulus of the medial pterygoid plate for the pterygomandibular ligament and the styloid process for the stylomandibular and stylohyoid ligaments.

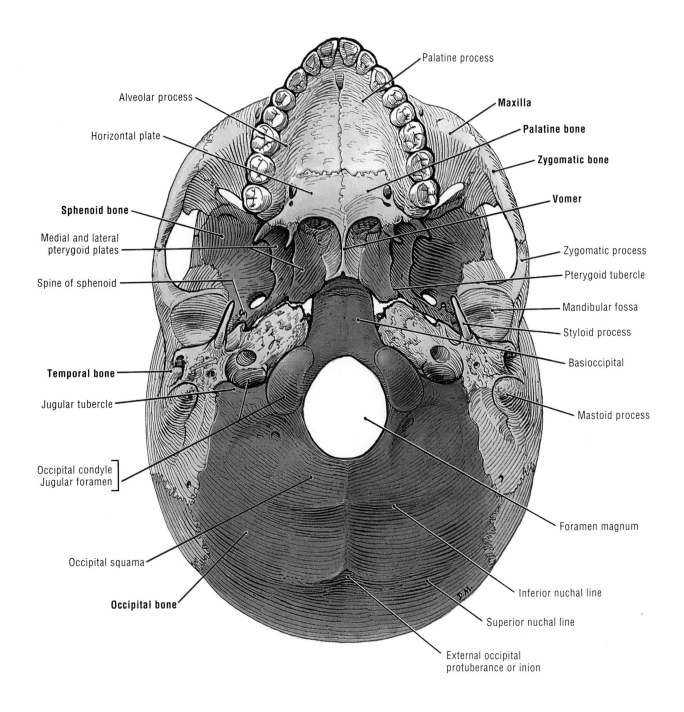

Alveolar process
Horizontal plate
Sphenoid bone
Medial and lateral pterygoid plates
Spine of sphenoid
Temporal bone
Jugular tubercle
Occipital condyle
Jugular foramen
Occipital squama
Occipital bone

Palatine process
Maxilla
Palatine bone
Zygomatic bone
Vomer
Zygomatic process
Pterygoid tubercle
Mandibular fossa
Styloid process
Basioccipital
Mastoid process
Foramen magnum
Inferior nuchal line
Superior nuchal line
External occipital protuberance or inion

8.53
Exterior of the base of the skull–II

A blow delivered to the side of the mandible does not drive the mandible under the cranium, because the head of the mandible would be required to descend the steep medial wall of the mandibular fossa and the spine of the sphenoid in which that wall ends. Like a sentinel, the spine "keeps guard over" four strategic points: anteriorly, the foramen spinosum for the middle meningeal artery; posteriorly, the entrance to the carotid canal; medially, the entrance to the bony auditory tube; and laterally, the mandibular fossa that lodges the head of the mandible, which therefore is the surface landmark to the spine.

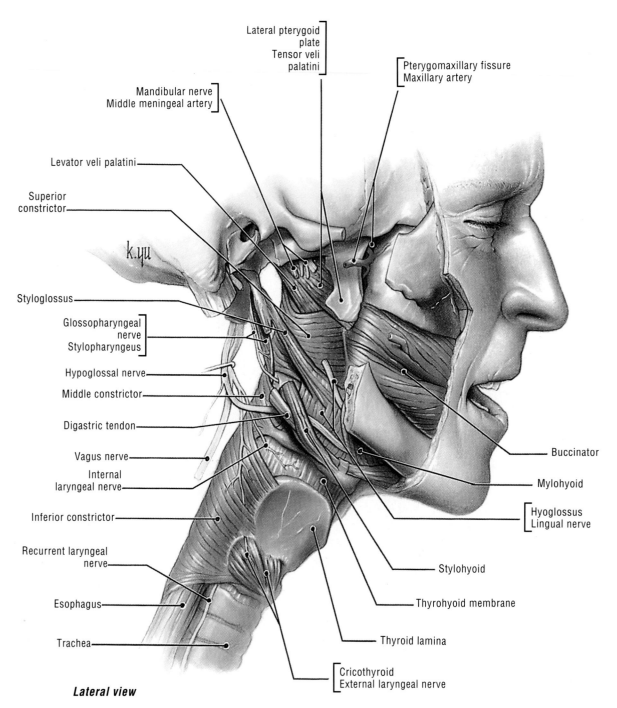

Lateral pterygoid plate
Tensor veli palatini

Pterygomaxillary fissure
Maxillary artery

Mandibular nerve
Middle meningeal artery

Levator veli palatini

Superior constrictor

k.yu

Styloglossus

Glossopharyngeal nerve
Stylopharyngeus

Hypoglossal nerve

Middle constrictor

Digastric tendon

Vagus nerve

Internal laryngeal nerve

Inferior constrictor

Recurrent laryngeal nerve

Esophagus

Trachea

Buccinator

Mylohyoid

Hyoglossus
Lingual nerve

Stylohyoid

Thyrohyoid membrane

Thyroid lamina

Cricothyroid
External laryngeal nerve

Lateral view

8.54
Pharynx

Observe:

1. The superior constrictor and buccinator muscles arising from opposite sides of the pterygomandibular raphe;

2. The middle constrictor muscle overlapped by the hyoglossus muscle, and the hyoglossus muscle, in turn, overlapped by the mylohyoid muscle;

3. The tensor and levator veli palatini muscles, posterior to the lateral pterygoid plate, helping to form the medial wall of the infratemporal region;

4. The styloid process and the three muscles that arise from it: styloglossus, stylopharyngeus, stylohyoid;

5. The styloglossus muscle interdigitating with the hyoglossus muscle on the side of the tongue;

6. The stylohyoid muscle split by the tendon of the digastric muscle and attached to the hyoid bone.

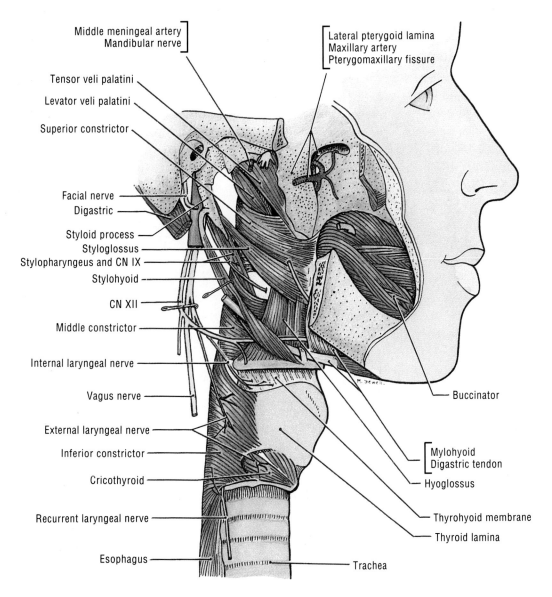

Lateral view

8.55
A diagram of the pharyngeal muscles and the buccinator muscle

Observe that there are four gaps in the pharyngeal musculature allowing the entry of structures:

1. *Superior to the superior constrictor muscle:* levator veli palatini muscle and auditory tube;

2. *Between the superior and middle constrictors:* the stylopharyngeus muscle, CN IX, and stylohyoid ligament;

3. *Between the middle and inferior constrictors:* the internal laryngeal nerve and superior laryngeal artery and nerve (not shown).

4. *Inferior to the inferior constrictor muscle:* the recurrent laryngeal nerve and inferior laryngeal artery and nerve (not shown).

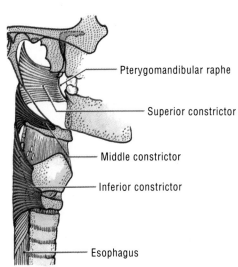

8.56
Constrictors of the pharynx

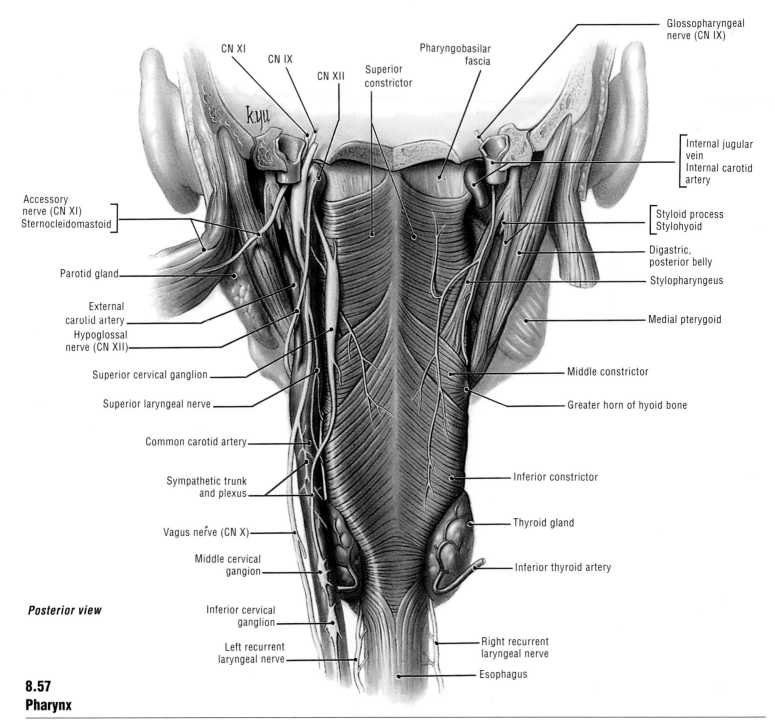

Glossopharyngeal
nerve (CN IX)

CN XI
CN IX
CN XII
Superior
constrictor
Pharyngobasilar
fascia

kyu

Internal jugular
vein
Internal carotid
artery

Accessory
nerve (CN XI)
Sternocleidomastoid

Styloid process
Stylohyoid

Digastric,
posterior belly

Parotid gland

Stylopharyngeus

External
carotid artery

Medial pterygoid

Hypoglossal
nerve (CN XII)

Superior cervical ganglion

Middle constrictor

Superior laryngeal nerve

Greater horn of hyoid bone

Common carotid artery

Sympathetic trunk
and plexus

Inferior constrictor

Vagus nerve (CN X)

Thyroid gland

Middle cervical
gangion

Inferior thyroid artery

Inferior cervical
ganglion

Posterior view

Right recurrent
laryngeal nerve

Left recurrent
laryngeal nerve

Esophagus

**8.57
Pharynx**

Observe:

1. The three pharyngeal constrictor muscles nestle within each
other; thus, the inferior overlaps the middle and the middle
overlaps the superior; the posterior aspect is flat or even slightly
concave;

2. *On the right side:* the stylopharyngeus muscle passing from the
medial side of the styloid process anteromedially to the interval
between the superior and middle constrictor muscles; stylohyoid
muscle passing from the lateral side anterolaterally to be split on
its way to the hyoid bone by the digastric; the glossopharyngeal
nerve making a spiral around the stylopharyngeus muscle and
both entering the pharyngeal wall;

3. *On the left side:* cranial nerves IX, X, XI and XII; the sympathetic trunk and the superior, middle and inferior sympathetic
ganglia; the common carotid artery branching into the internal
and external carotid arteries.

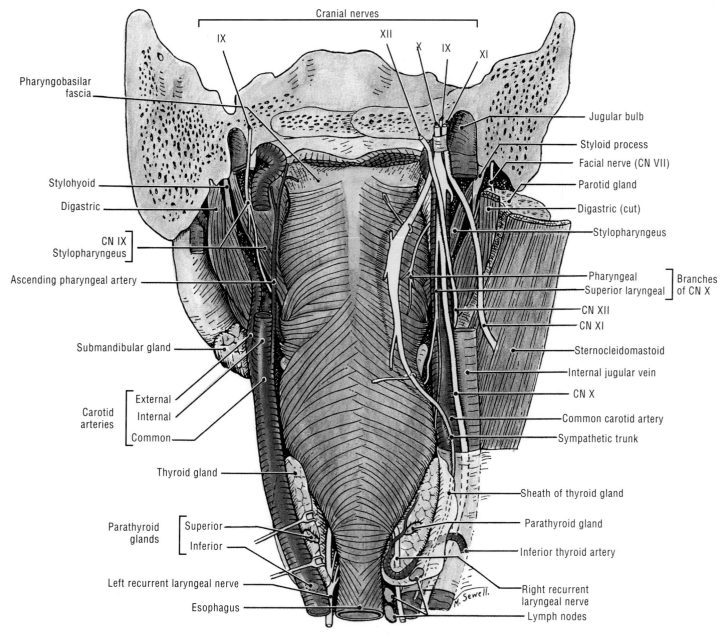

Cranial nerves

IX

XII

X IX

XI

Pharyngobasilar fascia

Jugular bulb

Styloid process

Facial nerve (CN VII)

Parotid gland

Stylohyoid

Digastric

Digastric (cut)

Stylopharyngeus

CN IX
Stylopharyngeus

Pharyngeal ⎤ Branches
Superior laryngeal ⎦ of CN X

Ascending pharyngeal artery

CN XII

CN XI

Submandibular gland

Sternocleidomastoid

Internal jugular vein

CN X

External

Internal

Common

Common carotid artery

Sympathetic trunk

Carotid arteries

Thyroid gland

Sheath of thyroid gland

Parathyroid gland

Parathyroid glands

Superior

Inferior

Inferior thyroid artery

Left recurrent laryngeal nerve

Right recurrent laryngeal nerve

Esophagus

Lymph nodes

M. Sewell.

Posterior view

8.58
Diagram of the pharynx and cranial nerves IX, X, XI, and XII

Observe:

1. The narrowest and least distensible part of the alimentary canal, where the pharynx becomes the esophagus;

2. The inferior constrictor muscle of the pharynx overlapping the middle constrictor, and the middle overlapping the superior;

3. Between the superior constrictor muscle and the base of the skull, the semilunar area on each side where the pharyngobasilar fascia can be seen attaching the pharynx to the basioccipital bone;

4. The nerves and vein that emerge from the foramina are: the facial nerve, the internal jugular vein, and the last four cranial nerves; of the four nerves: IX lies anterior to X and XI; and XII, which is the most medial, makes a half-spiral posterior to X;

5. Lying posterior to the internal carotid artery are the sympathetic trunk and the (elongated) superior cervical ganglion from which fibers, called the internal carotid nerve, accompany the artery into the skull.

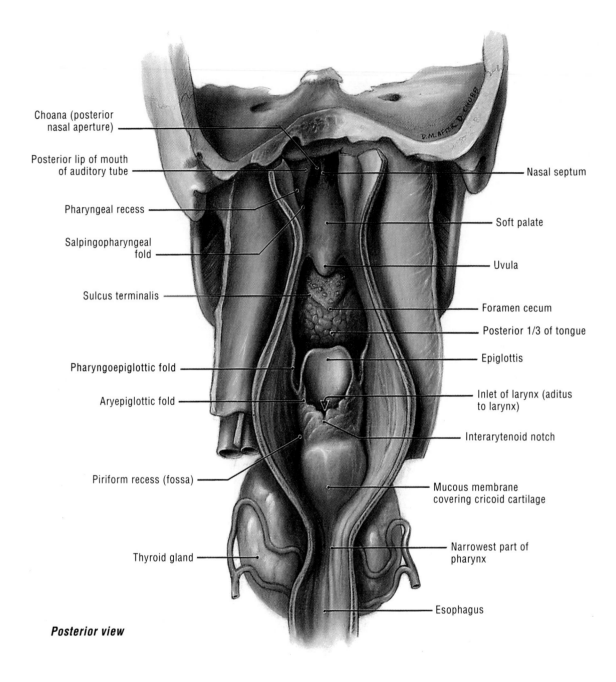

Choana (posterior nasal aperture)

Posterior lip of mouth of auditory tube

Pharyngeal recess

Salpingopharyngeal fold

Sulcus terminalis

Pharyngoepiglottic fold

Aryepiglottic fold

Piriform recess (fossa)

Thyroid gland

Nasal septum

Soft palate

Uvula

Foramen cecum

Posterior 1/3 of tongue

Epiglottis

Inlet of larynx (aditus to larynx)

Interarytenoid notch

Mucous membrane covering cricoid cartilage

Narrowest part of pharynx

Esophagus

Posterior view

8.59
Interior of the pharynx

Observe:

1. The pharynx extending from the base of the skull to the inferior border of the cricoid cartilage where it narrows to become the esophagus;

2. The soft palate ending posteroinferiorly in the uvula, and the larynx ending superiorly to the tip of the epiglottis;

3. The three parts of the pharynx: nasal, oral, laryngeal;

4. The nasal part (nasopharynx) lying superior to the level of the soft palate and continuous anteriorly, through the choanae, with the nasal cavities;

5. The oral part, lying between the levels of the soft palate and larynx, communicating anteriorly with the oral cavity, and having the posterior one-third of the tongue as its anterior wall; this part of the tongue is studded with lymph follicles (collectively called the lingual tonsil), and is demarcated from the anterior two-thirds by the foramen cecum and the V-shaped sulcus terminalis;

6. The laryngeal part lying posterior to the larynx, and communicating with the cavity of the larynx through the aditus; on each side of the inlet and separated from it by the aryepiglottic fold is a piriform recess.

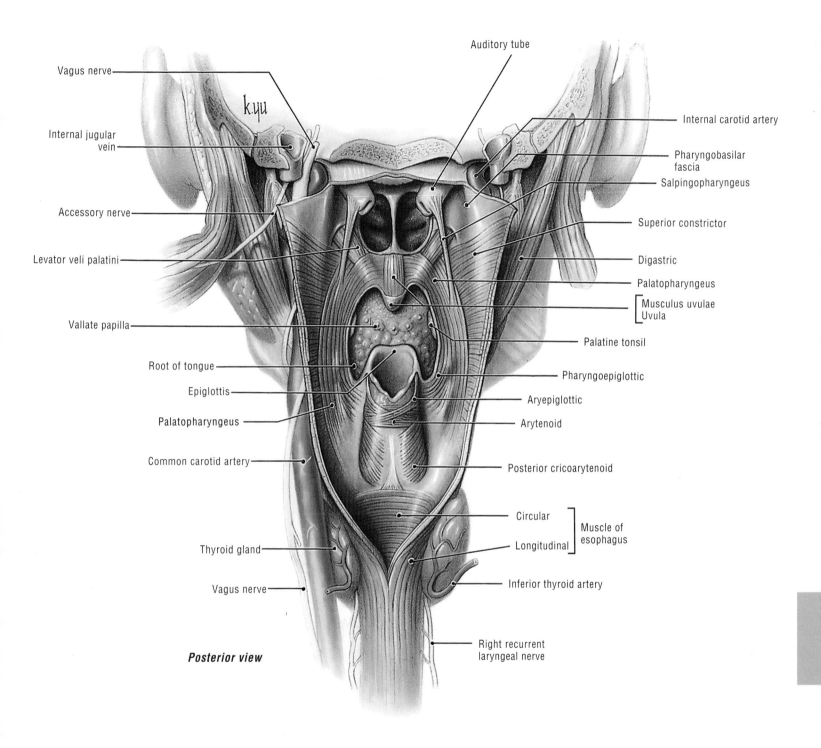

Vagus nerve

Internal jugular vein

Accessory nerve

Levator veli palatini

Vallate papilla

Root of tongue

Epiglottis

Palatopharyngeus

Common carotid artery

Thyroid gland

Vagus nerve

Posterior view

Auditory tube

Internal carotid artery

Pharyngobasilar fascia

Salpingopharyngeus

Superior constrictor

Digastric

Palatopharyngeus

Musculus uvulae
Uvula

Palatine tonsil

Pharyngoepiglottic

Aryepiglottic

Arytenoid

Posterior cricoarytenoid

Circular
Longitudinal Muscle of esophagus

Inferior thyroid artery

Right recurrent laryngeal nerve

8.60
Muscles of the soft palate and the interior of the larynx and pharynx

Note the posterior wall of the pharynx has been cut in the midline and reflected laterally to reveal the interior of the pharynx and the nasal, oral, and laryngeal orifices. The mucous membrane has been removed to expose the underlying musculature.

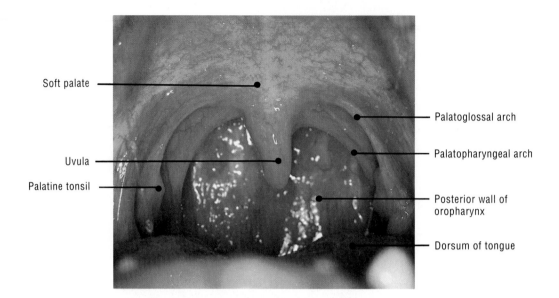

Soft palate

Uvula

Palatine tonsil

Palatoglossal arch

Palatopharyngeal arch

Posterior wall of oropharynx

Dorsum of tongue

8.61
Oral cavity and palatine tonsils

(From Liebgott B. *The Anatomical Basis of Dentistry*, Philadelphia, WB Saunders Co, 1982.)

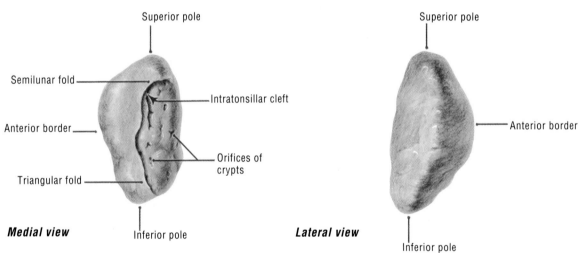

Superior pole

Semilunar fold

Intratonsillar cleft

Anterior border

Orifices of crypts

Triangular fold

Medial view

Inferior pole

Superior pole

Anterior border

Lateral view

Inferior pole

8.62
Palatine tonsil

Observe:

1. The long axis running vertically;

2. The fibrous capsule forming the lateral or attached surface of the tonsil; in removing the tonsil, the loose areolar tissue lying between the capsule and the thin pharyngobasilar fascia, which forms the immediate bed of the tonsil, was easily torn through;

3. The capsule extending around the anterior border and slightly over the medial surface as a thin, free fold, covered with mucous

membrane on both surfaces; the superior part of this fold is called the semilunar fold; the inferior, the triangular fold;

4. On the medial or free surface, the dozen stellate orifices of the test tube-like crypts, which extend right through the organ to the capsule; the intratonsillar cleft, which extends toward the superior pole.

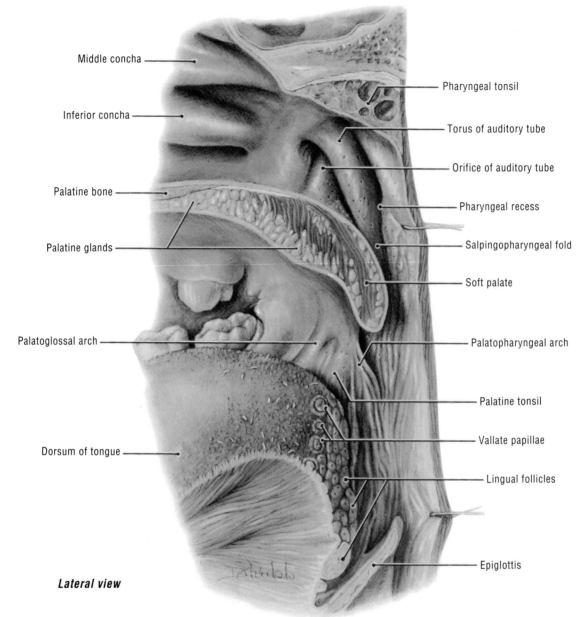

Middle concha

Inferior concha

Palatine bone

Palatine glands

Palatoglossal arch

Dorsum of tongue

Pharyngeal tonsil

Torus of auditory tube

Orifice of auditory tube

Pharyngeal recess

Salpingopharyngeal fold

Soft palate

Palatopharyngeal arch

Palatine tonsil

Vallate papillae

Lingual follicles

Epiglottis

Lateral view

8.63
Interior of the pharynx

Observe:

1. The prominent torus of the auditory tube and the salpingopharyngeal fold, which descends from the torus;

2. The location of the orifice of the auditory tube – about 1 cm posterior to the inferior concha;

3. The ridge produced by levator veli palatini muscle, which has the appearance of being poured out of the tube;

4. The deep pharyngeal recess posterior to the torus of the tube;

5. The numerous pinpoint orifices of the ducts of mucous glands about the torus and elsewhere;

6. The pharyngeal tonsil, where deep clefts extend into the lymphoid tissue;

7. The considerable proportion of glandular tissue in the soft palate and its disposition;

8. The palatoglossal and the palatopharyngeal arches that, in this specimen, are not the sharp folds commonly seen, and the somewhat inconspicuous palatine tonsil between them;

9. The lingual follicles, each with the duct of a mucous gland opening on to its surface; collectively, the follicles are known as the lingual tonsil;

10. Although not shown here, it is instructive to summarize the sensory supply of the pharynx; the pharyngeal branch of the maxillary nerve to the roof, the lesser palatine nerves to the anterior parts of the soft palate, and the internal laryngeal nerve to the inferior part of the pharynx and somewhat to the surroundings of the laryngeal orifice.

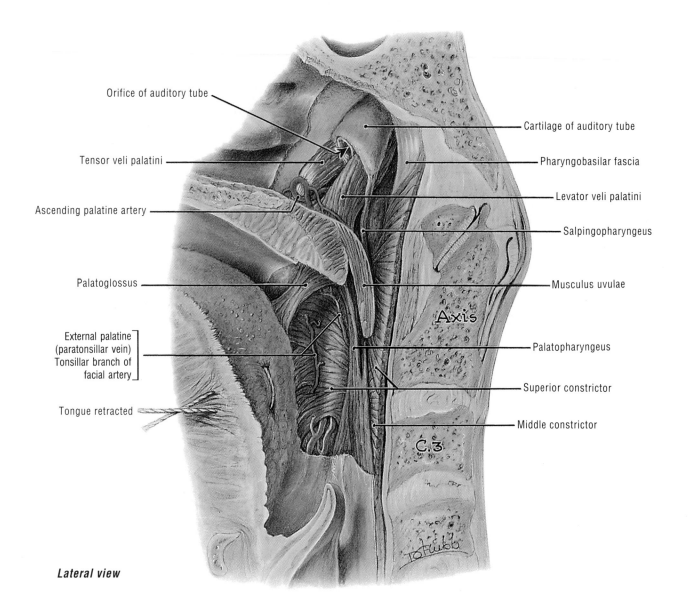

Orifice of auditory tube

Tensor veli palatini

Ascending palatine artery

Palatoglossus

External palatine
(paratonsillar vein)
Tonsillar branch of
facial artery

Tongue retracted

Cartilage of auditory tube

Pharyngobasilar fascia

Levator veli palatini

Salpingopharyngeus

Musculus uvulae

Axis

Palatopharyngeus

Superior constrictor

Middle constrictor

C.3

Lateral view

8.64
Interior of the pharynx dissected

The palatine and pharyngeal tonsils and the mucous membrane are removed. The submucous pharyngobasilar fascia, which attaches the pharynx to the basilar part of the occipital bone, is thick superiorly and thin posteriorly. It too has been removed, except at the superior arched border of superior constrictor.

Observe:

1. The curved cartilage of the auditory tube; its free superior and posterior lips and the pharyngeal orifice of the tube; and salpin-gopharyngeus muscle descending from the posterior lip to join palatopharyngeus muscle;

2. The ascending palatine branch of the facial artery descending with the levator veli palatini muscle to the soft palate;

3. The five paired muscles of the palate: tensor veli palatini;

levator veli palatini providing most of the muscle fibers seen in the sectioned soft palate; uvular muscle (musculus uvulae), a finger-like bundle, arising largely from the palatine aponeurosis at the posterior nasal spine; palatoglossus, here a substantial band, but commonly a wisp of muscle with free anterior and posterior borders; and palatopharyngeus;

4. The tonsil bed from which a thin sheet of pharyngobasilar fascia has been removed, thereby exposing the palatopharyngeus and superior constrictor muscles.

Note: The bed of the palatine tonsil extends far into the soft palate; the tonsillar branch of the facial artery is long and large; the paratonsillar vein, descending from the soft palate to join the pharyngeal plexus of veins, is a close lateral relation of the tonsil.

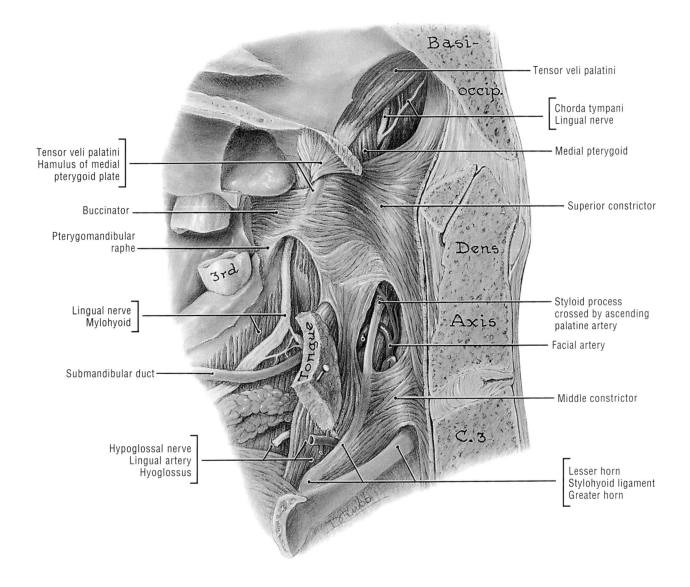

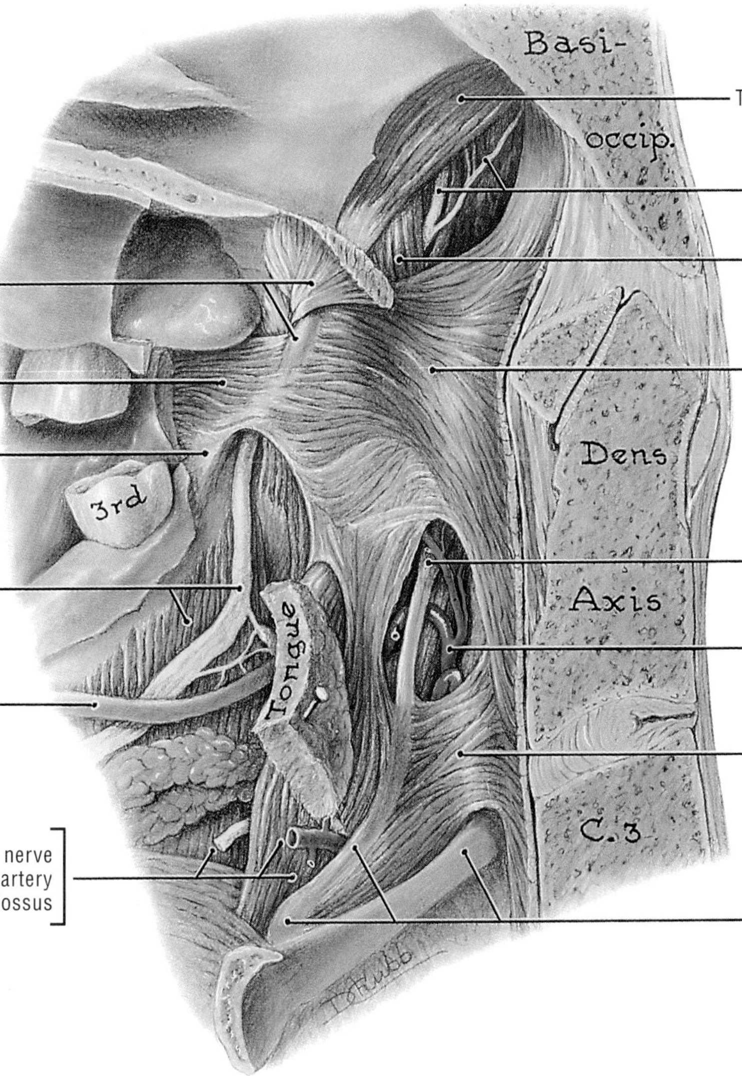
Basi-
occip.
Dens
Axis
C.3
3rd
Tongue
Tensor veli palatini
Chorda tympani
Lingual nerve
Medial pterygoid
Superior constrictor
Styloid process crossed by ascending palatine artery
Facial artery
Middle constrictor
Lesser horn
Stylohyoid ligament
Greater horn
Tensor veli palatini
Hamulus of medial pterygoid plate
Buccinator
Pterygomandibular raphe
Lingual nerve
Mylohyoid
Submandibular duct
Hypoglossal nerve
Lingual artery
Hyoglossus

8.65
Superior and middle constrictor muscles of the pharynx, from within

Observe:

1. The superior constrictor muscle arising from the pterygomandibular raphe, which unites it to the buccinator muscle, and from the bone at each end of the raphe (the hamulus of the medial pterygoid plate superiorly and the mandible inferiorly) and also from the root of the tongue;

2. The arched superior and inferior borders of the superior constrictor extending to the median plane where the muscle meets its fellow of the opposite side;

3. The middle constrictor muscle arising from the angle formed by the greater and lesser horns of the hyoid bone and from the stylohyoid ligament; in this specimen, the styloid process is long and is, therefore, a lateral relation of the tonsil;

4. The facial artery arching superior to the posterior belly of the digastric muscle, and the loop of the lingual artery just inferior to it;

5. The tendon of the tensor veli palatini muscle hooking around the hamulus and then ascending to blend with the palatine aponeurosis;

6. The lingual nerve joined by the chorda tympani, disappearing at the posterior border of medial pterygoid muscle, reappearing at the anterior border, and applied to the mandible.

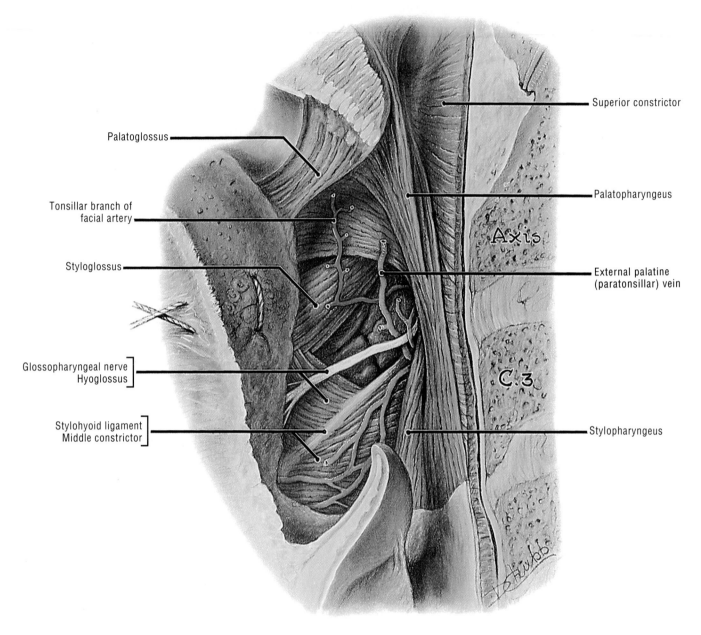

Palatoglossus

Tonsillar branch of
facial artery

Styloglossus

Glossopharyngeal nerve
Hyoglossus

Stylohyoid ligament
Middle constrictor

Superior constrictor

Palatopharyngeus

Axis

External palatine
(paratonsillar) vein

C.3

Stylopharyngeus

8.66
Deep dissection of the tonsil bed

The tongue is pulled anteriorly and the inferior part of the origin of the superior constrictor muscle is cut away.

Observe:

1. The styloglossus muscle passing to the anterior two-thirds of the tongue, where its bundles interdigitate with those of the hyoglossus muscle; the glossopharyngeal nerve, passing to the posterior one-third of the tongue and lying anterior to the stylopharyngeus muscle; the stylopharyngeus muscle descending along the anterior border of the palatopharyngeus muscle;

2. The tonsillar branch of the facial artery sending a branch (cut short) to accompany the glossopharyngeal nerve to the tongue;

lateral to the artery and the paratonsillar vein, the submandibular gland is seen;

3. The palatopharyngeus and stylopharyngeus muscles forming the longitudinal muscle coat of the pharynx; the constrictor muscles form the circular coat.

Note: In the region of the tonsil bed, the palatopharyngeus muscle is commonly not well differentiated from the superior constrictor muscle, which makes it difficult to decide where the inferior border of the palatopharyngeus muscle is; elsewhere, its borders are easily defined.

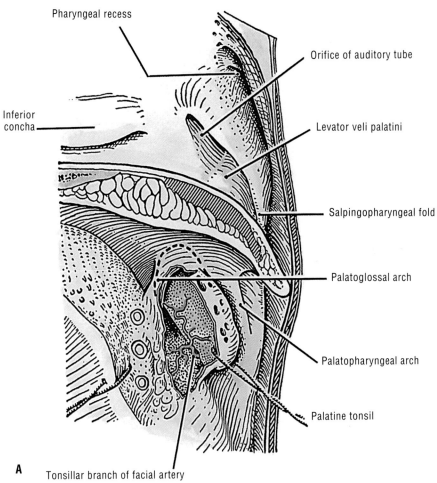

Pharyngeal recess

Inferior concha

Orifice of auditory tube

Levator veli palatini

Salpingopharyngeal fold

Palatoglossal arch

Palatopharyngeal arch

Palatine tonsil

A   Tonsillar branch of facial artery

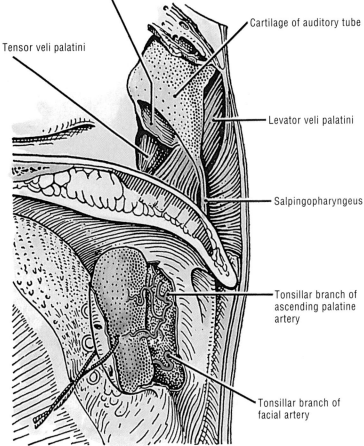

Membranous lateral wall

Tensor veli palatini

Cartilage of auditory tube

Levator veli palatini

Salpingopharyngeus

Tonsillar branch of ascending palatine artery

Tonsillar branch of facial artery

B

8.67
Removal of the tonsil – the arterial supply

A. First stage. **B**. Second stage. The mucous membrane has been incised along the palatoglossal arch, and the areolar space lateral to the fibrous capsule of the tonsil has been entered.

With the point and the rounded handle of the knife, the anterior border of the tonsil has been freed and the superior part, which extends far into the soft palate, has been shelled out. The mucous membrane along the palatopharyngeal arch is cut through.

8.68
The thyroid gland and the laryngeal nerves

Observe:

1. The superior parathyroid gland, here, as usual, fusiform in shape and lying in a crevice on the posterior border of the lobes of the thyroid gland; the inferior gland, more circular and applied to the inferior pole of the thyroid gland; on the right side, both parathyroid glands are low, the inferior gland being altogether inferior to the thyroid gland;

2. The internal laryngeal nerve, which innervates the mucous membrane superior to the vocal folds; the external laryngeal nerve, supplying the inferior constrictor and cricothyroid muscles; the recurrent laryngeal nerve, supplying the esophagus, trachea, and inferior constrictor muscle, and then accompanying the inferior laryngeal artery into the larynx; where it supplies sensory innervation to the area of the larynx inferior to the vocal folds and motor innervation to all the intrinsic muscles of the larynx except the cricothyroid muscle.

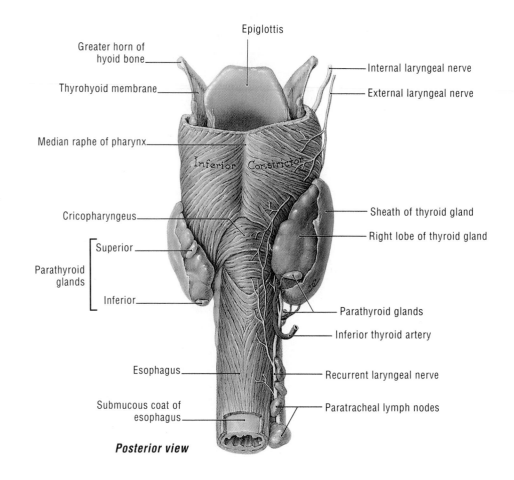

Posterior view

8.69
Skeleton of the larynx

Observe:

1. The thyroid cartilage, shielding the smaller cartilages of the larynx (epiglottic, arytenoid, corniculate, and cuneiform); the hyoid bone – although not a part of the larynx – likewise shields the superior part of the epiglottic cartilage;

2. The rounded posterior border of the thyroid cartilage, prolonged into a superior and an inferior horn: the inferior horn articulating with the cricoid cartilage at a synovial joint, the capsule of which is reinforced by two distinct ligaments (posterosuperior and anteroinferior);

3. The quadrangular membrane, connecting the border of the epiglottic cartilage to the arytenoid and corniculate cartilages, having a free superior border, and ending inferiorly as the vestibular ligament.

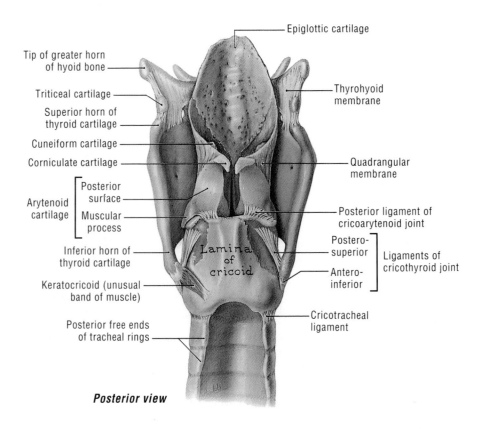

Posterior view

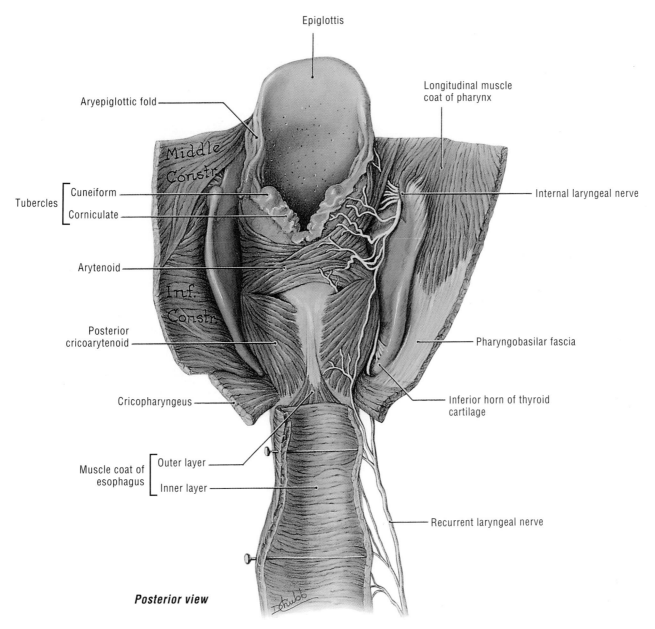

Epiglottis

Aryepiglottic fold

Longitudinal muscle
coat of pharynx

Middle
Constr

Tubercles
- Cuneiform
- Corniculate

Internal laryngeal nerve

Arytenoid

Inf.
Constr

Posterior
cricoarytenoid

Pharyngobasilar fascia

Cricopharyngeus

Inferior horn of thyroid
cartilage

Muscle coat of
esophagus
- Outer layer
- Inner layer

Recurrent laryngeal nerve

Posterior view

8.70
Muscles of the pharynx, larynx, and esophagus

The mucous membrane of the pharynx and esophagus is removed; the left palatopharyngeus muscle also is removed and the constrictor muscles are thereby uncovered.

Observe:

1. On the epiglottis, the pinpoint orifices of the glands that occupy the pits on the epiglottic cartilage;

2. The palatopharyngeus and stylopharyngeus muscles together constituting the inner or longitudinal muscle coat of the pharynx, and inserting into pharyngobasilar fascia and thyroid cartilage;

3. The esophagus, having inner or circularly arranged muscle fibers and outer or longitudinally arranged fibers, the latter suspending the esophagus from the cricoid cartilage;

4. The inferior constrictor muscle, attached not to the posterior border of the thyroid cartilage but to the oblique line and the

tubercles; its lowest fibers, called cricopharyngeus, which act as a sphincter, attached to the cricoid cartilage;

5. The fan shape of posterior cricoarytenoid muscle; its superior fibers rotate the arytenoid cartilage laterally; its lower fibers pull the cartilage inferiorly;

6. Arytenoid (interarytenoid) muscle, having transverse fibers and also oblique fibers that are continued into the aryepiglottic fold as aryepiglotticus muscle;

7. The recurrent laryngeal nerve (mixed – motor and sensory), entering the larynx as two branches, of which the anterior runs immediately posterior to the cricothyroid joint;

8. The internal laryngeal nerve (sensory) piercing the thyrohyoid membrane as several diverging branches.

8.71
Skeleton of the larynx

The larynx extends vertically from the tip of the epiglottis to the inferior border of the cricoid cartilage. The hyoid bone is not regarded as part of the larynx.

Observe:

1. The lesser horn of the hyoid bone, partly cartilaginous; the thyroid and cricoid cartilages, partly ossified;

2. The lamina of the thyroid cartilage, projecting anteriorly superior to the point of union with its fellow to form the laryngeal prominence; its posterior border, prolonged into superior and inferior horns;

3. The cricoid cartilage, having an arch anteriorly, and a lamina posteriorly; the superior border of the arch of the cricoid, inclined; and the inferior border, projecting anteriorly beyond the trachea;

4. The thyrohyoid membrane: attaching the whole length of the superior border of the thyroid lamina to the superior border of the body and greater horn of the hyoid bone; thickened posteriorly to form the thyrohyoid ligament; pierced by the internal laryngeal nerve and vessels.

Epiglottis

Greater horn of hyoid bone

Triticeal cartilage

Lesser horn of hyoid

Body of hyoid

Fat body

Thyrohyoid membrane

Thyroid cartilage
- Superior horn
- Superior tubercle
- Oblique line
- Inferior tubercle
- Inferior horn

Cricothyroid ligament

Laryngeal prominence

Median cricothyroid ligament

Arch of cricoid cartilage

Cricoid cartilage
- Lamina
- Lateral tubercle

Cricotracheal ligament

1st
2nd } Tracheal cartilages
3rd

Lateral view

8.72
Muscles and nerves of the larynx, cricothyroid joint

The thyroid cartilage is sawn through on the right of the median plane; the cricothyroid joint is laid open; the right lamina of the thyroid cartilage is turned anteriorly, stripping the cricothyroid muscle off the arch of the cricoid cartilage.

Observe:

1. The lateral cricoarytenoid muscle, arising from the superior border of the arch of the cricoid cartilage, and inserted with the posterior cricoarytenoid muscle into the muscular process of the arytenoid cartilage;

2. The thyroarytenoid muscle, inserted with the arytenoid muscle into the lateral border of the arytenoid cartilage; its superior fibers continue to the epiglottis as the thyroepiglottic muscle;

3. The internal and recurrent laryngeal nerves, described with Figure 8.68.

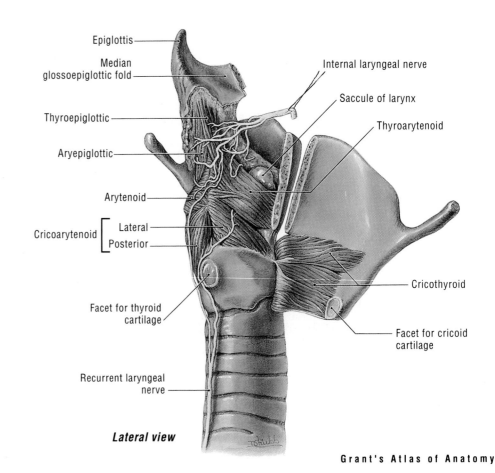

Epiglottis

Median glossoepiglottic fold

Thyroepiglottic

Aryepiglottic

Arytenoid

Cricoarytenoid
- Lateral
- Posterior

Facet for thyroid cartilage

Recurrent laryngeal nerve

Internal laryngeal nerve

Saccule of larynx

Thyroarytenoid

Cricothyroid

Facet for cricoid cartilage

Lateral view

8.73
Thyroid cartilage and cricothyroid muscle

The cricothyroid muscle arises from the outer surface of the arch of the cricoid cartilage and has two parts: a straight, which is inserted into the inferior border of the lamina of the thyroid cartilage, and an oblique, which is inserted into the anterior border of the inferior horn.

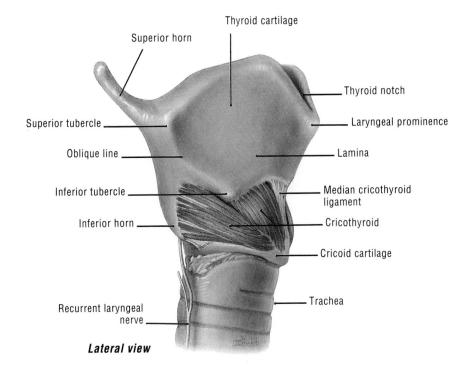

Superior horn — Thyroid cartilage
Thyroid notch
Laryngeal prominence
Superior tubercle
Oblique line — Lamina
Inferior tubercle — Median cricothyroid ligament
Inferior horn — Cricothyroid
Cricoid cartilage
Trachea
Recurrent laryngeal nerve

Lateral view

8.74
Larynx

Superior to the vocal folds (vocal cords), the larynx is sectioned near the median plane and the interior of its left side is seen. Inferior to this level, the right side of the larynx is dissected.

Observe:

1. The hyoepiglottic ligament and the thyrohyoid membrane, both attached to the superior part of the body of the hyoid bone;

2. The fatpad and the collection of glands (not labeled) filling the triangular space between ligament, membrane, and epiglottic cartilage;

3. The anterolateral surface of the arytenoid cartilage;

4. The lateral aspect of the cricoid cartilage – the raised circular facet for the inferior horn of the thyroid cartilage; superior to this, the sloping facet for the arytenoid cartilage; the nearly horizontal inferior border; and the oblique superior border of the arch;

5. The cricothyroid ligament, having the vocal ligament for its superior border, blending with the median cricothyroid ligament anteroinferiorly.

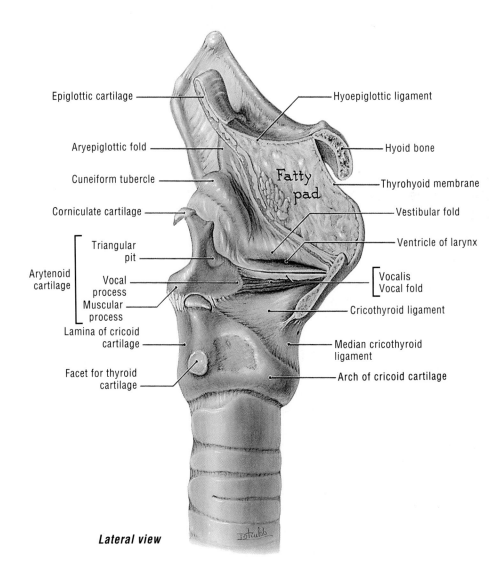

Epiglottic cartilage — Hyoepiglottic ligament
Aryepiglottic fold — Hyoid bone
Cuneiform tubercle — Thyrohyoid membrane
Fatty pad
Corniculate cartilage — Vestibular fold
Ventricle of larynx
Triangular pit
Arytenoid cartilage
Vocal process — Vocalis / Vocal fold
Muscular process — Cricothyroid ligament
Lamina of cricoid cartilage
Median cricothyroid ligament
Facet for thyroid cartilage — Arch of cricoid cartilage

Lateral view

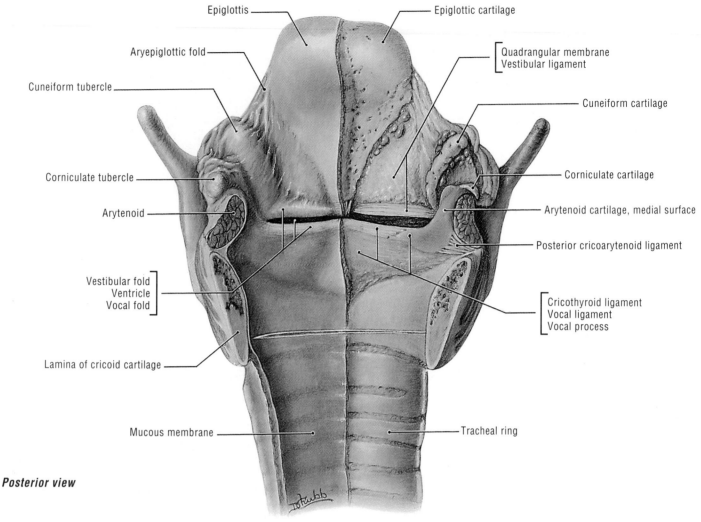

Epiglottis

Epiglottic cartilage

Aryepiglottic fold

Quadrangular membrane
Vestibular ligament

Cuneiform tubercle

Cuneiform cartilage

Corniculate tubercle

Corniculate cartilage

Arytenoid

Arytenoid cartilage, medial surface

Posterior cricoarytenoid ligament

Vestibular fold
Ventricle
Vocal fold

Cricothyroid ligament
Vocal ligament
Vocal process

Lamina of cricoid cartilage

Mucous membrane

Tracheal ring

Posterior view

8.75
Interior of the larynx

The posterior wall of the larynx is split in the median plane, and the two sides are held apart. On the *left side*, the mucous membrane, which is the innermost coat of the larynx, is intact; on the *right side*, the mucous and submucous coats are peeled off and the next coat, consisting of cartilages, ligaments, and fibroelastic membrane, is thereby laid bare.

Observe:

1. Arytenoid muscle and the lamina of the cricoid cartilage, divided posteriorly;

2. The entrance to the larynx is oblique; the inferior limit, at the inferior border of the cricoid cartilage where the trachea begins, is horizontal;

3. The three compartments of the larynx: (a) the superior compartment of vestibule, superior to the level of the vestibular folds; (b) the middle, between the levels of the vestibular and vocal folds, and having a right and a left canoe-shaped depression, the ventricles; and (c) the inferior or infraglottic cavity, inferior to the level of the vocal folds;

4. The mucous membrane, particularly smooth and adherent over the epiglottic cartilage and vocal ligaments; and particularly loose and wrinkled about the arytenoid cartilages, where movement is free;

5. The two parts of the fibroelastic membrane: (a) a superior quadrangular, and (b) an inferior triangular; the superior part, the quadrangular membrane, is thickened inferiorly to form the vestibular ligament; the inferior part, the cricothyroid ligament (conus elasticus), begins inferiorly as the strong median cricothyroid ligament and ends superiorly as the vocal ligament; between the vocal and the vestibular ligament, the membrane, lined with mucous membrane, is evaginated to form the wall of the ventricle;

6. The cuneiform cartilage, composed of elastic cartilage and pitted for, and surrounded with, glands, attached to the arytenoid cartilage beside the posterior end of the vestibular ligament;

7. The posterior ligament of the cricoarytenoid joint, anchoring the arytenoid cartilage; the flat, medial, submucous surface of the arytenoid cartilage.

8.76
Larynx

Observe:

1. The inlet or aditus to the larynx, bounded anteriorly by the epiglottis; posteriorly, by the arytenoid cartilages, the corniculate cartilages that cap them and the interarytenoid fold that unites them; and, on each side, by the aryepiglottic fold, which contains the superior end of the cuneiform cartilage;

2. The vocal folds, closer together than the vestibular folds (false cords).

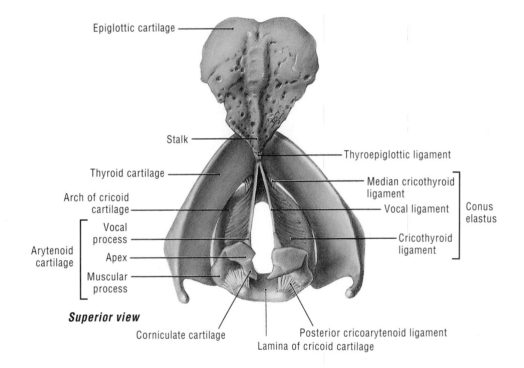

Greater horn of hyoid bone

Aryepiglottic fold

Piriform recess

Epiglottis

Epiglottic tubercle

Vestibular fold

Ventricle of larynx

Vocal fold (cord)

Superior view

Cuneiform tubercle

Corniculate tubercle

Rima glottidis

8.77
Skeleton of the larynx

Observe:

1. The right and the left lamina of the thyroid cartilage, united anteriorly (at an angle of about 60 degrees in the male and 90 degrees in the female);

2. The epiglottic cartilage, pitted for mucous glands, and attached at its apex by ligamentous fibers to the angle of the thyroid cartilage superior to the vocal ligaments;

3. The paired arytenoid cartilages, having a blunt apex prolonged as the corniculate cartilage; a rounded, lateral, basal angle called the muscular process; and a sharp, anterior basal angle called the vocal process, for the attachment of the vocal ligament;

4. The strong posterior cricoarytenoid ligament, which prevents the arytenoid cartilage from falling into the larynx;

5. The vocal ligament, which forms the skeleton of the vocal fold, extending from the vocal process to the "angle" of the thyroid cartilage, and there joining its fellow inferior to the thyroepiglottic ligament;

6. The cricothyroid ligament blending anteriorly with the median cricothyroid ligament, and sweeping superiorly from the superior border of the arch of the cricoid cartilage to the vocal ligament.

Epiglottic cartilage

Stalk

Thyroid cartilage

Arch of cricoid cartilage

Arytenoid cartilage

Vocal process

Apex

Muscular process

Thyroepiglottic ligament

Median cricothyroid ligament

Vocal ligament

Cricothyroid ligament

Conus elastus

Superior view

Corniculate cartilage

Lamina of cricoid cartilage

Posterior cricoarytenoid ligament

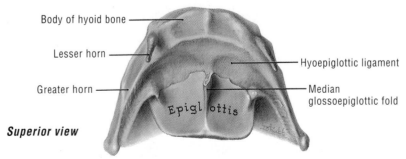

Body of hyoid bone

Lesser horn

Greater horn

Hyoepiglottic ligament

Median glossoepiglottic fold

Epiglottis

Superior view

8.78
Epiglottis and hyoepiglottic ligament

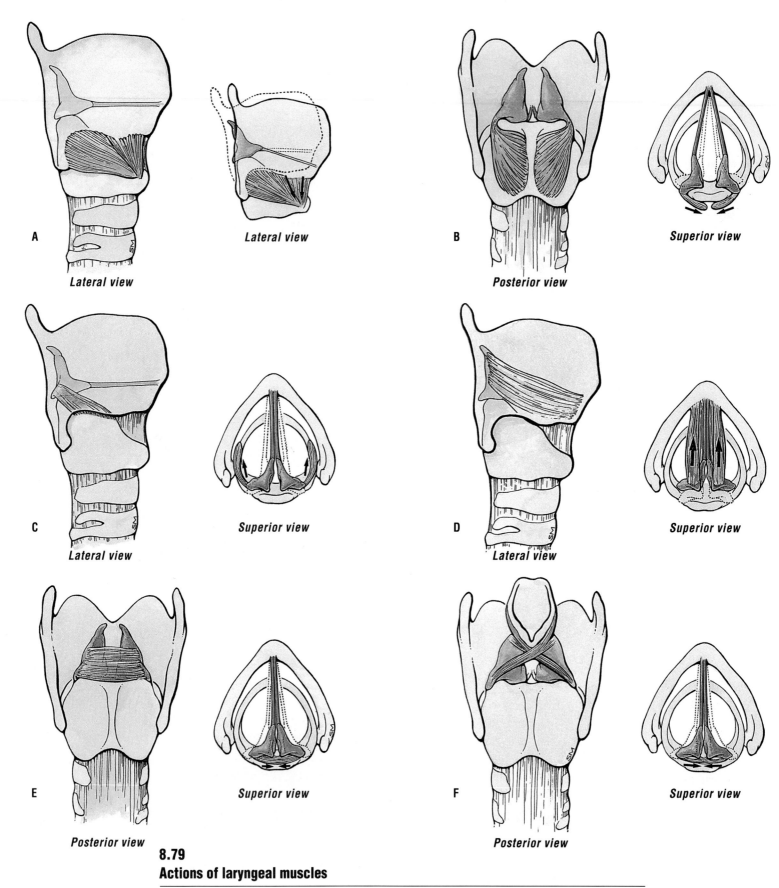

A. Lateral view   *Lateral view*

Lateral view

B. Posterior view   *Superior view*

Posterior view

C. Lateral view   *Superior view*

Lateral view

D. Lateral view   *Superior view*

Lateral view

E. Posterior view   *Superior view*

Posterior view

F. Posterior view   *Superior view*

Posterior view

8.79
Actions of laryngeal muscles

A. Cricothyroid. **B.** Posterior cricoarytenoid. **C.** Lateral cricoarytenoid. **D.** Thyroarytenoid.
E. Transverse arytenoid. **F.** Oblique arytenoid.

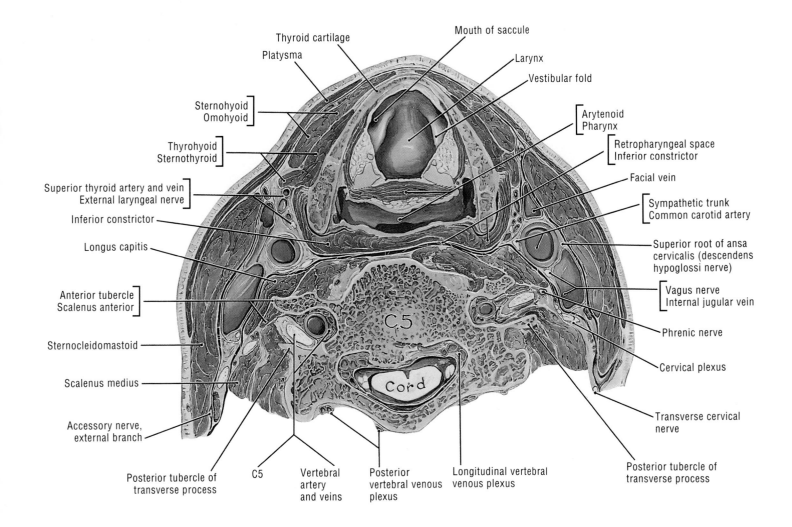

Thyroid cartilage
Platysma
Mouth of saccule
Larynx
Vestibular fold
Sternohyoid
Omohyoid
Arytenoid
Pharynx
Thyrohyoid
Sternothyroid
Retropharyngeal space
Inferior constrictor
Superior thyroid artery and vein
External laryngeal nerve
Facial vein
Inferior constrictor
Sympathetic trunk
Common carotid artery
Longus capitis
Superior root of ansa cervicalis (descendens hypoglossi nerve)
Anterior tubercle
Scalenus anterior
Vagus nerve
Internal jugular vein
Sternocleidomastoid
Phrenic nerve
Scalenus medius
Cervical plexus
Accessory nerve, external branch
Transverse cervical nerve
Posterior tubercle of transverse process
C5
Vertebral artery and veins
Posterior vertebral venous plexus
Longitudinal vertebral venous plexus
Posterior tubercle of transverse process

8.80
Transverse section of the neck, through the middle of the larynx

Observe:

1. The thyroid cartilage shielding the larynx and the pharynx;

2. The vestibular folds, seen inferiorly and, lateral to them, the mouths of the saccules of the larynx;

3. Arytenoid muscle (cut obliquely, hence appearing wide) attached to the posterior surface of the arytenoid cartilage and in continuity with thyroarytenoid muscle (not labeled);

4. The inferior constrictor muscle, curving around the posterior borders of the laminae of the thyroid cartilage to be attached to the oblique line; the sternothyroid and thyrohyoid muscles sharing the oblique line;

5. The superior thyroid vessels and the external laryngeal nerve applied to the inferior constrictor muscle;

6. The three contents of the carotid sheath: the common carotid artery, internal jugular vein, and, in the posterior angle between them, the vagus nerve;

7. The sympathetic trunk, posteromedial to the carotid artery and medial to the vagus nerve; the superior root of ansa cervicalis anterior to the carotid artery;

8. The retropharyngeal space, between the pretracheal fascia, which covers the inferior constrictor muscle, and the prevertebral fascia, which covers the longi colli and capitis muscles; the areolar space extending laterally to the carotid sheath and readily opened up beyond it; the phrenic nerve deep to the prevertebral fascia;

9. The vertebral artery, surrounded with a plexus of veins that inferiorly becomes the vertebral vein and the ventral ramus of a cervical nerve (C5) crossing posterior to it;

10. The internal and external parts of the vertebral venous plexus.

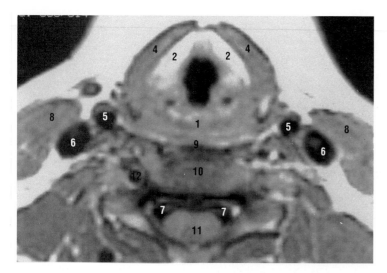

A

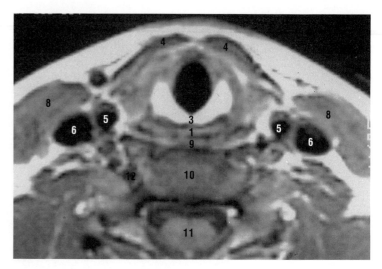

B

8.81
Transverse MRI (magnetic resonance image) of the larynx

A. Through the thyroid cartilage. **B.** Through the cricoid cartilage. *1* - Esophagus, *2* - Thyroid cartilage, *3* - Lamina of cricoid cartilage, *4* - Strap muscles, *5* - Common carotid artery, *6* - Internal jugular vein, *7* - Ventral root, *8* - Sternocleidomastoid, *9* - Inferior constrictor, *10* - Vertebral body, *11* - Spinal cord in cerebrospinal fluid, *12* - Vertebral artery. (Courtesy of Dr. W. Kucharczyk, Clinical Director of Tri-Hospital Resonance Centre, Toronto, Ontario, Canada.)

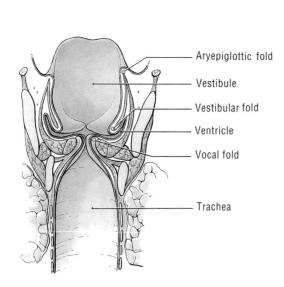

Aryepiglottic fold

Vestibule

Vestibular fold

Ventricle

Vocal fold

Trachea

8.82
Compartments of larynx, coronal section

These are: a vestibule, a middle compartment having a right and a left ventricle, and an infraglottic cavity.

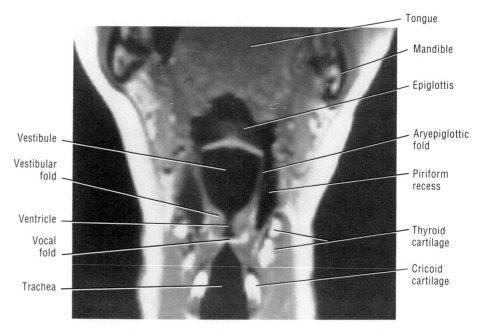

Tongue

Mandible

Epiglottis

Aryepiglottic fold

Piriform recess

Thyroid cartilage

Cricoid cartilage

Vestibule

Vestibular fold

Ventricle

Vocal fold

Trachea

8.83
Coronal MRI (magnetic resonance image) through the oropharynx, larynx, and trachea

(Courtesy of Dr. W. Kucharczyk, Clinical Director of Tri-Hospital Resonance Centre, Toronto, Ontario, Canada.)

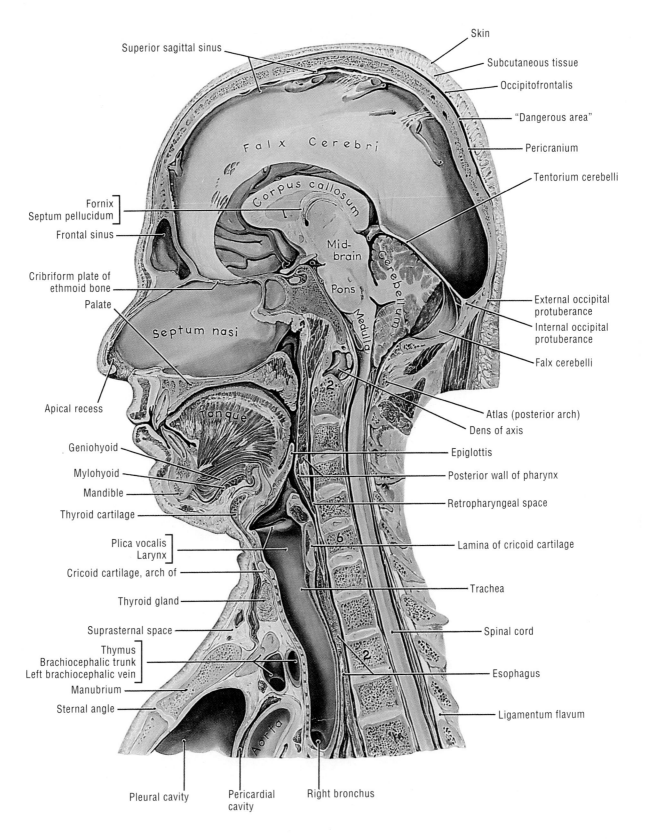

Superior sagittal sinus

Skin

Subcutaneous tissue

Occipitofrontalis

"Dangerous area"

Pericranium

Falx Cerebri

Corpus callosum

Tentorium cerebelli

Fornix
Septum pellucidum

Frontal sinus

Mid-
brain

Cerebellum

Pons

Cribriform plate of
ethmoid bone

Palate

Medulla

External occipital
protuberance

Internal occipital
protuberance

Septum nasi

Falx cerebelli

Apical recess

Tongue

Atlas (posterior arch)

Dens of axis

Geniohyoid

Epiglottis

Mylohyoid

Posterior wall of pharynx

Mandible

Retropharyngeal space

Thyroid cartilage

Plica vocalis
Larynx

Lamina of cricoid cartilage

Cricoid cartilage, arch of

Thyroid gland

Trachea

Suprasternal space

Thymus
Brachiocephalic trunk
Left brachiocephalic vein

Spinal cord

Manubrium

Esophagus

Sternal angle

Ligamentum flavum

Aorta

Pleural cavity

Pericardial
cavity

Right bronchus

8.84
Head and neck, median section

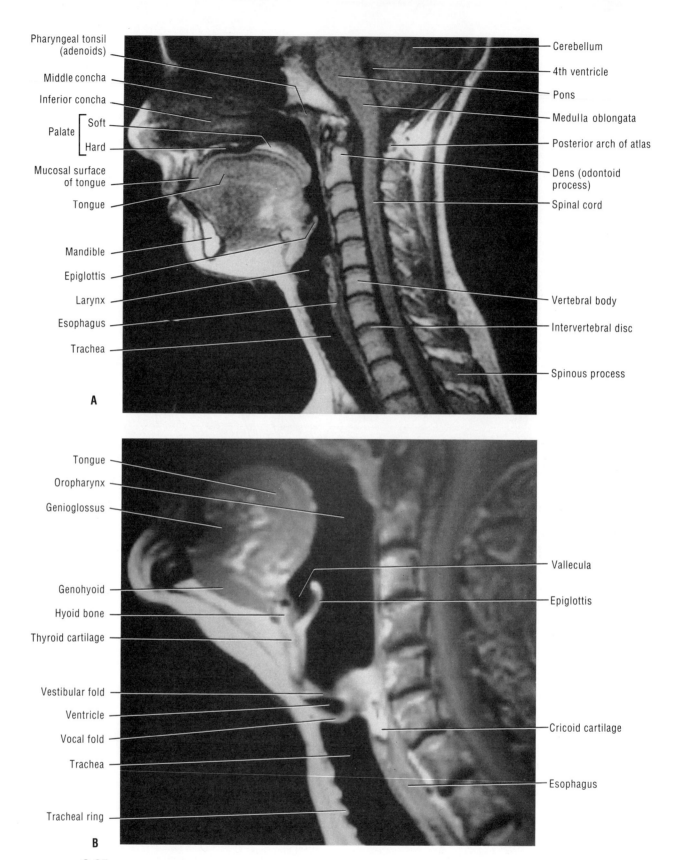

Pharyngeal tonsil
(adenoids)

Middle concha

Inferior concha

Palate — Soft

Palate — Hard

Mucosal surface
of tongue

Tongue

Mandible

Epiglottis

Larynx

Esophagus

Trachea

A

Cerebellum

4th ventricle

Pons

Medulla oblongata

Posterior arch of atlas

Dens (odontoid
process)

Spinal cord

Vertebral body

Intervertebral disc

Spinous process

Tongue

Oropharynx

Genioglossus

Genohyoid

Hyoid bone

Thyroid cartilage

Vestibular fold

Ventricle

Vocal fold

Trachea

Tracheal ring

B

Vallecula

Epiglottis

Cricoid cartilage

Esophagus

8.85
Median MRIs (magnetic resonance images) through the head and neck

(Courtesy of Dr. W. Kucharczyk, Clinical Director of Tri-Hospital Resonance Centre, Toronto, Ontario, Canada.)

9 The Cranial Nerves

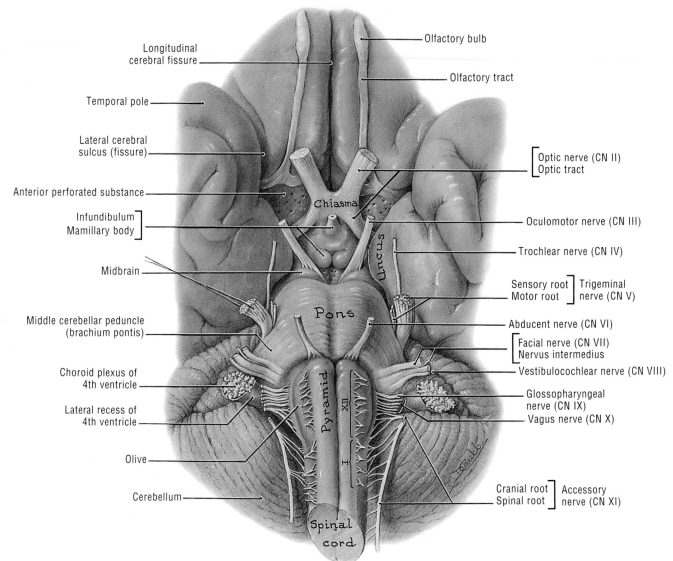

Longitudinal cerebral fissure

Temporal pole

Lateral cerebral sulcus (fissure)

Anterior perforated substance

Infundibulum
Mamillary body

Midbrain

Middle cerebellar peduncle (brachium pontis)

Choroid plexus of 4th ventricle

Lateral recess of 4th ventricle

Olive

Cerebellum

Olfactory bulb

Olfactory tract

Optic nerve (CN II)
Optic tract

Chiasma

Uncus

Oculomotor nerve (CN III)

Trochlear nerve (CN IV)

Sensory root   Trigeminal
Motor root   nerve (CN V)

Abducent nerve (CN VI)

Pons

Facial nerve (CN VII)
Nervus intermedius

Vestibulocochlear nerve (CN VIII)

Pyramid   XII   Glossopharyngeal
nerve (CN IX)

Vagus nerve (CN X)

II

Cranial root   Accessory
Spinal root   nerve (CN XI)

Spinal cord

9.1
Base of the brain: the superficial origins of the cranial nerves

9.2
Outline of the cranial nerves

Note that there are four modalities that may be carried by cranial nerves. Three cranial nerves (I, II, and VIII) carry special sense only and have no motor component. Four cranial nerves (III, VII, IX, and X) carry parasympathetic fibers to smooth muscles and glands.

There are four autonomic ganglia in the head: ciliary, pterygopalatine, otic, and submandibular. Each receives three types of fibers: (a) sensory: from a branch of the trigeminal nerve; (b) parasympathetic: from cranial nerves III, VII, or IX; these nerves synapse in the ganglion; (c) sympathetic: from the sympathetic trunk, hitchhiking on the wall of the closest artery.

No.	Name	Special Sense	Sensory	Motor	Para-sympathetic
I	Olfactory	•			
II	Optic	•			
III	Oculomotor			•	•
IV	Trochlear			•	
V	Trigeminal		•	•	
VI	Abducent			•	
VII	Facial	•	•	•	•
VIII	Vestibulocochlear	•			
IX	Glossopharyngeal	•	•	•	•
X	Vagus	•	•	•	•
XI	Accessory			•	
XII	Hypoglossal			•	

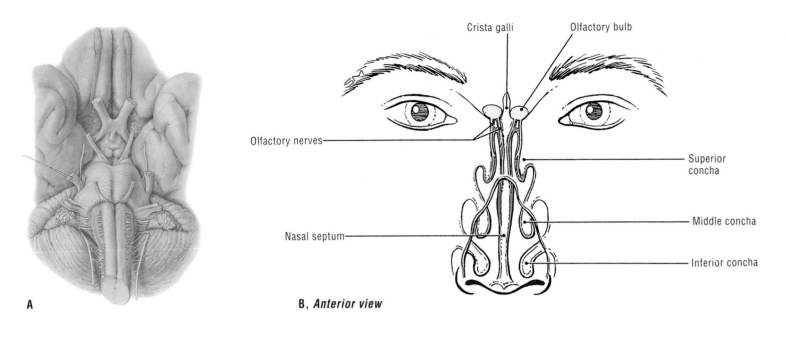

A

Crista galli   Olfactory bulb

Olfactory nerves

Superior
concha

Nasal septum

Middle concha

Inferior concha

B, *Anterior view*

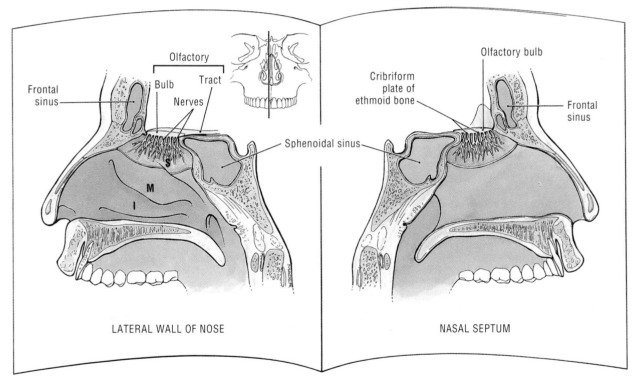

Olfactory

Frontal
sinus

Bulb   Tract

Nerves

Olfactory bulb

Cribriform
plate of
ethmoid bone

Frontal
sinus

Sphenoidal sinus

S

M

I

LATERAL WALL OF NOSE

NASAL SEPTUM

C

9.3
Distribution of the olfactory nerve – cranial nerve I

Observe:

1. In the roof of the nasal cavity, an area of yellowish brown mucous membrane contains the olfactory receptors; from here, 15 to 20 fine bundles of nerve fibers pierce the cribriform plate to enter the anterior cranial fossa and synapse in the olfactory bulb; the olfactory tract passes posteriorly to the brain;

2. The olfactory area is usually much smaller than that shown here, and it is irregular in outline as a result of streamer-like invasion by nonolfactory, ciliated, columnar epithelium; a study of the olfactory nerves in 143 adults (over 21 years of age) revealed

that only 12% had a full complement of olfactory nerve fibers, that 8% had lost all fibers on one side, and that 5% had lost all fibers on both sides. There is considerable variation in the number of olfactory nerve fibers in individuals of a given age but, on the average, there is a loss of 1% of fibers per year during postnatal life (see Smith CG. *Incidence of atrophy of the olfactory nerves in man.* Arch Otolaryngol 1941; 34:533). *S* - Superior concha, *M* - Middle concha, *I* - Inferior concha.

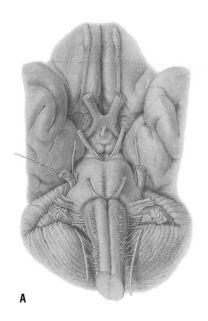

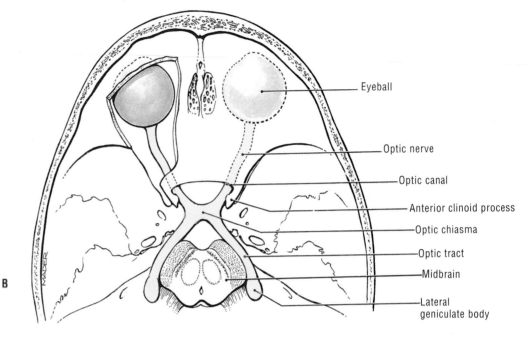

Eyeball

Optic nerve

Optic canal

Anterior clinoid process

Optic chiasma

Optic tract

Midbrain

Lateral geniculate body

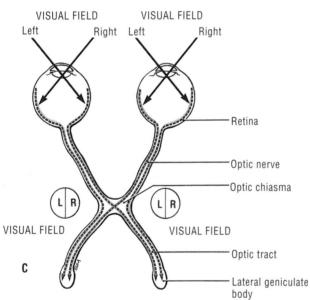

VISUAL FIELD
Left   Right

VISUAL FIELD
Left   Right

Retina

Optic nerve

Optic chiasma

VISUAL FIELD   VISUAL FIELD

Optic tract

Lateral geniculate body

C

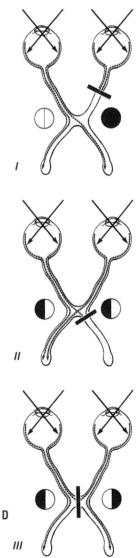

9.4
Distribution of the optic nerve – cranial nerve II

Diagram **C** of a horizontal section through the visual apparatus shows that neurons from the retina of the eyeball travel through the optic nerve to the optic chiasma, where the fibers from the nasal half of the retina cross the midline and join the optic tract of the opposite side. The *large arrows* represent rays of light from the right *(R)* and left *(L)* halves of this person's field of vision. Note that the rays of light from the right half of this person's field of vision would stimulate receptors in the left half of the retina of both eyes and reach the brain through the left optic tract.

Therefore in **D**, a section through the right optic nerve *(I)* would result in blindness of the right eye; a section through the right optic tract *(II)* would eliminate vision from left visual fields of both eyes; and a section through the optic chiasma *(III)* would reduce peripheral vision (tunnel vision). Remember that the pituitary gland lies just posterior to the optic chiasma and expansion of this gland by a tumor would put pressure on these crossing-over fibers.

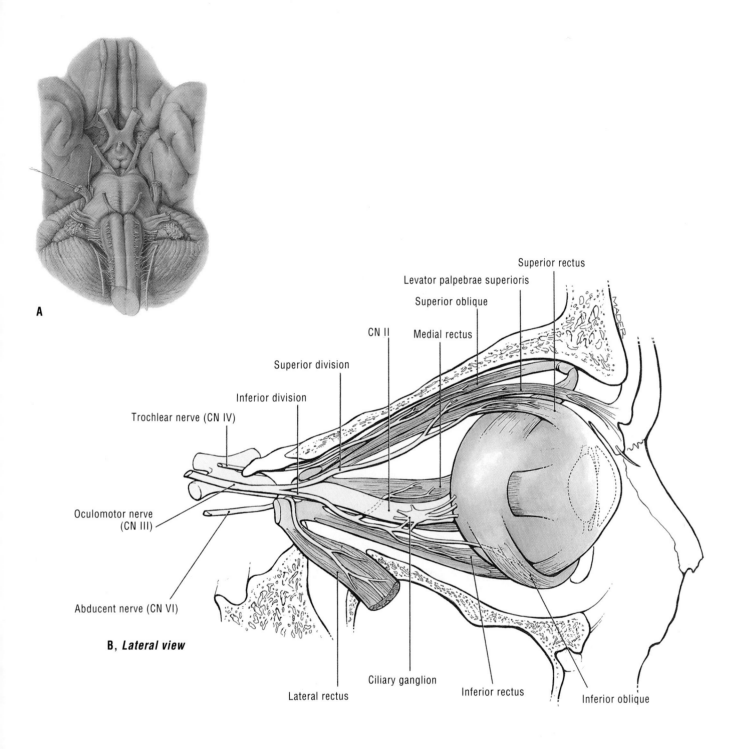

A

B, *Lateral view*

Labels in figure B:
- Superior rectus
- Levator palpebrae superioris
- Superior oblique
- CN II
- Medial rectus
- Superior division
- Inferior division
- Trochlear nerve (CN IV)
- Oculomotor nerve (CN III)
- Abducent nerve (CN VI)
- Lateral rectus
- Ciliary ganglion
- Inferior rectus
- Inferior oblique
- MADER

9.5
Distribution of the oculomotor, trochlear, and abducent nerves – cranial nerves III, IV, VI

A. Overview. **B**. Somatic motor and parasympathetic motor innervation of the orbit. These three motor nerves, after receiving proprioceptive fibers from the trigeminal nerve, supply the orbital (extraocular) muscles. Nerves IV and VI each supply one muscle and nerve III supplies the remaining five muscles.

The trochlear nerve supplies the superior oblique – the muscle that passes through a trochlea or pulley; the abducent nerve supplies the lateral rectus – the muscle that abducts; and the

oculomotor nerve supplies levator palpebrae superioris, superior rectus, medial rectus, inferior rectus, and inferior oblique muscles.

In addition, the oculomotor nerve carries fibers that are preganglionic, parasympathetic, and motor to smooth muscle. These fibers pass to the ciliary ganglion where they synapse and are distributed via short ciliary nerves to the sphincter pupillae (causing constriction of the pupil) and to the ciliary muscle (resulting in a more convex lens.)

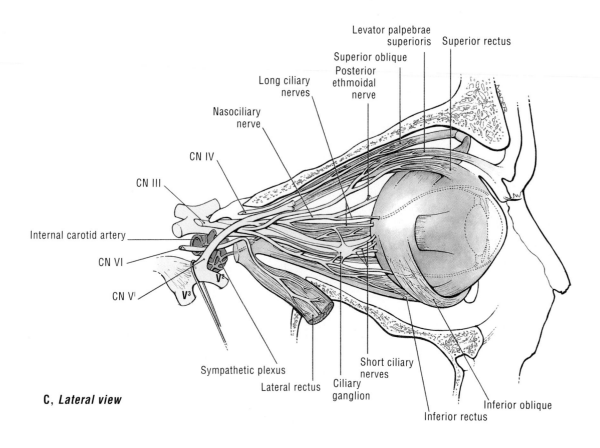

Levator palpebrae
superioris
Superior oblique
Posterior
ethmoidal
nerve
Superior rectus
Long ciliary
nerves
Nasociliary
nerve
CN IV
CN III
Internal carotid artery
CN VI
CN V¹
V³
V²
Sympathetic plexus
Lateral rectus
Ciliary
ganglion
Short ciliary
nerves
Inferior rectus
Inferior oblique

C, *Lateral view*

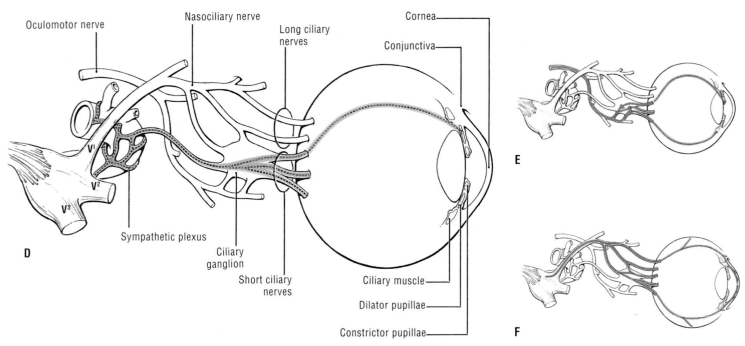

Oculomotor nerve
Nasociliary nerve
Long ciliary
nerves
Cornea
Conjunctiva
V¹
V²
V³
Sympathetic plexus
Ciliary
ganglion
Short ciliary
nerves
Ciliary muscle
Dilator pupillae
Constrictor pupillae
D
E
F

9.5
Distribution of the oculomotor, trochlear, and abducent nerves –
cranial nerves III, IV, VI *(continued)*

Innervation of the eye. **C**. Overview. **D**. Sympathetic. **E**. Parasympathetic. **F**. Sensory.

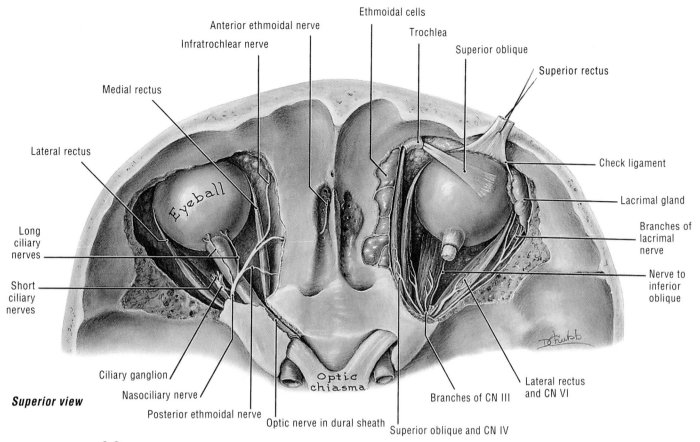

Superior view

Labels (clockwise from top):
Anterior ethmoidal nerve, Ethmoidal cells, Trochlea, Superior oblique, Superior rectus, Infratrochlear nerve, Medial rectus, Check ligament, Lacrimal gland, Lateral rectus, Branches of lacrimal nerve, Long ciliary nerves, Nerve to inferior oblique, Short ciliary nerves, Lateral rectus and CN VI, Ciliary ganglion, Branches of CN III, Nasociliary nerve, Superior oblique and CN IV, Posterior ethmoidal nerve, Optic nerve in dural sheath, Eyeball, Optic chiasma

9.6
Orbital cavity, dissected superiorly

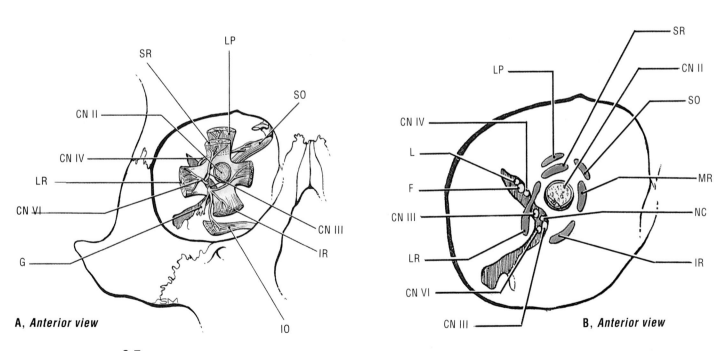

A, Anterior view

Labels: SR, LP, SO, CN II, CN IV, LR, CN VI, G, CN III, IR, IO

B, Anterior view

Labels: SR, CN II, SO, LP, CN IV, L, F, MR, CN III, NC, LR, IR, CN VI, CN III

9.7
Muscles and nerves of the orbit

L - Lacrimal nerve (CN V¹), *F* - Frontal nerve (CN V¹), *NC* - Nasociliary nerve (CN V¹), *LR* - Lateral rectus, *LP* - Levator palpebrae superioris, *SO* - Superior oblique, *SR* - Superior rectus, *MR* - Medial rectus, *IR* - Inferior rectus, *IO* - Inferior oblique, *G* - Ciliary ganglion.

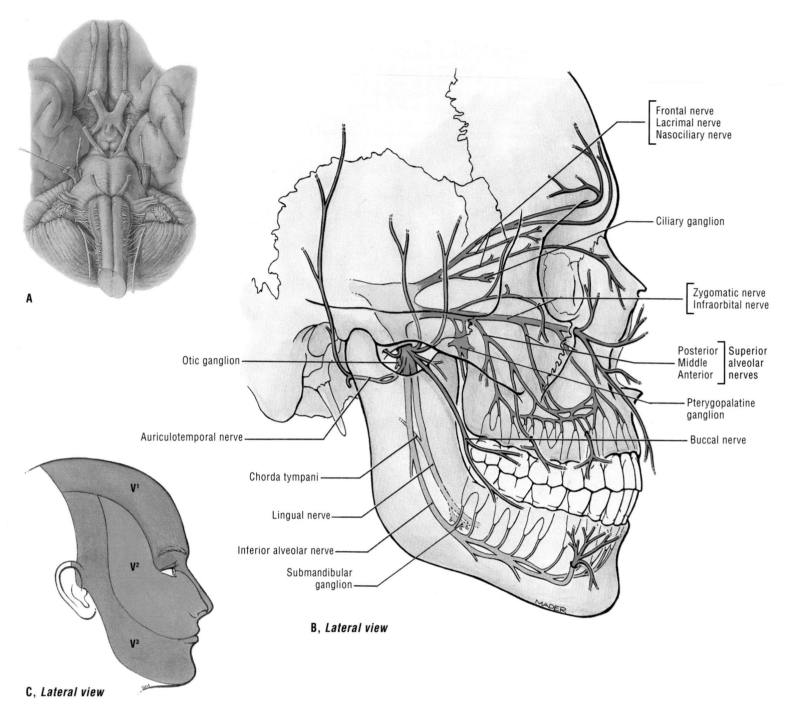

A

B, Lateral view

Frontal nerve
Lacrimal nerve
Nasociliary nerve

Ciliary ganglion

Zygomatic nerve
Infraorbital nerve

Posterior | Superior
Middle | alveolar
Anterior | nerves

Pterygopalatine ganglion

Buccal nerve

Otic ganglion

Auriculotemporal nerve

Chorda tympani

Lingual nerve

Inferior alveolar nerve

Submandibular ganglion

C, Lateral view

V¹

V²

V³

9.8
Distribution of the trigeminal nerve – cranial nerve V

The trigeminal nerve has three divisions: CN V¹, the ophthalmic nerve; CN V², the maxillary nerve; CN V³, the mandibular nerve.

All three divisions are sensory. Their cutaneous distribution is shown in **C**. However, each division supplies not only the skin surface, but the whole thickness of tissue from skin to mucous membrane. Each of the three divisions sends a twig to the dura mater: CN V¹ to the tentorium cerebelli, CN V² and CN V³ to the floor and side wall of the middle cranial fossa. Each of the three divisions provides the sensory component to an autonomic gan-

glion: CN V¹ to the ciliary, CN V² to the pterygopalatine, and CN V³ to the submandibular and otic.

In addition to its sensory component, CN V³ is motor to four pairs of muscles: (a) the two large elevators of the mandible – temporalis and masseter; (b) the two pterygoid muscles – medial and lateral; (c) the two tensors – veli palatini and tensor tympani; (d) the two muscles of the floor of the mouth – mylohyoid and anterior belly of the digastric.

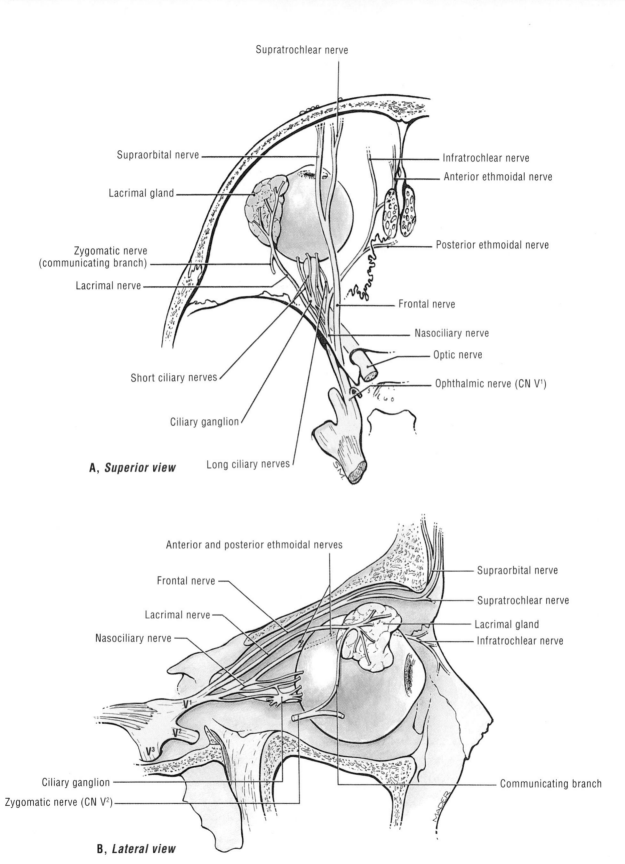

A, Superior view

Supratrochlear nerve

Supraorbital nerve

Lacrimal gland

Zygomatic nerve (communicating branch)

Lacrimal nerve

Short ciliary nerves

Ciliary ganglion

Long ciliary nerves

Infratrochlear nerve

Anterior ethmoidal nerve

Posterior ethmoidal nerve

Frontal nerve

Nasociliary nerve

Optic nerve

Ophthalmic nerve (CN V¹)

B, Lateral view

Anterior and posterior ethmoidal nerves

Frontal nerve

Lacrimal nerve

Nasociliary nerve

V¹

V²

V³

Ciliary ganglion

Zygomatic nerve (CN V²)

Supraorbital nerve

Supratrochlear nerve

Lacrimal gland

Infratrochlear nerve

Communicating branch

9.9
Ophthalmic nerve (CN V¹)

The ophthalmic nerve (CN V¹) is sensory: (a) to the eyeball and cornea via the ciliary nerves; hence, if paralyzed, the ocular conjunctiva is insensitive to touch; (b) to the frontal, ethmoidal, and sphenoidal sinuses via the supraorbital and ethmoidal nerves; and (c) to the skin and conjunctival surfaces of the upper eyelid and to the skin and mucous surfaces of the external nose.

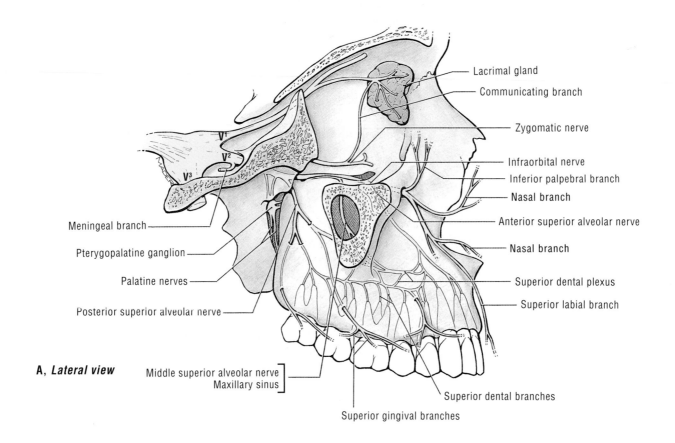

A, *Lateral view*

Labels (clockwise from top right):
- Lacrimal gland
- Communicating branch
- Zygomatic nerve
- Infraorbital nerve
- Inferior palpebral branch
- Nasal branch
- Anterior superior alveolar nerve
- Nasal branch
- Superior dental plexus
- Superior labial branch
- Superior dental branches
- Superior gingival branches

Labels (left side):
- Meningeal branch
- Pterygopalatine ganglion
- Palatine nerves
- Posterior superior alveolar nerve
- Middle superior alveolar nerve
- Maxillary sinus

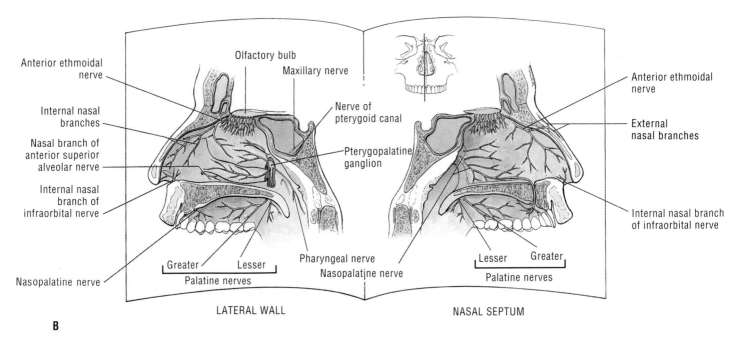

Labels (left side):
- Anterior ethmoidal nerve
- Internal nasal branches
- Nasal branch of anterior superior alveolar nerve
- Internal nasal branch of infraorbital nerve
- Nasopalatine nerve

Center labels:
- Olfactory bulb
- Maxillary nerve
- Nerve of pterygoid canal
- Pterygopalatine ganglion
- Pharyngeal nerve
- Nasopalatine nerve
- Greater / Lesser Palatine nerves

Right side labels:
- Anterior ethmoidal nerve
- External nasal branches
- Internal nasal branch of infraorbital nerve
- Lesser / Greater Palatine nerves

LATERAL WALL   NASAL SEPTUM

B

9.10
Maxillary nerve (CN V²)

Observe:

The maxillary nerve (CN V²) is sensory: (a) to the upper teeth and gums; (b) to the face, both surfaces of the lower lid, the skin of the side and vestibule of the nose, and both surfaces of the upper lip; (c) via the pterygopalatine ganglion to the mucoperiosteum of the nasal cavity, palate, and roof of the pharynx; and (d) to the maxillary, ethmoidal, and sphenoidal sinuses; secretory fibers from the pterygopalatine ganglion pass with the zygomatic nerve, and then with the lacrimal nerve to the lacrimal gland.

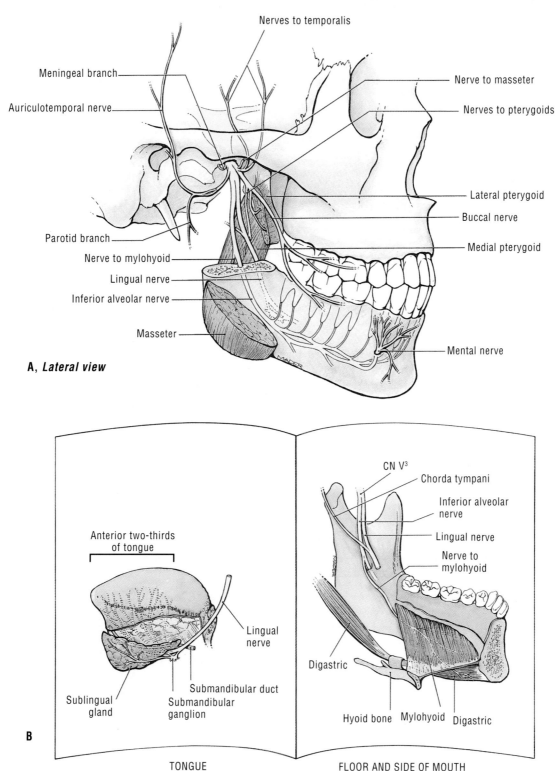

Nerves to temporalis

Meningeal branch

Auriculotemporal nerve

Nerve to masseter

Nerves to pterygoids

Lateral pterygoid

Buccal nerve

Parotid branch

Nerve to mylohyoid

Lingual nerve

Inferior alveolar nerve

Medial pterygoid

Masseter

Mental nerve

A, *Lateral view*

Anterior two-thirds of tongue

CN V³

Chorda tympani

Inferior alveolar nerve

Lingual nerve

Nerve to mylohyoid

Lingual nerve

Digastric

Sublingual gland

Submandibular ganglion

Submandibular duct

Hyoid bone **Mylohyoid** **Digastric**

B

TONGUE

FLOOR AND SIDE OF MOUTH

9.11
Mandibular nerve (CN V³)

The mandibular nerve (CN V³) is motor to: (a) the four muscles of mastication – but not to the buccinator; (b) the two tensors (tympani and veli palatini) via the otic ganglion; and (c) the mylohyoid and anterior belly of the digastric muscle. It is sensory to: (a) the lower teeth and gums; the territory of any of these gingival and dental nerves may either be extended or contracted; e.g., twigs of the mental and lingual nerves may cross the median plane to supply the gums of the opposite side, and the inferior alveolar nerves may decussate in the mandibular canal to supply the incisors of the opposite side; (b) both surfaces of the lower lip by the mental nerve; (c) the auricle and temporal region by the auriculotemporal nerve, which also sends twigs to the external meatus and outer surface of the eardrum, and conveys secretory fibers from the otic ganglion to the parotid gland; (d) the mucous membrane of the cheek by the buccal nerve; and (e) the anterior two-thirds of the tongue, floor of the mouth, and gums by the lingual nerve, which also distributes the chorda tympani.

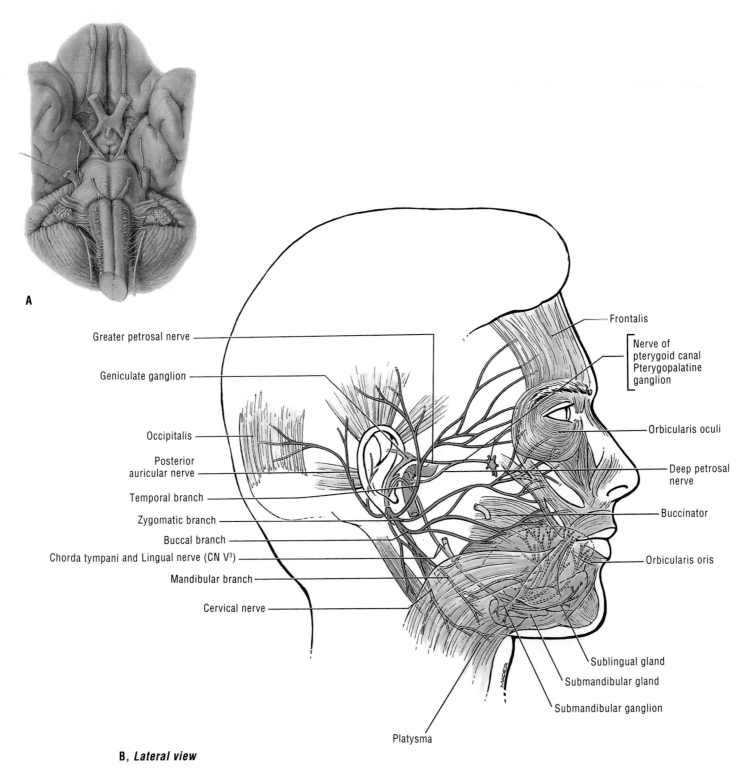

A

Greater petrosal nerve

Geniculate ganglion

Occipitalis

Posterior auricular nerve

Temporal branch

Zygomatic branch

Buccal branch

Chorda tympani and Lingual nerve (CN V³)

Mandibular branch

Cervical nerve

Frontalis

Nerve of pterygoid canal
Pterygopalatine ganglion

Orbicularis oculi

Deep petrosal nerve

Buccinator

Orbicularis oris

Sublingual gland

Submandibular gland

Submandibular ganglion

Platysma

B, *Lateral view*

9.12
Distribution of the facial nerve – cranial nerve VII

All four modalities are carried by the facial nerve.

Observe:

Motor: To the "muscles of expression," the superficial muscles around the eye, nose, mouth, and ear; of the scalp superiorly and the platysma inferiorly. It also supplies the stylohyoid and posterior belly of the digastric muscles, as well as the stapedius.

Special sense: Taste fibers, with cell stations in the geniculate ganglion, pass (a) from the palate nonstop through the pterygopalatine ganglion, nerve of the pterygoid canal, and greater petrosal nerve to the geniculate ganglion; and (b) from the anterior two-thirds of the tongue via the chorda tympani to the facial nerve and so to the geniculate ganglion.

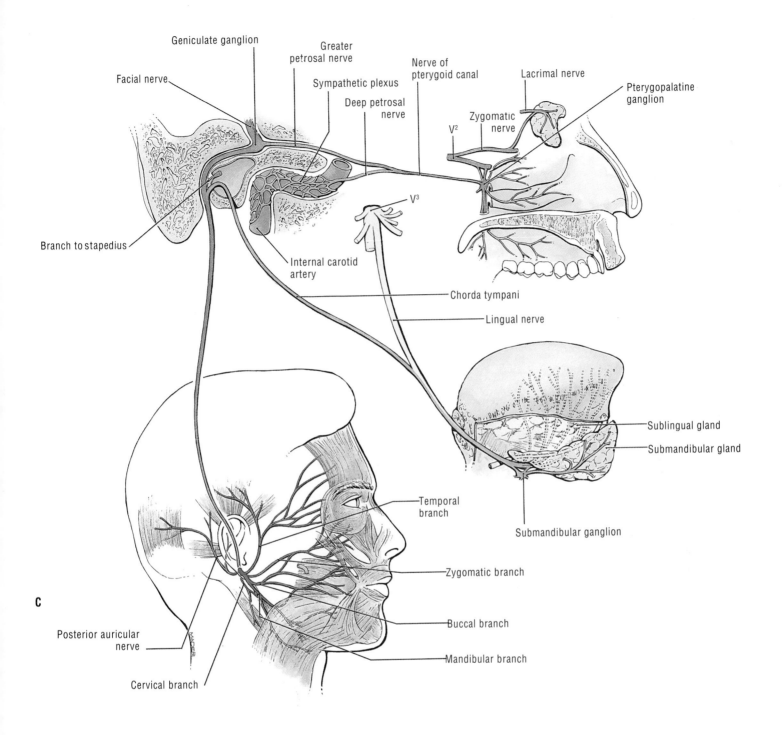

Geniculate ganglion

Greater petrosal nerve

Facial nerve

Sympathetic plexus

Nerve of pterygoid canal

Deep petrosal nerve

Lacrimal nerve

Pterygopalatine ganglion

V²

Zygomatic nerve

Branch to stapedius

Internal carotid artery

V³

Chorda tympani

Lingual nerve

Sublingual gland

Submandibular gland

Temporal branch

Submandibular ganglion

Zygomatic branch

Posterior auricular nerve

Buccal branch

Mandibular branch

Cervical branch

C

9.12
Distribution of the facial nerve – cranial nerve VII *(continued)*

Parasympathetic: Secretory (a) via the greater petrosal nerve and the nerve of the pterygoid canal to the pterygopalatine ganglion, then relayed by postsynaptic fibers to the glands of the nose and palate and to the lacrimal gland; (b) via the chorda tympani (1) to the submandibular ganglion, from which postsynaptic fibers are relayed to the submandibular and sublingual salivary glands;

and (2) via its connection with the otic ganglion, it innervates the parotid gland.

Sensory: supplies general sensation to a small area of the external acoustic meatus and the auricle.

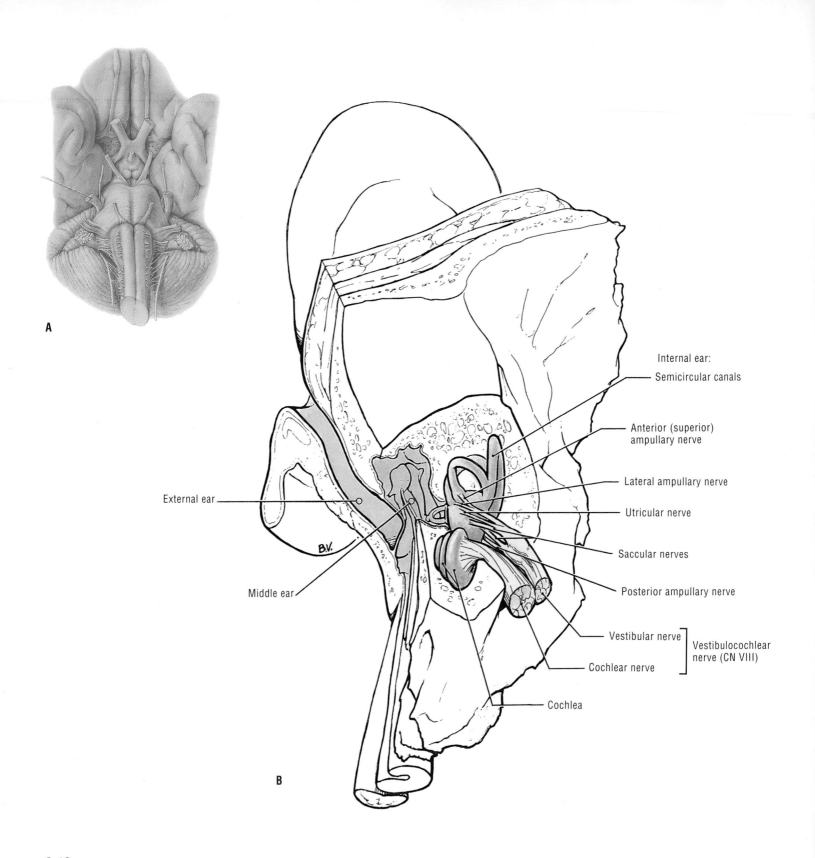

A

B

Internal ear:
Semicircular canals

Anterior (superior) ampullary nerve

Lateral ampullary nerve

Utricular nerve

Saccular nerves

Posterior ampullary nerve

Vestibular nerve ⎤ Vestibulocochlear
Cochlear nerve ⎦ nerve (CN VIII)

Cochlea

External ear

B.V.

Middle ear

9.13
Distribution of the vestibulocochlear nerve – cranial nerve VIII

This nerve has two parts: (a) the cochlear nerve, or nerve of hearing, whose fibers transmit impulses from the spiral organ of Corti in the cochlear duct; and (b) the vestibular nerve, or nerve of balancing, whose fibers transmit impulses from the maculae of the saccule and utricle and in the ampullae of the three semicircular ducts.

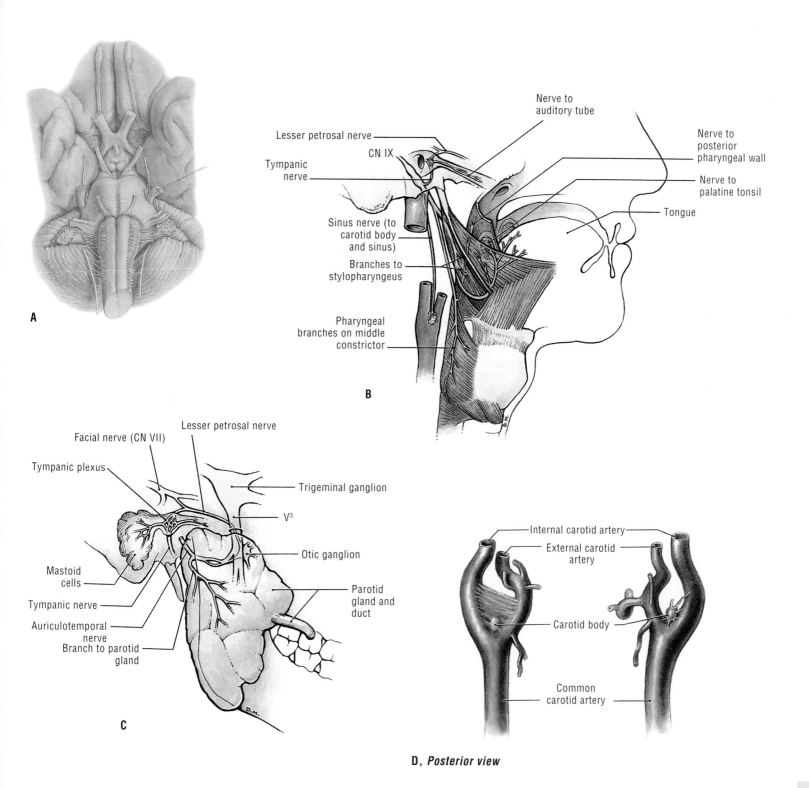

A

B

C

D, *Posterior view*

Labels in figure B:
- Nerve to auditory tube
- Lesser petrosal nerve
- CN IX
- Tympanic nerve
- Nerve to posterior pharyngeal wall
- Nerve to palatine tonsil
- Tongue
- Sinus nerve (to carotid body and sinus)
- Branches to stylopharyngeus
- Pharyngeal branches on middle constrictor

Labels in figure C:
- Facial nerve (CN VII)
- Lesser petrosal nerve
- Tympanic plexus
- Trigeminal ganglion
- V³
- Otic ganglion
- Mastoid cells
- Parotid gland and duct
- Tympanic nerve
- Auriculotemporal nerve
- Branch to parotid gland

Labels in figure D:
- Internal carotid artery
- External carotid artery
- Carotid body
- Common carotid artery

9.14
Distribution of the glossopharyngeal nerve – cranial nerve IX

This nerve does all four things, but sparingly; (a) it is motor to one muscle, the stylopharyngeus; (b) its parasympathetic component supplies secretory fibers through the otic ganglion to the parotid gland; (c) it provides the special sense of taste to the posterior one-third of the tongue including the vallate papillae; and (d) general sensory fibers supply almost the entire one-half of the pharyngeal wall, including the oropharyngeal isthmus (i.e., undersurface of the soft palate, tonsil, pharyngeal arches, and posterior one-third of the tongue). It also supplies the dorsum of the soft palate, the auditory tube, tympanum, medial surface of the eardrum, mastoid antrum, and mastoid cells. The sinus nerve is afferent from the carotid sinus (which responds to pressure changes within the artery) and the carotid body (**D**) (which responds to falling PO_2 or rising PCO_2 in the blood).

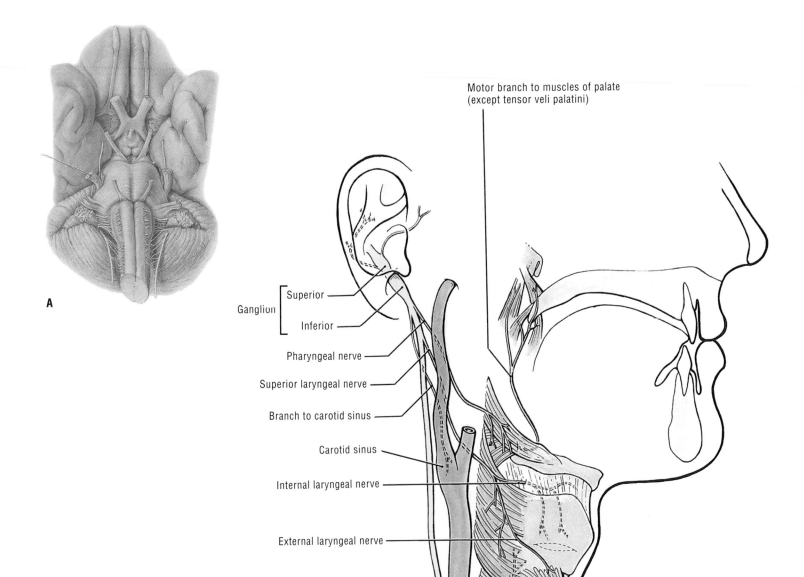

Motor branch to muscles of palate
(except tensor veli palatini)

Ganglion { Superior
Inferior

Pharyngeal nerve

Superior laryngeal nerve

Branch to carotid sinus

Carotid sinus

Internal laryngeal nerve

External laryngeal nerve

Recurrent laryngeal nerve

A

B, Lateral view

9.15
Distribution of the vagus nerve – cranial nerve X

Observe:

The vagus nerve, the wanderer, is:

1. Motor to all smooth muscle,

2. Secretory to all glands, and

3. Afferent from all mucous surfaces in the following parts – pharynx (lowest part), larynx, trachea, bronchi, and lungs; esophagus (entire), stomach, and gut down to the left colic (splenic) flexure; liver, gallbladder, and bile passages; pancreas and pancreatic ducts; and perhaps spleen and kidney,

4. Motor to all muscles of the larynx, all muscles of the pharynx (except the stylopharyngeus), and all muscles of the palate (except tensor veli palatini),

5. The conveyor of taste from the few taste buds about the epiglottis,

6. Inhibitory to cardiac muscle,

7. Sensory to the outer surface of the eardrum, the external acoustic meatus, and the back of the auricle.

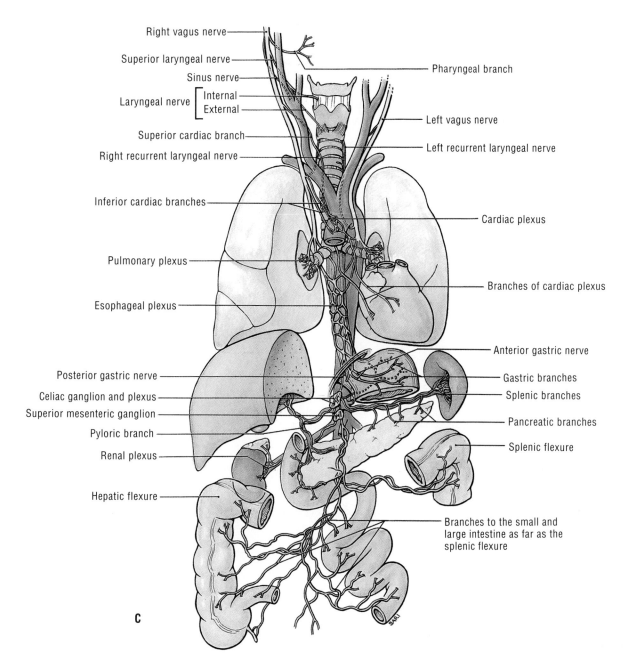

Right vagus nerve

Superior laryngeal nerve

Sinus nerve

Laryngeal nerve
- Internal
- External

Superior cardiac branch

Right recurrent laryngeal nerve

Inferior cardiac branches

Pulmonary plexus

Esophageal plexus

Posterior gastric nerve

Celiac ganglion and plexus

Superior mesenteric ganglion

Pyloric branch

Renal plexus

Hepatic flexure

Pharyngeal branch

Left vagus nerve

Left recurrent laryngeal nerve

Cardiac plexus

Branches of cardiac plexus

Anterior gastric nerve

Gastric branches

Splenic branches

Pancreatic branches

Splenic flexure

Branches to the small and large intestine as far as the splenic flexure

C

9.15
Distribution of the vagus nerve – cranial nerve X *(continued)*

Branches arise from the vagus:

In the jugular fossa: (a) a meningeal branch to the dura of the posterior cranial fossa; and (b) an auricular branch;

In the neck: (a) the pharyngeal branch is motor to the superior and middle constrictors and muscles of the soft palate; (b) the superior laryngeal nerve, via the internal laryngeal nerve, is sensory to the larynx superior to the vocal cords and to the most inferior part of the pharynx and, via the external laryngeal nerve, motor to the inferior constrictor and cricothyroid; (c) a twig (sinus nerve) to the carotid sinus; and (d) two cardiac branches.

In the thorax: (a) the recurrent nerve sends a motor branch to the

inferior constrictor, is motor to all the laryngeal muscles (excepting the cricothyroid), and is both afferent and efferent to the larynx inferior to the level of the cords, as well as to the superior part of the esophagus; (b) cardiac branches; (c) pulmonary branches; and (d) the esophageal plexus.

In the abdomen: (a) the posterior and anterior vagal trunks (formerly right and left vagus nerves) entering on the esophagus and supplying gastric branches; (b) the celiac branch of the posterior vagal trunk contributing to the preaortic plexuses; (c) the hepatic branches of the anterior vagal trunk, note the hepatic branch is cut.

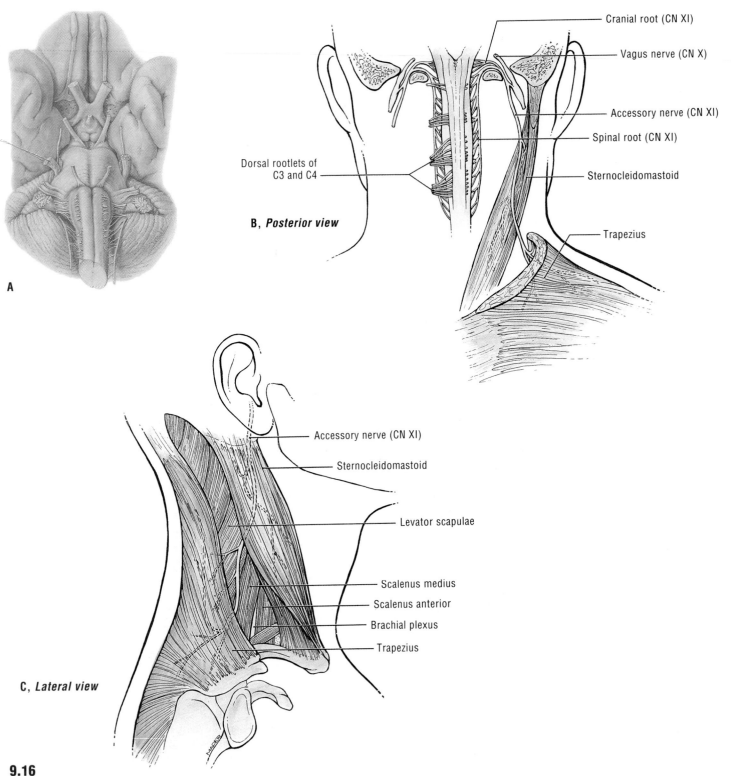

A

B, *Posterior view*

Cranial root (CN XI)

Vagus nerve (CN X)

Accessory nerve (CN XI)

Spinal root (CN XI)

Sternocleidomastoid

Dorsal rootlets of C3 and C4

Trapezius

Accessory nerve (CN XI)

Sternocleidomastoid

Levator scapulae

Scalenus medius

Scalenus anterior

Brachial plexus

Trapezius

C, *Lateral view*

9.16
Distribution of the accessory nerve – cranial nerve XI

The cranial root of this nerve is accessory to the vagus by providing part of its motor component.

The spinal root of the accessory nerve, joined by fibers from the ventral ramus of C2, supplies sternocleidomastoid and, joined by fibers from the ventral rami of C3 and C4, supplies the trapezius muscle. There is clinical evidence (both surgical and medical) that these contributions from C2, C3, and C4 convey motor as well as sensory fibers (see Haymaker W, Woodhall B. *Peripheral Nerve Injuries,* 2nd ed. Philadelphia, WB Saunders Company, 1953).

The spinal root of the accessory nerve usually passes through the dorsal root ganglion of C1 and may receive sensory fibers from it.

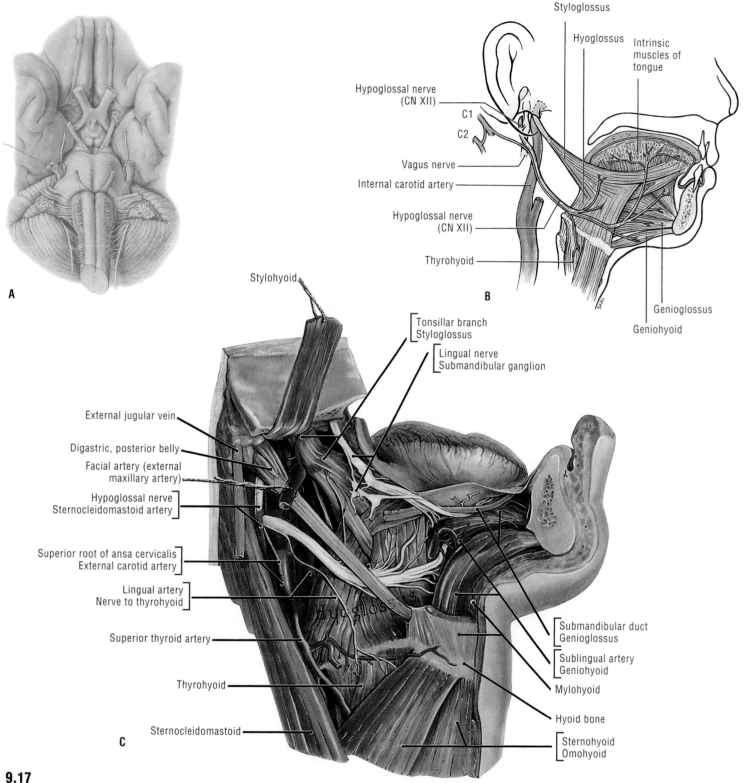

Styloglossus

Hyoglossus **Intrinsic muscles of tongue**

Hypoglossal nerve (CN XII)

C1

C2

Vagus nerve

Internal carotid artery

Hypoglossal nerve (CN XII)

Thyrohyoid

Genioglossus

Geniohyoid

B

A

Stylohyoid

Tonsillar branch
Styloglossus

Lingual nerve
Submandibular ganglion

External jugular vein

Digastric, posterior belly

Facial artery (external maxillary artery)

Hypoglossal nerve
Sternocleidomastoid artery

Superior root of ansa cervicalis
External carotid artery

Lingual artery
Nerve to thyrohyoid

Superior thyroid artery

Thyrohyoid

Submandibular duct
Genioglossus

Sublingual artery
Geniohyoid

Mylohyoid

Hyoid bone

Sternocleidomastoid

Sternohyoid
Omohyoid

C

9.17
Distribution of the hypoglossal nerve – cranial nerve XII

A. Overview. **B.** Distribution of the hypoglossal nerve. **C.** Suprahyoid region. This efferent nerve supplies all the intrinsic (longitudinal, transverse, and vertical) and extrinsic (styloglossus, hyoglossus, and genioglossus) muscles of the tongue, palatoglossus excepted.

It receives a mixed (motor and sensory) branch from the loop between the ventral rami of C1 and C2. The sensory or afferent fibers, in part, take a recurrent course and end in the dura mater of the posterior cranial fossa. The motor or efferent branch supplies the geniohyoid and thyrohyoid muscles, and it provides a descending branch that unites with a descending branch of C2 and C3 to form a loop, the ansa cervicalis. This and the ansa supply the remaining depressor (strap) muscles of the hyoid bone.

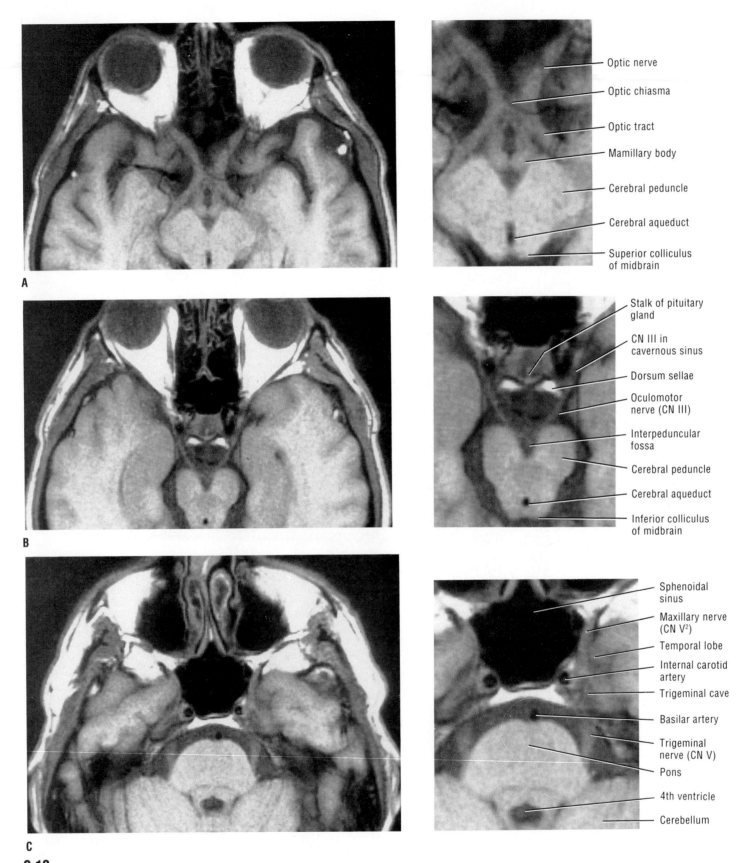

9.18
Transverse MRIs (magnetic resonance images) through the head, showing cranial nerves

(Courtesy of Dr. W. Kucharczyk, Clinical Director of Tri-Hospital Resonance Centre, Toronto, Ontario, Canada.)

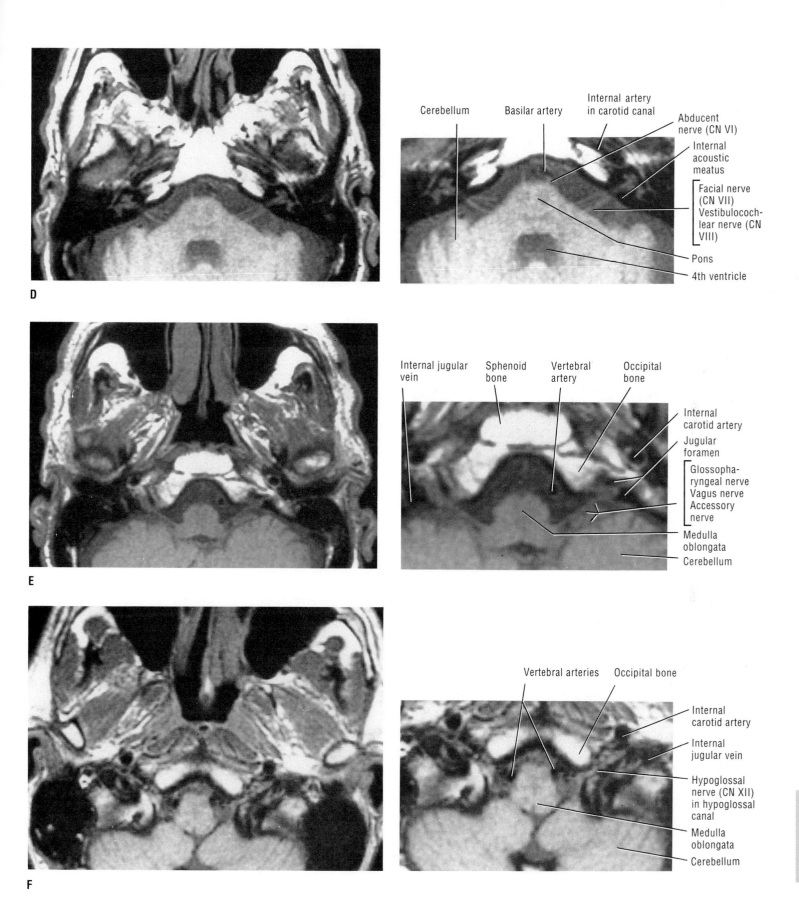

D

Cerebellum | Basilar artery | Internal artery in carotid canal

Abducent nerve (CN VI)

Internal acoustic meatus

Facial nerve (CN VII)
Vestibulocochlear nerve (CN VIII)

Pons

4th ventricle

E

Internal jugular vein | Sphenoid bone | Vertebral artery | Occipital bone

Internal carotid artery

Jugular foramen

Glossopharyngeal nerve
Vagus nerve
Accessory nerve

Medulla oblongata

Cerebellum

F

Vertebral arteries | Occipital bone

Internal carotid artery

Internal jugular vein

Hypoglossal nerve (CN XII) in hypoglossal canal

Medulla oblongata

Cerebellum

9.18
Transverse MRIs (magnetic resonance images) through the head, showing cranial nerves *(continued)*

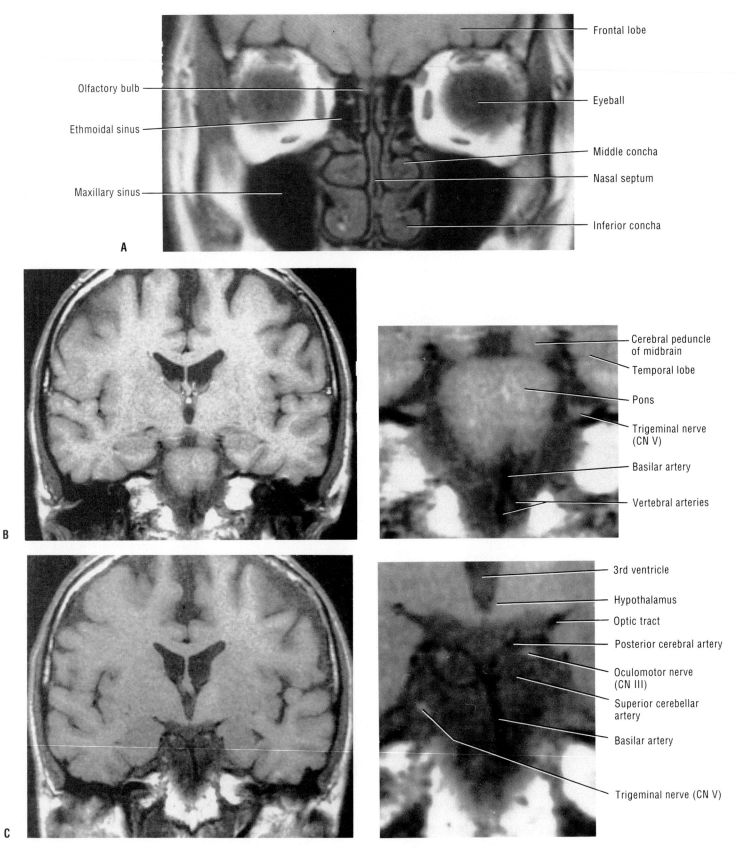

9.19
Coronal MRIs (magnetic resonance images) through the head, showing cranial nerves

(Courtesy of Dr. W. Kucharczyk, Clinical Director of Tri-Hospital Resonance Centre, Toronto, Ontario, Canada.)

INDEX

Page numbers in **bold** type indicate chief references.